Advanced Clinical MRI of the Kidney

Suraj D. Serai • Kassa Darge
Editors

Advanced Clinical MRI of the Kidney

Methods and Protocols

Springer

Editors
Suraj D. Serai
Department of Radiology
Children's Hospital of Philadelphia,
Perelman School of Medicine,
University of Pennsylvania
Philadelphia, PA, USA

Kassa Darge
Department of Radiology
Children's Hospital of Philadelphia,
Perelman School of Medicine,
University of Pennsylvania
Philadelphia, PA, USA

ISBN 978-3-031-40168-8 ISBN 978-3-031-40169-5 (eBook)
https://doi.org/10.1007/978-3-031-40169-5

This Springer imprint is published by the registered company Springer Nature Switzerland AG
The registered company address is: Gewerbestrasse 11, 6330 Cham, Switzerland

Paper in this product is recyclable.

Preface

Quantitative MRI techniques reveal promising markers for renal disease and could provide additional insights into kidney pathology characterization and disease progression in patients. The interest in renal MRI-derived biomarkers is driven by the potential to quantify morphological, microstructural, hemodynamic, and metabolic changes noninvasively and across the entire kidney parenchyma. Radiologists generally evaluate signal using intensity descriptors such as "hyperintense" or "hypointense" and use the expected signal appearance of various tissues and associated pathologies to render a differential diagnosis. However, this subjective analysis of relatively "weighted" images is only a fraction of the tissue property information that could be provided by MRI techniques. The very concept of "weighting" can start to break down when more than one tissue is being compared. In addition, limitations of current MRI technologies include variable image acquisition across scanners, limited reproducibility of images, and known inter-reader variability in image interpretation. Quantitative MRI provides a unique and discrete analysis of tissue parameters and holds promise in addressing some of these limitations. To date, the most common quantitative MRI properties used in clinical practice are diffusion-weighted imaging, fat fraction (FF) mapping, and perfusion mapping. Quantification and mapping of T1 and T2 relaxation times, which affect all MR signals, are not commonly performed given the additional significant scan time that would be required. In the past decade, it has become increasingly apparent that the biophysical quantities measurable by MRI can have a utility beyond generating image contrast. In particular, these biophysical quantities such as T1, T2, and T2* are sensitive to tissue type and should enable them to characterize changes "within" tissues caused by aging, disease, or intervention. This is a compelling hypothesis in the context of renal medicine because a range of MRI techniques is sensitive to the pathophysiological changes associated with the progression of renal disease. In that sense, MRI may open up a novel source of noninvasive biomarkers to inform about pathogenesis, improve predictions of disease progression, and evaluate treatment effects. These quantitative MR techniques could aid in a deeper understanding of the function and composition of a patient's renal tissue, which could provide a more accurate and earlier assessment of renal disease and facilitate earlier interventions to halt or slow down renal disease progression.

Despite considerable research effort and unique quantitative information available on clinical MRI scanners, integration of quantitative MRI methods into clinical practice has been limited. There are multiple reasons for this, including the fact that acquisition parameters and data analysis protocols have not yet been standardized. Other factors are limited vendor support, difficulties in interpretation, limited perceived "added-value" above conventional MRI, and lack of additional reimbursement. This book is intended to address some of these issues. It gives the reader a solid basis for understanding both the techniques and the applications of quantitative MRI biomarkers in kidney imaging.

We have now entered an era in which it is possible to obtain rapid quantitative measurements of numerous physiologically relevant tissue properties—diffusion, perfusion, fat content, iron content, blood oxygen level, tissue elasticity, T1, T2, etc. Each property has found scientific and clinical utility in various applications. With the advancement of the computing power of modern MRI scanners, the images can be post-processed and quantitative maps be generated on the scanner console, ready for review as soon as the acquisition is complete. Such quantitative MRI methods in kidney imaging are vital because they are relatively unbiased as compared with qualitative descriptions.

It is also becoming clear that no single tissue property or measurement technique is likely to be sufficient to resolve complex clinical and research questions. In order to achieve comprehensive tissue assessments that provide actionable information, many of these quantitative tissue parameters will need to be used together. The aim of this book is to provide a practical reference that covers all aspects of quantitative MRI for the kidney. This book addresses the measurement process with an emphasis on "how to," what these measures mean biologically, and image analysis methodology. We also provide relevant clinical applications of the techniques described in each chapter. Any physician looking to apply quantitative MRI biomarkers in clinical practice must be familiar with the concepts elucidated in this book. We hope that widespread adoption of quantitative biomarkers in renal imaging will lead to better diagnosis and improved outcomes for individual patients.

The purpose of this book is to openly share the protocols and post-processing methods of quantitative MRI methods for renal clinical applications. The book provides answers to common questions regarding how renal MRI technologies emerging from research can be translated to routine clinical practice. With this "from the community, to the community" approach, the book is designed to enhance training in renal MRI sciences, to improve the reproducibility of renal imaging research, and to boost the comparability of renal MRI studies.

The book is divided into three major parts. Chapters in the first part discuss general considerations and practical steps for kidney MRI. The second part is focused on the metrics themselves. This part covers the physics and applications of intrinsic MRI parameters (T1, T2, T2*), diffusion, perfusion, magnetization transfer, metabolic imaging, susceptibility mapping, elasticity, and gadolinium-based measurement methods. The third part is dedicated to emerging methods that are currently considered advanced. The topics covered in the chapters are interdisciplinary in nature and bridge the gaps between physics, physiology, and medicine. With this book, we hope to encourage more collaboration between nephrologists, urologists, computer scientists, biomedical engineers, and radiologists to accelerate the development and application of modern MRI tools in clinical practice.

Finally, we are grateful to all the authors for their outstanding contributions, passion, and dedication to renal MRI. We are hopeful this work will prove useful to clinicians and inspire another generation of researchers to pursue renal MRI.

Philadelphia, PA, USA Suraj D. Serai
Philadelphia, PA, USA Kassa Darge

Contents

Contributors

Menaka Ambarishan North Tyneside General Hospital, Newcastle-upon Tyne, UK

Susan J. Back Children's Hospital of Philadelphia, University of Pennsylvania, Philadelphia, PA, USA

Edwin J. Baldelomar Washington University School of Medicine in St. Louis, St. Louis, MO, USA

Biomedical MR Center—Mallinckrodt Institute of Radiology, Washington University School of Medicine in St. Louis, St. Louis, MO, USA

Octavia Bane, PhD Department of Radiology, Icahn School of Medicine at Mount Sinai, New York, NY, USA

BioMedical Engineering and Imaging Institute, Icahn School of Medicine at Mount Sinai, New York, NY, USA

Eric Bechler Department of Diagnostic and Interventional Radiology, Medical Faculty, Heinrich Heine University Düsseldorf, Düsseldorf, Germany

Diana Bencikova High Field MR Center, Department of Biomedical Imaging and Image-Guided Therapy, Medical University of Vienna, Vienna, Austria

Kevin M. Bennett Washington University School of Medicine in St. Louis, St. Louis, MO, USA

Biomedical MR Center—Mallinckrodt Institute of Radiology, Washington University School of Medicine in St. Louis, St. Louis, MO, USA

Anneloes de Boer Department of Radiology, University Medical Center Utrecht, Utrecht University, Utrecht, The Netherlands

Nikolaj Bøgh Department of Clinical Medicine, Aarhus University, Aarhus, Denmark

Anna Caroli Bioengineering Department, Istituto di Ricerche Farmacologiche Mario Negri IRCCS, Bergamo, Italy

Sanjeev Chawla Department of Radiology, University of Pennsylvania School of Medicine, Philadelphia, PA, USA

Yong Chen Department of Radiology, Case Western Reserve University, Cleveland, OH, USA

Rachelle Crescenzi Radiology and Radiological Sciences, Vanderbilt University Medical Center, Nashville, TN, USA

Vanderbilt University Institute of Imaging Science, Vanderbilt University Medical Center, Nashville, TN, USA

Biomedical Engineering, Vanderbilt University, Nashville, TN, USA

Ilona A. Dekkers Department of Radiology, Cardiovascular Imaging Group (CVIG), Leiden University Medical Center, Leiden, The Netherlands

Katherine M. Dell Department of Pediatrics, Case Western Reserve University, Cleveland, OH, USA

Center for Pediatric Nephrology, Cleveland Clinic Children's Hospital, Cleveland, OH, USA

Rajiv S. Deshpande Laboratory for Structural, Physiologic, and Functional Imaging, Department of Radiology, University of Pennsylvania, Philadelphia, PA, USA

Jonathan R. Dillman Department of Radiology, Cincinnati Children's Hospital Medical Center, Cincinnati, OH, USA

Department of Radiology, University of Cincinnati College of Medicine, Cincinnati, OH, USA

Alexey V. Dimov Department of Radiology, Weill Cornell Medicine, New York, NY, USA

Behzad Ebrahimi Department of Radiation and Cellular Oncology, University of Chicago, Chicago, IL, USA

Carolina C. Fernandes Perspectum Ltd., Oxford, Oxfordshire, UK

Maria A. Fernandez-Seara Radiology Department, Clínica Universidad de Navarra, University of Navarra, Pamplona, Spain

Chris A. Flask Department of Radiology, Case Western Reserve University, Cleveland, OH, USA

Department of Biomedical Engineering, Case Western Reserve University, Cleveland, OH, USA

Department of Pediatrics, Case Western Reserve University, Cleveland, OH, USA

Susan Francis Sir Peter Mansfield Imaging Centre, University of Nottingham, Nottingham, UK

Deep Gandhi Mayo Clinic, Rochester, MN, USA

Adarsh Ghosh Children's Hospital of Philadelphia, University of Pennsylvania, Philadelphia, PA, USA

Adriana V. Gregory Division of Nephrology and Hypertension, Mayo Clinic, Rochester, MN, USA

Mark A. Griswold Department of Radiology, Case Western Reserve University, Cleveland, OH, USA

Michael N. Hoff Department of Radiology and Biomedical Imaging, University of California San Francisco, San Francisco, CA, USA

J. M. Hoogduin Department of Radiology, University Medical Center Utrecht, Utrecht University, Utrecht, The Netherlands

Sherry Huang Department of Biomedical Engineering, Case Western Reserve University, Cleveland, OH, USA

Sachin Jambawalikar Department of Radiology, Columbia University Medical Center, New York, NY, USA

Kai Jiang Department of Radiation Oncology, University of Maryland School of Medicine, Baltimore, MD, USA

Jochen Keupp Philips Research, Hamburg, Germany

Dmitry Khrichenko Department of Radiology, Children's Hospital of Philadelphia, Philadelphia, PA, USA

Timothy L. Kline Department of Radiology, Mayo Clinic, Rochester, MN, USA

Orpheus Kolokythas Department of Radiology, University of Washington, Seattle, WA, USA

Valentina Kon Department of Pediatrics, Vanderbilt University Medical Center, Nashville, TN, USA

Ramkumar Krishnamurthy Medical and Scientific Affairs, ICON Medical Imaging, Philadelphia, PA, USA

Sila Kurugol Harvard Medical School, Boston, MA, USA

Hildo J. Lamb Department of Radiology, Cardiovascular Imaging Group (CVIG), Leiden University Medical Center, Leiden, The Netherlands

Michael C. Langham Laboratory for Structural, Physiologic, and Functional Imaging, Department of Radiology, University of Pennsylvania, Philadelphia, PA, USA

Christoffer Laustsen Department of Clinical Medicine, Aarhus University, Aarhus, Denmark

Lilach Lerman Division of Nephrology and Hypertension, Mayo Clinic, Rochester, MN, USA

Sara Lewis, MD Department of Radiology, Icahn School of Medicine at Mount Sinai, New York, NY, USA

Lu-Ping Li Department of Radiology, NorthShore University HealthSystem, Evanston, IL, USA

Alexandra Ljimani Department of Diagnostic and Interventional Radiology, Medical Faculty, Heinrich Heine University Düsseldorf, Düsseldorf, Germany

Christina J. MacAskill Department of Radiology, Case Western Reserve University, Cleveland, OH, USA

Ananth J. Madhuranthakam Department of Radiology, UT Southwestern Medical Center, Dallas, TX, USA

Michael T. McMahon F.M. Kirby Research Center for Functional Brain Imaging, Kennedy Krieger Institute, Baltimore, MD, USA

Russell H. Morgan Department of Radiology and Radiological Science, Johns Hopkins University School of Medicine, Baltimore, MD, USA

Iosif A. Mendichovszky Department of Radiology, University of Cambridge, Cambridge, UK

Department of Radiology, Addenbrooke's Hospital, Cambridge University Hospitals NHS Foundation Trust, Cambridge, UK

G. J. Metzger Center for Magnetic Resonance Research, University of Minnesota, Minneapolis, MN, USA

Bastien Milani Department of Medicine, Service of Nephrology and Hypertension, Lausanne University Hospital and University of Lausanne, Lausanne, Switzerland

Ewald Moser High Field MR Center, Center for Medical Physics and Biomedical Engineering, Medical University of Vienna, Vienna, Austria

Mohana Sopanahalli Narasimhamurthy Department of Pathology, University of Pennsylvania Health System, Philadelphia, PA, USA

Thoralf Niendorf Berlin Ultrahigh Field Facility (B.U.F.F.), Max-Delbrück Center for Molecular Medicine in the Helmholtz Association, Berlin, Germany

Experimental and Clinical Research Center, A Joint Cooperation Between the Charité Medical Faculty and the Max-Delbrück Center for Molecular Medicine in the Helmholtz Association, Berlin, Germany

Dominik Nörenberg Department of Radiology and Nuclear Medicine, University Medical Center Mannheim, Heidelberg University, Mannheim, Germany

Levy C. Onyango Children's Hospital of Philadelphia, Philadelphia, PA, USA

Perelman School of Medicine, University of Pennsylvania, Philadelphia, PA, USA

Hansel J. Otero Department of Radiology, Children's Hospital of Philadelphia, Philadelphia, PA, USA

Perelman School of Medicine at the University of Pennsylvania, Philadelphia, PA, USA

Pottumarthi V. Prasad Department of Radiology, NorthShore University HealthSystem, Evanston, IL, USA

Martin R. Prince Department of Radiology, Weill Cornell Medicine, New York, NY, USA

Menno Pruijm Department of Medicine, Service of Nephrology and Hypertension, Lausanne University Hospital and University of Lausanne, Lausanne, Switzerland

Pim Pullens University of Antwerp, Antwerp University Hospital, Edegem, Belgium

Erika A. Rincon-Escobar Department of Radiology, Children's Hospital of Philadelphia, Philadelphia, PA, USA

Matthew D. Robson Perspectum Ltd., Oxford, Oxfordshire, UK

Kai Ruppert Department of Radiology, University of Pennsylvania School of Medicine, Philadelphia, PA, USA

Suraj D. Serai Perelman School of Medicine, University of Pennsylvania, Philadelphia, PA, USA

Children's Hospital of Philadelphia, University of Pennsylvania, Philadelphia, PA, USA

Department of Radiology, Children's Hospital of Philadelphia, University of Pennsylvania School of Medicine, Philadelphia, PA, USA

Eric Sigmund NYU Langone Health, New York, NY, USA

Elizabeth Silvestro Children's Hospital of Philadelphia, University of Pennsylvania, Philadelphia, PA, USA

Julia Stabinska F.M. Kirby Research Center for Functional Brain Imaging, Kennedy Krieger Institute, Baltimore, MD, USA

Russell H. Morgan Department of Radiology and Radiological Science, Johns Hopkins University School of Medicine, Baltimore, MD, USA

Judd Storrs Nationwide Children's Hospital, Columbus, OH, USA

Rui Teixeira Perspectum Ltd., Oxford, Oxfordshire, UK

Sree H. Tirumani Department of Radiology, University Hospitals Cleveland Medical Center, Cleveland, OH, USA

Elizabeth M. Tunnicliffe The University of Oxford Centre for Clinical Magnetic Resonance Research (OCMR), University of Oxford, Oxford, Oxfordshire, UK

Shyam Sunder B. Venkatakrishna Children's Hospital of Philadelphia, Philadelphia, PA, USA

Sudhakar K. Venkatesh Mayo Clinic, Rochester, MN, USA

Giulia Villa Bioengineering Department, Istituto di Ricerche Farmacologiche Mario Negri IRCCS, Bergamo, Italy

Bernarda Viteri Children's Hospital of Philadelphia, Philadelphia, PA, USA

Perelman School of Medicine, University of Pennsylvania, Philadelphia, PA, USA

Yi Wang Department of Radiology, Weill Cornell Medicine, New York, NY, USA

Zhen Jane Wang University of California San Francisco, San Francisco, CA, USA

Felix W. Wehrli Laboratory for Structural, Physiologic, and Functional Imaging, Department of Radiology, University of Pennsylvania, Philadelphia, PA, USA

Marcos Wolf High Field MR Center, Center for Medical Physics and Biomedical Engineering, Medical University of Vienna, Vienna, Austria

Frank G. Zöllner Computer Assisted Clinical Medicine, Mannheim Institute for Intelligent Systems in Medicine, Medical Faculty Mannheim, Heidelberg University, Mannheim, Germany

Part I

General Considerations for Kidney MRI

1 Kidney Anatomy and Physiology

Shyam Sunder B. Venkatakrishna,
Levy C. Onyango, Suraj D. Serai,
and Bernarda Viteri

The kidneys are a pair of bean-shaped organs located retroperitoneally on either side of midline, between the transverse processes of T12–L3 vertebrae. Kidneys are involved in the maintenance of the fluid and electrolyte levels, acid-base balance, filtration and excretion of metabolic waste such as urea and ammonium, stimulate red blood cell (RBC) synthesis, and regulation of blood pressure through the renin-angiotensin-aldosterone system and other mechanisms. The maintenance of homeostasis is required for optimum performance by the cells and organs. The kidneys also play a vital endocrine role in hormone production such as renin, erythropoietin, and calcitriol (1,25-dihydroxycholecalciferol).

S. S. B. Venkatakrishna
Children's Hospital of Philadelphia,
Philadelphia, PA, USA
e-mail: venkatakrs@chop.edu

L. C. Onyango · S. D. Serai (✉) · B. Viteri
Children's Hospital of Philadelphia,
Philadelphia, PA, USA

Perelman School of Medicine, University of Pennsylvania, Philadelphia, PA, USA
e-mail: onyangol@chop.edu; serais@chop.edu; viterib@chop.edu

Anatomy

The kidneys are located between the transverse processes of T12–L3 vertebrae, in the retroperitoneum, on either side of the midline. Each kidney has an upper pole and a lower pole with a minor concave medial border and major lateral border, which is convex. They consist of three regions: the outer cortex, the medulla subdivided into outer and inner medulla, and the innermost papilla. About the size of a closed fist, each kidney's usual dimensions [in cm] are 5–7 width and 3–5 thickness with 10–12 length in adults [1]. Initial development of the kidney is opposite future S2 vertebra, but it finally settles opposite the L1/L2 vertebra [2, 3]. Usual orientation of the upper poles of the kidney is slightly medial and posterior with respect to the lower poles of the kidneys. Most likely due to the presence of the liver, the right kidney is typically positioned slightly below the left kidney [1, 4]. Lateral orientation of the upper kidney poles may be suggestive of the **horseshoe kidney** or renal mass of superior pole. The normal kidney's medial border is more anterior compared to the lateral border when lying supine; thus the kidneys are at an angle of around 30° from the horizontal [3, 5].

Anatomical relations of the kidneys with respect to their surroundings [1, 3, 6, 7] are the following:

S. D. Serai, K. Darge (eds.), *Advanced Clinical MRI of the Kidney*,
https://doi.org/10.1007/978-3-031-40169-5_1

- Anteriorly, the left kidney has relations with the spleen, tail of the pancreas, stomach, left colon and left colic flexure, small intestine, and ligament of Treitz.
- Anteriorly, the right kidney has relations with the inferior surface of the liver, second part of the duodenum, the right colic flexure, and the small intestine.
- The posterior surface of both kidneys have relations with the diaphragm, psoas major muscle, quadratus lumborum, transversus abdominis, medial and lateral arcuate ligaments, subcostal vessels, and subcostal, iliohypogastric, and ilioinguinal nerves [right kidney related to 12th rib and left kidney to 11th and 12th ribs due to its higher position].
- The following structures are posterior to the right kidney: the liver is separated from the right kidney by the hepatorenal recess, and the right kidney is also posterior to the second part of the duodenum [medial] and ascending colon.
- The upper poles of each kidney, superiorly, have relation with the suprarenal glands [adrenal glands].
- Splenorenal ligament [vertical] and transverse mesocolon [horizontal] are two main peritoneal reflections over the left kidney.
- Location of the kidneys is above the psoas muscles [medially] and quadratus lumborum muscles [lateral aspect].
- The upper part of each kidney is covered by the diaphragm posteriorly, and the upper pole is most frequently crossed by the 12th rib.
- Each kidney, on its medial margin, has a deep fissure, where there is entry of renal artery and the renal vein and pelvis exit the renal sinus and this is the "renal hilum" (Fig. 1.1), and its projection is at L2 vertebra level.
- From deep to superficial, complex layers of fascia and fat enclose the kidney as follows: renal capsule (fibrous and firm), perinephric fat, renal fascia (or perirenal fascia or Gerota's fascia, which covers the suprarenal glands and kidneys), and the paranephric fat.

Figures 1.1 and 1.2 represent the schematic representation of an overview on kidney anatomy. The internal structural anatomy of the kidney is unique and complex (Fig. 1.2). Outer renal cortex and inner medulla forms the renal parenchyma. Cortical lobules [caps over pyramid base] and renal columns [dips between pyramids] are the two parts of the renal cortex. A lobe of kidney is formed by a single pyramid and the cortical arch that is overlying. Around 1–3 million uriniferous tubules make up the kidney, and each one consists of two parts that are different embryologically. The structural and functional units of the kidneys are the nephrons [1–1.5 million nephrons in each kidney]. Each nephron consists of a filter (renal corpuscle) and a renal tubule (Fig. 1.4). Renal corpuscles contain a tuft of capillaries called the glomerulus which refers to as "Latin ball" that are surrounded by Bowman (glomerular) capsule; here the blood is filtered. Each renal tubule helps return to the blood nutrients needed (as a blood vessel runs alongside each tubule) and continues to remove excess waste products from the filtered fluid through the proximal and distal convoluted tubules [PCT and DCT], located in the renal cortex (Fig. 1.3), and through the loops of Henle [descending and ascending tubules] and collecting tubules, located in the medulla. The medulla is formed by the renal pyramids [around 8–12 in number] and the loops of Henle and collecting tubules. Renal pyramid's apex is the renal papilla and they extend into the minor calyx. Fluid filtered from the collecting tubules becomes urine and is received by the minor calyces and is then emptied to [around 2 or 3 in number] major calyces. The urine collected here is later emptied into the renal pelvis, which is the dilated upper portion of the ureter. It travels via the ureter to the urinary bladder, which stores urine until it is time for micturition.

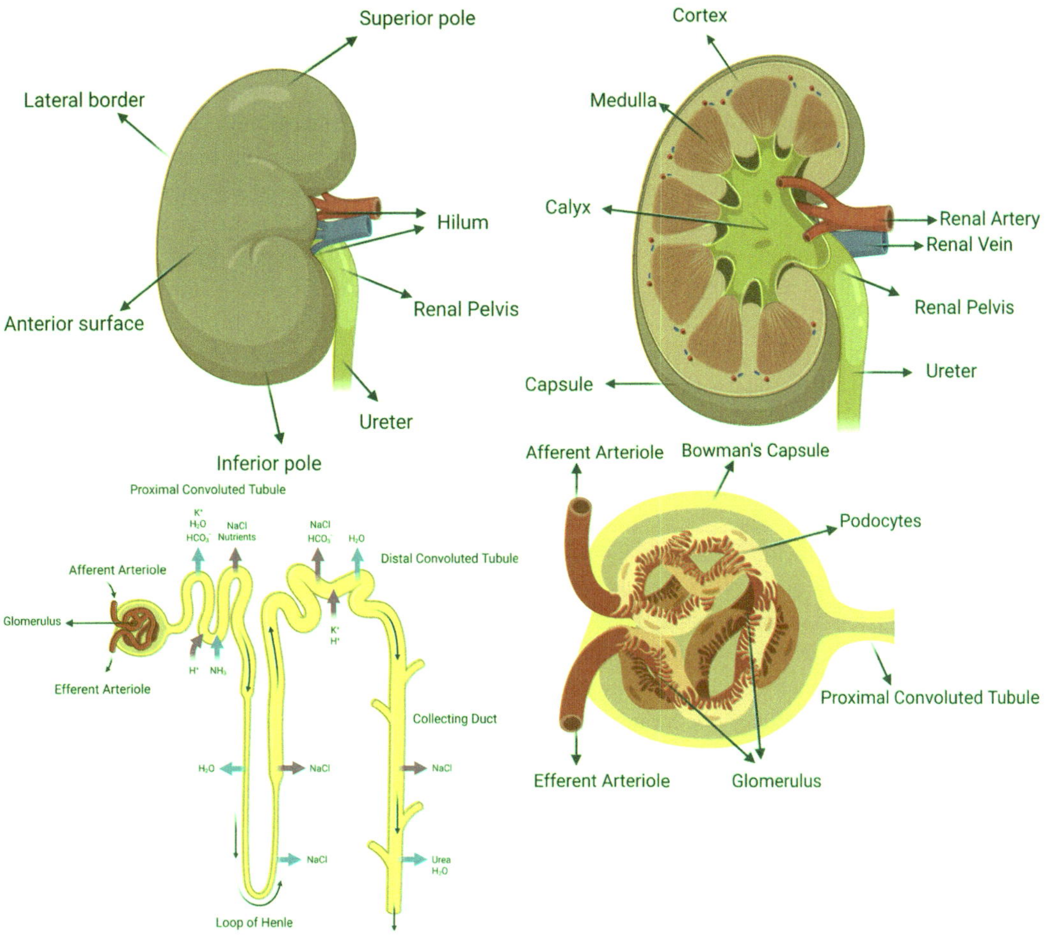

Figs. 1.1–1.4 Schematic representation of the anatomy of the kidney (1) with an overview on cross-sectional anatomy (2), nephron structure [*also showing reabsorption and secretion; purple arrow, active transport, and blue arrow, passive transport*] (3), and renal corpuscle (4) [*Created with* BioRender.com]

Blood Supply, Innervation, and Lymphatics

Kidneys are highly vascular organs with around 20% of cardiac output received by the kidneys. Right and left renal arteries are the main blood supply of the kidneys, and these are direct lateral branches of the abdominal aorta, and the artery is immediately distal to the superior mesenteric artery (SMA) origin. The right renal artery is longer due to the abdominal aorta's anatomical position situated slightly to the left of the midline with its crossing of vena cava posteriorly. Five segmental branches [end arteries with no collaterals or anastomosis] arise from the renal artery, where in anterior division it supplies four segments and just one from the posterior division. The following areas are supplied by the segmental arteries of the same name from anterior division, the superior segment, the anterosuperior segment, the anteroinferior segment, and the inferior segment, whereas the posterior segment is supplied by the posterior segmental artery. Renal artery branches and renal vein tributaries are in the renal sinus, which is a space extending from the hilus into the kidney. This is also of surgical importance. In case of vessel degeneration failure, accessory renal arteries may originate from the aorta or renal artery and typically enter the poles, and these arteries are left over embryologically, in around 25% of patients [1, 3, 8–10].

Detection of renal lymphatics using microradiography at autopsy was done in humans [11]. There is abundance of lymphatic vessels around intrarenal vessels, but as the lymphatic starts in the cortical interstitium, there is scarcity around the glomeruli or between the tubules [3, 12]. The renal hilar nodes and the abdominal para-aortic nodes, with the interaortocaval, paracaval, precaval, retrocaval, preaortic, and retroaortic lymph nodes, are the lymph nodes for the kidneys [3, 13]. Renal hilar and paracaval lymph node groups are primarily responsible for draining the ureters [3].

The nerve supply to the kidney is via *renal plexus* and it consists of sympathetic and parasympathetic fibers. The spinal cord, at the level of T8–L1, is the origin of the preganglionic sympathetic neural innervation of the kidneys. Parasympathetic innervation of the kidney is provided by the renal branches of the vagus nerve [3]. The sympathetic fibers in the spinal ganglia and cord segments [T11–L2] receive pain signals from visceral afferent fibers [1, 14, 15]. Corresponding dermatomes sense the pain as a result of which referred pain from the kidney can be felt in the corresponding flank region.

Embryology

The nephrogenic cord, along with the pronephros, mesonephros, and metanephros, starts to develop in week four of gestation, and this marks the beginning of the embryological development of the urinary tract [1, 3, 16–18]. Intermediate mesoderm is the source of development of the kidney. The urinary system and reproductive system both develop from the same origin, which is frequently referred to as the "urogenital ridge." Due to this reason, anomalies in one system may also be present in the other. The nephrogenic cord, which develops into the urinary system, and the gonadal ridge, which develops into the reproductive tract, separate from the urogenital ridge during the fourth week of pregnancy. The three embryonic kidneys (the pronephros, mesonephros, and metanephros) begin rostral in position and progress to caudal in position sequentially. Around fourth week of gestation, the development of pronephros begins, but in utero, they regress and in humans will not be functioning kidneys. The development of mesonephros in the next caudal region to pronephros forms the mesonephric tubules and glomeruli. At the end of the first trimester, there is regression of mesonephros. Metanephric kidney starts to develop in gestation of fifth week and later on forms the permanent kidneys after differentiation. Around the sixth week, there is presence of two bilateral organs [17]. Ureter develops from the ureteric bud stalk. The development of renal pelvis, calyces, and collecting tubules is from the ureteric bud branching [18]. Development of nephrons occurs in the metanephric blastema.

Bladder is formed from the superior portion of urogenital sinus, and by the fourth month of gestation, there is completion of both ureter and bladder development.

If there is degeneration of ureteric bud early or metanephros involution, it can lead to metanephric blastema regression and renal agenesis. Partial duplication of collecting system can be caused due to ureteric bud bifurcation [18]. Ureteral ectopia and/or VUR (vesicoureteral reflux) may develop due to an abnormality in the ureteric bud origin or maldevelopment [3, 18, 19].

Around 32–36 weeks of gestation, the kidney structure is complete, and the initial location of the permanent kidneys is in the pelvis. However, even after birth, the maturation of nephron continues. There is ascension of the kidneys in the growing embryo to a lumbar position, and the convex borders are oriented laterally due to the undergoing of a 90° rotation. The course of the ureter is inferior along the psoas muscles and into the pelvis via the retroperitoneum, crossing anterior to iliac vessels and finally linking to the bladder. On the posterolateral side of the bladder

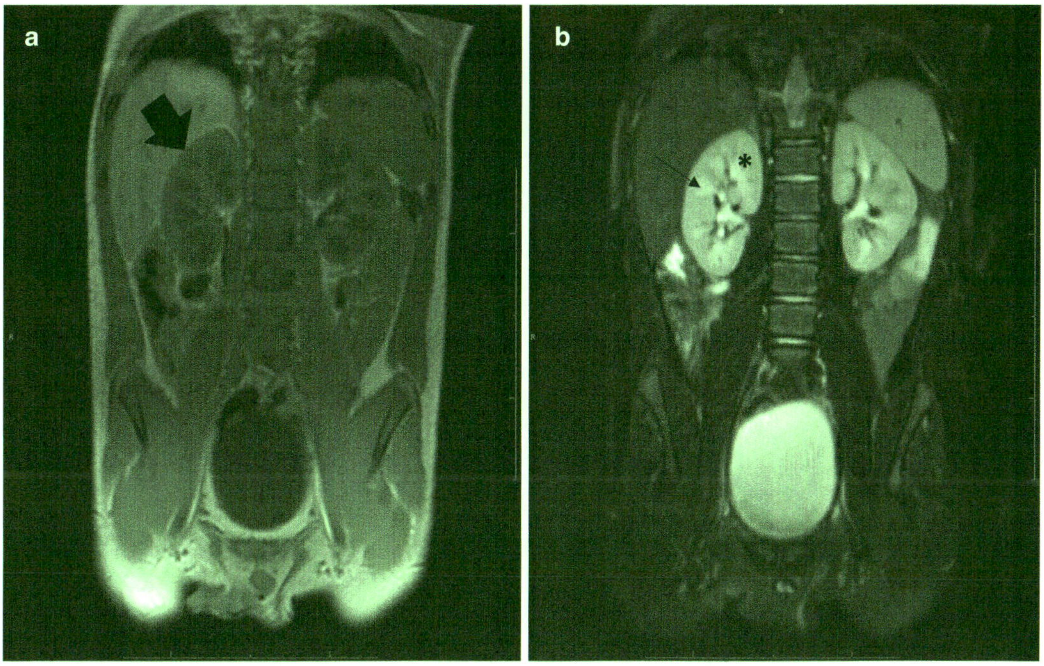

Fig. 1.5 (**a**) Coronal T1-weighted MR image of a nine-year-old boy demonstrating expected normal T1 hyperintense cortex (*black arrow*) and (**b**) normal coronal T2-weighted fat-suppressed MR image demonstrating the expected T2 prolongation within the cortex (*asterisk*) and medulla (*black arrow*)

trigone is the location of insertion of the normal ureter [18]. On T1- and T2-weighted MR images, hyperintense appearance of the renal cortex [normal] is seen compared to the medulla [18, 20]. Corticomedullary differentiation which is distinct should be observed, and early in life, normal fetal lobulations may be observed; while they often regress, there may be persistence as a normal variant to adult life [18].

Figures 1.5 and 1.6 show examples of normal MR imaging appearance of the kidney. Complete absence of one or both kidneys refers to renal agenesis, and estimated associated reproductive tract anomalies are at 30% [females] and 20% [males] [18, 21]. Complete absence of renal tissue on one side ranging from the pelvis to renal fossa is seen on MRI (Fig. 1.7).

The most frequent fusion anomaly is the horseshoe kidney where the kidneys are fused by an isthmus of renal parenchyma or fibrous tissue and the kidneys are on either side of the spine and the depiction of fused right- and left-sided kidneys is seen on MRI (Fig. 1.8).

Due to developmental anomalies associated with an issue in the caudal to cranial migration, the location of a kidney or both kidneys are abnormal and is referred to as renal ectopia. If the location of both kidneys is on the same side of the spine, it is referred to as crossed renal ectopia, and it may be unfused or fused [18, 22]. Figure 1.9 represents the MR imaging appearance of cross fused renal ectopia.

Developmental anomalies in the ureteric bud can lead to duplex kidney, and the urinary tract's most common anomaly is ureteral duplication. Its incidence rate is estimated at 0.8–5% and more common is incomplete duplication compared to complete duplication [18, 23, 24]. Figures 1.10 and 1.11 represent examples of MR imaging appearance of duplicated systems.

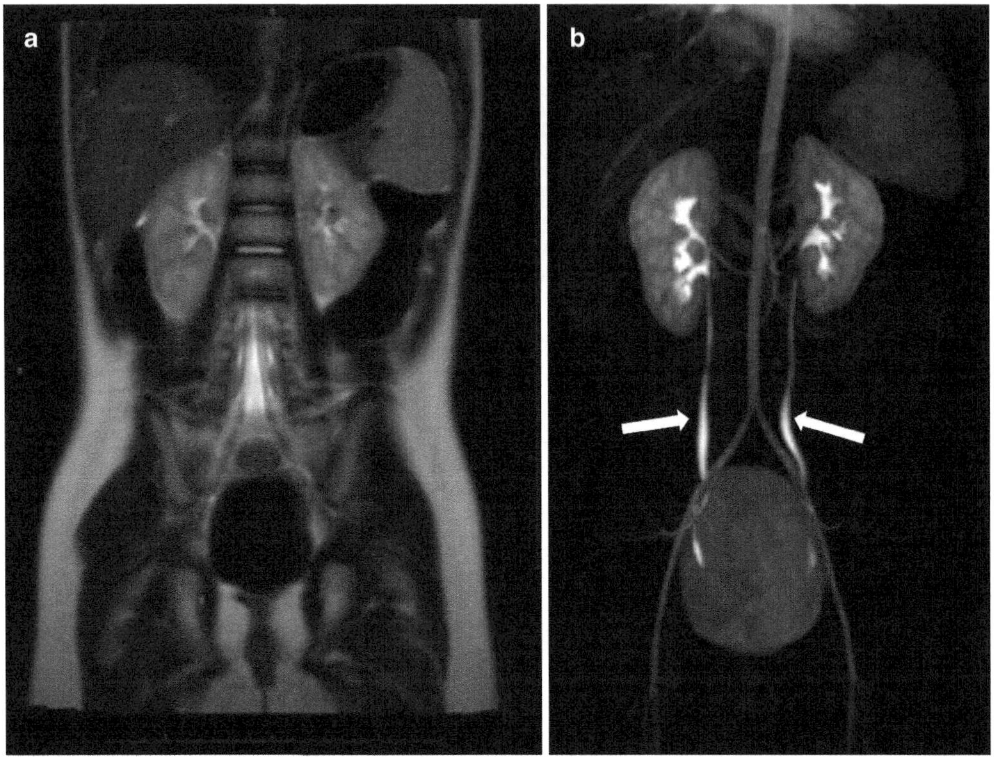

Fig. 1.6 (**a**) Coronal T2-weighted MR image of a three-year-old girl demonstrating an expected increased T2 signal of the cortex relative the medulla and (**b**) three-dimensional subtraction coronal MR image demonstrating bilateral kidneys in the secretory phase. Note opacification of the bilateral ureters (*white arrows*)

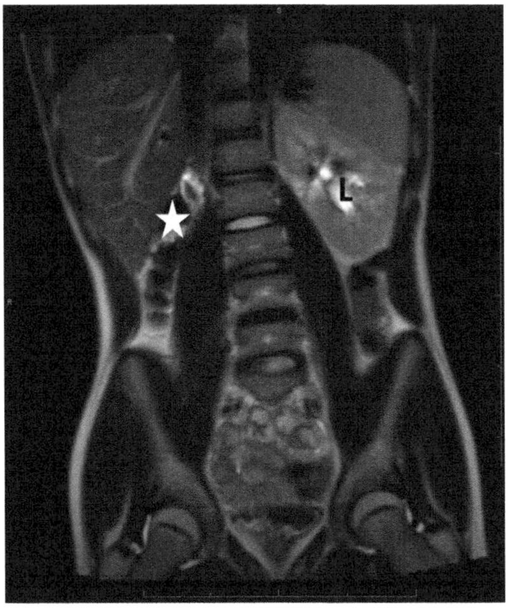

Fig. 1.7 Coronal T2-weighted MR image of a 13-year-old boy with **right renal agenesis** demonstrating a normal left kidney (*L*). Note the absence of the right kidney in the right renal fossa (*white star*)

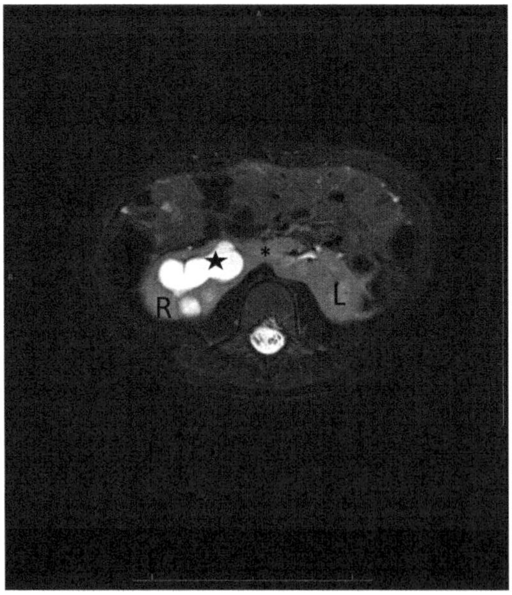

Fig. 1.8 Axial T2-weighted fat saturated MR image of a three-year-old girl demonstrating **horseshoe kidney**. Note the fusion of the right (*R*) and left (*L*) moieties at the isthmus (*black asterisk*) as well as mild calyceal dilation (*black star*) of the right moiety collecting system

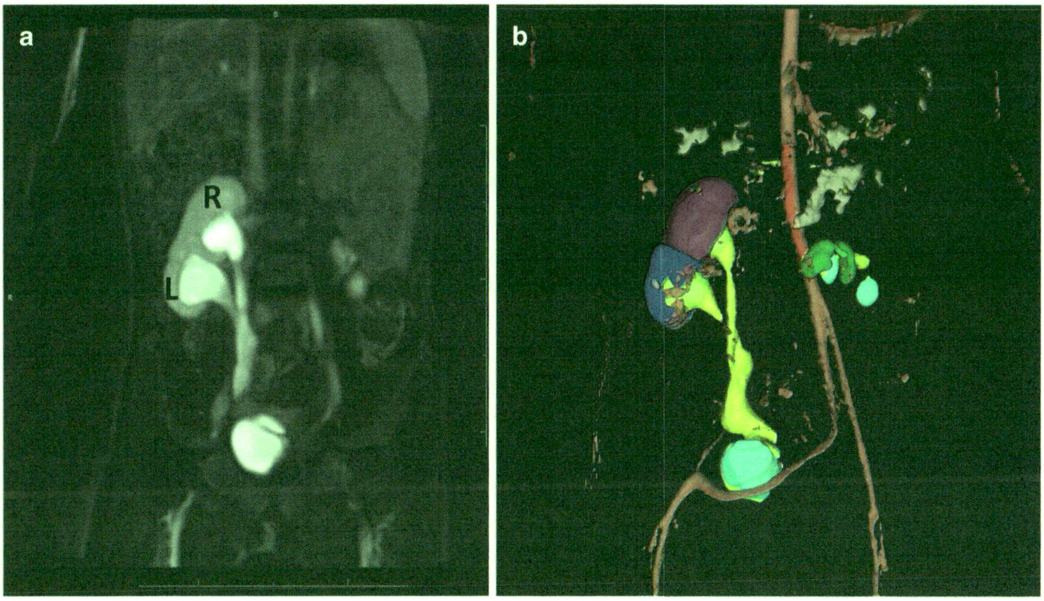

Fig. 1.9 (**a**) Coronal T2-weighted fat-suppressed MR image of an eight-year-old girl with history of **cross fused renal ectopia demonstrates the fusion of the left kidney** (*L*) to the right kidney (*R*) at the lower pole with respective ureters mildly prominent and coursing inferiorly. (**b**) Three-dimensional rendered post processed image with purple representing the native right kidney. Blue represents the ectopic left kidney, yellow represents bilateral ureters, and light blue represents the urinary bladder

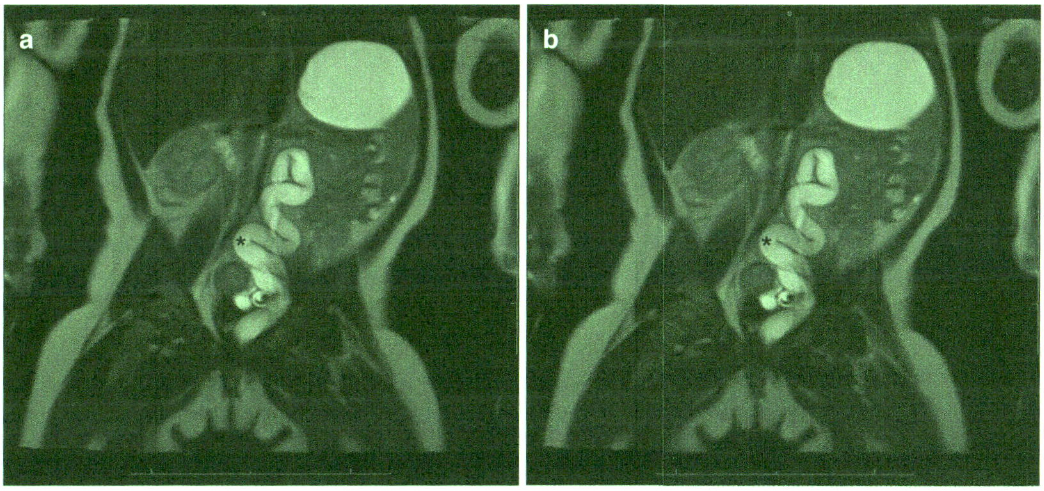

Fig. 1.10 MRI of a five-month-old girl shows duplicating system with hydroureteronephrosis of the upper moiety. (**a**) Coronal T2 image demonstrating a **duplication of the right collecting system** (*black and white asterisks*). (**b**) **Ureterectasis of the upper moiety** with tortuosity of the ureter (*black asterisk*) related to distal obstruction and characteristic of the upper moiety in duplication systems

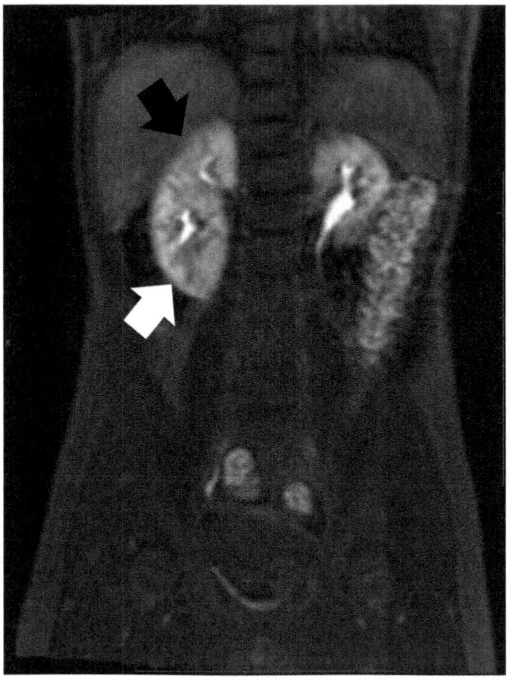

Fig. 1.11 Coronal postcontrast T1-weighted MR image of a four-year-old girl showing a **duplicated system** with the *black arrow* demonstrating the upper moiety and *white arrow* representing lower moiety

Physiology

Kidneys are essential in the homeostasis of blood pressure, electrolyte, bone minerals, and fluid [25–32]. Another important function of the kidneys is filtering and excreting metabolic waste products from the body. Kidneys also play vital endocrinology role in the production of erythropoietin and 1,25-dihydroxycholecalciferol. The kidneys have a high blood supply with normal renal blood flow of about 1.25 L/min, around 20–25% of the cardiac output. Filtration of around 20% of the plasma passing through the kidneys occurs [25]. The three main primary steps for filtration of blood and maintenance of electrolyte balance are as follows: glomerular filtration, tubular reabsorption, and tubular secretion.

In the process of production of urine, glomerular filtration is the first step. Capillary endothelial cells, glomerular basement membrane, and podocytes form the glomerular filtration barrier. Endothelial cells have 70–100 nm fenestrations. Collagen, glycoproteins, peptidoglycan, and laminin make up the glomerular basement membrane. The glomerular membrane is composed of one electronic dense layer sandwiched between two electron lucent layers when viewed under an electron microscope. Interdigitating foot processes with 20–30 nm filtration slits are seen on podocytes. Water and small- and medium-sized plasma solutes, including insulin, can freely pass through the filtration barrier. Based on their sizes and charges, other solutes are filtered. The amount of water and solutes that can pass the filtration membrane is determined by the outward and inward force of the capillaries. The primary filtration force, with a pressure of 55 mmHg, comes from the glomerular capillaries' hydrostatic pressure [33]. The colloid osmotic pressure in the capsular space, which is another possible filtration force, is zero since the capsular space typically lacks proteins. The net Starling forces across the glomerular capillary wall are responsible for glomerular ultrafiltration. Glomerular filtration rate (GFR) is a main parameter to indicate the renal function, and it corresponds to the volume of water filtered out of the plasma via the glomerular capillary walls and into Bowman's capsules per unit of time [3]. GFR is determined by the net filtration pressure, the total amount of surface area that is accessible for filtration, and the permeability of the filtration membrane. The normal GFR ranges from 120 to 125 mL/min. A process called autoregulation is involved in holding the glomerular filtration constant despite changes of systemic and renal artery pressures. The macula densa, which lies next to the glomerulus, regulates the constriction and dilation of the afferent arteriole. The macula densa detects the movement of sodium chloride via the adjacent tubule. The macula densa causes the afferent arteriole to constrict, when this flow is increased, hence decreasing the glomerular filtration rate [25]. In contrast, if there is decrease in the pressure of blood entering the kidney, the resistance in the afferent arteriole decreases in order to maintain the pressure inside the glomerulus. In case the inflow pressure continues to decrease, angiotensin II forces the efferent arteriole to constrict, thus maintaining the pressure of filtration in the glomerulus [25]. Renin-angiotensin-aldosterone mechanism and sympathetic nervous system are responsible for the extrinsic control mechanisms in maintaining GFR and systemic blood pressure [33].

Each of the four tubular segments have absorptive properties that are unique (Fig. 1.3). PCT is the first segment with highest capability of absorption. Sixty-five percent of Na and water along with all glucose and amino acids is absorbed by the PCT [33]. Urea is reabsorbed in the PCT by passive paracellular diffusion driven by a chemical gradient [33, 34]. Non-reabsorbed filtrates proceed to the loop of Henle which has a descending [water reabsorption through osmosis] and ascending limb, where there is passive movement of Na (sodium) down the concentration gradient in thin segment of the ascending limb with reabsorption of sodium, potassium, and chlorides in the thick segment [33]. Reabsorption of water does not occur in the ascending limb [33, 35]. Primary and secondary active sodium transport occurs via Na-Cl symporters and channels in DCT, and at the distal portion, it is regulated by aldosterone [33]. Parathyroid hormone-controlled reabsorption of calcium through passive uptake occurs. The final reabsorption stage occurs in the collecting tubule [33, 36]. Removal of waste metabolites, drugs, and unwanted substances that were passively reabsorbed [e.g., urea, uric acid] occurs in tubular secretion. The urine, after its production, travels to the urinary bladder via the ureter, and the unique structure of the bladder allows it to store urine until it is time to void the urine [micturition] where there is contraction of the detrusor muscle and urethral sphincter [internal and external] relaxation.

Summary

Kidneys are complex and vital organs that serve in various capacities such as excretory, regulatory, and endocrine organs. Through various biochemical mechanisms that are exquisite, the kidneys regulate blood pressure, electrolytes, water, and acid-base balance along with its main role of excretion of metabolic waste products.

References

1. Soriano RM, Penfold D, Leslie SW. Anatomy, abdomen and pelvis, kidneys. Treasure Island: StatPearls Publishing; 2020.
2. Federle MP. Embryology of the abdomen. In: Federle MP, Rosado-de-Christenson ML, Woodward PJ, et al., editors. Diagnostic and surgical imaging anatomy. Chest, abdomen, pelvis. Altona: Amirsys; 2006. p. 446–83.
3. Quaia E, Martingano P, Cavallaro M, Zappetti R. Normal radiological anatomy and anatomical variants of the kidney. In: Quaia E, editor. Radiological imaging of the kidney. Berlin: Springer Berlin Heidelberg; 2011. p. 17–77.
4. El-Reshaid W, Abdul-Fattah H. Sonographic assessment of renal size in healthy adults. Med Princ Pract. 2014;23:432–6.
5. Nino-Murcia M, DeVries PA, Friedland GW. Congenital anomalies of the kidneys. Clin Uroradiol. 2000;1:690–763.
6. Coffin A, Boulay-Coletta I, Sebbag-Sfez D, Zins M. Radioanatomy of the retroperitoneal space. Diagn Interv Imaging. 2015;96:171–86.
7. Tirkes T, Sandrasegaran K, Patel AA, Hollar MA, Tejada JG, Tann M, et al. Peritoneal and retroperitoneal anatomy and its relevance for cross-sectional imaging. Radiographics. 2012;32:437–51.
8. Lung K, Lui F. Anatomy, abdomen and pelvis, arteries. Treasure Island: StatPearls Publishing; 2021.
9. Wright N, Burns B. Anatomy, abdomen and pelvis, posterior abdominal wall arteries. Treasure Island: StatPearls Publishing; 2020.
10. Jamkar AA, Khan B, Joshi DS. Anatomical study of renal and accessory renal arteries. Saudi J Kidney Dis Transpl. 2017;28:292–7.
11. Cuttino JT, Clark RL, Jennette JC. Microradiographic demonstration of human intrarenal microlymphatic pathways. Urol Radiol. 1989;11:83–7.
12. Ishikawa Y, Akasaka Y, Kiguchi H, Akishima-Fukasawa Y, Hasegawa T, Ito K, et al. The human renal lymphatics under normal and pathological conditions. Histopathology. 2006;49:265–73.
13. Russell PS, Hong J, Windsor JA, Itkin M, Phillips ARJ. Renal lymphatics: anatomy, physiology, and clinical implications. Front Physiol. 2019;10:251.
14. Frame AA, Carmichael CY, Wainford RD. Renal afferents. Curr Hypertens Rep. 2016;18:69.
15. Kopp UC. Role of renal sensory nerves in physiological and pathophysiological conditions. Am J Physiol Regul Integr Comp Physiol. 2015;308:R79–95.
16. Zweyer M. Embryology of the kidney. In: Quaia E, editor. Radiological imaging of the kidney. Berlin: Springer Berlin Heidelberg; 2014. p. 3–15.
17. Rehman S, Ahmed D. Embryology, kidney, bladder, and ureter. Treasure Island: StatPearls Publishing; 2022.
18. Tutman JJ, Lee EY, Shabani A, Paltiel HJ. Kidney, ureter, and bladder. In: Lee EY, Liszewski MC, Gee MS,

Daltro P, Restrepo R, editors. Pediatric body MRI: a comprehensive, multidisciplinary guide. Cham: Springer International Publishing; 2020. p. 327–54.
19. Bedard MP, Wildman S, Dillman JR. Embryology, anatomy, and variants of the genitourinary tract. In: Coley BD, editor. Caffey's pediatric diagnostic imaging. 12th ed. Philadelphia: Elsevier; 2013. p. 1163–73.
20. Leung AW, Bydder GM, Steiner RE, Bryant DJ, Young IR. Magnetic resonance imaging of the kidneys. AJR Am J Roentgenol. 1984;143:1215–27.
21. Shapiro E, Goldfarb DA, Ritchey ML. The congenital and acquired solitary kidney. Rev Urol. 2003;5:2–8.
22. Solanki S, Bhatnagar V, Gupta AK, Kumar R. Crossed fused renal ectopia: challenges in diagnosis and management. J Indian Assoc Pediatr Surg. 2013;18:7–10.
23. Williams H. Renal revision: from lobulation to duplication—what is normal? Arch Dis Child Educ Pract Ed. 2007;92:ep152–8.
24. Fernbach SK, Feinstein KA, Spencer K, Lindstrom CA. Ureteral duplication and its complications. Radiographics. 1997;17:109–27.
25. Rayner HC, Thomas ME, Milford DV. Kidney anatomy and physiology: the basis of clinical nephrology. Understanding kidney diseases. Cham: Springer International Publishing; 2020. p. 1–9.
26. Hoenig MP, Zeidel ML. Homeostasis, the milieu intérieur, and the wisdom of the nephron. Clin J Am Soc Nephrol. 2014;9:1272–81.
27. Pluznick JL, Caplan MJ. Chemical and physical sensors in the regulation of renal function. Clin J Am Soc Nephrol. 2015;10:1626–35.
28. Subramanya AR, Ellison DH. Distal convoluted tubule. Clin J Am Soc Nephrol. 2014;9:2147–63.
29. Palmer LG, Schnermann J. Integrated control of Na transport along the nephron. Clin J Am Soc Nephrol. 2015;10:676–87.
30. Danziger J, Zeidel ML. Osmotic homeostasis. Clin J Am Soc Nephrol. 2015;10:852–62.
31. Curthoys NP, Moe OW. Proximal tubule function and response to acidosis. Clin J Am Soc Nephrol. 2014;9:1627–38.
32. Blaine J, Chonchol M, Levi M. Renal control of calcium, phosphate, and magnesium homeostasis. Clin J Am Soc Nephrol. 2015;10:1257–72.
33. Ogobuiro I, Tuma F. Physiology, renal. Treasure Island: StatPearls Publishing; 2022.
34. Agnoli GC, Garutti C. [Renal water-electrolyte excretion and its control mechanisms. Current status of knowledge]. Minerva Med. 1976;67:3673–3702.
35. Mount DB. Thick ascending limb of the loop of Henle. Clin J Am Soc Nephrol. 2014;9:1974–86.
36. Roy A, Al-bataineh MM, Pastor-Soler NM. Collecting duct intercalated cell function and regulation. Clin J Am Soc Nephrol. 2015;10:305–24.

2 MR Physics, Hardware Considerations, and Practical Steps for Clinical MRI of the Kidney

Suraj D. Serai, Kai Ruppert, Sanjeev Chawla, and Sachin Jambawalikar

Introduction

Magnetic resonance imaging (MRI) is a comprehensive diagnostic imaging modality with high soft tissue contrast capable of generating multiparametric images based on anatomical, metabolic, chemical, or physiological information from inside the body—noninvasively and without the use of ionizing radiation. It is a highly versatile tomographic imaging technique that acquires data as multiple slices or sections in any orientation, including oblique planes. An MRI system is composed of four main hardware components: (1) a primary, high-field strength magnet that is large enough to encompass the body of an adult subject, (2) the gradient subsystem, (3) the radiofrequency (RF) subsystem, and (4) computer systems that interface with and control the various components (Figs. 2.1, 2.2, 2.3, and 2.4). Understanding the interplay of these key components of the MRI system is foundational to acquiring diagnostic-quality MR images.

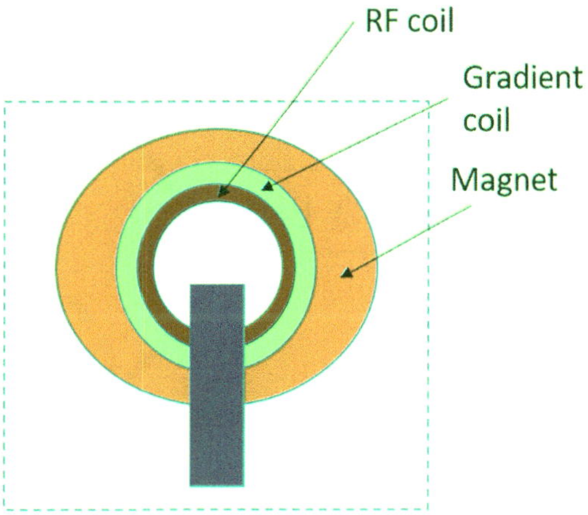

Fig. 2.1 Block diagram of a typical MRI system. (© [Suraj D. Serai, 2023. All Rights Reserved])

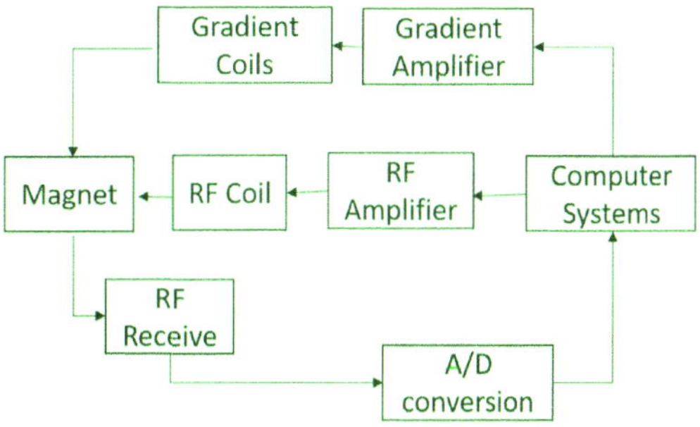

Fig. 2.2 A functional block diagram of MRI data flow

S. D. Serai (✉)
Department of Radiology, Children's Hospital of Philadelphia, University of Pennsylvania School of Medicine, Philadelphia, PA, USA
e-mail: serais@chop.edu

K. Ruppert · S. Chawla
Department of Radiology, University of Pennsylvania School of Medicine, Philadelphia, PA, USA
e-mail: kai.ruppert@pennmedicine.upenn.edu; Sanjeev.Chawla@pennmedicine.upenn.edu

S. Jambawalikar
Department of Radiology, Columbia University Medical Center, New York, NY, USA
e-mail: sj2532@cumc.columbia.edu

S. D. Serai, K. Darge (eds.), *Advanced Clinical MRI of the Kidney*,
https://doi.org/10.1007/978-3-031-40169-5_2

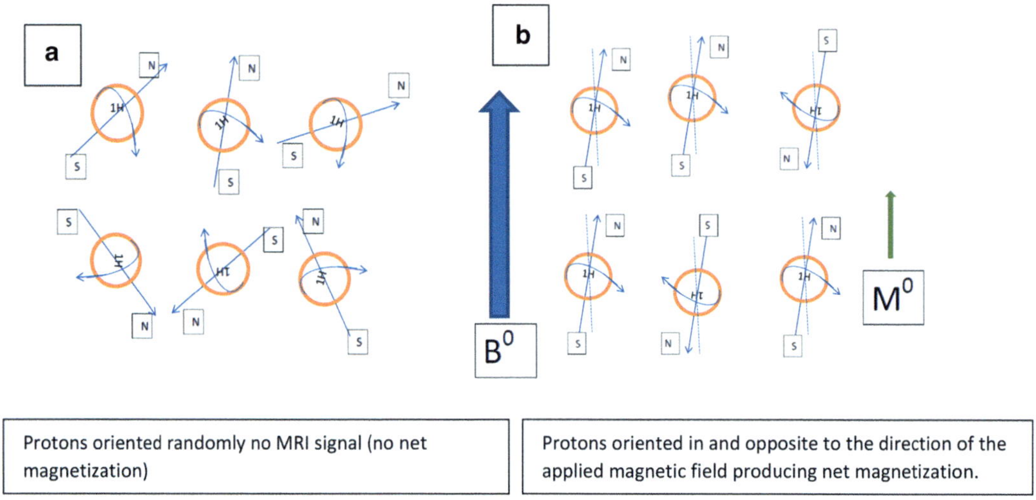

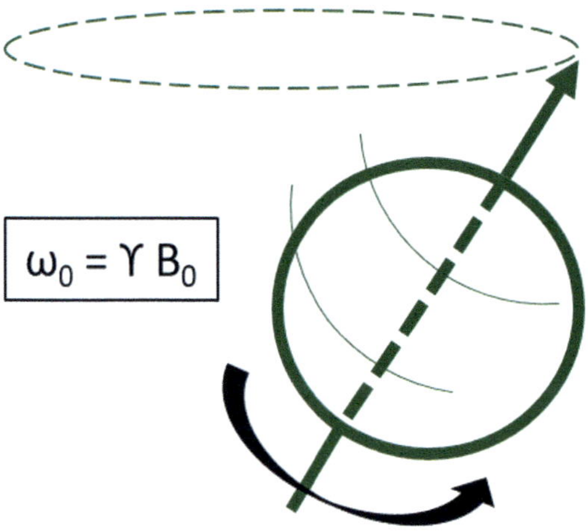

Fig. 2.3 Schematic representation of a spinning proton. The frequency of hydrogen nuclei precession is known as the Larmor frequency (ω_0), where ϒ is the gyromagnetic ratio (42.5 MHz/T) and B_0 is the external magnetic field. (© [Suraj D. Serai, 2023. All rights reserved])

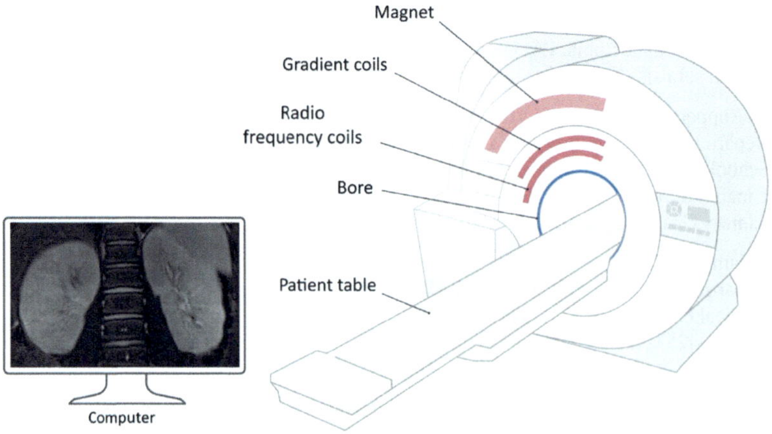

Fig. 2.4 Schematic of a clinical MRI scanner. (© [Suraj D. Serai, 2023. All rights reserved])

The most dominant, and usually also the most expensive, component of a closed-bore clinical MRI scanner is the powerful superconducting magnet that generates the strong static, stable, and homogenous magnetic field (denoted by B_0) in which the subject is placed for the scan. In general, the higher the field strength, the stronger the resulting signal but also the higher price tag of the system. The second component is a set of three concentric gradient coil systems (oriented orthogonally in X, Y, and Z directions) close to the walls of the bore of the main coil. During the MRI scan, the gradient coils superimpose approximately linear, time-varying magnetic field variations upon the static B_0 field used for spatial encoding and localization of the MR signal [1]. These oscillations are also the source of the characteristic knocking sounds that accompany MRI acquisitions. The third component is the RF system. Most notably, it consists of one or more coils near the subject that transmit the megahertz range electromagnetic field oscillations (B_1) at the resonant frequency of the imaged nucleus (usually protons) to be excited. In response, the excited nuclei then emit the MRI signal that is detected by a receiver coil. Since transmitting and receiving RF signals are implemented as sequential events, they can be performed by the same coil although many MRI coil arrangements have separate transmit and dedicated receive elements for different anatomy locations to improve MRI image quality and signal to noise. Finally, the fourth component consists of multiple interconnected computer systems that provide the user interface, perform the digital-to-analog conversion for generating the gradient waveforms and the RF-excitation field B_1, conduct the analog-to-digital conversion of the collected signals from the patient, and calculate the resulting images that can be displayed and interpreted on the console.

A unique feature of MRI is the intricate dependence of the obtained image information and quality on the temporal arrangement and variation of the applied RF fields and image-encoding gradients in the form of so-called pulse sequences. Over the decades, countless pulse sequences have been developed that are optimized for measuring relevant information about all the main organs and structures in the body. The focus of this book is the detection, staging, and monitoring of kidney diseases (KD) using measurements of renal function and structure that is critical in clinical nephrology as accessible with the help of MRI. In addition to established anatomical imaging techniques, novel pulse sequences such as dynamic contrast-enhanced MRI (DCE-MRI), arterial spin labeling (ASL), blood-oxygen-level-dependent (BOLD) MRI, and diffusion-weighted imaging (DWI) can provide a broad characterization of the kidney, including renal vascular perfusion, oxygenation, and glomerular filtration rate. The high spatial and temporal resolution provided by this modality is essential for functional MR urography techniques, and they can be performed longitudinally even in pediatric population as there is no exposure to ionizing radiation. This chapter is intended to outline the key hardware components and operational features of an MRI scanner and to provide an overview of currently employed renal MR imaging technologies and is written for a target audience of clinicians and MR technicians. The basic concepts and terminologies are explained, and a broad overview of the applications is given. An in-depth explanation of current state-of-the-art kidney imaging methods is provided, followed by novel technologies, approaches, and current advances in the field of kidney MRI in the final sections.

The MRI Signal

The principles of MRI physics can be conceptualized by envisioning that those nuclei of certain atoms produce nuclear magnetic resonance signal. Several different types of nuclei are suitable for MR imaging, but hydrogen nuclei, that is, protons, which are overly abundant in the human body as part of water and fat molecules, are by far the most commonly used. The hydrogen atom, consisting of single proton (nucleon), forms the MRI signal source in routine clinical MR images. Nucleons behave as small current-carrying loop and give rise to a small magnetic field, that is, they behave like tiny little bar magnets. Without an external magnetic field, these tiny magnets are randomly oriented, thereby producing no net magnetization as shown in Fig. 2.3a. However, once a subject is immersed in a magnetic field, these 1H protons align in two energy favorable states either in the direction of the external field or opposite to the direction as shown in Fig. 2.3b. As a consequence, at the field strength of a typical clinical MRI scanner for every million atoms, there is only approximately one atom more aligned than anti-aligned with the field, but due to the huge number of atoms in the human body, this tiny excess provides enough net magnetization to give rise to an easily measurable signal. There are two options available for increasing the number of nuclei that are aligned with the external magnetic field: (1) cooling the sample close to absolute zero, which for obvious reasons would be impractical for human subjects, and (2) increasing the field strength of the external magnetic field B_0. Hence the interest lies in imaging at higher field strength to obtain images with higher signal-to-noise ratios.

At equilibrium, the vector of the generated net magnetization ***Mo*** is aligned with the direction of the magnetic field vector $\boldsymbol{B_0}$ such that, by definition, only its M_z component, that is, the longitudinal magnetization, is nonzero. Similar to a spinning top that starts to wobble in the Earth's gravitational field when tipped, this magnetization begins to precess about $\boldsymbol{B_0}$ when tipped by the magnetic vector component $\boldsymbol{B_1}$ of an RF pulse perpendicular to the direction of ***Mo***. Once ***Mo*** is tipped out of its complete alignment with $\boldsymbol{B_0}$ its M_x and M_y components, the so-called transverse magnetization M_{xy} are no longer zero. As ***Mo*** precesses about $\boldsymbol{B_0}$, its transverse magnetization components oscillate, which in turn induces an electric current in an appropriately oriented RF receiver coil as described in more detail below. The frequency of the precession f_0 is proportional to the strength of the magnetic field and the gyromagnetic ratio γ, an intrinsic property specific to each type of nucleus. This relationship was reported by Sir Joseph Larmor, summarizing it in what is now called the *Larmor equation*:

$$f_0 = \frac{\gamma}{2\pi} B_0. \tag{2.1}$$

Under the condition that the frequency of an applied RF pulse with a magnetic field $\boldsymbol{B_1}$ perpendicular to $\boldsymbol{B_0}$ matches the precession frequency f_0, it is called to be "on resonance," the origin of the term magnetic "resonance" imaging. This has the effect that ***Mo*** is simultaneously precessing about $\boldsymbol{B_0}$ with frequency f_0 and $\boldsymbol{B_1}$ with frequency f_1, where f_1 can be calculated equivalent to Eq. 2.1. For as long as the RF pulse is turned on, ***Mo*** continues to be tipped toward the transverse M_{xy} plane and then becomes inverted before returning to its original alignment with $\boldsymbol{B_0}$ and so on. Therefore, the temporal modulation and amplitude of the applied $\boldsymbol{B_1}$ allow the user to control the tipping angle or flip angle α the magnetization ***Mo*** experiences and which fraction of the total available magnetization ends up in the transverse plane, forming the MRI signal amplitude S_0 as described by

$$S_0 \propto M_0 \sin\alpha. \tag{2.2}$$

In the following section, we will describe the hardware that is required to generate, spatially localize, and measure this MR signal.

MRI Hardware

The Primary Magnet

Usually, low magnetic fields are measured using the standard unit Gauss (G). The most familiar and ubiquitous magnetic field we experience, the Earth's magnetic field, measures about 0.5 G, while most refrigerator magnets fall in the 500–1000 G range. The majority of current clinical MRI scanners are cylindrical closed-bore superconducting magnets, which can produce magnetic fields that are thousands of times more powerful than the Earth's magnetic field. Because of their very strong magnetic fields, medical magnets are usually measured using a larger unit, much like pounds and tons, called Tesla (T), with 1.0 T equal to 10,000 G. Within the MRI suite, the location of the 5 G line surrounding the periphery of the MRI scanner should have controlled access, that is, the distance from the main magnet where the magnetic field drops to below

5 G is considered to be a safe level of field exposure for the general, unscreened public to move around freely.

MRI scanners can be described by the magnetic field strength of their primary magnet or by the precession frequency of the hydrogen nuclei within the magnet. For example, a 1.5 T scanner can also be referred to as a 63 MHz scanner based on the *Larmor frequency* of hydrogen at this field strength because $\frac{\gamma_H}{2\pi} = 42.58\,\text{MHz}/\text{T}$ (see Eq. 2.1). Strong magnets are an essential component of all MRI scanners, and in the decades since the introduction of clinical MRI, all three types of magnets, that is, permanent, resistive, and superconducting, have been used. Superconducting magnets have the advantage of producing strong and stable magnetic fields, and once the superconducting windings are energized with electrical power, no additional current is required to maintain the magnetic field produced by superconducting coils. In superconducting and permanent MR scanners, the magnetic field is *always on* as compared to the resistive electromagnet design where the field can be switched off.

Clinical scanners using superconducting magnets of 3 T and research scanners with even stronger magnetic fields have become commonplace. While there are some theoretical and practical limitations to medical imaging at 3 T, the motivation behind this migration to higher field strengths is to maximize the available MR signal by recruiting a larger proportion of the available hydrogen nuclei in the body for imaging. The linear increase in the signal-to-noise ratio based on field strength that follows can in principle be used to provide some combination of better resolution, faster imaging, or thinner sections. However, there are some disadvantages to utilizing MR scanners with higher field strengths such as 3 T: greater RF power deposition in the body of the patient in the form of heat could pose a safety challenge for patients with implants, decreased T_1 contrast, dielectric shading effects due to nonuniform RF penetration especially during body imaging, increased risk of projectile effects from magnetic metal in the room, and larger chemical shift image artifacts. The latter are caused by the spatial misregistration of signals originating from water and fat protons, which have slightly different Larmor frequencies caused by the differences in their chemical environment as will be discussed below in Sect. 2.3.2. A less common, but still potentially problematic, issue is the increased level of signal blowout (loss) artifacts caused by susceptibility differences in air-tissue interfaces or the local magnetic field changes due to the presence of metallic objects inside the body. As shown in Eq. 2.1, such field variations result in changes in resonance frequency which gives rise to signal cancelations in the affected volumes. For some applications, however, like magnetic resonance angiography (MRA), functional MRI, and MR spectroscopy, or for detailed structural imaging, the benefits outweigh these drawbacks. Modern 3 T scanner designs and pulse sequence techniques alleviate many of the negative effects and harness the higher field for advanced imaging applications.

Gradients

The gradient system is a key component of the MRI machine, being responsible for the spatial encoding in image generation and integral to controlling a range of physiological imaging contrasts, most notably diffusion-weighted MRI. The design and performance of the gradient system have substantial influence on the overall quality of the acquired images and have been the focus of intense engineering efforts over the last three decades in the quest for better image quality and ever-faster imaging speed. Gradient performance is parameterized by the maximum gradient amplitude, which is measured in mT/m, and the slew rate, which describes how fast a gradient can attain a desired amplitude within a given amount of time and is measured in T/m/s. Since the inception of MRI, gradient amplitudes and slew rates have increased by orders of magnitude, roughly doubling every 10 years since the 1990s. For localization of the MRI signal, three additional sets of coils called gradients are incorporated in the scanner bore. Gradient coils produce time-varying magnetic fields across the field of view (FOV) to be imaged that linearly increase or decrease the main magnetic field in a spatially dependent manner along the X, Y, and Z directions. Depending on their position along the gradient, the nuclei inside the body are temporarily exposed to magnetic fields of different strength and hence differ in their precessional frequencies. This behavior is exploited during MRI acquisitions in two different ways. For one, as will be explained in more detail in Sect. 2.3.3, the RF pulses used to tip the magnetization vectors are only effective over a certain range of frequencies. Thus, it is possible to excite transverse magnetization and thereby signal, only in specific, well-defined regions of the body, usually in the form of a thin imaging slice. Secondly, once a slice has been selected in this manner, additional spatially encoding with the gradient coils is now required within the slice to obtain a two-dimensional (2D) image.

In MRI, each imaging dimension is encoded separately. In a typical two-dimensional image acquisition, one direction, for example, along the *x*-axis, is termed the *frequency-encoding* direction while the other, in this example the *y*-axis, is called the *phase-encoding* direction (Fig. 2.5). If no slice selection with an RF pulse was performed, spatial encoding along the *z*-axis, the second phase-encoding direction, would be necessary and yield a three-dimensional image data set. Encoding the MR signal along the frequency-encoding direction can be easily understood by picturing a piano keyboard. Each of the keys is associated with a specific note: low frequencies on the left and high frequencies on the right. Upon hearing a particular note, a trained listener can exactly identify which key along the length of the keyboard had been pressed by the pianist even without being able to see the keyboard. Similarly, for as long as the frequency-encoding gradient is activated, all the transverse magnetization at a particular location along the *x*-axis is precessing with a specific frequency. The receiver coil integrates all the signals with their characteristic frequencies, individually weighted by the strength of the signal originating from the associated spatial location and measures the combined oscillations. This would be equivalent to all keys on our imaginary piano being pressed simultaneously but with a force that differs from key to key such that some notes are louder while others much softer. Of course, regardless how well trained, no human observer would now be able to still identify the amplitude of each note in the resulting cacophony. Fortunately, mathematics offers a tool for analyzing a signal consisting of the superposition of many different frequencies by means of the *Fourier transform.* Applying a one-dimensional (1D) Fourier transform to a frequency-encoded signal reveals the amplitudes of the different signal frequencies as vertical bands in our two-dimensional image matrix. However, to resolve the image information along the *y*-axis, this information needs to be first encoded during additional steps in the MR data acquisition process.

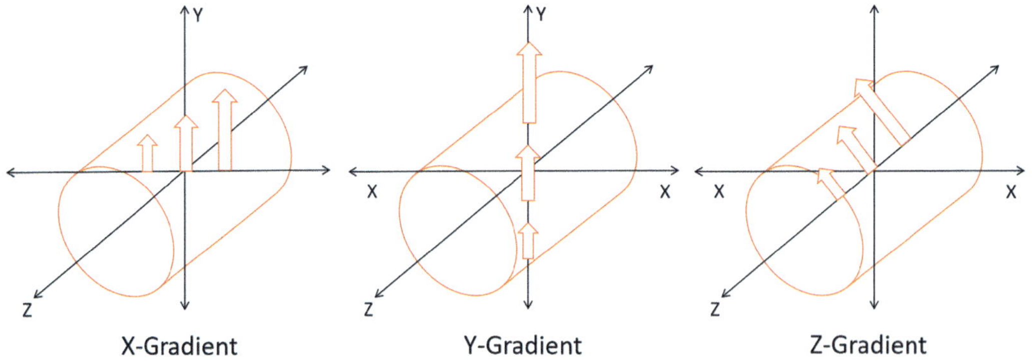

Fig. 2.5 Diagrams illustrate the field gradients generated in each of the X, Y, and Z directions. (© [Suraj D. Serai, 2023. All rights reserved])

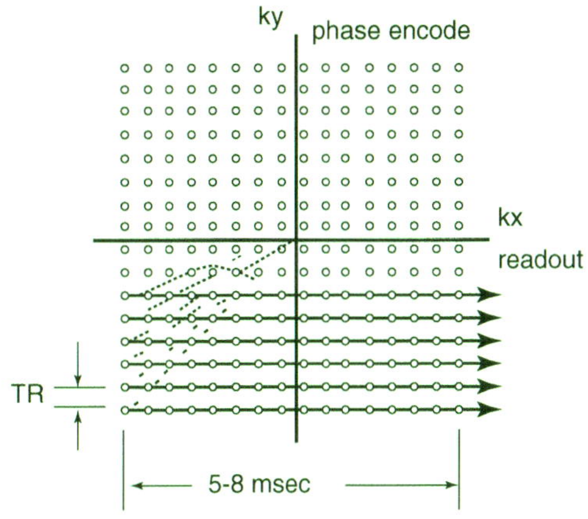

Fig. 2.6 A single phase-encoding line is collected per TR. Collecting less phase-encoding lines increases acquisition speed at the expense of spatial resolution

Unfortunately, simply applying frequency encoding along the *y*-axis again will not suffice because, after Fourier transform along the *y*-direction, the image matrix would now only contain horizontal bands, and combining them with the vertical bands of the first frequency encoding will not result in an image. Instead, encoding along the *y*-direction has to be performed in a multistep phase-encoding procedure (Fig. 2.6). This is achieved by activating the magnetic field gradient along the *y*-axis just like the frequency-encoding gradient along the *x*-axis. However, while the frequency-encoding gradient is active for the entire duration of data sampling, the phase-encoding gradient is only turned on for a short amount of time and before data sampling begins. As during frequency encoding, the transverse magnetization precesses with a frequency that is a function of its location but this time as a function of its location along the *y*-axis. Although no measurements are conducted during phase encoding, spatial information is imprinted on the transverse magnetization in the form of a location-dependent phase shift because the higher the precession frequency at any given y-position, the faster the transverse magnetization at this location is precessing and the more phase is accumulated while the phase-encoding gradient is turned on. Then the signal is measured again while only the frequency-encoding gradient is active. This phase-encoding procedure is repeated once for each line in the measured image but with a higher amplitude of the *y*-gradient such that each phase-encoding step imparts a steeper linear phase shift along the *y*-axis. Returning to our piano analogy one last time, phase encoding is the equivalent of adding a position-dependent, linearly increasing delay until any given key is pressed. Once all keys are activated, the sound is recorded in the same manner as before but for each phase-encoding step the rate with which the delay time increases also increases, resulting in a slightly different modulation of the combined notes for each phase-encoding step. Following a two-dimensional Fourier transform, all these modulations in the MRI measurement reveal the signal contributions of each y-position for each of the vertical one-dimensional bands along the x-position, that is, the complete two-dimensional image information. In a three-dimensional measurement, for each phase-encoding step along the *z*-axis, all phase-encoding steps along the *y*-axis have to be repeated prior to frequency encoding, lengthening the total acquisition time proportionally.

The final step of image computation, a Fourier transform of the measured raw data, has the interesting and often confusing implication that MRI measurements are actually not performed in image space, such as taking a photograph or acquiring a CT image, but in the spatial frequency space, or *k-space*, created by the encoding of spatial positions as phase and frequency shifts by the application of magnetic field gradients. This peculiar characteristic has a tremendous impact on how various choices in measurement parameters affect image contrast, signal-to-noise ratios, acquisition speeds, and image artifacts that are highly nonintuitive without this important insight. Further, the concept of phase and frequency encoding provided above, assumes a Cartesian acquisition scheme in which a square (2D) or cube (3D) in k-space is filled with lines of sampled data from left to right, top to bottom, and front to back. However, while the number and location of points in k-space that should be filled with measurement data are dictated by the FOV and spatial resolution of the final image, the order in which they are filled is, in principle, arbitrary. This circumstance is exploited by several advanced acquisition techniques that employ a variety of sampling orders, such as radial or spiral trajectories to name two of the most popular ones, each with their own advantages and disadvantages.

RF Coils

While advances in the MRI hardware such as higher field strengths and improved gradient performance have been substantial, recent progress in RF technology has led to increased spatial and temporal image resolution, improved signal uniformity, and shortened MRI scan durations. MRI RF coils are essential components for every MRI examination, as they are the "antennas" of the MRI system. RF coils have two functions: first, to excite and manipulate transverse magnetization by transmitting RF power (Tx coil), and second, to detect the precessing transverse magnetization of the excited nuclei as an electric current via electromagnetic induction (Rx coil).

RF coils serving both as transmitter and receiver, especially for head and extremity imaging, used to be the norm on older MRI systems. These days, modern scanners mostly utilize the integrated body coil for RF transmission and receive-only RF coils close to the imaged body part for signal reception. These Rx coils are commonly constructed with multiple smaller coil elements, each with its own receive chain, called phased array coils. The combination of multiple surface coils into an array allows for a good signal-to-noise ratio over a large FOV. The signals from each coil in the array are subsequently combined to create a single image. In addition, phased array volume coils can greatly accelerate image acquisition by collecting data from different regions of k-space in parallel.

As mentioned before, the RF transmit coil generates a $\boldsymbol{B}_1$ field vector perpendicular to which the net magnetization vector $\boldsymbol{M}$ is precessing. A typical MRI data acquisition begins with the application of an RF excitation pulse that tips $\boldsymbol{M}$ toward the transverse plane and thereby generates a signal (see Eq. 2.2). However, depending on the size and the design of the transmit coil, the created B_1 amplitude can be very location dependent and affects a poorly defined volume of the body. One way to address the problem is the use of field gradients to spatially encode all the excited volume as described in Sect. 2.3.2. The drawback of this approach is that, for a given image resolution, the larger the FOV, the more phase-encoding steps are required and the longer the total acquisition time. In fact, long scan times make the collected image data sets highly susceptible to patient motion, and a full three-dimensional measurement covering a large volume may even be completely unnecessary for the diagnostic objective of the scan. A more practical solution is to limit the effect of the RF pulse to specific, user-selectable thin slices using the same gradient coils as for spatial encoding.

For an RF pulse to tip $\boldsymbol{M}$, its frequency has to match the precession frequency f_0 of $\boldsymbol{M}$ in the transverse plane (see Sect. 2.2). However, an RF pulse never consists of just a single frequency, but rather a band of frequencies around its center frequency and, depending on the amplitude modulation of the pulse, multiple frequency side lobes. Nevertheless, RF excitation pulses optimized for two-dimensional slice selection will have a sharp center frequency band that determines the bandwidth of the pulse and only low-amplitude side lobes. By applying, for instance, a magnetic field gradient along the z-axis, f_0 varies linearly in the patient's head-to-toe direction. Therefore, changing the center frequency of the RF excitation pulse will move the center of the targeted slice up or down the z-axis. The thickness of the selected slice is dictated by the bandwidth of the pulse and the steepness of the field gradient. The smaller the bandwidth and the larger the slope, the thinner the slice and vice versa. Nevertheless, because the slice location and profile are dependent on an appropriate matching of the RF pulse parameters with the spatial precession frequency distribution, any imperfections in the RF pulse amplitude or the linearity of the magnetic field gradients can result in slice distortions and out-of-slice excitations that give rise to image artifacts.

In addition to generating signal in specific locations, RF excitation pulses also have an important function in removing unwanted signal from images. Since in an MR image acquisition, spatial locations are identified by the precession frequencies of the transverse magnetization in the associated volume, the implicit assumption is that, in the absence of frequency-encoding gradients, all magnetization precesses with the same f_0. However, the resonance frequency of a nucleus does not truly depend on the applied external field strength B_0 but rather on the field strength at the nucleus itself. These two quantities are usually almost identical except for a tiny shielding effect by the electron cloud surrounding the nucleus. It is the size and the shape of this electron cloud as dictated by the type of nucleus and its chemical environment that causes the magnetic field at the nucleus to be slightly lower than B_0. For conventional proton MRI of the human body, only the protons in water and fat molecules give rise to strong signals but with water having a 3.5 ppm higher resonance frequency than fat, which translates into a frequency difference of approximately 224 Hz at 1.5 T or 447 Hz at 3 T. Since the MRI acquisition and reconstruction do not "know" about the presence of two resonance frequencies in the signal, the final image will consist of a superposition of a fat and a water image that are shifted along the frequency-encoding direction relative to each other, potentially obscuring important pathological abnormalities.

While there are many techniques available for suppressing the undesirable fat signal in MR images, some of the simplest ones take advantage of the 3.5 ppm difference in resonance frequency of fat and water. By applying a narrow-bandwidth RF pulse with a 90° flip angle centered at the fat resonance frequency, the fat magnetization vector can be tipped into the transverse plane and then be dephased with the help of so-called spoiler gradients (Sect. 2.4.5). Once the fat signal has been thereby saturated, the acquisition of the water signal can begin. Depending on the specifics of the image acquisition, this procedure may need to be performed only once at the start of the measurements or repeatedly for each phase-encoding step.

A Walk Through k-Space

k-space is a raw data matrix which is essentially an array of number representing spatial frequencies in MRI image [2]. The letter "K" represents a wavenumber defined as reciprocal of wavelength of a wave. Wavenumber is a number of waves or cycles per unit distance.

The concept of wavelength was first introduced by Heinrich Kayser, a German physicist when he was working on the emission spectra of elementary substances [3]. Unlike temporal frequency, which is defined as number of cycles per unit time, spatial frequency is defined as number of cycles per unit distance [4].

General Properties of K-Space

1. In general, the K-space grid is usually square and evenly spaced. Regular spacing makes data acquisition and processing easier, faster, and more efficient. The cells of K-space are commonly displayed on rectangular grid with principal axes *kx* and *ky*. The *kx* and *ky* axes of K-space correspond to the horizontal (*x*-) and vertical (*y*-) axes of the image. The K-axes represent spatial frequencies in the *x*- and *y*-directions.
2. Each point (kx, ky) in the K-space does not correspond with individual pixel (x,y) in the image. In fact, each point in K-space contains information about spatial frequency and phase about every pixel in the image. Equally, each pixel in the image maps to every point in the K-space.
3. While the data near the center of K-space corresponds to low spatial frequencies and provide information about image signal, brightness, contrast, general shapes, and contours of the object, data from the periphery corresponds to high spatial frequencies and provide information about image resolution (details), edges, and sharp transitions (Fig. 2.7).
4. Center of the K-space has the highest signal intensity because the central row is acquired with no phase-encoding gradient, and therefore no destructive wave interference occurs and no signal loss occurs. Additionally, the central column of K-space coincides with the peak of an echo of a pulse sequence.
5. The K-space have an important property known as conjugate or Hermitian symmetry.

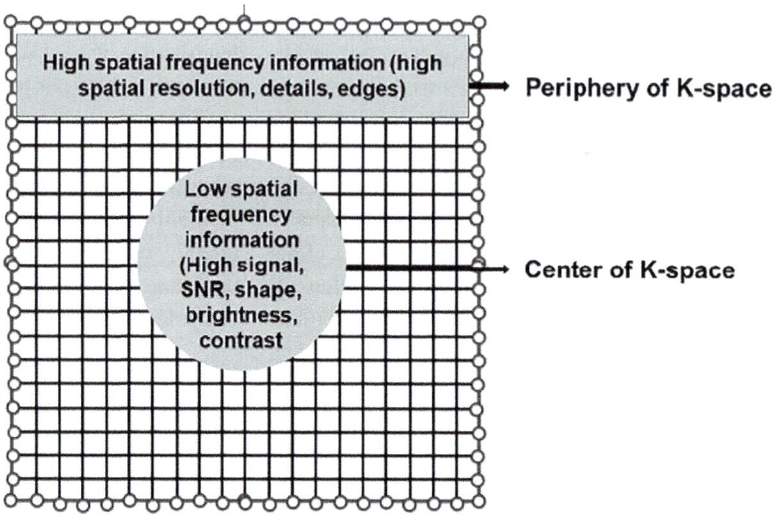

Fig. 2.7 Location of spatial frequencies in K-space. The center of K-space contains low spatial frequency information which determines overall image signal, general shape, brightness, and contrast. The periphery of K-space contains high spatial frequency information which determines image resolution (general details)

It refers to pairs of points that are located diagonally from each other across the origin of K-space. Two data points, which are mirror images across the origin of K-space, possesses identical amplitudes but opposite phases. However, conjugate symmetry may not always be perfect because of the presence of phase errors. The sources of these phase errors include B_0 inhomogeneity, susceptibility effects, eddy currents, physiologic motion, and spatial variations in transmit RF uniformity.

6. The distance between adjacent rows and columns is denoted as ΔK. The distance from the center of K-space to the edge is called Kmax.

While the reciprocal of ΔK determines field of view (FOV) in the image as $\Delta K = 1/\text{FOV}$, the Kmax determines the pixel size (ΔW) as $\Delta W = 1/K_{\text{FOV}}$ where $K_{\text{FOV}} = (+k\text{max}) - (-k\text{max}) = 2k\text{max}$.

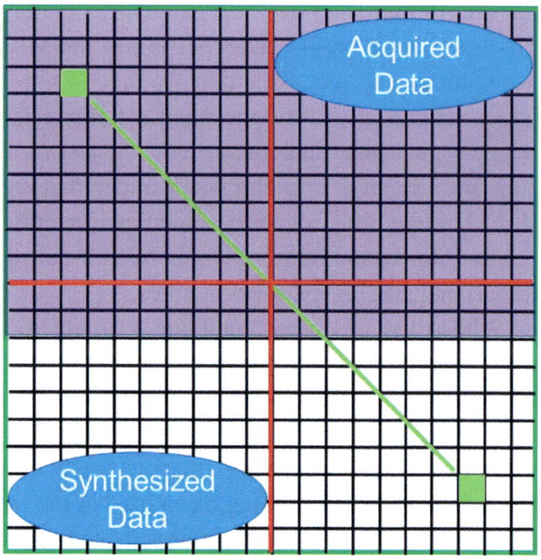

Fig. 2.8 Phase-conjugate symmetry allows acquisition of data using only half the normal number of phase-encoding steps. This potentially reduces the imaging time while preserving spatial resolution. However, SNR of the image decreases

Partial Fourier Techniques and K-Space

Phase-Conjugate Symmetry

Phase-conjugate symmetry is also known as half Fourier or half scan. In this case, top half of the data is actually acquired and lower half of the data is synthesized using the property of conjugate (Hermitian) symmetry. Phase-conjugate symmetry allows acquisition of data using only half the normal number of phase-encoding steps, therefore potentially reducing scanning time by 50%. However, in the actual practice, more than half the lines of K-space (approximately 60%) are acquired (Fig. 2.8). These extra lines are then used to generate phase correction maps of K-space. Using phase-conjugate symmetry, spa-

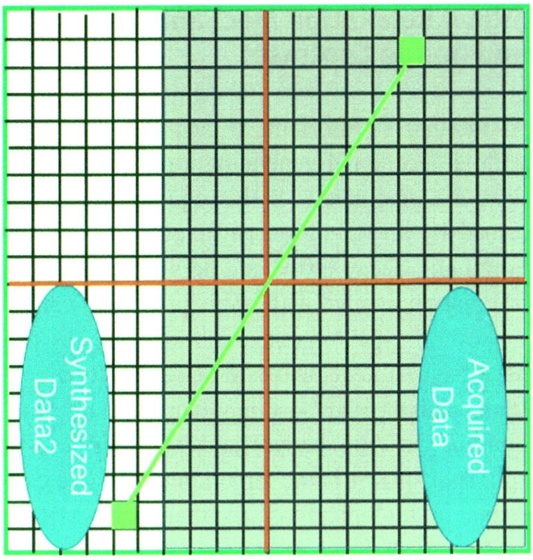

Fig. 2.9 Read-conjugate symmetry allows sampling of data from right half of K-space and estimating data from left half of K-space resulting in shorter echo time

tial resolution is preserved. However, scanning time is reduced at expense of lower signal-to-noise ratio (SNR).

Read-Conjugate Symmetry

Read-conjugate symmetry is also known as partial-echo or half-echo imaging. In this case, right half of the K-space is acquired and left half of the K-space is synthesized (Fig. 2.9). Unlike phase-conjugate symmetry, the full number of phase-encoding steps are acquired in read-conjugate symmetry. Hence, there is no direct scan time saving. However, the advantage in read-conjugate symmetry is that only a part of echo is sampled, thus reducing the echo time (TE). Both read-conjugate and phase-conjugate symmetry techniques are useful but these two techniques cannot be used together.

K-Space Trajectories and Image Reconstruction

There are different sampling methods of filling K-space by digitized MR signals, and these methods include Cartesian (row by row, also known as rectilinear), radial, spiral, and zigzag. Cartesian filling of K-space can be sequential filling of K-space lines from one end to another end of K-space or centric ordering of K-space lines starting from the center to periphery or starting from periphery to center of K-space.

Cartesian data acquisition method is very popular. The main advantage of using Cartesian sampling is that the data elements are regularly spread out and can be placed directly into the standard array processors which are used for efficient fast Fourier transform (FFT).

However, radial or spiral sampling of K-space data is fast gaining momentum. Unlike Cartesian methods, radial sampling does not have unique frequency and phase-encoding directions. Noise arising from moving anatomic structures does not propagate as discrete ghosts along a particular phase-encoding direction, but the noise is simply distributed more diffusely across the entire image. Therefore, radial imaging is relatively less sensitive to motion artifacts. Moreover, the center of K-space is oversampled, and this redundancy is usually exploited to detect and correction for any motion artifacts, if any. The reduction in motion and aliasing artifacts are some of the advantages of using radial sampling. The disadvantage includes nonuniform collection of data points, thus requiring an iterative process known as gridding in which data points are morphed into a Cartesian arrangement prior to performing FFT. In addition to the Fourier transform and iterative reconstruction techniques, newer reconstruction algorithms are developed to improve speed of acquisition or generate higher spatial resolution from limited samples ok K-space data collected. Compressed sensing (CS) reconstruction is a type of MRI reconstruction that uses mathematical algorithms to reduce the amount of data required to produce an image, thus reducing the scan time. For compressed sensing to work, underdamping of the data must be performed in an incoherent (semi-random) manner. CS requires that the acquired image is compressible. In other words, it needs to have a sparse representation in a well-known transform domain. If this condition is met, and K-space is undersampled such that the undersampling artifacts have a noise-like appearance in this transform domain, the image can be reconstructed using a nonlinear iterative optimization. Current CS reconstruction approaches employ variable density random Poisson disk and golden-angle radial semi-random acquisition of data with preferential sampling near the center of K-space. The level of scan acceleration is governed by the compressibility of the image rather than the factors that affect standard parallel imaging and may highly depend on the application and the basic SNR conditions at hand. While CS is typically suited to three-dimensional applications and excellent results are obtained in two-dimensional functional studies, the sparsity requirements are often not met with static two-dimensional sequences. The most recent innovation and potentially the most exciting is the use of artificial intelligence (AI) image reconstruction techniques to denoise and sharpen our data in our quest to reduce scan times. We know from the literature and every MR lecture we attend that the final MR image is a compromise between three tightly associated factors: SNR, resolution, and acquisition time. Minor modifications of one factor significantly affect the others—and AI or deep learning (DL) reconstruction methods have the potential to minimize these effects. DL-based reconstruction is a type of MRI reconstruction that uses artificial neural networks trained on lots of prior data to reconstruct the images. Deep learning reconstructions have been successfully employed by vendors to perform image denoising and artifact removal. By using deep learning, we can increase the resolution, introduce higher parallel acceleration factors, or reduce the number of averages. We can intentionally create an image with more noise present in the data and use DL in the reconstruction phase to produce images of diagnostic quality. These techniques have enabled us to reduce the scan times of our two-dimensional acquisitions that were previously not suitable for iterative reconstruction techniques. These DL techniques have gained popularity in recent years due to their ability to produce higher SNR images with reduced scan time or generate higher spatial resolution images at clinically acceptable scan times.

Signal Relaxation Mechanisms and Image Contrasts

At thermal equilibrium, $\boldsymbol{M}$ and $\boldsymbol{B}_0$ are aligned without any signal-generating transverse magnetization components. If this equilibrium is disturbed by an RF pulse, any created signal will eventually decay away, and $\boldsymbol{M}$ will return to its original alignment again. This process is caused by several types of relaxation mechanisms that have environment- and tissue-specific time constants with the two most important being: T_1 (longitudinal or spin lattice) and T_2 (transverse or spin/spin) [1]. It is the large range of these constants in biological tissues that gives MR its excellent soft tissue contrast.

T_1 Relaxation

T_1 relaxation describes the recovery of the longitudinal magnetization M_z back to its thermal equilibrium value M_0 following a perturbation by an RF pulse (Fig. 2.10) with an exponential recovery time constant T_1:

$$M_z(t) = M_0\left(1 - e^{-t/T1}\right), \tag{2.3}$$

where t is the time after an ideal 90° RF excitation pulse. Thus, T_1 is the time at which $M_z(t)$ has returned from 0 to 1/e (~63%) of M_0. In the process, the excited nuclei transfer the absorbed RF energy to surrounding water and macromolecules, the "lattice," realigning $\boldsymbol{M}$ with $\boldsymbol{B}_0$. Hence, T_1 relaxation is also called longitudinal, thermal, or spin-lattice relaxation [1].

T1 relaxation is stimulated by the presence of local magnetic fields oscillating at the resonance frequency f_0 of the nuclei. The main source for these fields is the dipole moment of nearby protons attached to the same or other molecules. As the molecules tumble around due to thermal motion, their dipole moments create rapidly fluctuating magnetic fields in their vicinity. Because of their small size, free water molecules at body temperature rotate, on average, at a much higher rate than f_0 even for the strongest clinical MRI systems. As a result, only a relatively small number of water molecules happen to generate magnetic field fluctuations at f_0 at any given point in time, and T_1 in

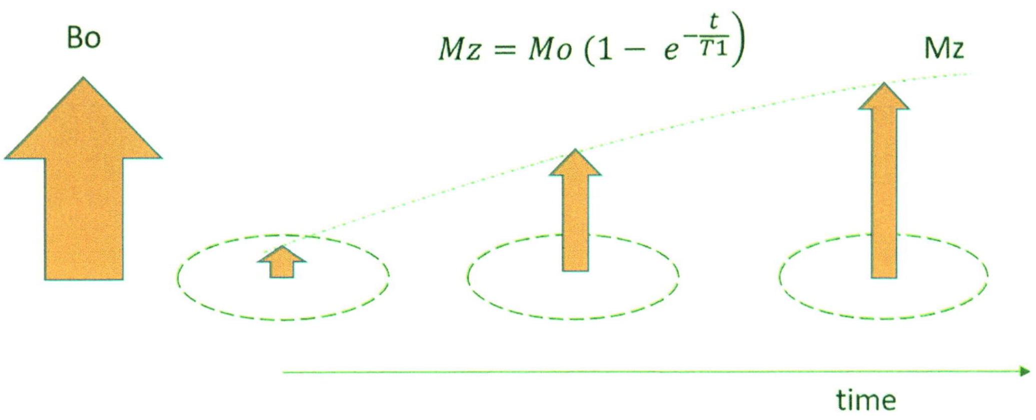

Fig. 2.10 The rate at which the spin magnetization (Mz) at time t recovers to the original magnetization (M_0) at time $t = 0$ is called T_1 relaxation time, where B_0 is the external magnetic field. T_1 relaxation time measured is the time for the longitudinal magnetization to re-grow to about 63% of its final value (the flipped nuclei realign with the main magnetic field). (© [Suraj D. Serai, 2023. All rights reserved])

pure water is quite long (~4 s). The motion of large protein molecules or lipid chains, on the other hand, is much slower than that of water molecules, and their mean rotational frequency is much closer to f_0, giving rise to a much shorter T_1 relaxation. It is, therefore, the ratio of free water to protons bound to macromolecules that determines the T_1 of a given tissue type. As a rule of thumb, the more "water-like" the tissue, the longer the T_1 and the more protein dense or fatty the shorter the T_1. For instance, the T_1 of cerebrospinal fluid is close to that of water (4 s) while the T_1 of body fat is only about 250 ms with all other body tissues falling somewhere in between.

How to Measure T_1 Relaxation Time for Body Imaging

According to Eq. 2.3, T_1 maps could be generated by saturating M_z with a 90° excitation pulse and then, after a certain delay time, perform an image acquisition. If the transverse magnetization has been sufficiently spoiled (see Sect. 2.4.5), then the resulting images for very short delay times would have very low signal intensities but would rapidly brighten as the delay increases until reaching their normal intensities for delay times that are much longer than T_1 (>~3 * T_1). Tissues with short T_1 would thereby appear brighter sooner than those with long T_1, and by fitting Eq. 2.3 to the signal intensity in each pixel as a function of the delay time, T_1 maps could be calculated. Although this approach would be most accurate, it is also so time consuming that it is impractical for diagnostic studies.

The preferred way of measuring T_1 relaxation in body MR imaging is the look-locker method. For a more accurate measurement, it applies a 180° inversion pulse such that M_z recovers according to

$$M_z(t) = M_0\left(1 - 2e^{-t/\mathrm{T1}}\right). \tag{2.4}$$

Instead of waiting after each inversion pulse until a specific delay time is reached before beginning with the image acquisition, the recovery of M_z is sampled by a series of RF excitations with small flip angles. In other words, not just one but multiple delay times are measured as a train of signals after each saturation. Although the additional RF excitations interfere with the T_1 relaxation process toward thermal equilibrium by tipping part of the regrowing longitudinal magnetization back into the transverse plane, for low flip angles, the effect is sufficiently small to still permit fitting with Eq. 2.4. In clinical settings, liver T_1 is measured using a modified look-locker inversion recovery (MOLLI) pulse sequence that allows measurement of T_1 times in a single breath-hold (Fig. 2.11). This has become the most popular T_1-mapping method for abdomen and cardiac imaging.

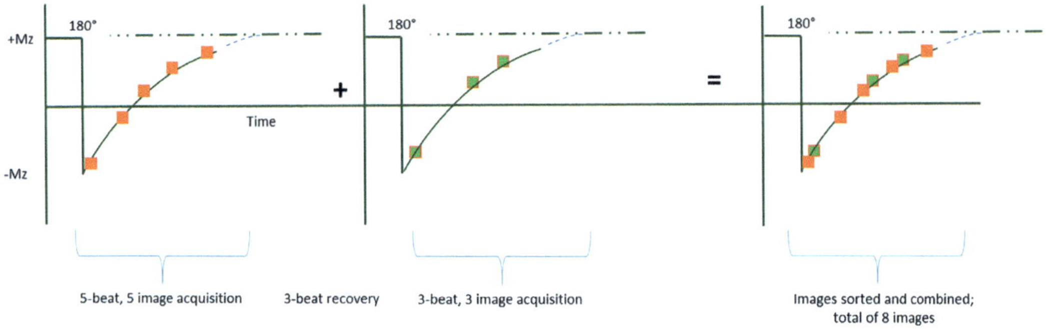

Fig. 2.11 Acquisition strategy for the modified look-locker (MOLLI) sequence. In this example, after a 180° inversion pulse, images are acquired in diastole over five heartbeats, followed by a rest period of three heartbeats. Then, after another inversion, another three images are acquired with slightly offset inversion times (TI) to sample more points along the inversion recovery curves. Based on the number of heartbeats for acquiring images after each inversion pulse, and on a rest period of three heartbeats between the two cycles, this MOLLI acquisition scheme is termed 5(3)3

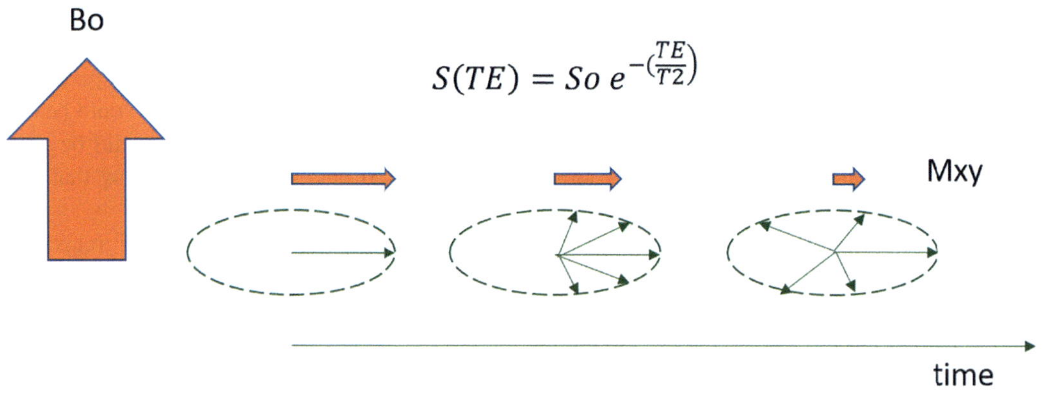

Fig. 2.12 T_2 relaxation. Following turning off of the radiofrequency pulse, differences in magnetic fields experienced by the spins cause them to precess at slightly different frequencies and fan out about the transverse plane. T_2 relaxation time is the time for the transverse magnetization to decay to about 37% of its initial value (the flipped nuclei that started spinning together become incoherent). S(TE) is the signal intensity measured at each individual echo time (TE) and S_0 is the initial signal intensity at time $t = 0$. Mxy is the magnetization in the transverse plane.

T2 Relaxation

Equivalently to T_1 relaxation, T_2 relaxation is the exponential return of the transverse magnetization to its thermal equilibrium value in the absence of static magnetic field inhomogeneities following a 90° RF excitation pulse (Fig. 2.12):

$$M_{xy}(t) = M_0 e^{-t/\mathrm{T2}}. \tag{2.5}$$

Under equilibrium conditions, $M_{xy} = 0$, which is clearly fulfilled when $M_z = M_0$, and therefore T_2 is always shorter than T_1 but this is not the only possibility. It is important to keep in mind that the magnetization measured macroscopically by the MRI scanner is generated by a myriad of nuclei such that the net magnetization vector for even the smallest pixel in a high-resolution scan still consists of the superposition of a huge number of microscopic magnetization vectors. Following an ideal 90° excitation pulse, all of these microscopic vectors are in phase, that is, having the same orientation in the transverse plane, and add up to the largest possible transverse net magnetization vector. However, as phase coherence disappears and the microscopic magnetization vectors begin to point in different directions, the net magnetization decreases until, at the point of complete phase randomization, the magnetization vectors cancel each other out and the macroscopic transverse magnetization reaches zero despite $M_z < M_0$. Still, it is noteworthy that the microscopic transverse magnetization is not zero, though, and that it can be further manipulated by the scanner, which is both a feature of MRI and the source of various kinds of image artifacts that are beyond the scope of this book.

There are multiple mechanisms that give rise to phase randomization and, thus, relaxation of transverse magnetization beyond that caused by T_1 relaxation. One of them, static field inhomogeneities cause a recoverable phase coherence loss that is not attributed to T_2 relaxation and will be discussed in more detail in Sects. 2.5.4–2.5.6. Two irrecoverable T_2 relaxation mechanisms are dipole-dipole interactions and nanoscale field inhomogeneities. In the case of the former, also referred to as spin-spin relaxation, two nuclei in very close proximity, one of them with its magnetic moment aligned with $\boldsymbol{B}_0$ and the other one anti-aligned, switch their alignments. While the net magnetic moment remains unaffected, the phase is randomized during the switching. The latter case, nanoscale field inhomogeneity, is the dominant factor of T_2 relaxation. As already mentioned in Sect. 2.5.1, thermal motion causes nuclei in solution to tumble around at a wide range of frequencies. The magnetic moments of those that move the slowest generate sufficiently stationary magnetic field inhomogeneities to slightly change the value of B_0 in their immediate vicinity and thereby alter the precession frequencies of other nuclei as they enter the affected volume. This results in a small, random phase change for those other nuclei that, over time, dephases the net transverse magnetization. As for T_1 relaxation, T_2 is longest in pure water because the number of slowly moving molecules is much smaller than in solutions with a high concentration of macromolecules.

How to Measure T_2 Relaxation Time for Body Imaging

Since T_2 mapping measures the decay of the transverse magnetization without the contributions from static magnetic field inhomogeneities, the signal dephasing by the latter needs to be undone before the signal is measured. Static magnetic fields alter the precession frequencies of nuclei at a specific location, which means that the associated transverse magnetization in this area accumulates phase at a different rate than in other locations, resulting in a net signal cancellation over time. However, the phase accumulation can be reversed again with the help of 180° RF refocusing pulses. While the 180° RF inversion pulses described in Sect. 2.4.2 act on the longitudinal magnetization, refocusing pulses are designed to flip the entire transverse plane by 180° about an axis within the plane. This in effect turns the direction of phase accumulation around such that the different magnetization vectors are in phase again and form a spin echo for t = TE, where TE is the so-called echo time, with the refocusing pulses being activated at t = TE/2. The mechanism can be pictured as runners sprinting down a track at different but constant speeds. If, once the first runner reaches the halfway point of the track, all runners turn around, sprinting back the way they came with the same speed as before, all runners will return to the starting line at the same time.

Although the transverse magnetization will peak at the echo time, its peak amplitude decreases as *TE* is increased because of irreversible T_2 relaxation processes. Therefore, T_2 can be quantified by applying a 90° RF excitation pulse at t = 0 s, followed by a refocusing pulse at t = TE/2, measuring the signal at t = TE, and then fitting the pixel intensity S as a function of TE to the mono-exponential decay curve

$$S(\mathrm{TE}) = S_0 e^{-\mathrm{TE}/\mathrm{T2}}, \tag{2.6}$$

with $S_0 = S(0)$. In practice, the T_2 decay is measured by applying a train of refocusing pulses spaced apart by Δt = TE, in the form of multi-echo spin-echo (MSME) and fast spin-echo (FSE) MRI pulse sequences. T_2 relaxation times are routinely used in the clinic for liver and musculoskeletal applications [5–8].

T_2* Relaxation

T_2* relaxation is the decay of the transverse magnetization following an RF excitation pulse including all contributions from static magnetic

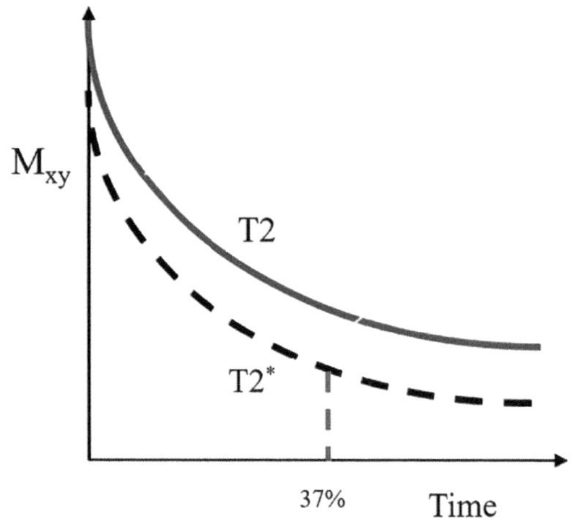

Fig. 2.13 T_2* measurement. While T_2 relaxation time is the "true" T_2 caused by spin-spin molecular interactions, T_2* relaxation time is the "observed" T_2, reflecting true T_2 as well as the effect of magnetic and gradient inhomogeneity. T_2 or T_2* as measured is the time required for the transverse magnetization to fall to approximately 37% of its initial value

field inhomogeneities [1]. Similar to Eq. 2.5, it is described by a mono-exponential decay function:

$$M_{xy}\left(t\right) = M_0 e^{-t/T2^*}. \quad (2.7)$$

The relationship between T_2 and T_2* can be expressed as

$$\frac{1}{T2^*} = \frac{1}{T2'} + \frac{1}{T2}, \quad (2.8)$$

where T2' is the relaxation time constant exclusively tied to the static field inhomogeneities. Therefore, the three main relaxation time constants can be ordered as $T_2^* < T_2 < T_1$ (Fig. 2.13).

There are numerous causes for magnetic field inhomogeneities in the human body that can give rise to image distortions (see Sect. 2.4.2) and rapid signal decay due to the associated short T_2*. The most common one is a difference in magnetic susceptibility between neighboring tissue types. This effect is particularly pronounced at air-tissue interfaces such as around the ear canal, the sinuses, and the oral cavity and in the lungs. Other field inhomogeneities are created by implants or metallic objects in or near the body (dental fillings, jewelry, zippers, belt buckles, etc.), which is one of the reasons that patients need to be screened and should remove such objects prior to an MRI scan whenever possible. As discussed in Sect. 2.5.4, the impact of magnetic field inhomogeneities can be partially or completely alleviated by the application of RF refocusing pulses in the form of spin-echo MRI measurements. However, these types of acquisitions have their own shortcomings in the form of increased acquisition times, decreased T_1 weighting, and much higher RF power deposition in the body due to the large number of high flip angle pulses required.

While a short T_2* can cause considerable problems for MRI acquisitions, a reduction of T_2*, in a controlled manner, can also be very beneficial under certain circumstances. For instance, ferromagnetic nanoparticles can cause signal voids in the image even at extremely low concentrations, making them an excellent marker for molecular imaging applications. However, the most mundane use of T_2* shortening is the application of spoiling gradients during MR imaging [6]. A single MRI acquisition can contain hundreds or even thousands of RF pulses, each creating additional transverse magnetization. If RF excitation pulses could only be applied after the transverse magnetization from the pulse before had decayed away due to T_2 relaxation to prevent interference between the magnetization components from different excitations, such scans might take hours. Fortunately, this problem can be mitigated by applying a spoiling gradient using the built-in gradient coils once the data from any given excitation pulse has been spatially encoded and sampled. If the amplitude of the spoiling gradient is chosen such that the phase of the transverse magnetization increases by a multiple of 360° over the width of a pixel, then the net transverse magnetization within each pixel, under ideal conditions, is zero. Of course, care needs to be taken that subsequent RF pulses do not refocus the spoiled transverse magnetization until it has been irrecoverably dephased due to T_2 relaxation.

How to Measure T_2* Relaxation Time for Body Imaging

MRI acquisitions that do not contain RF refocusing pulses, so-called gradient-recalled echo (GRE) pulse sequences, are inherently T_2* weighted. Like the quantification of T_1 and T_2, T_2* can be measured by fitting the signal intensity S of each pixel from multiple data sets to the associated exponential decay function:

$$S(\mathrm{TE}) = S_0 e^{-\mathrm{TE}/T2^*}, \tag{2.9}$$

with each data set acquired at a different TE and $S_0 = S(\mathrm{TE} = 0)$. In a GRE pulse sequence, TE is defined as the time from the center of the RF excitation pulse to the point in time when the gradient moment, that is, the gradient amplitude integrated over time, along the frequency-encoding axis has been refocused to zero. T_2*-based methods have been validated and are frequently used to measure iron in body organs such as the liver and heart [6, 9–13].

$T_1\rho$ Relaxation

$T_1\rho$, or spinlock T_1 relaxation time, is the time constant for magnetic relaxation in the presence of continuous RF irradiation [1, 14]. When a long, on-resonance RF pulse, a so-called spinlock pulse, is applied, it generates a magnetic field vector $\boldsymbol{B}_1$ in the transverse plane. Throughout the activation of this spinlock pulse, its B_1 field is in all respects equivalent to the main B_0 field, except that its amplitude is only on the order of a few microtesla. As described in Sect. 2.4.1, magnetic field fluctuations at the resonance frequency associated with B_0 in the tens of Megahertz range give rise to T_1 relaxation along $\boldsymbol{B}_0$. An equivalent T_1 relaxation effect, that is, $T_1\rho$, can be observed along $\boldsymbol{B}_1$ in the transverse plane, but it is induced by field fluctuations in the Kilohertz range, the resonance frequency associated with B_1. However, the increase of transverse magnetization due to $T_1\rho$ relaxation is counteracted the simultaneous process of T_2 relaxation. Hence, $T_1\rho$ relaxation is detectable as a lengthening of T_2. $T_1\rho$ is believed to be sensitive to the slow interactions between free water and proton nuclei in large macromolecules, such as collagen and proteoglycans. For instance, because fibrosis involves the accumulation of extracellular macromolecules, including collagen and proteoglycans, it is hypothesized that $T_1\rho$ imaging ρ is a direct measure of fibrosis.

How to Measure $T_1\rho$ Relaxation in Body Imaging

$T_1\rho$ mapping is the most common form of $T_1\rho$ imaging and is frequently used for various applications [1, 14, 15]. It requires measurements for at least two but usually several different spinlock times (TSL), the time during which the spinlock RF pulse is activated, to obtain a series of images with different levels of $T_1\rho$-weighted contrast. An efficient way of acquiring such images is the application of a 90° excitation pulse followed by the spinlock pulse for a duration of TSL. The transverse magnetization is then flipped back to the longitudinal axis with a −90° pulse. The now $T_1\rho$-weighted longitudinal magnetization is subsequently imaged with a rapid acquisition using RF excitation pulses with low flip angles. The image voxel intensities at different TSLs, $S(\mathrm{TSL})$, are then fitted to a mono-exponential decay function to calculate the $T_1\rho$ values, yielding a $T_1\rho$ map ρ, using

$$S(\mathrm{TSL}) = S_0 e^{-\mathrm{TSL}/\mathrm{T1}\rho}, \tag{2.10}$$

where and $S_0 = S(\mathrm{TSL} = 0)$.

Diffusion-Weighted Imaging

MRI permits turning the molecular diffusion of the nuclei into an image contrast. Section 2.4.2 describes the use of frequency-encoding gradients to spatially localize the excited transverse magnetization. While the gradient is activated, the precession frequency of the transverse magnetization is modified according to the amplitude of the frequency-encoding gradient at that position, changing the phase of the magnetization as a function of the gradient duration. If, after this gradient is switched off, a second gradient identical to the first except that its amplitude is reversed

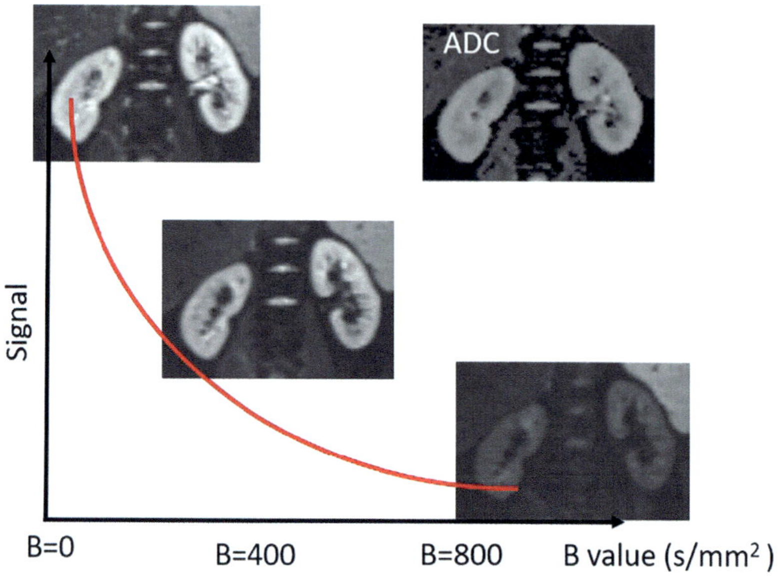

Fig. 2.14 In diffusion-weighted imaging, a progressive decrease in image signal intensity is evident and can be measured with increasing *b*-values, as in these three representative axial images obtained at $b = 0$ s/mm^2, $b = 400$ s/mm^2, and $b = 800$ s/mm^2 in a 14-year-old boy. The signal intensity can be measured and fitted to a mono-exponentially decaying curve to generate an apparent diffusion coefficient (ADC) map (top-right). ()

is turned on the entire effect of the first gradient is undone, the phase of the transverse magnetization returns to its original value. Hence, the MRI signal with and without these gradients is the same. However, the rephasing of the magnetization is contingent upon the nuclei being completely stationary while such a gradient pair is applied. If, on the other hand, the nuclei are diffusing around, they will move into regions with different gradient amplitudes, changing their precession frequency and, therefore, their rate of phase accumulation. As a consequence of the random nature of the diffusion process, the phase change of the transverse magnetization after the first gradient will no longer be completely reversed by the second gradient, and part of the transverse magnetization within a pixel will cancel out. The faster the diffusion of the nuclei, the larger the phase discrepancy and the lower the resulting signal compared to a measurement without diffusion-weighting gradients.

The sensitivity of the diffusion weighting, the so-called *b*-value (measured in units of s/mm^2), depends on the amplitude of the applied gradients, their duration, and the delay time between the two bipolar gradients comprising the diffusion-weighting gradient pair. The higher the b-value, the stronger the diffusion weighting (Fig. 2.14). Strong gradients and high slew rates are important hardware requirements for diffusion-weighted imaging (DWI) because they reduce the diffusion encoding time, which improves the signal-to-noise ratio (SNR) by shortening the TE. High slew rates also enable faster image encoding, which can further decrease TE and help mitigate distortions by shortening the echo spacing. On clinical scanners, DWI is typically performed with single-shot K-space trajectories, most commonly using the echoplanar imaging (EPI) technique [1]. For additional imaging acceleration, diffusion images are often under-sampled to minimize the effective TE and length of the echo train. Parallel imaging techniques are employed to restore the unaliased images by using spatial information inherent in the coil sensitivity profiles of a multichannel receiver coil.

How to Measure Apparent Diffusion Coefficients for Body Imaging

The application of diffusion-weighting gradients prior to data sampling will generate a qualitative diffusion-weighted image contrast in which the signals from regions with more rapid diffusion will appear more attenuated than those from regions with slower diffusion relative to the signal from an equivalent acquisition without diffusion gradients [1]. Nevertheless, the self-diffusion D constant of the nuclei, typically that of water, can principally be quantified based on the relative signal difference in just two images measured with different b-values because in the case of unrestricted diffusion, the signal decreases exponentially with increasing b-value:

$$\frac{S_2}{S_1} = e^{-(b_2 - b_1)D}, \quad (2.11)$$

where S_1 and S_2 are the pixel intensities in the measurements with diffusion weightings of b_1 and b_2, respectively. Although this relation holds for any b-value combination, b_1 is usually chosen to be 0 s/mm^2, that is, no diffusion gradients are applied. However, in biological specimen, pure water diffusing without restrictions is rarely encountered. Rather, water exists as a solvent containing numerous macromolecules that slow down the diffusion of water molecules. Further, various structural obstacles such as cell membranes block the diffusion pathways. As a result, MR diffusion measurements yield an apparent diffusion coefficient (ADC) that tends to be considerably smaller than D and that depends on the selected acquisition parameters.

In clinical practice, measurements with 3–5 different b-values are typically used. The number of signal averages is usually increased for higher b-values to ensure a sufficient SNR while maintaining clinically acceptable scan times. The ADC is calculated by fitting the measured signal intensities $S(b)$ to a mono-exponential decay curve:

$$S(b) = S_0 e^{-b(ADC)}, \quad (2.12)$$

where $S_0 = S(b = 0)$.

Pulse Sequence and Imaging Parameters

1. **Echo time (TE):** It is the time interval between application of radiofrequency pulse and measurement of an echo.
2. **Field of view (FOV):** It is the image area that contains the object of interest to be measured. The smaller is the FOV, the higher is the image resolution and smaller is the voxel size and hence lower signal-to-noise ratio.

   FOV is expressed as

   $$\mathrm{FOV} = \mathrm{BW} / \gamma G$$

   where BW, receiver bandwidth (Hz); γ, gyromagnetic ratio of a nucleus (MHz/T); and G, amplitude or strength of a gradient (mT/m).
3. **Flip angle:** It is the extent of rotation experienced by the net magnetization during the application of a RF pulse. The flip angle over an image depends on B_0 inhomogeneity, type of RF pulse, pulse profile, slice select gradient, and off-resonance effects.

   For a strong and rectangular RF pulse of constant amplitude (B_1) and duration (τ), the flip angle (α) is given by

   $$\alpha = \gamma^* B_1^* \tau$$

4. **Image contrast:** It is the relative difference in signal intensities between two adjacent regions of an image. Image contrast depends upon tissue properties such as T_1, T_2, proton density, susceptibility, chemical shift, diffusion, perfusion, and flow. It also depends upon type of pulse sequences, several sequence parameters, and factors such as temperature and pH of the tissues.
5. **Image resolution**: Resolution is an ability of the human eyes to distinguish one structure from another; in other words, the resolution is the level of detail of an image. The resolution is defined by number of pixels in a given FOV. The higher the number of pixels, the greater the image resolution. The pixel size is measured by dividing the FOV by matrix size. There are two types of image resolution used in MRI.

(a) Base resolution is defined as the number of pixels in the frequency encoding-direction. Base resolution is directly proportional to scan time and inversely proportional to pixel size and hence the SNR. Increasing the base resolution more than an acceptable range results in grainy image due to low SNR, and decreasing the base resolution more than an acceptable range produces a blurry image due to increased SNR.

(b) Phase resolution is defined as the number of pixels in the phase-encoding direction. Phase resolution is generally expressed a percentage of base resolution. Decreasing phase resolution will increase the pixel size in one direction resulting in rectangular pixel shape. Phase resolution is directly proportional to scan time and inversely proportional to pixel size and hence SNR (Fig. 2.15).

6. **Inversion time (TI):** It is the time interval between applications of 180° and 90° RF pulses.
7. **Number of excitations (NEX):** It is defined as the number of times each line of K-space is acquired. Doubling the NEX increases the SNR by a factor of $\sqrt{2}$ because random noise is also sampled. However, it increases the scan time.
8. **Receiver bandwidth:** It is also known as digitization rate of MR signal. It is reciprocal of dwell time (time interval between digitized samples). The dwell time is defined as the number of complex sample points multiplied by sampling time. Different MRI vendors express the receiver bandwidth in different ways. While Siemens and Canon scanners use bandwidth per pixel, GE scanners use the total bandwidth across an entire image. The receiver bandwidth is also defined as range of frequencies from $-f$max to $+f$max.

$$\mathrm{BW} = \pm f\,\mathrm{max}\;\mathrm{or}\;2f\,\mathrm{max}$$

BW is also defined as $1/\Delta Ts$ or Nx/Ts

where ΔTs is a dwell time (time interval between complex data points), Nx is the number of frequency-encoding steps, and Ts is the sampling time ($Nx * \Delta Ts$).

9. **Repetition time (TR):** It is the time interval between two successive applied radiofrequency pulses.
10. **Scan time for conventional spin-echo sequence**: TR * NEX * number of phase-encoding steps
11. **Scan time for fast spin-echo sequence:** TR * NEX * number of phase-encoding steps/echo train length
12. **Scan time for gradient recalled echo sequence:** TR * NEX * number of phase-encoding steps * number of slices
13. **Scan for three-dimensional imaging:** TR * NEX * number of phase-encoding steps * number of phase-encoding steps (partitions) in *z*-direction
14. **Signal-to-noise ratio (SNR)**

    A digital MR image consists of signal and noise. The parameter signal-to-noise ratio (SNR) is used to describe the image quality. A number of factors affect the SNR of an image, and these factors are the following:

FOV Read (mm)	FOV Phase	Phase resolution	Matrix size	Pixel size (mm)
256	100%	100%	256 x 256	1 x 1
256	100%	75%	256 x 192	1 x 1.33
256	100%	50%	256 x 128	1 x 2
256	100%	25%	256 x 64	1x 4

Fig. 2.15 Decreasing phase resolution increases the pixel size and the SNR

(a) SNR depends upon the composition and characteristics of a biological tissue being imaged. Tissues with higher number of proton spins produce higher signal intensities and hence possess higher SNR.
(b) SNR varies with primary magnetic field as SNR α $B_0^{7/4}$. High magnetic field strength tends to align a greater number of spins along the direction of magnetic field. Henceforth, high field strength increases the net longitudinal magnetization and SNR.
(c) To achieve high SNR, the RF receiver coil should be placed as close as possible to the anatomical structure being imaged. Therefore, a coil with smaller radius will produce higher SNR. Additionally, the greater the number of receiver channels, the greater the SNR.
(d) SNR increases with increase in TR as a high TR will allow longitudinal magnetization to recover back to high values and will produce high signal.
(e) SNR decreases with increase in TE as a high TE will allow transverse magnetization to decay to low values and will result in signal loss
(f) SNR decreases with increasing matrix size as voxel size is inversely proportional to matrix size.
(g) SNR increases with increasing FOV as voxel size is proportional to FOV
(h) SNR is directly proportional to square root of number of phase-encoding steps. Therefore, doubling the NEX causes 1.44 times increase in SNR.
(i) SNR increases with increasing interslice gap which is the distance between two adjacent slices and is usually described as percentage of slice thickness. Slice gap reduces or eliminates slice overlapping and cross-talk that may be caused by imperfect slice profiles. This crosstalk causes a saturation effect (signal loss) in the area of slice overlap, resulting in lower SNR.
(j) SNR increases with increasing voxel size. A larger voxel contains a greater number of proton spins per unit volume.
(k) SNR increases with increasing slice thickness.
(l) SNR is directly proportional to square root of number of excitations (NEX). Therefore, doubling the NEX causes 1.44 times increase in SNR.
(m) SNR is inversely proportional to square root of receiver bandwidth, and hence, SNR decreases as receiver bandwidth increases.
(n) The use of lower receiver bandwidth increases SNR and allows selection of a smaller FOV for scanning small tissues of interest. However, lower receiver bandwidth causes more chemical shit artefacts, susceptibility artifacts, and more spatial distortion of an image.
(o) Application of any saturation pulses decreases the overall SNR in the image. For example, nullifying the fat proton signals reduces the overall signal intensity from anatomical structure being imaged.
(p) Partial filling of K-space lines in the phase-encoding direction decreases SNR.

15. **Transmitter bandwidth:** Range of frequencies (measured in Hz) is involved in transmitted radiofrequency pulse. It is expressed as

$$\Delta F = \gamma^* \text{Gss}^* \Delta z$$

where ΔF is the transmitter bandwidth (Hz), γ the gyromagnetic ratio of a nucleus (MHz/T), Gss the amplitude/strength of slice select gradient (mT/m), and Δz the slice thickness (mm).

16. **Voxel:** It is a volume element representing a value in the three-dimensional space, corresponding to a pixel (pictorial element) for a given slice thickness.

Kidney MRI

Image Acquisition

MR image acquisition requires four basic steps: (1) place the patient in a uniform magnetic field generated by the combination of the MRI components, (2) displace the equilibrium magnetization vector with an RF pulse, (3) collect the signal as the magnetization vector returns to equilibrium, and (4) convert the collected signals into images using the computer's signal processing algorithms.

With MR, smaller picture elements mean that there are fewer hydrogen nuclei per "voxel." This three-dimensional projection of the pixel (voxel) is defined by the face of the pixel and the slice thickness. Decreasing either the slice thickness or the pixel size results in fewer protons per voxel (Fig. 2.16). With fewer hydrogen protons in each voxel, and assuming the noise stays the same, the signal-to-noise ratio decreases, which may decrease image contrast. The scan time for a simple spin-echo acquisition is based on the facts that a 90° pulse is necessary for each gradient step and that one gradient step is necessary for each line of information in the phase-encoding direction. As a result, a 512 × 512 matrix requires twice as much time to acquire as a 256 × 256 scan, but the pixels at 512 × 512 will be one-fourth the size. While it might seem that this would decrease the signal by one-fourth, since each phase-encoding step contributes to the signal of the entire image, the signal loss decreases by only one-half since there are twice as many phase-encoding steps in a 512 versus a 256 square matrix. The decrease in the signal-to-noise ratio can be corrected in part by repeating the entire pulse sequence more than once and averaging the results. This variable is sometimes abbreviated as NEX, meaning "number of excitations." Each excitation adds time, of course, so using a NEX of 2 doubles the scan time (Fig. 2.17). You might think that one would double the signal by doubling the scan time. Unfortunately, you still will not come out even because when you double the scan time, the signal-to-noise ratio increases only by a factor of 1.4 (square root of 2), not 2. To double the signal, you would need to use a NEX of 4 or a scan time four times as long (square root of 4 = 2) to break even. For this reason, it is prudent to avoid an extremely fine matrix unless your scanner provides signal to burn (remember the drive to high field strength) or the indications warrant this added time. One compromise commonly used is an asymmetric matrix such as 128 × 256. In MRI

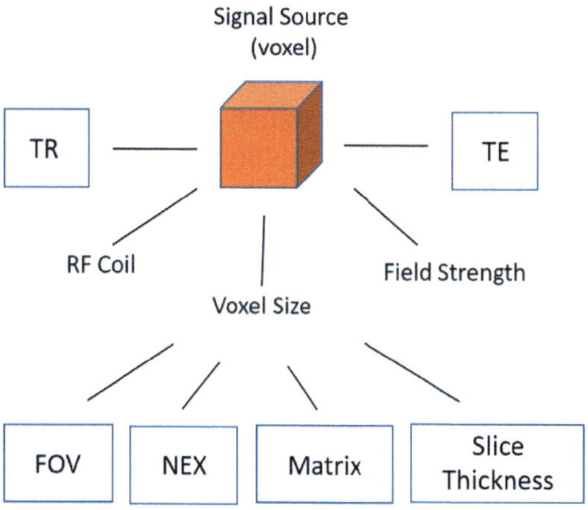

Fig. 2.16 Diagram shows the interplay of protocol parameters directly affecting signal in MRI. FOV field of view, NEX number of excitations, RF radiofrequency, TE echo time, and TR repetition time

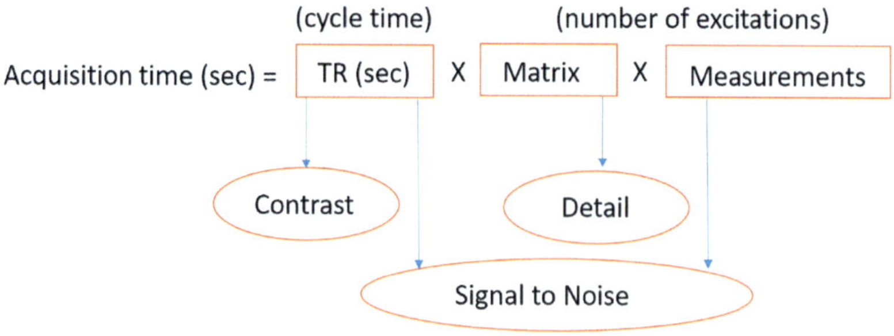

Fig. 2.17 Image quality and acquisition time optimization

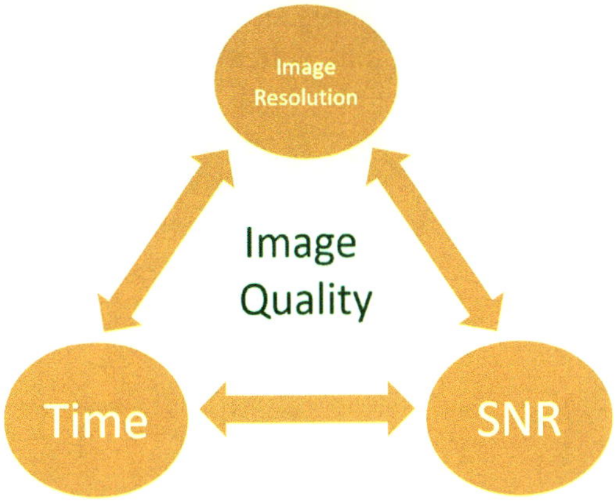

Fig. 2.18 The scan time, image resolution, and signal-to-noise ratio (SNR) are interdependent on each other

image acquisition, the scan time, image resolution, and signal-to-noise ratio (SNR) are interdependent on each other (Fig. 2.18). Increasing the matrix size in the frequency direction requires applying a stronger gradient that does not add time. In addition, using phase encoding for the short side of this rectangular matrix will take the same time as a scan with a 128 × 128 matrix while still providing a finer detail.

Physiological Monitoring and Motion Consideration

One of the main challenges that continues to drive innovation in pediatric imaging is motion. Much time and effort are devoted to reducing the numerous sources of motion and their resultant artifacts (Fig. 2.19). These sources of motion include gross body (i.e., voluntary) motion, respiratory motion, cardiac contractions, vascular pulsations, and bowel peristalsis. Obtaining diagnostic-quality images requires the patient to "lie still" during image acquisition; however, many patients and especially children are unable to comply with this request for various reasons. Physiology-synchronized acquisition techniques (e.g., triggering, gating, and tracking) may mitigate respiratory and cardiac motion at the expense of additional scan time.

There are clinically established and emerging MRI techniques for the abdominal imaging. These techniques fall under two general categories: undersampling the K-space for accelerated imaging and motion compensation and correction techniques. Some of the newer methods combine the two as self-navigating accelerated imaging techniques. Most of the techniques can be employed with physiological motion compensation strategies such as breath-holding and respiratory synchronized acquisition.

Respiratory Synchronization

Respiratory motion can be monitored and tracked in real time using pneumatic respiratory bellows placed on the abdomen or two-dimensional radiofrequency (RF) excitation pulses, known as RF pulse navigators, positioned at the lung/diaphragm interface in foot to head direction. Data acquisition can be synchronized to the respiratory motion in three different modes: (1) triggering, where typically data is acquired at certain delay after the detection of expiration; (2) gating, where data is acquired during a prescribed acceptable diaphragmatic displacement; and (3) tracking, where upon detection of expiration, the slice offset is adjusted in real time prior to data acquisition.

The bellows track the body wall motion as a surrogate to abdominal organ motion. The RF navigator tracks the diaphragmatic movement directly and allows slice offset correction in real time. Respiratory gating restricts data acquisition to a designated phase of the respiratory cycle, typically expiration (Fig. 2.20). While physiologically more accurate, RF navigator may not be effective in patients with extremely shallow breathing due to the inability to pick up synchronous signal and in patients with iron overload due to low signal to noise ratio. Similarly, the respiratory gating may not work well in older children with heavy chest breathing and larger diaphragmatic excursions, which cause larger abdominal organ motion (Fig. 2.21). Generally, respiratory gating also results in an approximately threefold increase in total scan time. To reduce scan time to a reasonable duration, a single-shot acquisition with a triggered approach is employed.

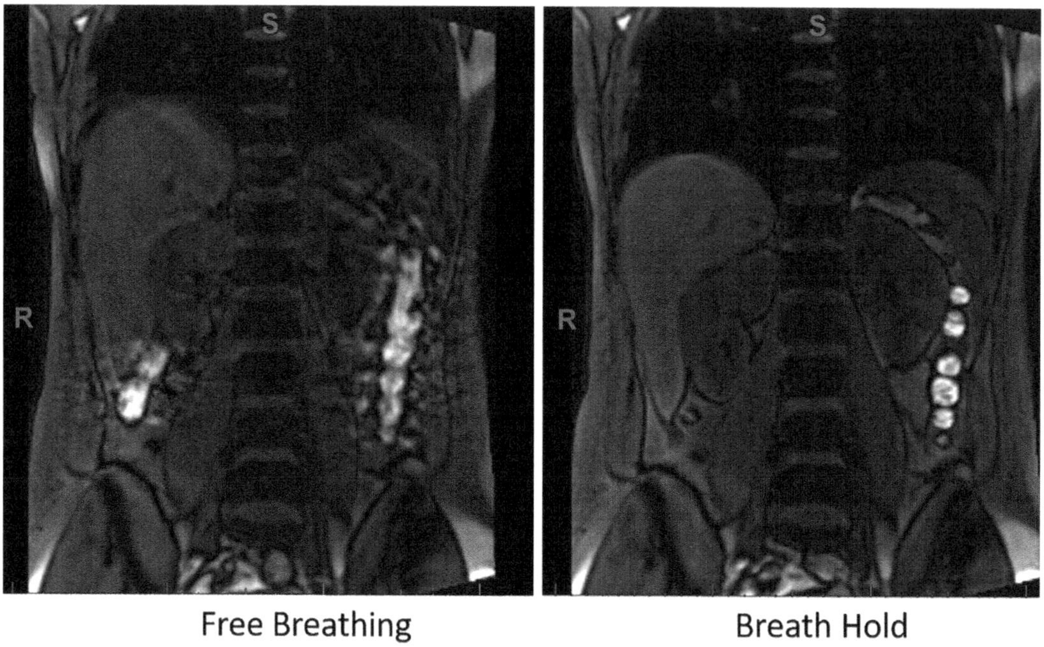

Fig. 2.19 Free-breathing versus breath-holding

Fig. 2.20 Respiratory-triggered scan

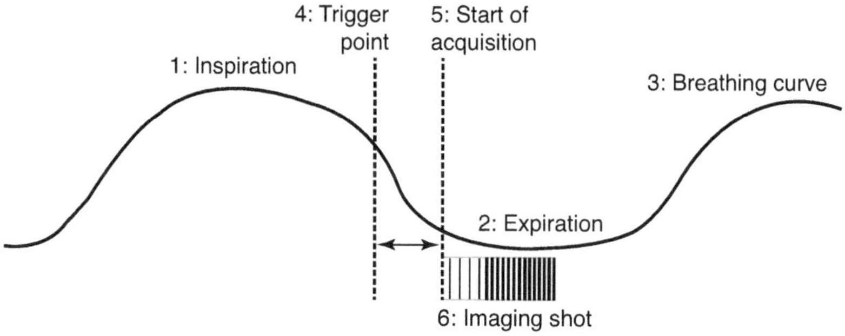

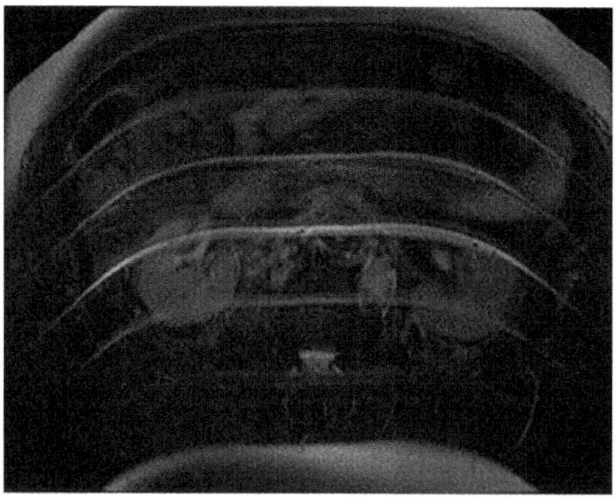

Fig. 2.21 Note that the motion has a pattern—they mostly occur along the phase-encoding direction, since adjacent lines of phase encode are separated by TR interval that can last 3000 ms or longer. ()

Signal Averaging

When breath-hold and respiratory synchronization is not feasible, averaging the signal over multiple number of excitations (NEX) may help reduce motion artifacts. This technique cohesively adds up the signal intensity in the static anatomy and reduces the signal intensity of ghosts caused by the anatomy moving out of synchronization with the acquisition. Increasing NEX also increases the SNR by a factor of the square root of the NEX value. To achieve adequate artifact reduction, the NEX is often set to 3 or greater, resulting in a threefold or proportional increase in total scan time. Careful attention should be paid to increase in total RF deposition with higher NEX values.

Swapping Encoding Direction and Saturation Bands

Motion artifacts are predominant in the phase-encoding direction. Typically, because the anterior to posterior (AP) dimension is the smallest and most favorable for coil topology, phase encoding is prescribed in AP direction. In certain cases, by swapping the phase-encoding direction, motion artifacts can be constrained to outside the anatomy of diagnostic interest. Subcutaneous abdominal fat generates a higher signal in almost all types of contrasts (T_1W, T_2W, and PDW) and, being closer to coil elements, dominates the signal intensity spectrum. Therefore, respiratory artifacts from the moving anterior abdominal wall are generated distinctly over the rest of the abdomen. The signal from moving tissue, especially abdominal fat, can be suppressed with fat saturation techniques or by placing a regional saturation band over the anterior abdominal wall.

Practical Points to Consider When Performing a Kidney MRI Study

Scheduling a Renal MRI Scan

Renal MRI studies are typically scheduled into timeslots of between 30 min and 1 h depending on the complexity of the study and capabilities of the MRI scanner and/or if contrast will need to be injected. Examinations that need sedation or anesthesia may require more time for patient preparation and recovery. Either at the time of the appointment or when confirming the appointment time with the patient, it is prudent for the staff to briefly review the patient's reason for the scan and perform a prescreening of metallic implants, pacemakers, or other electronic implants and inquire about claustrophobia, allergies, or any other special needs the patient may have. This is a good opportunity for staff to also give some information to the patient about the length of the visit, how a patient should dress (e.g., no jewelry, hair clips, makeup, etc.), or if they will need to change into a hospital gown for the study. It is quite costly to an MRI facility to have an unexpected open time slot if the patient does not arrive for an appointment or arrives late. A late arrival will cause stress to the delays for the rest of the day. After the study is scheduled, the radiologist reviews the indication for the requested study and decides on the scanning protocol. The team then determines if the examination is scheduled appropriately based on the time of the day, available staff, resources, and the length of the exam. Most scheduled exams will need few alterations when handled by experienced personnel. Renal MRI studies are becoming more complex, and certain examinations require detailed clinical information for the MRI team to plan properly the scanning protocol. Continuous flow of communication is essential among all team members. An adequately prepared team reduces the chance of unanticipated problems, allowing for smooth execution of the examination.

Patient Positioning

In order to obtain images, an MRI technologist must first select the appropriate RF coil and position the patient. The patient should be made as comfortable as possible to achieve cooperation. For most renal MRI scans, the patient lies supine. Prone positioning may help reduce claustrophobia since the patient can look outside the bore, but it is less comfortable than supine position. Phased array receive coils with posterior elements must be positioned on the table before the patient lies down. Most new MRI scanners now have the posterior elements built into the table, which simplifies the positioning workflow. The anterior portion of the phased array coil is then positioned and stabilized using Velcro straps. Adequate cushioning must be placed between the patient and the coil to ensure that the patient will be comfortable for the duration of the study.

Physiological Monitoring

Depending on the MR system, and as described in Sect. 2.5.3, available respiratory gating methods include using mechanical bellows and navigator gating. While these methods are highly effective in many patients, the results vary according to the regularity and depth of the patient's breathing. Extra time is required to position the bellows optimally and to choose the thresholds for accepting the data or, in case of navigator echoes, to position the navigator appropriately and obtain baseline data about respiratory patterns. With respiratory gating methods, some data gets rejected, so the scan times are increased, typically by a factor of 2.

Coil Selection and Image Acquisition

The first step for image acquisition is to choose the appropriate receiver coil. Recollect that our receiver coil acts like an antenna for the radio signal tuned to the specific frequency, and choosing the correct coil for the anatomy of interest can make a big difference in SNR. A series of surface coils are combined to form a phased array coil; individual coils are magnetically decoupled, thus providing sensitivity for imaging over a large volume that is often required for renal imaging. Depending on the scanner capabilities, phased array coils nowadays may have as few as 4 to as many as 32 or more elements. The development of phased array technology is partly driven by the development of parallel imaging methods. In general, higher acceleration factors work most effectively with coils that have larger number of elements. It is important to know the number of receive channels available on the scanner hardware and the number of elements on the coil being used. With certain phased array coil combinations, there may be more coil elements, than the number of receive channels. The scanning MR technologist should prefer to activate only those coil elements that are needed to image the specific anatomy of interest. If too many elements are activated, multiple elements are multiplexed into a single receiver channel. Moreover, some elements might be located relatively far away from the magnet isocenter. The result is a worsening SNR along with the potential to introduce artifacts into the image. Moreover, image reconstruction time increases with the number of elements as does the amount of space needed to store raw data. Long reconstruction times can limit the practical application of some advanced imaging techniques such as compressed sensing, particularly when large amount of data is rapidly acquired in conjunction with the use of phased array coils with numerous elements. For body imaging, coil centering and imaging on isocenter are equally important for better image quality and uniformity. The magnetic field is most uniform at the magnet isocenter. The magnet uniformity and linearity of the gradients decline as we move away from the isocenter. Therefore, the coil should be centered, and imaging should be performed at isocenter. In general, image quality will not suffer greatly if the body part is a few centimeters away from the isocenter. However, with large displacements, SNR may degrade, and shim may worsen resulting in poor fat suppression that is often done for renal imaging. For a clinical renal MRI scan, and especially for quantitative imaging, a good SNR is essential for image quality. A higher SNR means image will appear to be less grainy and fine details will be more apparent. Consequently, a low SNR results in a grainy image in which fine details are obscured. Although a high SNR is desirable, increasing the SNR often requires more scan time, and a balance needs to be played between acceptable image quality and image acquisition time. Figure 2.22 provides a summary of factors that affect image quality and acquisition time.

Finally, there are several practical ways to optimize and adjust the imaging parameters during a renal MRI scan to maximize SNR or spatial resolution in an attempt to produce high-quality MR images. The overview of the physics and the details of the currently employed image acquisition techniques are included in this chapter, and in subsequent chapters in this section, we intend to familiarize the reader on how different various configurations impact image quality in state-of-the-art clinical kidney MRI. Ultimately, with this background information, the user can experiment with different imaging parameters and decide what suits the needs of the particular MRI study. The power of MRI lies in its flexibility, and its clinical potential will continue to grow with developments in the underlying technology.

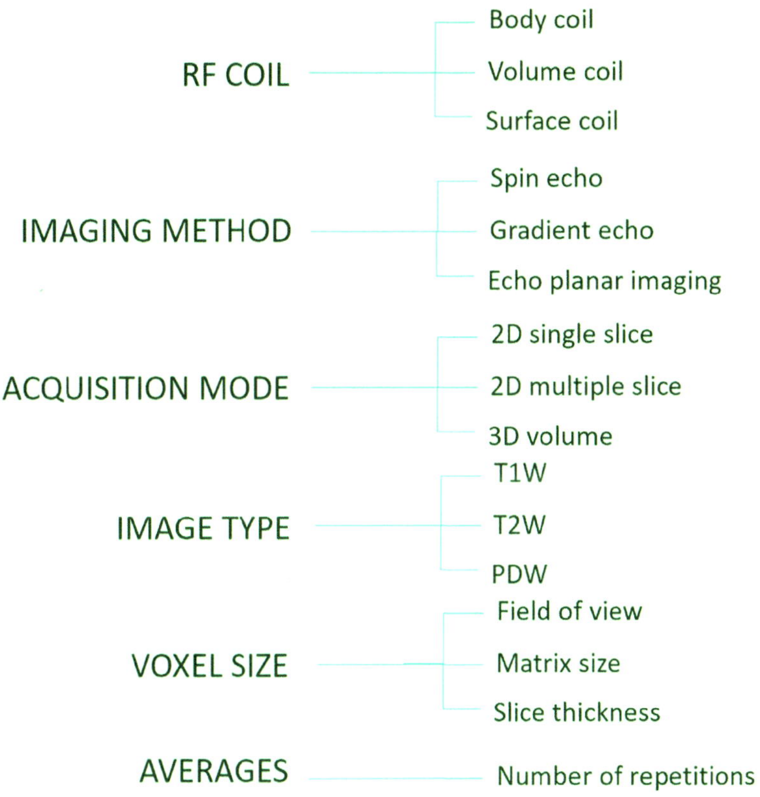

Fig. 2.22 MRI factors that affect image quality and acquisition time. (© [Suraj D. Serai, 2023. All rights reserved])

Fat Suppression Methods

Due to short relaxation times, fat has a high signal on MRI. This high signal due to fat may be responsible for artifacts such as ghosting and chemical shift. Moreover, a contrast-enhancing tumor may be hidden by the surrounding fat. These problems have led to the development of fat suppression techniques in MRI [16, 17]. Fat suppression depends on different magnetic properties of water and fat protons differ in two ways:

1. The T_1 values for fat protons are much shorter than those of water protons.
2. The water protons resonate slightly faster than those of fat protons. This difference in resonance frequency is known as water-fat chemical shift.

These differences in relaxation and chemical shift-dependent magnetic properties can be used to selectively suppress the signals of fat-bound protons.

Inversion Recovery (STIR, Short TI Inversion Recovery)

This technique is based on the different relaxation behavior of water and fat tissues. Because fat has a much shorter T_1 relaxation time than other tissues, its signal can be selectively nulled using a magnitude-reconstructed inversion recovery (IR) sequence. Prior to the excitation pulse of the sequence, an inversion pulse (α = 180°) is applied which inverts the spins of all the tissues, which subsequently undergo T_1 relaxation. By choosing intervention time (TI) such that the longitudinal magnetization of fat at that time is zero, fat spins will not contribute to the MR signal. STIR images have an inverted T_1 contrast: tissue with long T_1 appears brighter than tissue with short T_1.

Advantages

It is relatively insensitive to B_0 inhomogeneities and can be used near metallic implants and over large fields of view.

Disadvantages

Additional inversion pulse increases minimal TR and hence total scan time. It can also increase the specific absorption rate (SAR) due to additional 180° pulse.

The signal suppression is not specific to fat tissues. In fact, any material with short T_1 value such as melanin, methemoglobin, and mucus will be nulled. Signal-to-noise ratio can decrease as tissues of interest may have lower net magnetization recovery at null point.

Spectral Fat Saturation

This is the most widely used fat suppression technique. It is based on the difference in resonance frequencies (~3.5 ppm) between fat and water protons. In this technique, a frequency-selective RF pulse tuned to the resonance frequency of fat protons is applied in association with a crusher gradient to excite and then dephase the fat protons (Fig. 2.23). Thus, no fat magnetization is left for imaging and only water protons are present to produce an MR signal.

Advantages

The technique is simple and versatile and can be added to any pulse sequence.

Tissue contrast is not affected.

Disadvantages

It is sensitive to B_0 and B_1 inhomogeneities.

It works better on higher field strengths because of larger chemical shift dispersion between water and fat protons at higher field strength.

It requires homogeneous B_0 field and does not work properly around the metallic implants or around the air-tissue interfaces.

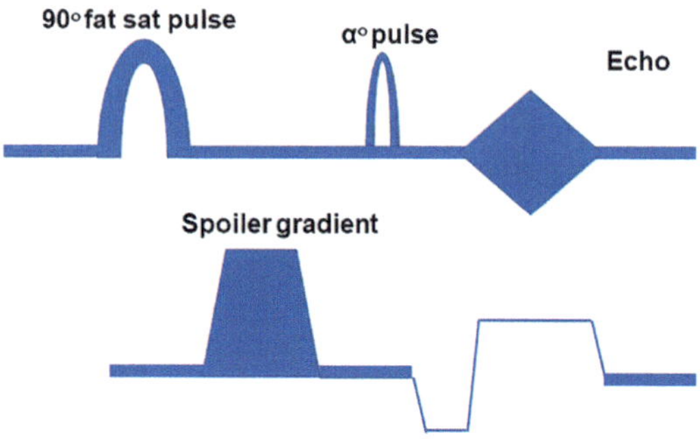

Fig. 2.23 Typical fat saturation/CHESS pulse sequence and spoiler gradient used in a GRE sequence

Dixon Technique

The Dixon technique is based on the difference in resonance frequencies between fat and water-bound protons. In this technique, signals from water and fat protons in the same voxel can be made to interfere constructively or destructively by changing TE [18, 19]. This method is routinely used in body applications for fat quantification [19–22].

Advantages

It is insensitive to B_0 and B_1 inhomogeneities.

Four contrast images (in-phase, opposed-phase, water, and fat images) are obtained in a single measurement.

Fat quantification is also possible.

Disadvantages

It increases minimal TR because in and opposed phase data must be acquired.

Typical Body Imaging Artifacts and Tips to Mitigate Them

An imaging artifact is a feature appearing in an image that is not usually present in the original object. Many different artifacts can occur during MRI affecting the diagnostic quality and mimicking with a pathological condition [23].

Motion Artifacts

Motion artifact is one of the most common artifacts observed on MR images that is generally present along the phase-encoding direction. The reason for mainly affecting data sampling in the phase-encoding direction is the significant difference in the time of acquisition in the frequency and phase-encoding directions [23]. Frequency-encoding sampling in all the rows of the matrix takes place during a single echo (milliseconds). On the other hand, phase-encoded sampling takes several seconds or even minutes because of the collection of all the K-space data. The most of physiological movements are of the order of milliseconds to seconds duration and thus too slow to affect the frequency-encoded sampling, but they have a pronounced effect in the phase-encoding direction. Periodic movements such as cardiac movement and blood vessel or CSF pulsation produce ghost images, while nonperiodic movements result in diffused image noise.

Several methods can be used to reduce motion artifacts including patient immobilization (by using foam pads, taping, bite bars, etc.), employing cardiac and respiratory gating, increasing the number of excitations/averaging, and using ultrafast sequences, radial/spiral sampling of K-space, flow compensation, and fat, spatial, and flow saturation pulses or techniques. The swapping of frequency and phase-encoding directions will displace the artifact out of the tissue of interest but will not eliminate it.

Chemical Shift Artifact

The chemical shift refers to change in resonance frequencies of two biological tissues owing to different in chemical environment of nuclei. The chemical shift artifact occurs at the water and fat interface especially along the frequency-encoding direction (Figs. 2.24 and 2.25). These artifacts arise due to the difference in resonance frequency

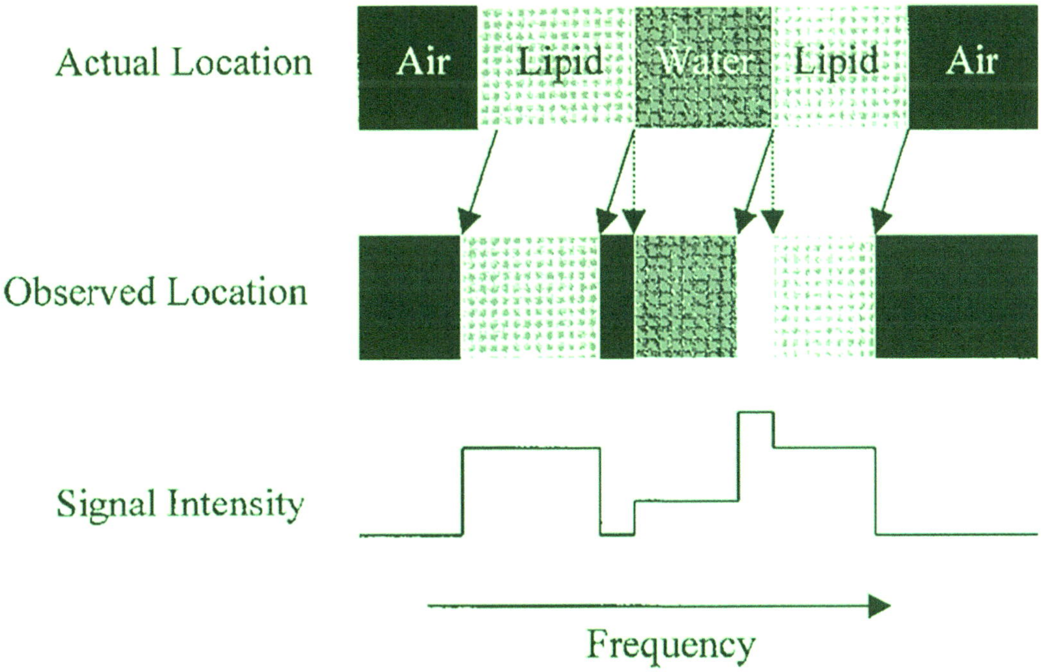

Fig. 2.24 Chemical shift artifacts arise because of spatial mismapping of water and fat signals due to their different resonance frequencies. Alternative bright and dark bands are observed along the frequency-encoding direction on a conventional spin-echo and gradient-echo images

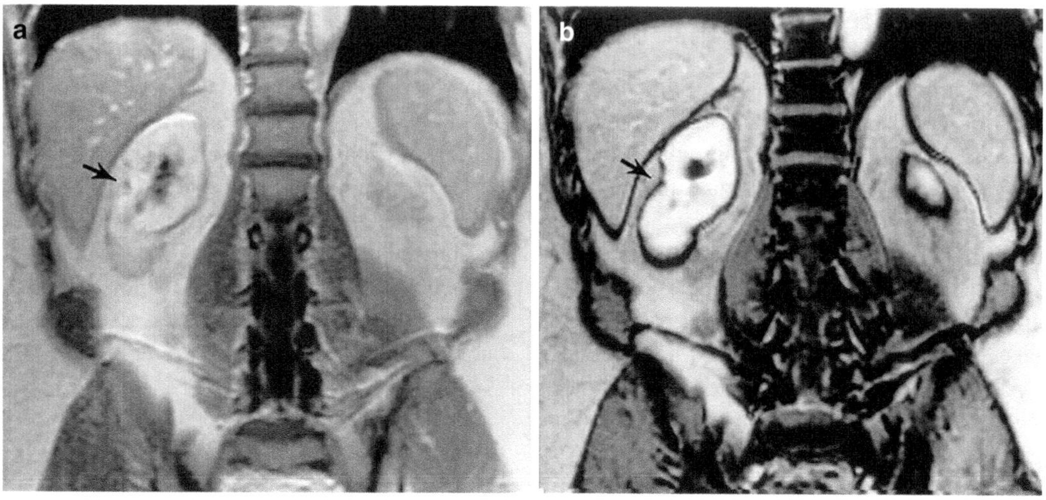

Fig. 2.25 Chemical shift artifacts seen on (**a**) in-phase and (**b**) out-of-phase kidney MR images

of water and fat protons, which causes spatial mismatching of fat and water pixels. These artifacts are reflected as alternative bright and dark bands along the frequency-encoding direction. The chemical shift distance is defined as

Chemical shift distance (mm) = Frequency shift (Hz) × FOV (mm)/receiver bandwidth (Hz).

The best strategy to reduce chemical shift artifact is to use fat suppression technique for reducing the signal from fat and thereby minimize this artifact. The other method is to increase total receiver bandwidth by reducing the field of view or increasing the strength of the frequency-encoding gradient. Swapping the frequency and phase-encoding directions prior to imaging will not eliminate the chemical shift artifact but will shift it to a different anatomical region.

Magnetic Susceptibility and Magnetic Susceptibility Artifact

The degree to which a substance gets magnetized when placed in an externally applied magnetic field is called magnetic susceptibility (χ). While diamagnetic substances are feebly repelled by magnetic field, paramagnetic substances are feebly attracted by magnetic field. Almost all biological tissues are diamagnetic in nature. The presence of metallic ions (Mn, Gd) in tissues produces weak paramagnetism. The globular non-heme iron protein complexes such as ferritin and hemosiderin create strong positive paramagnetic effect known as super-paramagnetism. The most powerful magnetic field susceptibility occurs in solid materials containing Fe, Co, or Ni and is called ferromagnetism (Fig. 2.26).

The magnetic susceptibility effects create magnetic field distortions resulting in variations in precessional frequency within a voxel. This frequency shift, in turn, produces signal loss from T_2*-dephasing and spatial mismapping of the MR signal. The susceptibility artifacts are usually present at the air-tissue interfaces and around the metallic objects and implants.

The intensity of susceptibility artifact depends on difference in magnetic susceptibilities between tissues, magnetic field strength (B_0), echo time (TE), and receiver bandwidth. This relationship is expressed as

Size of susceptibility artefact $\propto$ [(Δ*suceptibility*) $*$ *B0* $*$ *TE*]/receiver bandwith.

The swapping of the frequency and phase-encoding does not eliminate the susceptibility artifacts but changes the shape of artifact. The susceptibility artifacts can be reduced by using shorter TE values, increasing receiver bandwidth, increasing gradient strength for a given FOV, and using smaller voxel size, thinner slices, and parallel imaging. The susceptibility artifacts are most prominent on echo planar sequences and

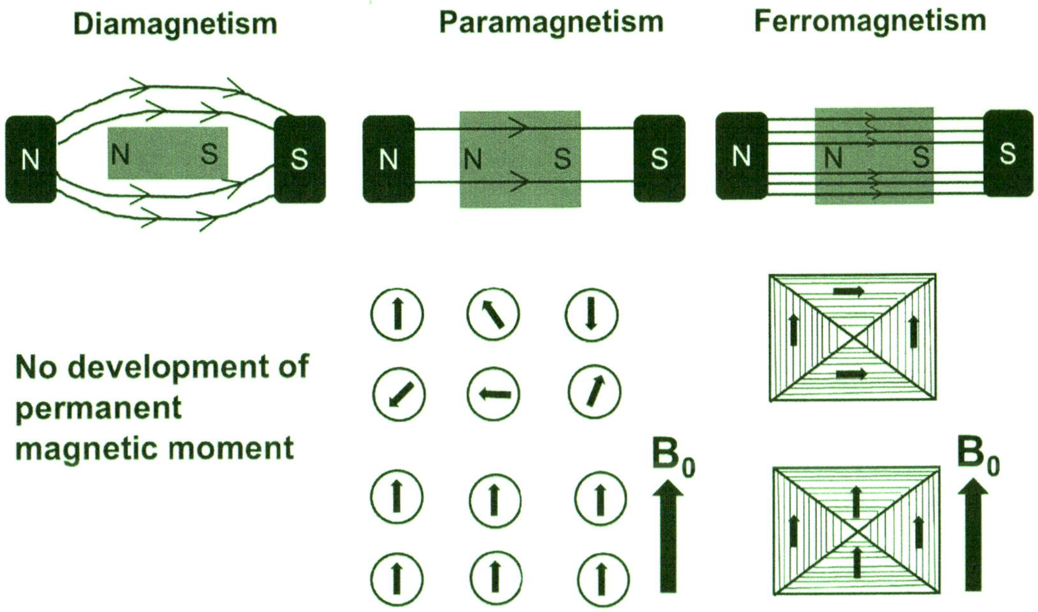

Fig. 2.26 Magnetic properties of materials. Diamagnetic materials (almost all biological tissues, oxyhemoglobin, and calcium) are feebly repelled by magnetic fields. These materials do not have permanent magnetic dipole moments (MDMs). Paramagnetic materials (deoxyhemoglobin, methemoglobin) and superparamagnetic materials (ferritin, hemosiderin) are attracted by magnetic field. In the absence of externally applied magnetic field, permanent MDMs of paramagnetic/superparamagnetic materials are randomly oriented. However, these MDMs become oriented in the presence of magnetic field along its direction. Ferromagnetic materials (iron, cobalt, and nickel) are strongly attracted by magnetic field. The MDMs in ferromagnetic materials exert strong forces on their neighbors and appear to be groped magnetically into domains. In the absence of magnetic field, all MDMs within a domain are aligned, but the direction of alignment varies from domain to domain. In the presence of magnetic field, all these domains are aligned along the direction of magnetic field

decrease in the order of using gradient-echo, conventional spin-echo, and fast spin-echo sequences.

Dielectric (Standing Wave) Artifacts

These artifacts arise because of interaction between electric field components of electromagnetic radiation with matter. RF wavelengths in a biological tissue vary as a function of field strength as shown in the following equation:

$$\lambda \propto 1 / B_0 \sqrt{\varepsilon}$$

where λ = wavelength, B_0 = magnetic field strength, and ε = dielectric constant of the medium.

In fact, RF wavelength is known to decrease as field strength increases and becomes similar or smaller than the anatomical dimension. When this happens, a standing wave pattern of electric current occurs, creating constructive and destructive interference and producing alternate bright and dark bands separated by one-fourth wavelength across an anatomical region. The dielectric artifacts can be reduced by using dielectric pads (which are filled with conducting solutions) between a patient and a receiver RF coil. The usage of multi (dual) transmitter RF coil also known as parallel transmission, especially at 7 T field strength, has been shown to reduce dielectric artifacts.

Gibbs/Ringing or Truncation Artifact

This artifact occurs near the sharp boundaries, where high contrast transitions occur between the tissues (brain/CSF, meniscus/fluid in the knee). It appears as multiple, regularly spaced parallel

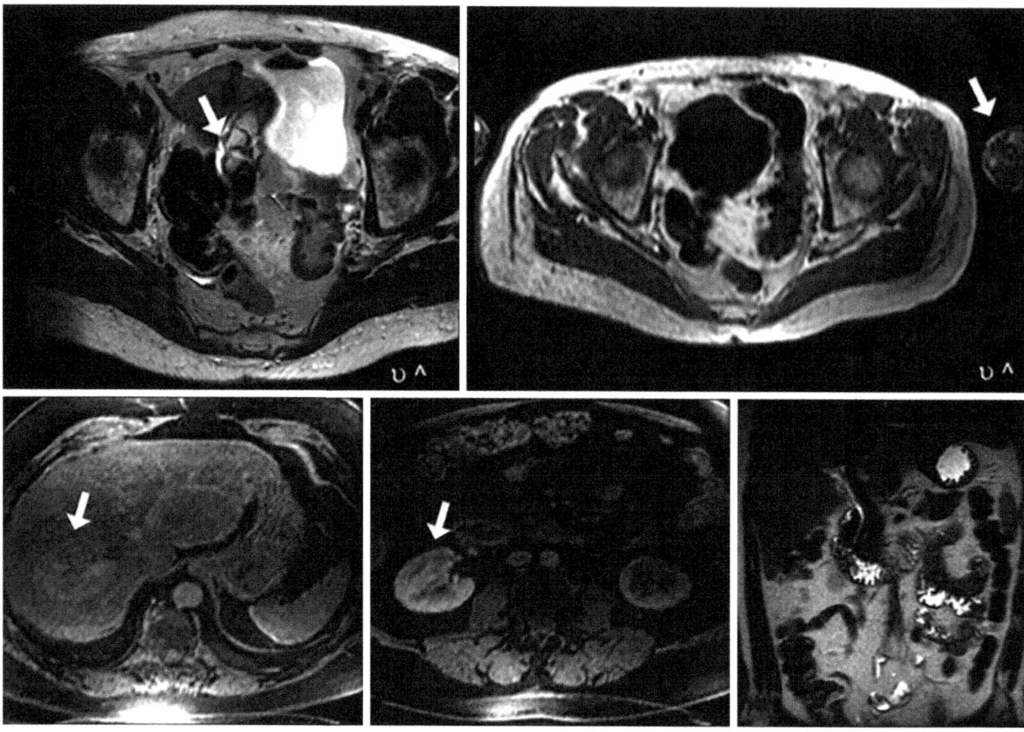

Fig. 2.27 Body structures outside the FOV seen as wraparound artifacts pointed by arrows

bands of alternating bright and dark signal intensities. An MR signal is defined as an infinite summation of sine waves of different amplitudes, phases, and frequencies. However, due to time constrains, only a finite number of frequencies are sampled. In fact, Gibbs artifact is caused by under sampling of high spatial frequencies at sharp boundaries in the image. Lack of appropriate high-frequency components leads to an oscillation at a sharp transition known as a ringing artifact. Since fewer samples are typically taken in the phase-encoding direction, this artifact is mostly noticeable along the phase-encoding direction. Gibbs artifact can be minimized by increasing the number of phase-encoding steps or by reducing the FOV.

Aliasing or Wraparound Artifact

Aliasing or wraparound occurs when the dimension of an objects exceeds the defined FOV and FOV = BW/$\gamma G_f$where FOV = field of view, BW = receiver bandwidth, γ = gyromagnetic ratio, and G_f = amplitude of frequency-encoding gradient.

Also, receiver bandwidth is defined as BW = 2*f*max = ±*f*max

where fmax is the Nyquist frequency or the highest frequency that a computer system can recognize. As a result, a computer system cannot recognize the portion of object present outside the defined BW or FOV. This portion of the object is wrapped around to the opposite side of the image, presenting as low-frequency signals. The perceived frequency is given by

$$f(\text{perceived}) = f(\text{actual}) - 2f\,\text{max}$$

Although aliasing or wraparound artifact may occur along the frequency-encoding direction, it generally occurs along the phase-encoding direction. These artifacts may also occur between end slices in three-dimensional imaging (Fig. 2.27). Phase wraparound artifacts can be reduced by increasing FOV along the phase-encoding direction so that the entire anatomic dimension of the object can be encompassed in that direction. If the FOV is increased, spatial resolution will suffer. To maintain the spatial resolution, the number of phase-encoding steps is increased, however at the cost of increased scanning time. Using surface coil or applying saturation bands outside the FOV may also reduce the wraparound artifacts.

Partial Volume Artifacts

This artifact occurs when portions of several tissue components are averaged together in a voxel or slice of interest. Imperfect RF pulse profiles may cause partial volume effects by exciting tissues outside the desired slice. Partial volume artifacts are reduced by selecting higher imaging matrix sizes, smaller FOVs, and thinner slices. The use of longer duration RF pulses improves slice profiles resulting in precisely defined voxels with less excitation of adjacent tissues, thereby reducing the partial volume artifacts.

Slice Overlapping

When multiple overlapping oblique slices are used to cover a tissue of interest, dark bands appear. It is because protons in the overlapped slices receive multiple RF irradiation and their steady-state magnetization is reduced due to magnetic saturation, resulting in signal loss or appearance of dark bands [23]. The possible solution is to obtain multiple oblique slices in concatenated rather than in sequential acquisition mode.

Summary

In this chapter, we reviewed the basics of MRI, outlined the key hardware components of an MRI scanner, and provided an overview of currently employed image acquisition techniques, with the goal of familiarizing the reader on how different hardware configurations impact image quality in state-of-the-art clinical kidney MRI. We also included some clinical examples of image artifacts, troubleshooting methods, and tips to mitigate them.

References

1. Serai SD. Basics of magnetic resonance imaging and quantitative parameters T1, T2, T2*, T1rho and diffusion-weighted imaging. Pediatr Radiol. 2022;52(2):217–27.
2. Moratal D, Vallés-Luch A, Martí-Bonmatí L, Brummer M. k-Space tutorial: an MRI educational tool for a better understanding of k-space. Biomed Imaging Interv J. 2008;4(1):e15.
3. Jacobs MA, Ibrahim TS, Ouwerkerk R. AAPM/RSNA physics tutorials for residents: MR imaging: brief overview and emerging applications. Radiographics. 2007;27(4):1213–29.
4. Plewes DB. The AAPM/RSNA physics tutorial for residents. Contrast mechanisms in spin-echo MR imaging. Radiographics. 1994;14(6):1389–404; quiz 1405.
5. Calle-Toro JS, Barrera CA, Khrichenko D, Otero HJ, Serai SD. R2 relaxometry based MR imaging for estimation of liver iron content: a comparison between two methods. Abdom Radiol (NY). 2019;44(9):3058–68.
6. Serai SD, Fleck RJ, Quinn CT, Zhang B, Podberesky DJ. Retrospective comparison of gradient recalled echo R2* and spin-echo R2 magnetic resonance analysis methods for estimating liver iron content in children and adolescents. Pediatr Radiol. 2015;45(11):1629–34.
7. Towbin AJ, Serai SD, Podberesky DJ. Magnetic resonance imaging of the pediatric liver: imaging of steatosis, iron deposition, and fibrosis. Magn Reson Imaging Clin N Am. 2013;21(4):669–80.
8. Xia W, Zhang Y, Liu C, Guo Y, He Y, Shao J, et al. Quantitative T2 mapping magnetic resonance imaging of articular cartilage in patients with juvenile idiopathic arthritis. Eur J Radiol. 2023;160:110690.
9. Reeder SB, Yokoo T, França M, Hernando D, Alberich-Bayarri Á, Alústiza JM, et al. Quantification of liver iron overload with MRI: review and guidelines from the ESGAR and SAR. Radiology. 2023;307:221856.
10. Venkatakrishna SSB, Otero HJ, Ghosh A, Khrichenko D, Serai SD. Rate of change of liver iron content by MR imaging methods: a comparison study. Tomography. 2022;8(5):2508–21.
11. Barrera CA, Khrichenko D, Serai SD, Hartung HD, Biko DM, Otero HJ. Biexponential R2* relaxometry for estimation of liver iron concentration in children: a better fit for high liver iron states. J Magn Reson Imaging. 2019;50(4):1191–8.
12. Barrera CA, Otero HJ, Hartung HD, Biko DM, Serai SD. Protocol optimization for cardiac and liver iron content assessment using MRI: what sequence should I use? Clin Imaging. 2019;56:52–7.
13. Serai SD, Trout AT, Fleck RJ, Quinn CT, Dillman JR. Measuring liver T2* and cardiac T2* in a single acquisition. Abdom Radiol (NY). 2018;43(9):2303–8.
14. Hectors SJ, Bane O, Kennedy P, El Salem F, Menon M, Segall M, et al. T1ρ mapping for assessment of renal allograft fibrosis. J Magn Reson Imaging. 2019;50(4):1085–91.

15. Serai SD, Trout AT, Miethke A, Diaz E, Xanthakos SA, Dillman JR. Putting it all together: established and emerging MRI techniques for detecting and measuring liver fibrosis. Pediatr Radiol. 2018;48(9):1256–72.
16. de Kerviler E, Leroy-Willig A, Clément O, Frija J. Fat suppression techniques in MRI: an update. Biomed Pharmacother. 1998;52(2):69–75.
17. Kalovidouri A, Firmenich N, Delattre BMA, Picarra M, Becker CD, Montet X, et al. Fat suppression techniques for breast MRI: dixon versus spectral fat saturation for 3D T1-weighted at 3 T. Radiol Med. 2017;122:731.
18. Yokoo T, Serai SD, Pirasteh A, Bashir MR, Hamilton G, Hernando D, et al. Linearity, bias, and precision of hepatic proton density fat fraction measurements by using MR imaging: a meta-analysis. Radiology. 2018;286(2):486–98.
19. Serai SD, Dillman JR, Trout AT. Proton density fat fraction measurements at 1.5- and 3-T hepatic MR imaging: same-day agreement among readers and across two imager manufacturers. Radiology. 2017;284(1):244–54.
20. Navaratna R, Zhao R, Colgan TJ, Hu HH, Bydder M, Yokoo T, et al. Temperature-corrected proton density fat fraction estimation using chemical shift-encoded MRI in phantoms. Magn Reson Med. 2021;86(1):69–81.
21. Hu HH, Yokoo T, Bashir MR, Sirlin CB, Hernando D, Malyarenko D, et al. Linearity and bias of proton density fat fraction as a quantitative imaging biomarker: a multicenter, multiplatform, multivendor phantom study. Radiology. 2021;298(3):640–51.
22. Joshi M, Dillman JR, Singh K, Serai SD, Towbin AJ, Xanthakos S, et al. Quantitative MRI of fatty liver disease in a large pediatric cohort: correlation between liver fat fraction, stiffness, volume, and patient-specific factors. Abdom Radiol (NY). 2018;43(5):1168–79.
23. Zhuo J, Gullapalli RP. AAPM/RSNA physics tutorial for residents: MR artifacts, safety, and quality control. Radiographics. 2006;26(1):275–97.

Managing Motion in Kidney MRI

3

Michael N. Hoff and Orpheus Kolokythas

Introduction

Kidney Motion

MR imaging of the kidneys and nearby abdominal regions is often impaired by motion. Accurate relaxometric contrast is essential for discrimination of focal kidney lesions. T2-weighted fluid signal intensity in simple and septated cysts cant be differentiated from lesser signal intensity in proteinaceous or hemorrhagic cysts or solid masses. Contrast-enhanced T1-weighted signal can allow distinction between a solid neoplasm, benign or malignant lesions, complex cysts, or abscesses. If motion such as bowel peristalsis and breathing occurs, these processes may be corrupted by artifacts. Arterial pulsation and random bulk motion may also contribute to image artifacts but tend to play minor roles in kidney imaging. Breathing and pulsation are considered periodic with a predictable pattern and direction, while peristalsis and bulk motion have unpredictable frequency and intensity. Due to the kidney's proximity to organs displaced by respiration, breathing tends to be the greatest cause of kidney imaging motion artifacts.

M. N. Hoff (✉)
Department of Radiology and Biomedical Imaging, University of California San Francisco, San Francisco, CA, USA
e-mail: michael.hoff2@ucsf.edu

O. Kolokythas
Department of Radiology, University of Washington, Seattle, WA, USA

Kidney Motion Artifacts

The effects of motion on kidney imaging can be described in terms of the artifacts generated. MR images are not acquired in a spatially contiguous manner. Instead, each data sample contributes signal to the entire corresponding image. Motion modulates the data, contaminating this sensitive relationship. Image artifacts may then arise along the phase-encoding (PE) direction, although fast motion may also cause artifacts along the frequency-encoding (FE) direction. Periodic motion such as arterial pulsation and respiration repeat at regular time intervals on a timescale comparable to or faster than the MRI pulse sequence repetition times, ghosting artifacts can appear across the imaging field of view. Ghosting artifacts appear as replicas of image features that may overlap with true anatomical structures. Blur occurs when motion is random, aperiodic, or slowly periodic as with most bulk motion and peristalsis. Other motion artifacts include intravoxel dephasing signal loss common to flow, misregistration due to flow oblique to the slice prescription, and dark banding that can occur due to signal region boundaries that interfere with ghosting and blur. The prevalence of ghosting and blur here inspires a focus on periodic and aperiodic/random

S. D. Serai, K. Darge (eds.), *Advanced Clinical MRI of the Kidney*,
https://doi.org/10.1007/978-3-031-40169-5_3

motion artifacts in terms of their appearance, causation, and methods of avoidance.

Avoiding Kidney Motion Artifacts

A variety of methods to mitigate motion artifacts exist. Sequence modifications are commonly employed, including radial and spiral k-space data acquisition schemes, swapping phase and frequency-encoding directions, or selective saturation or gradient compensation of moving tissue. Sequence timing may be manipulated using gating, where signal acquisition is triggered to occur during motionless periods, or by interleaving the acquisition to coincide with motion. Breath-holds can isolate motion, and navigator echoes can serve as a record of motion for later correction. Such techniques may also employ methods that manipulate the sequence to cause ghosts to overlap and be easily identified. Random motion often requires more advanced techniques to circumvent motion artifacts. Tracking cameras can permit correction of artifacts, while fast imaging, sedation, and patient immobilization can minimize or prevent motion altogether.

Periodic Motion Effects

Physics of Periodic Motion

When motion repeats at regular time intervals on a timescale comparable to or faster than the MRI pulse sequence repetition time, ghosting artifacts can appear across the imaging field of view. Appearing as replicas of image features, ghosting artifacts may overlap with true anatomical structures. Periodic motion such as arterial pulsation and respiration generates ghosts due to motion-induced coherent phase shifts to the acquired data. Ghost intensity depends on the signal intensity of the moving structure and the extent to which data is modulated. Ghost separation depends on the motion frequency and the imaging repetition time. These artifacts can resemble pathology and degrade diagnostic image quality and thus should be mitigated to ensure accurate radiological diagnoses.

Respiration

Regular breathing is characterized by a periodic variation of inspiration and expiration phases followed by a temporal pause during which motion is minimal. Each of these three phases lasts 1–2 s, but the lack of chest and abdominal wall motion during the pause indicates its specific suitability for MRI k-space data acquisition. However, respiration periodicity can vary substantially between individuals due to breathing amplitude variations (deep versus shallow breaths) or respiration frequency irregularities. A sleeping patient is a common example of such variation: while asleep, the patient's breathing frequency decreases; upon waking abruptly, periodicity may be disrupted. Certain neurological or cardiopulmonary conditions may also cause similar breathing irregularities. Irregularities in respiratory periodicity can disrupt the MRI sequence timing and spoil accurate gating of the acquired data to the pause phase.

Respiration tends to be the leading cause of kidney MRI motion artifacts. The kidneys reside in the retroperitoneum and move predominantly in a craniocaudal direction, as their anteroposterior displacement is limited posteriorly by the back wall and anteriorly by the posterior peritoneal reflection. The kidneys lack ligaments to affix them within the retroperitoneum. Instead they are kept in place by the vascular pedicles at their hilum and by the surrounding adipose tissue; this structural stability leads to minimal kidney motion and associated image artifacts. Intraperitoneal organs such as the liver and spleen undergo a more complex, pronounced motion pattern, where the few ligaments stabilizing them within the abdominal cavity lead to their displacement if the superiorly adjacent diaphragm, abdominal wall, and other intestinal organs move. Since phase encoding is typically applied anteroposteriorly, motion in this direction yields ghosting artifacts that can often overlap and obfuscate kidney images, as shown in Fig. 3.1.

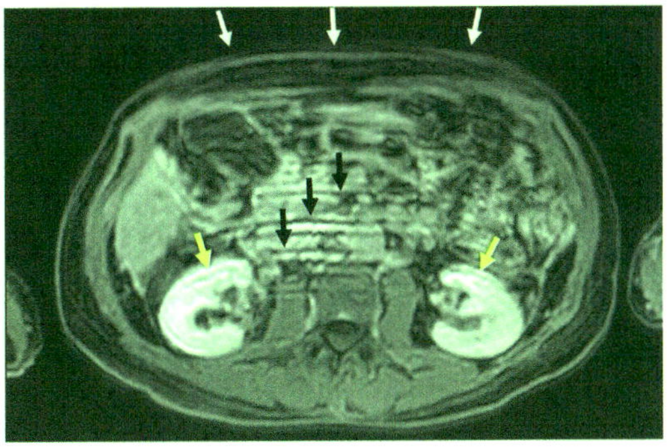

Fig. 3.1 A 62-year-old woman with clinically suspected cirrhosis: axial T1-weighted gradient echo Dixon-based fluid image of the abdomen. Despite using breath-holds, ghost artifacts (black arrows) are evident along the anteroposterior phase-encoding direction that overlay the kidneys (yellow arrows), and are caused by motion of the anterior wall (white arrows)

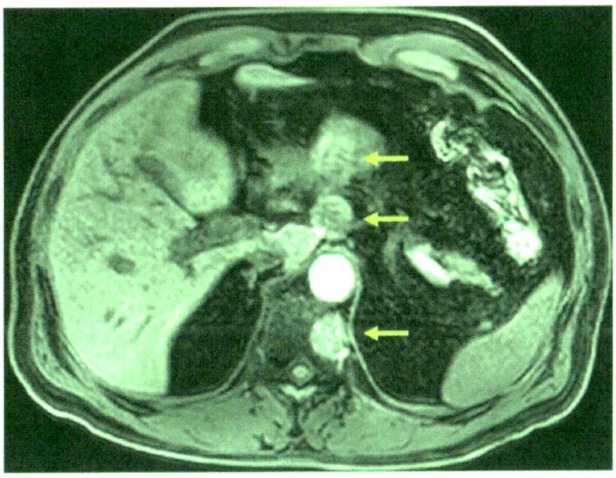

Fig. 3.2 Axial T1-weighted gradient echo Dixon-based fluid image indicates ghost artifacts (arrows) caused by aortic pulsation. Artifacts extend along the anteroposterior, phase-encoding direction

Arterial Pulsation

Another form of periodic physiological motion is arterial pulsation, although this motion typically has minimal effect on kidney imaging. Ghost artifacts often emanate from the aorta and heart and contaminate perception of the pancreas and the liver, specifically the left hepatic lobe due to its proximal location anterior to the abdominal aorta and inferior to the heart. As shown in Fig. 3.2, phase encoding is typically applied in the anteroposterior direction, such that circular and disc-shaped ghost artifacts appear along the same direction. These ghosts can mimic focal liver lesions but only obscure the laterally located kidneys in scenarios where phase-encoding direction is applied right to left.

Periodic Artifact Mitigation

Breath-Holds

Breath-holds are a useful mitigation strategy for respiration artifacts (although not for arterial pulsation). Patients are instructed to arrest movement and breathing during data acquisition periods to prevent motion artifacts from occurring. In order for breath-holds to be successful, data must be acquired in the short intervals during which the patient is assumed to remain motionless. Imaging is typically executed during end-exhalation due to its longer duration relative to end-inspiration.

Gating and Navigation Techniques

Gating, or signal acquisition timing alteration, is a popular method for dealing with respiration (and other types of periodic motion) artifacts. Data acquisition is typically triggered by an electrocardiogram signal, and data corrupted by excessive motion is discarded [1]. Prospective gating acquires the data at the same moment of each motion cycle and requires extra scan time, preparation, and processing [2]. Data is typically acquired during the relatively static pause following exhalation, when minimal chest and abdominal wall motion can cause imaging artifacts. Disruptions to breathing periodicity and consistency due to sleep and pathological conditions can contaminate accurate prospective gating. Retrospective gating involves imaging during the entire motion cycle [3] with data reorganization during image reconstruction. This is often combined with navigator echoes [4] that monitor and adjust the acquired image data to the patient's position within the scanner.

Phase-Encoding Gradient Orientation

Orienting the phase-encoding gradient perpendicular to the motion displacement direction can prevent artifacts caused by motion that has a timescale on the order of phase-encoding pulses and scan repetition time. However, very fast motion may still cause artifacts along the frequency-encoding gradient direction.

Signal Saturation

Saturating moving tissue or selective excitation is an option when imaging of dynamic anatomical regions is unnecessary. For example, vascular regions with blood flow may be saturated to avoid pulsation artifacts. While spatially saturating flow and moving tissue is possible, spectral saturation of fat is more common in kidney imaging.

Alternate K-Space Trajectories

Radial Approaches

Radial imaging techniques [5] lack unique frequency and phase-encoding directions, and thus coherent ghosts typically will not manifest. Rather, artifacts will be smeared and blurred across the image in a manner nearly indistinguishable from the gridding blur artifacts common to non-Cartesian k-space trajectories. Motion during any one radial k-space acquisition may be discarded since other k-space lines also pass through the key central part of k-space. Since radial spokes overlap at the center of k-space, the redundant data may also be used to correct motion artifacts.

Radial acquisitions are often acquired sequentially along the through-plane slice direction using the stack-of-stars (SoS) technique, as shown in Fig. 3.3. In kidney MRI, these acquisitions are frequently T1-weighted and stacked in three-dimensional fashion with phase-encoding applied along the through-plane direction. This sequence can mitigate ghosting in three-dimensional image blocks in

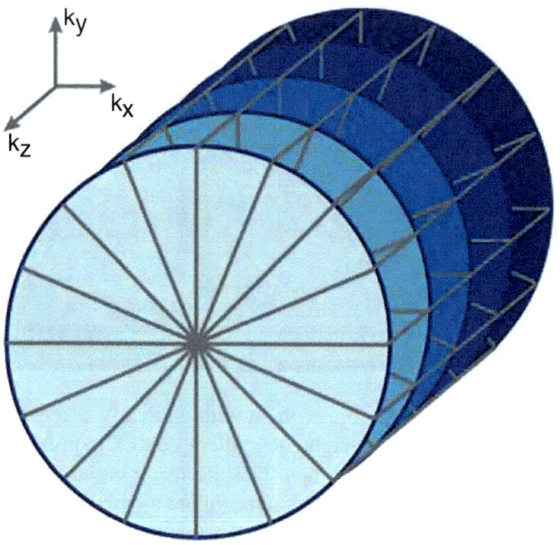

Fig. 3.3 Stack-of-stars (SoS) acquisition: in-plane kx and ky axis data are acquired using radial trajectories, while through-plane data (kz) are acquired using a low-high Cartesian profile order. (With permission from the Philips Healthcare)

an efficient manner and may include contrast agent administration.

The time efficiency of stack-of-stars minimizes the likelihood of motion during acquisition as shown in Fig. 3.4 and may be combined with other methods such as golden angle sampling and respiratory gating to increase motion compensation efficiency [6, 7] or compressed sensing for further scan time minimization [8]. Like other fast imaging methods that minimize motion exposure, these efficient sequences can achieve the needed temporal resolution (8–10 s) to permit dynamic imaging with adequate separation of arterial and venous contrast agent uptake (as shown in Fig. 3.5).

The PROPELLER (periodically rotated overlapping parallel lines with enhanced reconstruction, from GE, called BLADE and MultiVane by Siemens and Philips, respectively) sequence [9] acquires multiple parallel radial k-space lines for added central k-space redundancy and then rotates these groups of lines (blades) for further data acquisition as shown in Fig. 3.6.

Its main application is for T2-weighted imaging with or without spectral fat suppression, with the capacity to differentiate simple/septated cysts from proteinaceous/hemorrhagic cysts or solid

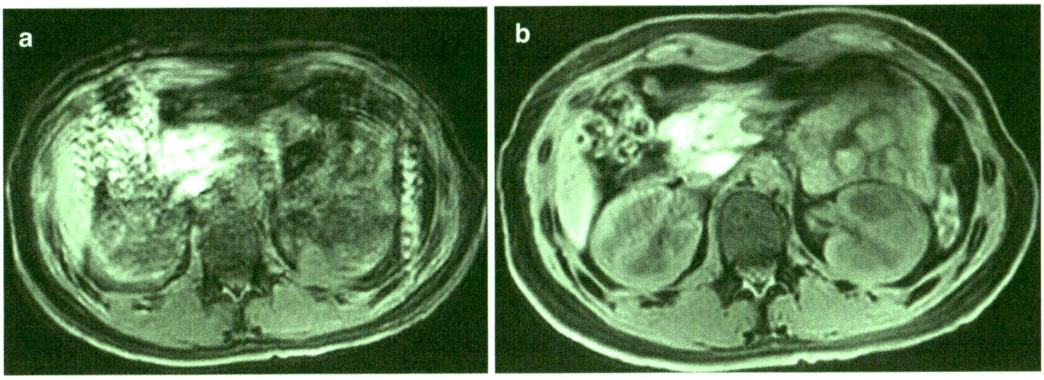

Fig. 3.4 Axial T1-weighted (T1w) gradient echo Dixon-based fluid kidney images of a volunteer with a 6-s breath-hold, followed by free breathing. (**a**) Cartesian trajectory, assessment rendered nondiagnostic by severe ghosting artifacts in anteroposterior orientation due to breathing motion of the abdominal intraperitoneal organs and bowel peristalsis. (**b**) Stack-of-stars radial k-space trajectory with respiratory gating largely eliminates ghosting artifacts

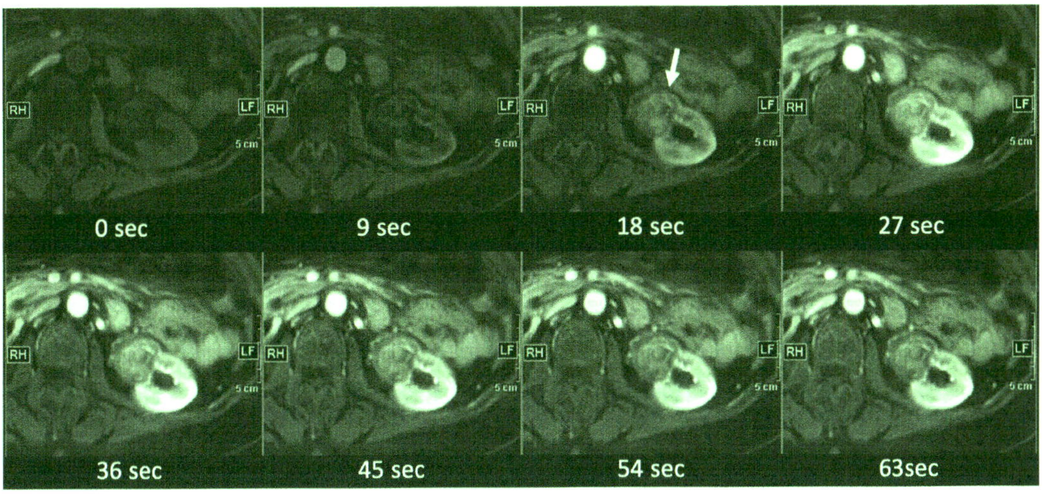

Fig 3.5 A 37-year-old woman with incidental left renal mass on ultrasound performed for abdominal pain assessed by gadolinium contrast-enhanced dynamic T1-weighted stack-of-stars gradient echo axial MRI. Eight free-breathing images were acquired over 63 s (temporal resolution = 9 s) from the unenhanced phase to the late-uptake phase, demonstrating an exophytic mass of the upper pole of the left kidney (arrow) with fat content on the unenhanced phase and an enhancement that follows the strong hypervascular intensity of the renal cortex between 18 and 27 s, after which enhancement decreases in relation to the kidney as is typical for benign angiomyolipoma (confirmed with an ultrasound-guided biopsy)

masses. The highly oversampled central k-space region can be employed to remove motion-induced data inconsistencies as shown in Fig. 3.7, prevent motion-induced volume shifts that may yield an incomplete anatomic representation as shown in Fig. 3.8, and correct pulsation and flow artifacts as shown in Fig. 3.9.

Spiral Approaches

Spiral k-space trajectories [10] can achieve similar benefits to radial trajectories due to the lack of coherent ghosts that normally stem from Cartesian trajectories with fixed phase/frequency-encoding directions. The varied encoding indicates that ghosts are smeared

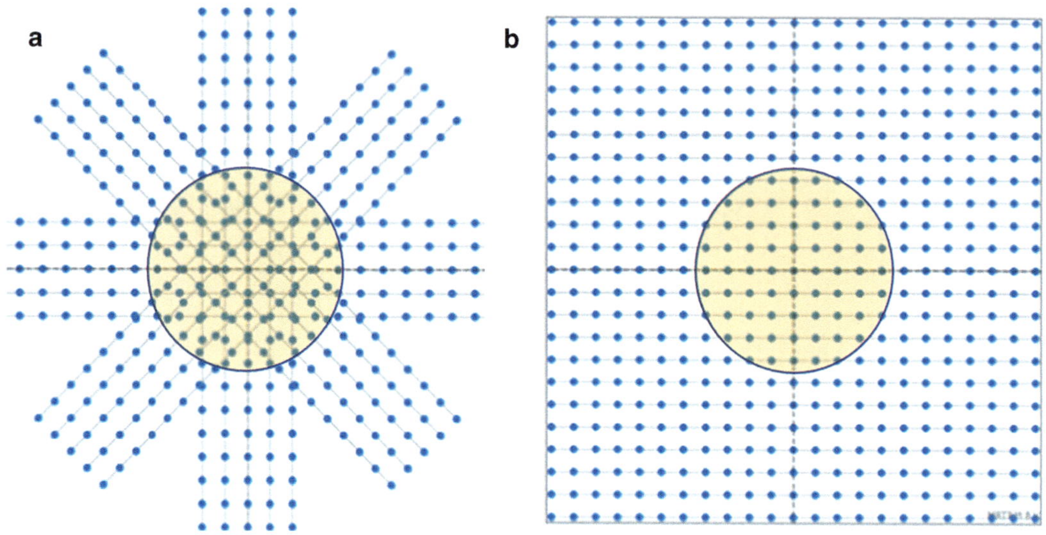

Fig. 3.6 PROPELLER k-space readout: parallel lines are grouped in bands/blades that rotate about the center of k-space. Note that a large region of central k-space is oversampled. (With permission from the Philips Healthcare, Best, Netherlands)

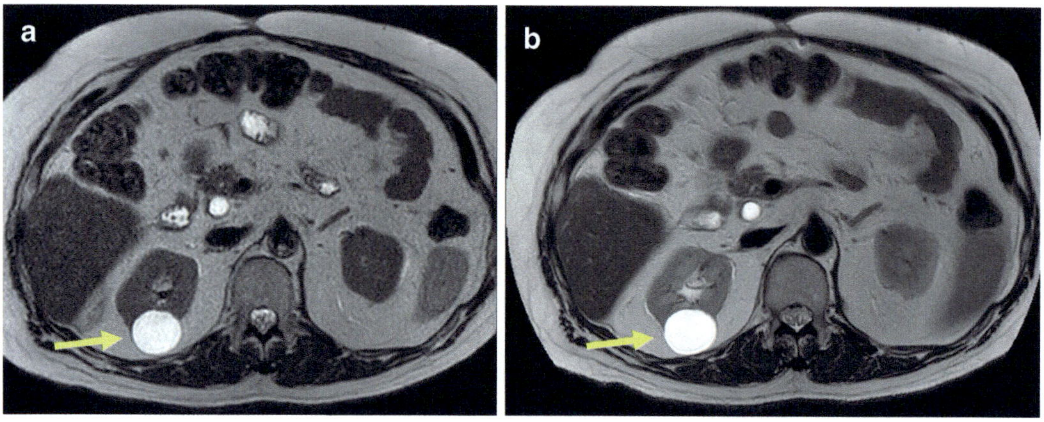

Fig. 3.7 Simple renal cyst: (**a**) Cartesian k-space trajectory, axial breath-hold T2-weighted (T2w) single-shot turbo spin echo (TSE) image, with a simple fluid-filled subcapsular cyst of the right kidney indicated by a yellow arrow. (**b**) A T2w TSE PROPELLER (100% radial oversampling) axial free-breathing respiratory-gated images with fat saturation demonstrates improved signal-to-noise ratio and a more homogeneous appearance of the cyst's simple fluid content

across the image, causing blur but minimizing obfuscation of anatomy and pathology. These techniques also similarly oversample the center of k-space to ensure data redundancy for motion correction [11]. While both radial and spiral sequences mitigate motion artifacts, spiral trajectories can theoretically improve upon radial imaging due to the continuous and rapid k-space acquisition readout that minimizes the time for motion to occur.

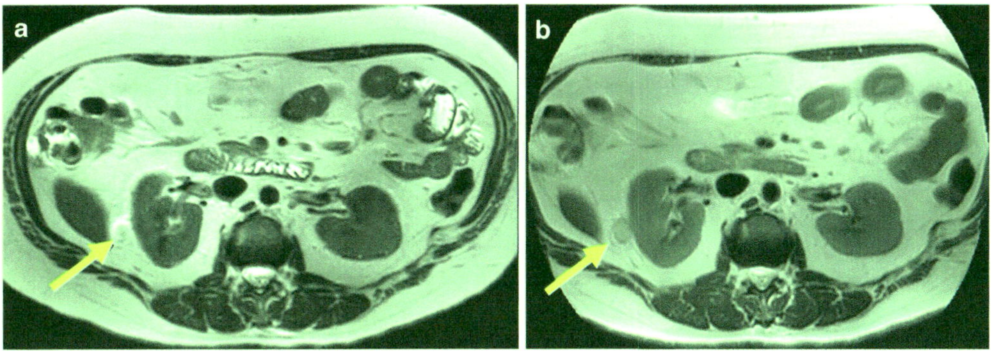

Fig. 3.8 Axial images of capsular complex cyst of the right kidney (arrow): (**a**) Cartesian T2-weighted (T2w) turbo spin echo (TSE) single-shot breath-hold image at the level of a capsular cyst is poorly seen due to partial volume averaging of moving tissue. (**b**) T2w TSE PROPELLER free-breathing acquisition with respiratory gating permits clear characterization of cyst filled with proteinaceous content

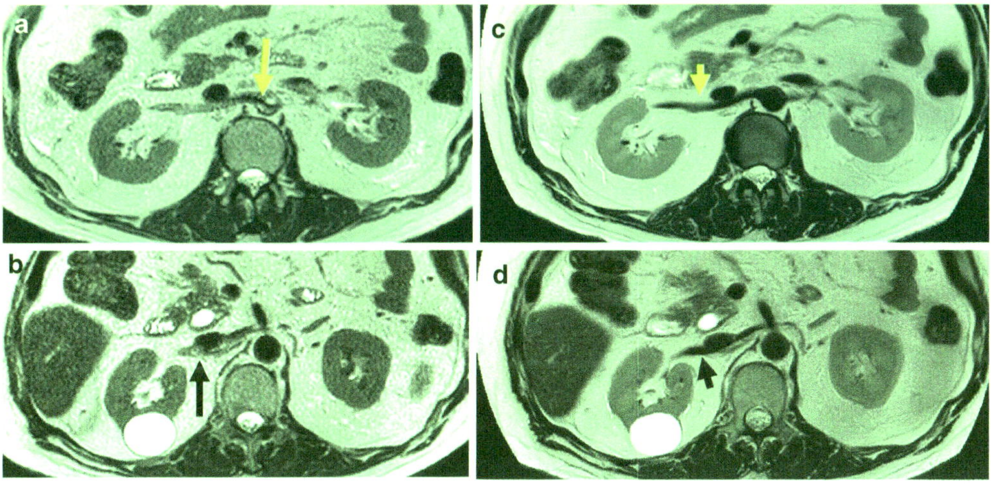

Fig. 3.9 A 59-year-old man 6 months after cryoablation of small renal cell carcinoma of the upper pole (ablation zone not shown): axial T2-weighted turbo spin echo single-shot images at the level of the renal arteries (top) and veins (bottom), with left images employing Cartesian and right images employing PROPELLER k-space trajectories. (**a**) Linear hypointense pulsation and flow artifacts from the right renal artery projecting into the lumen of the aorta (long yellow arrow) are resolved in (**c**); (**b**) hyperintense flow artifact in the right renal vein indistinguishable from a tumor thrombus (arrow) is resolved in (**d**)

Random Motion Effects

Physics of Random Motion

Random, aperiodic motion such as bulk motion and peristalsis causes blurring or smearing of signal across the image field of view. All motion yields ghost artifacts in MRI, but unpredictable motion adds random phase shifts to sampled data such that ghosts are incoherent with random separation and appear as image blur. While blur is generally preferable to the periodic motion-induced coherent, discrete ghosts that can be mistaken for anatomy or pathology, blur can be more difficult to correct due to the unpredictability of the source motion and subsequent artifacts. Some of the mitigation strategies described above to combat periodic motion ghosting, such as alternate k-space trajectories, may still show some efficacy in reducing artifacts caused by random motion. However, successful artifact correction depends on the complexity and periodicity of the movements as well as the applicability of the technique. Generally, correction of all motion artifacts is desirable for optimal kidney imaging.

Patient Bulk Motion

Patient bulk motion can occur due to a variety of underlying conditions. These include somatic disorders involving pain and discomfort due to positioning, neurological conditions such as tremor, mental developmental conditions, psychological disorders such as anxiety and claustrophobia, general discomfort, and a general lack of focus or control. Bulk motion artifacts can be problematic since they are unpredictable, and advanced mitigation strategies are often necessary to avoid associated artifacts.

Peristalsis

Peristalsis is a series of smooth muscle contractions typically within the digestive and urinary tracts that act to move food, urine, and bile through the gastrointestinal system. Although repetitive, peristalsis causes motion that is autonomic, sporadic and can endure beyond the imaging time; consequentially artifacts manifest as blurry diffuse ghosts (similar to those caused by random motion) that are difficult to predict and avoid via the standard methods discussed above.

Bowel Peristalsis

While its motion is unidirectional, bowel peristalsis results in random overall motion of bowel loops due to the relatively loose attachment to the mesenteric root. Bowel peristalsis impacts intraperitoneal organs more than the kidneys since the retroperitoneal fat anterior to the kidneys functions as a motion buffer. There is thus minimal effect on kidney image quality as demonstrated in Fig. 3.10; however, if bowel motion is excessive and body habitus is small and/or thin with less perinephric cuffing by adipose tissue compared to patients with larger body habitus, MR image quality of kidneys and ureters may be obscured as shown in Fig. 3.4.

Ureter Peristalsis

Ureteral peristalsis usually occurs in unpredictable phases of several seconds to minutes. This unpredictable cycle ensures difficulty in avoiding a peristaltic wave during imaging, where a lack of motion is usually needed to visualize small masses, calculi, and fluid within the ureters and to distinguish peristalsis from fixated strictures. Antiperistalsis of several minutes can allow for sufficient time to generate T1- or T2-weighted images of the ureters free of motion as depicted in Fig. 3.11.

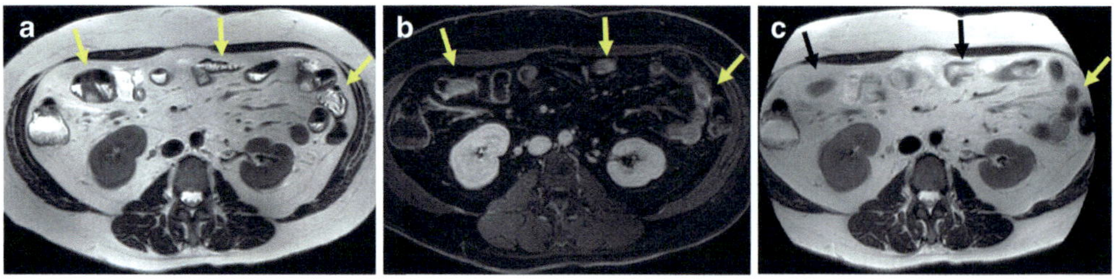

Fig. 3.10 A 53-year-old woman with moderately obese body habitus, effects of fast imaging and breath-holds on peristalsis artifact (arrows): (**a**) breath-hold Cartesian T2-weighted (T2w) turbo spin echo single-shot technique freezes bowel motion. (**b**) Breath-hold contrast-enhanced Cartesian gradient echo Dixon-based fluid image displays mild peristaltic motion artifact. (**c**) Free-breathing radial T2w image with visible peristaltic motion artifacts

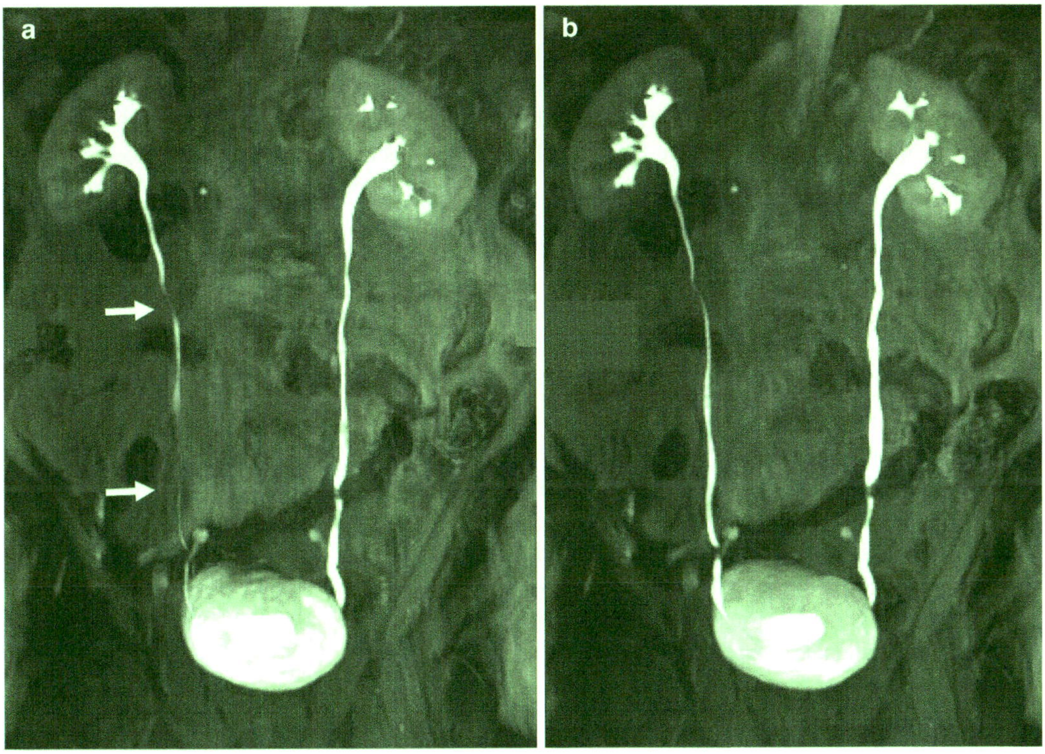

Fig. 3.11 A 71-year-old man 2 years after resection of a small bladder cancer for surveillance: MR intravenous urogram demonstrates (**a**) contracted right ureter due to ureteral peristalsis with suboptimal assessment for masses (arrows); (**b**) spasmolytic medication (0.25 mg sublingual hyoscyamine sulfate) improved depiction of the lumen of the gadolinium contrast-filled right ureter. Note that the left ureter, which was slightly patulous prior to administration of medication due to scarring at the ureteropelvic junction, is somewhat more distended after spasmolysis

Random Motion Artifact Mitigation

Sedation

Patient tranquility is essential for successful MRI devoid of random motion artifacts. While patient coaching before and during the exam may be sufficient to overcome anxiety and claustrophobia, more severe forms of these conditions or restlessness due to other etiologies may require a light form of anxiolysis or sedation. Mild sedation of a low dose of orally administered benzodiazepine medication may be sufficient to increase compliance and help the patient to endure the exam without moving. Patients with more severe pain, claustrophobia, or restlessness often require general anesthesia with intubation and ventilation, as administration of higher doses of benzodiazepines or opiates without intubation and ventilation can decrease breath-hold compliance. General noncompliance and young children may need special attention and customized sedation protocols with anesthesia support to minimize patient motion and subsequent artifacts.

Anticholinergic medications such as hyoscine butylbromide, hyoscyamine sulfate/dicyclomine, and glucagon are sometimes given for antiperistalsis intramuscularly (IM), intravenously (IM), and sublingually. The spasmolytic effect lasts 25–30 min and 10 min for IM and IV administrations, respectively. While more effective, the IV approach requires that medication is administered immediately prior to a motion-sensitive T1w MRI pulse sequence in order to manifest the antiperistaltic action desired [12, 13]. Figure 3.11 demonstrates how MR urograms can benefit from anticholinergic medication by mitigating peristalsis in both the ureter and the anteriorly adjacent bowel loops. Glucagon is not used for antiperistalsis of the ureters due to its limited antiperistaltic effect, although contraindications to the use of anticholinergic medications could inspire glucagon administration to reduce bowel motion.

Motion Tracking

Recently, position tracking using small RF coils [14, 15] has shown promise for correcting motion-related artifacts. This technique prospectively tracks patient motion, which can prove especially useful for the difficult correction of aperiodic, unpredictable motion artifacts. Generally speaking, this exciting approach to motion artifact correction could avoid both periodic and aperiodic motion artifacts, which has inspired significant research in the area.

Fast Imaging Techniques

Acquiring signal before motion can disrupt the encoding process is useful for preventing all types of kidney imaging motion artifacts but is especially useful for aperiodic motion due to the unpredictability of peristalsis. Parallel imaging [16–18], view sharing [19], compressed sensing [20–22], simultaneous multi-slice imaging [23], machine learning [24, 25], synthetic MR [26, 27], and MR fingerprinting [28] approaches may all speed up the imaging process to avoid motion. This is especially important for kidney imaging, where 15–20 motion-free seconds may be required to image the arterial contrast behavior of a kidney tumor.

Summary

While kidneys are unlikely to be directly moved by breathing and peristalsis given their position in the retroperitoneum, nearby abdominal organ and wall motion can cause artifacts that render kidney imaging nondiagnostic. Generally, motion may be periodic and aperiodic, and motion inconsistencies can compromise image quality and integrity to the extent that a comprehensive artifact correction tool is desired. Various basic and advanced mitigation strategies exist to address these artifacts. Clinically, careful sequence timing manipulation and alternate k-space trajectories are employed to reduce artifacts, since breath-hold sequences may be contaminated by noncompliant patients and generally extend scan time. Ultimately, examination protocols should be patient-specific without reliance on breath-holds or any specific imaging or workflow parameters to ensure consistent imaging with minimal artifacts.

References

1. Runge VM, Clanton JA, Partain CL, James AE. Respiratory gating in magnetic resonance imaging at 0.5 tesla. Radiology. 1984;151(2):521–3.
2. Liu YL, Riederer SJ, Rossman PJ, Grimm RC, Debbins JP, Ehman RL. A monitoring, feedback, and triggering system for reproducible breath-hold MR-imaging. Magn Reson Med. 1993;30(4):507–11.
3. Lenz GW, Haacke EM, White RD. Retrospective cardiac gating—a review of technical aspects and future-directions. Magn Reson Imaging. 1989;7(5):445–55.
4. Ehman RL, Felmlee JP. Adaptive technique for high-definition MR imaging of moving structures. Radiology. 1989;173(1):255–63.
5. Lauterbur PC. Image formation by induced local interactions: examples employing nuclear magnetic resonance. Nature. 1973;242:190–1.
6. Hedderich DM, Weiss K, Spiro JE, Giese D, Beck GM, Maintz D, Persigehl T. Clinical evaluation of free-breathing contrast-enhanced T1w MRI of the liver using pseudo golden angle radial k-space sampling. Rofo. 2018;90(7):601–9.
7. Kajita K, Goshima S, Noda Y, Kawada H, Kawai N, Okuaki T, Honda M, Matsuo M. Thin-slice free-breathing pseudo-golden-angle radial stack-of-stars with gating and tracking T1-weighted acquisition: an efficient gadoxetic acid-enhanced hepatobiliary-phase imaging alternative for patients with unstable breath holding. Magn Reson Med Sci. 2019;18(1):4–11.
8. Budjan J, Riffel P, Ong MM, Schoenberg SO, Attenberger UI, Hausmann D. Rapid Cartesian versus radial acquisition: comparison of two sequences for hepatobiliary phase MRI at 3T in patients with impaired breath-hold capabilities. BMC Med Imaging. 2017;17(1):32.
9. Pipe JG. Motion correction with PROPELLER MRI: application to head motion and free-breathing cardiac imaging. Magn Reson Med. 1999;42(5):963–9.

10. Ahn CB, Kim JH, Cho ZH. High-speed spiral-scan echo planar NMR imaging-I. IEEE Trans Med Imaging. 1986;5(1):2–7.
11. Liu C, et al. Self-navigated interleaved spiral (SNAILS): application to high-resolution diffusion tensor imaging. Magn Reson Med. 2004;52:1388–96.
12. Gutzeit A, Binkert CA, Koh DM, Hergan K, von Weymarn C, Graf N, et al. Evaluation of the anti-peristaltic effect of glucagon and hyoscine on the small bowel: comparison of intravenous and intramuscular drug administration. Eur Radiol. 2012;22(6):1186–94.
13. Froehlich JM, Daenzer M, von Weymarn C, Erturk SM, Zollikofer CL, Patak MA. Aperistaltic effect of hyoscine N-butylbromide versus glucagon on the small bowel assessed by magnetic resonance imaging. Eur Radiol. 2009;19(6):1387–93.
14. Dumoulin CL, Souza SP, Darrow RD. Real-time position monitoring of invasive devices using magnetic resonance. Magn Reson Med. 1993;29(3):411–5.
15. Ooi MB, Krueger S, Thomas WJ, Swaminathan SV, Brown TR. Prospective real-time correction for arbitrary head motion using active markers. Magn Reson Med. 2009;62(4):943–54.
16. Sodickson DK, Manning WJ. Simultaneous acquisition of spatial harmonics (SMASH): fast imaging with radiofrequency coil arrays. Magn Reson Med. 1997;38:591–603.
17. Pruessmann KP, et al. SENSE: sensitivity encoding for fast MRI. Magn Reson Med. 1999;42(5):952–62.
18. Griswold MA, et al. Generalized autocalibrating partially parallel acquisitions (GRAPPA). Magn Reson Med. 2002;47(6):1202–10. 18(VIEW).
19. Riederer SJ, et al. MR fluoroscopy: technical feasibility. Magn Reson Med. 1988;8(1):1–15.
20. Candes EJ, Romberg J, Tao T. Robust uncertainty principles: exact signal reconstruction from highly incomplete frequency information. IEEE Trans Inf Theory. 2006;52(2):489–509.
21. Donoho DL. Compressed sensing. IEEE Transactions on Information Theory, 2006;52:1289–1306.
22. Lustig M, Donoho D, Pauly JM. Sparse MRI: the application of compressed sensing for rapid MR imaging. Magn Reson Med. 2007;58:1182–95.
23. Muller S. Multifrequency selective rf pulses for multislice MR imaging. Magn Reson Med. 1988;6(3):364–71.
24. Hammernik K, et al. Learning a variational network for reconstruction of accelerated MRI data. Magn Reson Med. 2018;79(6):3055–71.
25. Akcakaya M, et al. Scan-specific robust artificial-neural-networks for k-space interpolation (RAKI) reconstruction: database-free deep learning for fast imaging. Magn Reson Med. 2019;81(1):439–53.
26. Bobman SA, et al. Cerebral magnetic resonance image synthesis. AJNR Am J Neuroradiol. 1985;6(2):265–9.
27. Gulani V, et al. Towards a single-sequence neurologic magnetic resonance imaging examination: multiple-contrast images from an IR TrueFISP experiment. Invest Radiol. 2004;39(12):767–74.
28. Ma D, et al. Magnetic resonance fingerprinting. Nature. 2013;495(7440):187–92.

4 Gadolinium-Based Contrast Agent Safety with Focus on Kidney MRI

Jonathan R. Dillman

Introduction

Gadolinium-based contrast materials (GBCMs) are essential to the modern-day clinical practices of radiology and magnetic resonance imaging (MRI), including evaluation of the brain and spinal cord, body, and musculoskeletal system. While primarily used to improve the visualization of anatomy and pathology due to both intravascular and extra-cellular enhancements (shortening of T1 relaxation times), they also can be used to assess a variety of physiologic processes, including dynamic blood flow, tissue perfusion, kidney and liver function, and kidney and hepatobiliary excretion. In general, these contrast agents are very well tolerated in the vast majority of patients, and, unlike iodinated contrast agents used for computed tomography, there is no association with acute kidney injury (AKI) following exposure to routine clinical doses.

GBCMs are composed of a gadolinium ion (Gd^{3+}), a rare Earth's element with seven unpaired electrons, and a carrier molecule referred to as a ligand or chelate [1]. The chelate is used to protect patients from free gadolinium's potential toxic effects, as gadolinium ions can interfere with calcium-dependent biological processes [1]. Gadopentetate dimeglumine (Magnevist) was the first GBCM available for use in the US, approved in 1988 [2]. This was followed by the approval of gadoteridol (ProHance) in 1992. Since then, numerous other GBCMs have become available for use, some of which have unique pharmacokinetic properties that can be taken advantage of when performing MRI (e.g., hepatobiliary excretion, increased blood pool dwell time due to reversible albumin binding with minimal of extracellular distribution) [3, 4]. Over the past decade, some approved GBCMs also have left the US market, with reasons cited including poor sales (gadofosveset [Ablavar] in 2017) or "evolving market trends" and the availability of an alternative agent from the same manufacturer (gadopentetate dimeglumine in 2019) [5].

GBCMs' intrinsic paramagnetic properties shorten both T1 and T2 relaxation times, with T1 effects dominating at standard extracellular concentrations [6]. Thus, these agents are most often associated with increased signal intensity on T1-weighted images when administered at US Food and Drug Administration (FDA)-approved doses. Upon concentration of these contrast agents, as occurs upon excretion into the renal collecting systems and bladder, however, T2 shortening effects may dominate with urine appearing markedly hypointense on both T1-weighted and T2-weighted images (Fig. 4.1).

J. R. Dillman (✉)
Department of Radiology, Cincinnati Children's Hospital Medical Center, Cincinnati, OH, USA

Department of Radiology, University of Cincinnati College of Medicine, Cincinnati, OH, USA
e-mail: jonathan.dillman@cchmc.org

S. D. Serai, K. Darge (eds.), *Advanced Clinical MRI of the Kidney*,
https://doi.org/10.1007/978-3-031-40169-5_4

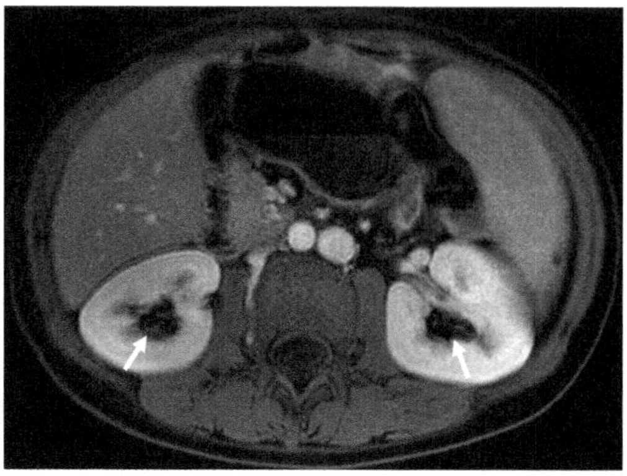

Fig. 4.1 Axial postcontrast T1-weighted fat-suppressed MR image shows dark signal (signal voids) in the renal collecting systems (arrows) due to concentrated gadolinium-based contrast material and its impact on T2 relaxation

In this chapter, we will review currently used GBCM in the US and related safety considerations, including nephrogenic systemic fibrosis (NSF), gadolinium retention, and physiologic- and allergic-like adverse reactions. We will also discuss the various tasks GBCM can perform when evaluating the kidneys with MRI.

Properties of Currently Used Contrast Agents

There are now five commonly used GBCMs in the US, as the four previously used agents are either no longer available, no longer marketed, or decreasingly used. These latter agents include the gadodiamide (Omniscan), gadopentetate dimeglumine (Magnevist), gadoversetamide (OptiMARK), and gadofosveset (Ablavar). The five contrast agents that are most often used today generally have differing structural, ionicity, and pharmacokinetic properties and include gadobenate dimeglumine (MultiHance), gadoxetate disodium (Eovist), gadoteridol, gadobutrol (Gadavist), and gadoterate (Dotarem, Clariscan) [7]. Gadopiclenol, marketed as Vueway and Elucirem, is recently available in the US.

First, these agents are either linear (gadobenate dimeglumine, gadoxetate disodium) or macrocyclic (gadoteridol, gadobutrol, gadoterate, gadopiclenol) with regard to chelate structure, with macrocyclic agents generally considered more stable with decreased rates of gadolinium dissociation (i.e., transmetallation). Second, these agents are either ionic (gadobenate dimeglumine, gadoterate, gadoxetate disodium) or nonionic (gadoteridol, gadobutrol), with ionic agents generally considered more stable with regard to transmetallation. Finally, two of the five commonly used agents, gadoxetate disodium and gadobenate dimeglumine (both of which have linear chelates), have noteworthy hepatobiliary excretion (in addition to renal excretion). This may in part explain why these agents have not been associated with nephrogenic systemic fibrosis (NSF, infra vide) despite their linear structure.

Nephrogenic Systemic Fibrosis

Nephrogenic fibrosing dermopathy was first described in 2000 as a scleroderma-like thickening of the skin and soft tissues [8, 9]. This condition was noted to occur in patients with considerably impaired renal function, and, in 2006, the association was made between the development of this condition and exposure to gadodiamide [10, 11]. Eventually renamed nephrogenic systemic fibrosis (NSF), this condition was observed to cause considerable morbidity in some patients, including joint contractures and visceral involvement.

Further investigations went on to show that nearly all unconfounded cases of NSF were associated with exposure to one of three linear GBCMs, gadodiamide, gadopentetate dimeglumine, or gadoversetamide, subsequently termed Group I agents by the American College of Radiology (ACR) [12], in the setting of AKI or chronic kidney disease (CKD) with an estimated glomerular filtration rate (eGFR) of less than 30 mL/min/1.73 m^2. The linear contrast agent gadobenate dimeglumine as well as the three macrocyclic GBCMs were classified as Group II agents, with few if any associated unconfounded cases of NSF. The ACR classification system, which is risk based, breaks down at least in part based on chelate structure and ionicity, with macrocyclic and ionic agents imparting greater GBCM stability and lower NSF risk, in general. Group I agents are hypothesized to undergo transmetallation in patients with severely impaired renal function due to increased GBCM dwell time in the body, thereby increasing the odds of developing NSF.

Following the recognition of the association between NSF and GBCMs, the US FDA and ACR Committee on Drugs and Contrast Material recommended avoiding GBCM in at-risk patients unless absolutely necessary for patient care. In the latter setting, patients should then only receive a Group II contrast agent. Based on this intervention as well as the shift from primarily linear to macrocyclic GBCM contrast agents, the incidence of NSF has markedly decreased with few if any cases still occurring in the US. Interestingly, the risk of NSF also seems to be higher in adults than children, with a systematic review demonstrating only 23 pediatric cases, and no child is affected under the age of 6 years [13].

The ACR describes two Group III GBCM agents, one of which is off the market (gadofosveset). Gadoxetate disodium, while linear and nonionic, has not been associated with NSF, perhaps due to both renal and hepatobiliary excretions (nearly 50/50 in healthy children and adults). Historically, this contrast agent has been considered a Group III agent due to the relatively small number of patient administrations compared to more conventional extra-cellular GBCM. Recently, however, a systematic review and meta-analysis that included 17 studies from nearly 15,000 patients documented an upper bound 95% confidence interval for the risk of NSF of 2.8% when gadoxetate disodium was administered [14]. Starekova et al. described 7820 gadoxetate disodium administrations that included 299 examinations in 242 patients with an eGFR between 30 and 44 mL/min/1.73 m^2 and 183 examinations in 157 patients with an eGFR less than 30 mL/min/1.73 m^2, with no associated cases of NSF identified over an average of approximately 4.2 years [15].

Furthermore, there is increasing evidence that ACR Group II contrast agents may be safe in the setting of severe CKD. A systematic review and meta-analysis by Woolen et al. that included 16 studies and 4931 patients found no cases of NSF in patients receiving this class of GBCM [16]. The authors concluded that the risk of NSF from Group II GBCM administration in CKD stages 4 and 5 is less than 0.07%. Based on this data, the ACR Manual on Contrast Media has indicated that measuring eGFR prior to contrast-enhanced MRI when using a Group II contrast agent is now optional [12].

Gadolinium Retention

The retention of gadolinium in the body following contrast-enhanced MRI came to the attention of the radiology community as well as its patients in 2015. It was at that time Kanda et al. first recognized the association between signal hyperintensity involving the dentate nucleus on

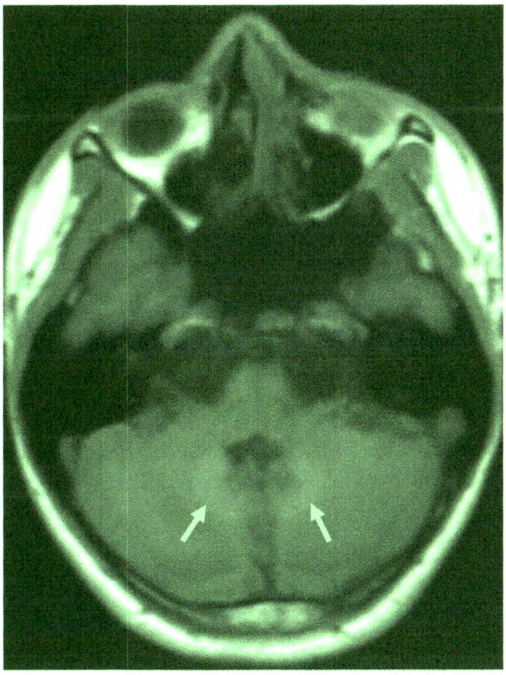

Fig. 4.2 Unenhanced T1-weighted MR image of the brain in an adult patient who had received more than 30 doses of linear (ACR Group I) gadolinium-based contrast material. The dentate nuclei appear hyperintense (arrows), suggesting gadolinium retention

unenhanced T1-weighted MR images and the previous administration of linear GBCM (Fig. 4.2) [17]. Since that time, numerous pediatric and adult imaging and pathology-based studies have confirmed the deposition or retention of gadolinium in certain portions of the brain and elsewhere in the body, including the bone [18–21].

Based on the most recent literature, all GBCMs have demonstrated some degree of retention in the brain, including in the settings of both normal and abnormal renal function. However, despite this phenomenon, there have been no widely accepted associated adverse clinical signs or symptoms to date. Histologic and electron microscopy assessments of human brain tissue following GBCM exposure have demonstrated that the gadolinium is located in the capillary endothelium and neuronal interstitium and that there is no apparent associated inflammation or tissue destruction [18]. However, based on the increasing amount of medical literature showing gadolinium retention in the brain, the US FDA indicated that all "… MRI centers should provide a Medication Guide the first time an outpatient receives a GBCA injection…" [22]. A recent study by O'Donohue et al. has shown that these FDA-inspired handouts informing patients about gadolinium retention do not significantly change the frequency of GBCM cancellation [23].

Physiologic Contrast Reactions

The intravascular administration of GBCM can elicit a number of physiologic adverse contrast reactions, the majority of which are mild and short-lived [24]. Examples of such reactions can be found in the Package Inserts of the various GBCMs and are likely due to a variety of factors, including osmolality and viscosity. The majority of physiologic reactions resolve quickly without particular intervention. The exact frequencies of these nonallergic-like reactions are not well documented in the literature. However, such reactions are more common than allergic-like contrast reactions [25, 26]. Physiologic adverse reactions do not require prior GBCM exposure, and they are likely dose-dependent, at least to a degree.

Allergic-Like Contrast Reactions

Like physiologic reactions, allergic-like, or anaphylactoid, adverse contrast reactions do not require prior GBCM exposure. One possible cause is mast cell degranulation and histamine release as contrast agent passes through the lungs [27]. Allergic-like reactions range in severity from mild to severe. Mild reactions may require only observation with no specific medical therapy, whereas moderate and severe reactions may require epinephrine administration, transfer to the emergency department, or inpatient hospitalization. While very rare, deaths related to allergic-like contrast reactions to GBCM have been described [28]. Hence, when GBCMs are being administered, a physician or other knowledgeable health care prover (as allowed by regulatory authorities) should be immediately available to respond to and treat allergic-like reactions.

So, how common are allergic-like reactions to GBCM? First, it is worth noting that they are much less common than physiologic reactions. Second, such reactions are considerably less common that reactions to modern iodinated contrast agents commonly used for computed tomography. Third, multiple studies have demonstrated that the frequency of allergic-like reactions is lower in children than adults [29]. Finally, a systematic review and meta-analysis of immediate allergic-like contrast reactions to GBCM concluded that the nonionic linear agents have the lowest rates of such reactions and that a higher rate of such adverse events is associated with ionic structure, greater protein binding, and macrocyclic chelate structure [30]. However, a recent large pediatric study that compared the frequencies of allergic-like reactions between gadopentetate dimeglumine and gadoterate showed no significant difference in allergic-like reaction occurrence [31].

In a recent very large single-center study of 281,945 GBCM injections in 158,100 children and adults, 442 allergic-like contrast reactions were observed for a reaction frequency of 0.16% [26]. These authors also found that patients receiving ACR Group II GBCM (gadobenate dimeglumine, gadobutrol) had higher frequencies of allergic-like reactions compared to patients receiving gadodiamide, a Group I agent. Dillman et al. documented 54 allergic-like reactions in adults and 6 allergic-like reactions in children following 65,009 and 13,344 GBCM administrations, respectively, for adult and pediatric reaction frequencies of 0.07% and 0.04% [29]. Forbes-Amrhein et al. documented 21 allergic-like reactions in children over a total of 32,365 administrations, for a reaction frequency of 0.06% [31]. Gadopentetate dimeglumine demonstrated a reaction frequency of 0.08%, gadoterate had a reaction frequency of 0.06%, and no reactions were observed following 672 injections of gadoxetate disodium. Only 1 of 21 (4.8%) reactions was severe.

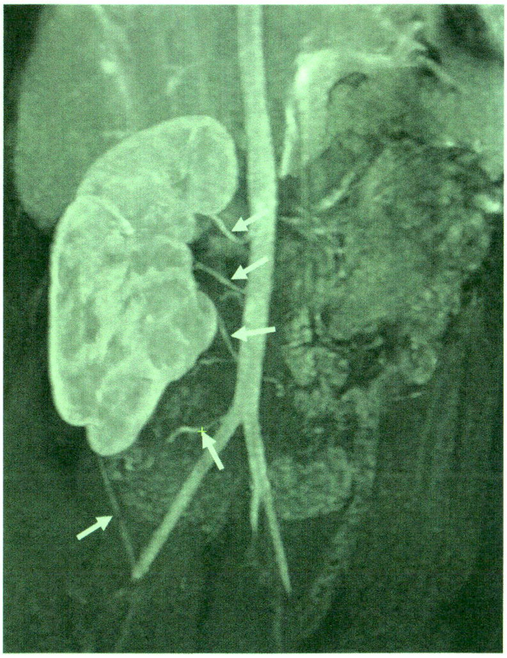

Fig. 4.3 Teenage patient with cross-fused renal ectopia. The right and "left" kidneys are located in the right retroperitoneum and form a conglomerate kidney. Contrast-enhanced T1-weighted maximum intensity projection MR image shows five renal arteries, with three arising from the abdominal aorta, one arising from the aortic bifurcation, and one arising from the right common iliac artery (arrows)

GBCM and MRI of the Kidneys

GBCMs are often used when evaluating of the kidneys by MRI, playing several important roles based on their pharmacokinetic properties. First, these contrast agents can aid in the evaluation of vascular anatomy. Specifically, the renal arteries and veins can be thoroughly assessed using a contrast-enhanced three-dimensional magnetic resonance angiography (MRA) sequence, aiding in the evaluation of living-related kidney donors and accessory renal arteries (Fig. 4.3) [32, 33]. Contrast-enhanced MRA also can be used to detect aortic and renal artery narrowing in the setting of renovascular hypertension (Fig. 4.4) [34]. Contrast-enhanced three-dimensional gradient echo and steady-state-free precession sequences can be used to evaluate the renal veins, including suspected nutcracker syndrome where the left renal vein narrows and becomes obstructed as it passes between the abdominal aorta and superior mesenteric artery and is associated collateral vessels (Fig. 4.5) [35]. Second, GBCM can aid in the assessment of the renal parenchyma, including renal mass characterization and staging, evaluation for recurrent tumor following kidney tumor ablation, and renal scarring (Fig. 4.6) [36–38].

Third, contrast-enhanced MRI can be used to obtain a detailed depiction of the upper urinary tracts (renal collecting systems and ureters) using so-called MR urography (MRU) technique. MRU entails obtaining delayed excretory phase post-contrast T1-weighted images through the kidneys and urinary tract, often following the prehydration with intravenous fluid and diuretic administration (Fig. 4.7) [39]. Prehydration and diuretic administration improve urinary tract distention and visualization as well as decrease the concentration of GBCM in the urinary tract, with a resultant increase in T2 relaxation, thereby allow-

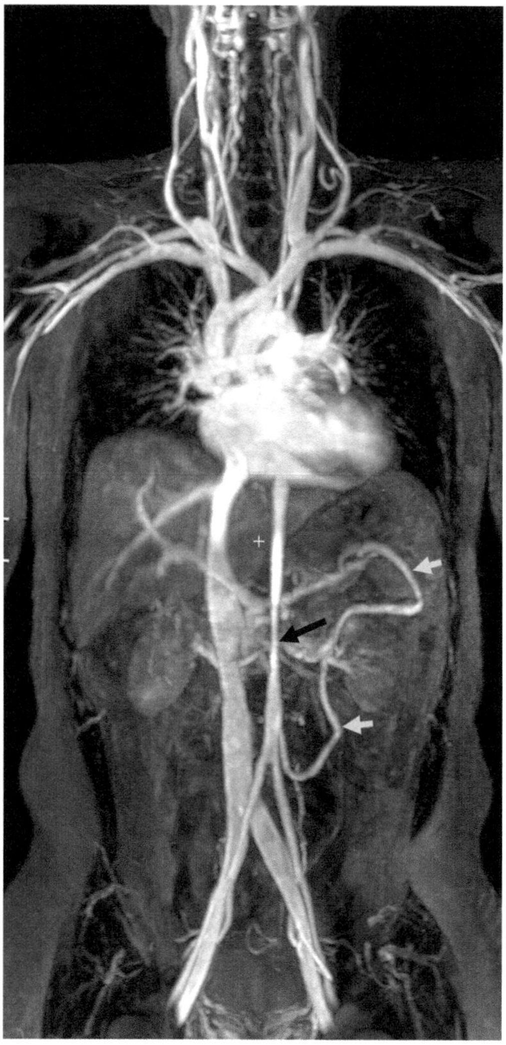

Fig. 4.4 Young adult with Williams syndrome and renin-mediated hypertension. Coronal postcontrast MR angiography maximum intensity projection image shows narrowing of the abdominal aorta above, at, and below the left of the renal arteries. The origins of the renal arteries are stenotic (black arrow). A large collateral artery is present in the small bowel mesentery (short arrows)

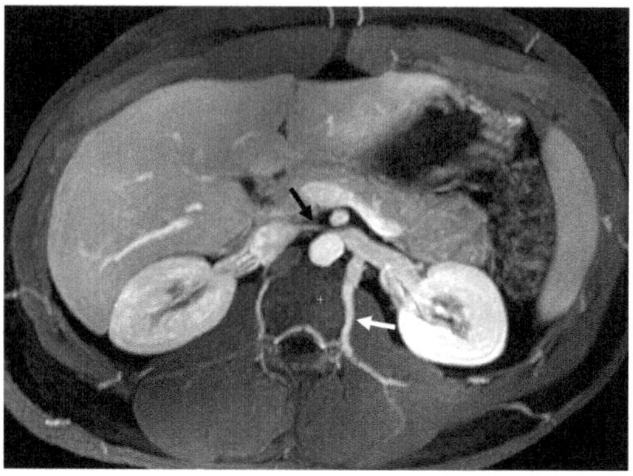

Fig. 4.5 Young adult with nutcracker syndrome. There is narrowing of the left renal vein as it passes between the abdominal aorta and superior mesenteric artery (black arrow). There is a prominent left paraspinal vein that is serving as a collateral pathway (white arrow)

ing urine to remain hyperintense with improved image contrast resolution. Jones et al. employed a standardized MRU technique to objectively document urinary tract obstruction using diuretic renal scintigraphy as reference standard [40].

Finally, contrast-enhanced MRI can be used to evaluate renal function and perfusion. There are both simple and much more complex methods for assessing renal function. The simplest method for establishing differential (right versus left) renal function is based on taking a ratio of the volume (ml) of right kidney versus left kidney enhancing parenchyma. More complicated methods for estimating renal function, including single kidney glomerular filtration rate (GFR), involve performing dynamic contrast-enhanced MRI and using more complex mathematical modeling that divides the kidney into multiple compartments (e.g., two or three, including the two-compartment Patlak-Rutland method) (Fig. 4.8) [41]. Bokacheva et al. concluded that GFR estimates vary based on the model used and that two and three compartment models produce similar correlations with the GFR reference standard [41]. MRI perfusion using GBCM has been utilized to characterize and grade a variety of kidney masses [42]. These techniques allow assessment of vascular permeability or transfer constant, volume of the extravascular extracellular space, and rate constant (K^{trans}, v_e, and k_{ep}, respectively) [43]. Michaely et al. demonstrated that dynamic contrast-enhanced MRI perfusion parameters can also be used to assess the effect of renal artery stenosis on renal parenchymal perfusion [44].

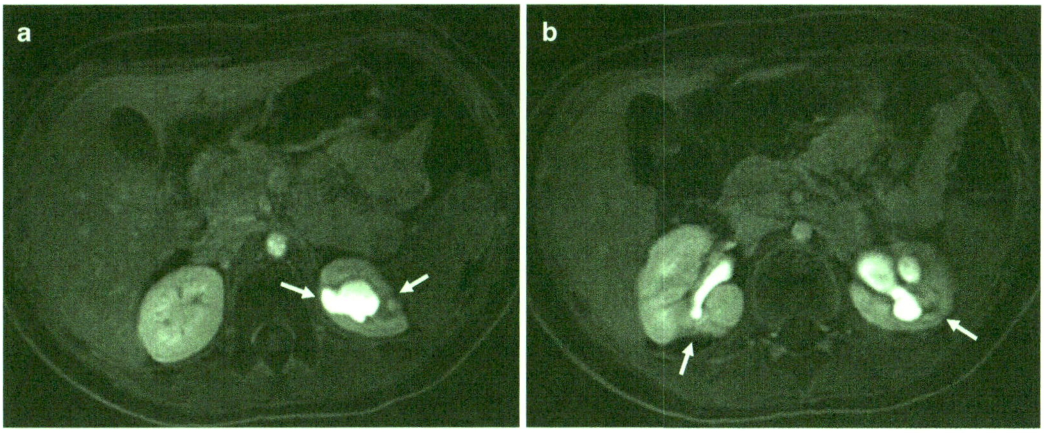

Fig. 4.6 A 10-year-old boy with left hydroureteronephrosis and recurrent pyelonephritis. (**a** and **b**) Axial postcontrast T1-weighted fat-suppressed MR images show bilateral areas of renal parenchymal thinning, consistent with multifocal scarring (arrows)

Fig. 4.7 A 3-year-old girl with known right hydronephrosis. Coronal postcontrast MR urography maximum intensity projection image shows excreted contrast material in the renal collecting systems, ureters, and bladder. There is right greater than left pelvocaliectasis, and there is abrupt narrowing of the right ureteropelvic junction (arrow). Imaging findings are consistent with right ureteropelvic junction obstruction. There is no evidence for renal scarring

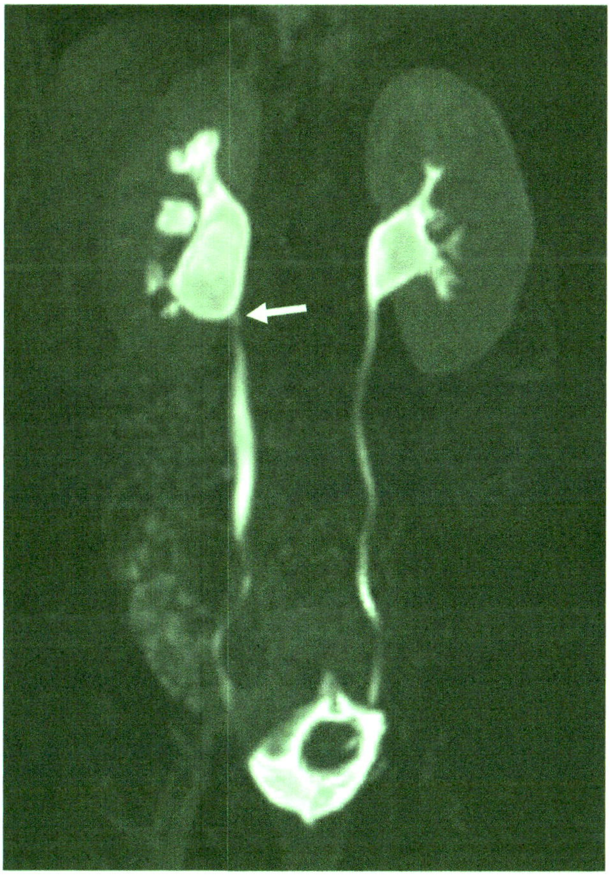

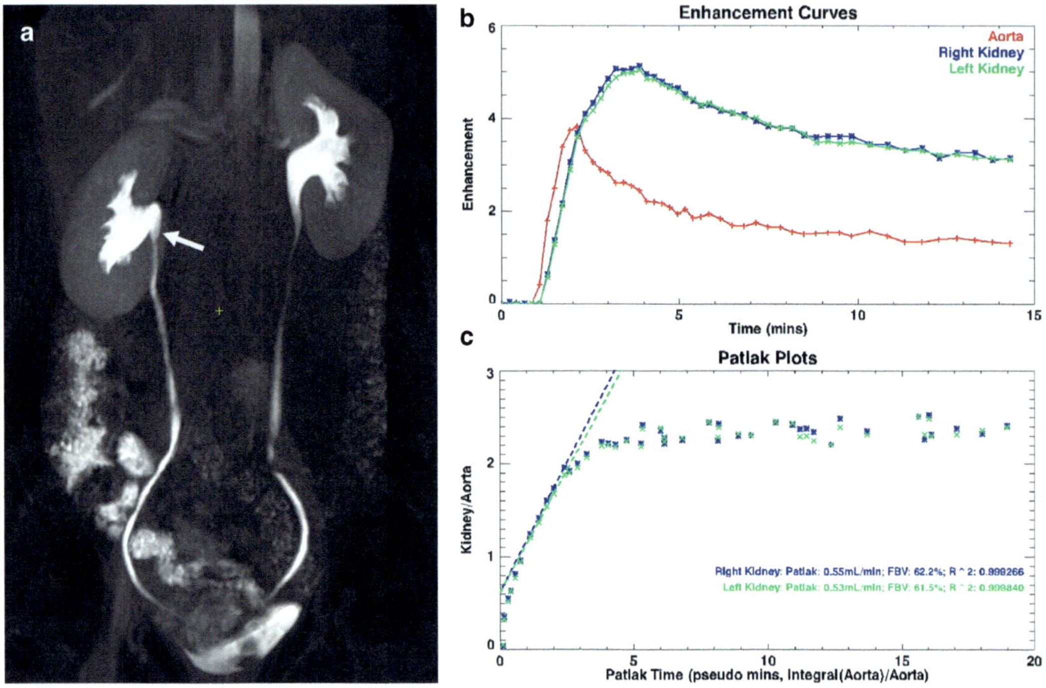

Fig. 4.8 A 16-year-old girl with recurrent urinary tract infections. (**a**) Coronal postcontrast MR urography maximum intensity project image shows high insertion of the right ureteropelvic junction (arrow). The kidneys and upper urinary tracts are otherwise normal with symmetric gadolinium-based contrast material excretion. (**b**) Time versus signal intensity plots for the abdominal aorta and kidneys show symmetric renal perfusion, concentration of contrast material, and contrast material excretion. (**c**) Patlak-Rutland plot demonstrates symmetric differential renal function/single kidney glomerular filtration rates using a two-compartment model

Disclosures Contrast material-related grant funding from the Guerbet and Bracco Imaging.

References

1. Rogosnitzky M, Branch S. Gadolinium-based contrast agent toxicity: a review of known and proposed mechanisms. Biometals. 2016;29(3):365–76. https://doi.org/10.1007/s10534-016-9931-7.
2. https://www.accessdata.fda.gov/drugsatfda_docs/label/2014/019596s057lbl.pdf. Accessed 20 Apr 2021.
3. Seale MK, Catalano OA, Saini S, Hahn PF, Sahani DV. Hepatobiliary-specific MR contrast agents: role in imaging the liver and biliary tree. Radiographics. 2009;29(6):1725–48. https://doi.org/10.1148/rg.296095515.
4. Rapp JH, Wolff SD, Quinn SF, Soto JA, Meranze SG, Muluk S, Blebea J, Johnson SP, Rofsky NM, Duerinckx A, Foster GS, Kent KC, Moneta G, Middlebrook MR, Narra VR, Toombs BD, Pollak J, Yucel EK, Shamsi K, Weisskoff RM. Aortoiliac occlusive disease in patients with known or suspected peripheral vascular disease: safety and efficacy of gadofosveset-enhanced MR angiography—multicenter comparative phase III study. Radiology. 2005;236(1):71–8. https://doi.org/10.1148/radiol.2361040148.
5. https://www.radiologysolutions.bayer.com/sites/g/files/kmftyc641/files/PP-MAG-US-0017-1%20Magnevsit%20Withdrawal%20Customer%20Letter%20%28web%20page%29%20Promotional%20Labeling%2020190815%20Clean.pdf. Accessed 20 Apr 2021.
6. Rohrer M, Bauer H, Mintorovitch J, Requardt M, Weinmann HJ. Comparison of magnetic properties of MRI contrast media solutions at different magnetic field strengths. Invest Radiol. 2005;40(11):715–24. https://doi.org/10.1097/01.rli.0000184756.66360.d3.
7. Mathur M, Jones JR, Weinreb JC. Gadolinium deposition and nephrogenic systemic fibrosis: a radiologist's primer. Radiographics. 2020;40(1):153–62. https://doi.org/10.1148/rg.2020190110.
8. Cowper SE, Su LD, Bhawan J, Robin HS, LeBoit PE. Nephrogenic fibrosing dermopathy. Am J Dermatopathol. 2001;23(5):383–93. https://doi.org/10.1097/00000372-200110000-00001.
9. Cowper SE, Robin HS, Steinberg SM, Su LD, Gupta S, LeBoit PE. Scleromyxoedema-like cuta-

neous diseases in renal-dialysis patients. Lancet. 2000;356:1000–1.
10. Grobner T. Gadolinium—a specific trigger for the development of nephrogenic fibrosing dermopathy and nephrogenic systemic fibrosis? Nephrol Dial Transplant. 2006;21(4):1104–8. https://doi.org/10.1093/ndt/gfk062.
11. Marckmann P, Skov L, Rossen K, Dupont A, Damholt MB, Heaf JG, Thomsen HS. Nephrogenic systemic fibrosis: suspected causative role of gadodiamide used for contrast-enhanced magnetic resonance imaging. J Am Soc Nephrol. 2006;17(9):2359–62. https://doi.org/10.1681/ASN.2006060601.
12. https://www.acr.org/-/media/ACR/Files/Clinical-Resources/Contrast_Media.pdf#page=85. Accessed 20 Apr 2021.
13. Nardone B, Saddleton E, Laumann AE, Edwards BJ, Raisch DW, McKoy JM, Belknap SM, Bull C, Haryani A, Cowper SE, Abu-Alfa AK, Miller FH, Godinez-Puig V, Dharnidharka VR, West DP. Pediatric nephrogenic systemic fibrosis is rarely reported: a RADAR report. Pediatr Radiol. 2014;44(2):173–80. https://doi.org/10.1007/s00247-013-2795-x.
14. Schieda N, van der Pol CB, Walker D, Tsampalieros AK, Maralani PJ, Woo S, Davenport MS. Adverse events to the gadolinium-based contrast agent gadoxetic acid: systematic review and meta-analysis. Radiology. 2020;297(3):565–72. https://doi.org/10.1148/radiol.2020200073.
15. Starekova J, Bruce RJ, Sadowski EA, Reeder SB. No cases of nephrogenic systemic fibrosis after administration of gadoxetic acid. Radiology. 2020;297(3):556–62. https://doi.org/10.1148/radiol.2020200788.
16. Woolen SA, Shankar PR, Gagnier JJ, MacEachern MP, Singer L, Davenport MS. Risk of nephrogenic systemic fibrosis in patients with stage 4 or 5 chronic kidney disease receiving a group II gadolinium-based contrast agent: a systematic review and meta-analysis. JAMA Intern Med. 2020;180(2):223–30. https://doi.org/10.1001/jamainternmed.2019.5284.
17. Kanda T, Osawa M, Oba H, Toyoda K, Kotoku J, Haruyama T, Takeshita K, Furui S. High signal intensity in dentate nucleus on unenhanced T1-weighted MR images: association with linear versus macrocyclic gadolinium chelate administration. Radiology. 2015;275(3):803–9. https://doi.org/10.1148/radiol.14140364.
18. McDonald RJ, McDonald JS, Kallmes DF, Jentoft ME, Murray DL, Thielen KR, Williamson EE, Eckel LJ. Intracranial gadolinium deposition after contrast-enhanced MR imaging. Radiology. 2015;275(3):772–82. https://doi.org/10.1148/radiol.15150025.
19. McDonald RJ, McDonald JS, Dai D, Schroeder D, Jentoft ME, Murray DL, Kadirvel R, Eckel LJ, Kallmes DF. Comparison of gadolinium concentrations within multiple rat organs after intravenous administration of linear versus macrocyclic gadolinium chelates. Radiology. 2017;285(2):536–45. https://doi.org/10.1148/radiol.2017161594.
20. Stanescu AL, Shaw DW, Murata N, Murata K, Rutledge JC, Maloney E, Maravilla KR. Brain tissue gadolinium retention in pediatric patients after contrast-enhanced magnetic resonance exams: pathological confirmation. Pediatr Radiol. 2020;50(3):388–96. https://doi.org/10.1007/s00247-019-04535-w.
21. Towbin AJ, Zhang B, Dillman JR. A retrospective cohort evaluation of the effect of multiple administrations of gadopentetate dimeglumine on brain magnetic resonance imaging T1-weighted signal. Pediatr Radiol. 2021;51(3):457–70. https://doi.org/10.1007/s00247-020-04860-5.
22. https://www.fda.gov/drugs/drug-safety-and-availability/fda-drug-safety-communication-fda-warns-gadolinium-based-contrast-agents-gbcas-are-retained-body. Accessed 20 Apr 2021.
23. O'Donohue LS, Shankar PR, Stein EB, Davenport MS. Characteristics of gadolinium-based contrast media cancellation at the point of care: a 15-month assessment of FDA-inspired medication guides on gadolinium retention. Abdom Radiol (NY). 2021;46(2):799–804. https://doi.org/10.1007/s00261-020-02670-9.
24. https://www.acr.org/-/media/ACR/Files/Clinical-Resources/Contrast_Media.pdf#page=81. Accessed 20 Apr 2021.
25. Uhlig J, Lücke C, Vliegenthart R, Loewe C, Grothoff M, Schuster A, Lurz P, Jacquier A, Francone M, Zapf A, Schülke C, Thomas D, May MS, Bremerich J, Lotz J, Gutberlet M, ESCR MRCT Registry Contributors. Acute adverse events in cardiac MR imaging with gadolinium-based contrast agents: results from the European Society of Cardiovascular Radiology (ESCR) MRCT Registry in 72,839 patients. Eur Radiol. 2019;29(7):3686–95. https://doi.org/10.1007/s00330-019-06171-2.
26. McDonald JS, Hunt CH, Kolbe AB, Schmitz JJ, Hartman RP, Maddox DE, Kallmes DF, McDonald RJ. Acute adverse events following gadolinium-based contrast agent administration: a single-center retrospective study of 281 945 injections. Radiology. 2019;292(3):620–7. https://doi.org/10.1148/radiol.2019182834.
27. Kun T, Jakubowski L. Influence of MRI contrast media on histamine release from mast cells. Pol J Radiol. 2012;77(3):19–24. https://doi.org/10.12659/pjr.883370.
28. Franckenberg S, Berger F, Schaerli S, Ampanozi G, Thali M. Fatal anaphylactic reaction to intravenous gadobutrol, a gadolinium-based MRI contrast agent. Radiol Case Rep. 2017;13(1):299–301. https://doi.org/10.1016/j.radcr.2017.09.012.
29. Dillman JR, Ellis JH, Cohan RH, Strouse PJ, Jan SC. Frequency and severity of acute allergic-like reactions to gadolinium-containing i.v. contrast media in children and adults. AJR Am J Roentgenol. 2007;189(6):1533–8. https://doi.org/10.2214/AJR.07.2554.
30. Behzadi AH, Zhao Y, Farooq Z, Prince MR. Immediate allergic reactions to gadolinium-

based contrast agents: a systematic review and meta-analysis. Radiology. 2018;286(2):471–82. https://doi.org/10.1148/radiol.2017162740.
31. Forbes-Amrhein MM, Dillman JR, Trout AT, Koch BL, Dickerson JM, Giordano RM, Towbin AJ. Frequency and severity of acute allergic-like reactions to intravenously administered gadolinium-based contrast media in children. Invest Radiol. 2018;53(5):313–8. https://doi.org/10.1097/RLI.0000000000000444.
32. Adamis MK, Goldszer RC, Pulde MF, Sax EJ, Edelman RR. Renal vasculature in potential renal transplant donors: comparison of MR imaging and digital subtraction angiography. Radiology. 1995;197(2):467–72. https://doi.org/10.1148/radiology.197.2.7480695.
33. Steffens JC, Link J, Grässner J, Mueller-Huelsbeck S, Brinkmann G, Reuter M, Heller M. Contrast-enhanced, K-space-centered, breath-hold MR angiography of the renal arteries and the abdominal aorta. J Magn Reson Imaging. 1997;7(4):617–22. https://doi.org/10.1002/jmri.1880070402.
34. Hany TF, Pfammatter T, Schmidt M, Leung DA, Debatin JF. Wertigkeit der kontrastverstärkten 3D-MR-Angiographie der Nierenarterien [Value of contrast-enhanced 3D magnetic resonance angiography of the renal arteries]. Radiologe. 1997;37(7):547–53. German. https://doi.org/10.1007/s001170050252.
35. Ananthan K, Onida S, Davies AH. Nutcracker syndrome: an update on current diagnostic criteria and management guidelines. Eur J Vasc Endovasc Surg. 2017;53(6):886–94. https://doi.org/10.1016/j.ejvs.2017.02.015.
36. Elkassem AA, Allen BC, Sharbidre KG, Rais-Bahrami S, Smith AD. Update on the role of imaging in clinical staging and restaging of renal cell carcinoma based on the AJCC 8th edition, from the *AJR* special series on cancer staging. AJR Am J Roentgenol. 2021;217:541. https://doi.org/10.2214/AJR.21.25493.
37. Davenport MS, Caoili EM, Cohan RH, Ellis JH, Higgins EJ, Willatt J, Fox GA. MRI and CT characteristics of successfully ablated renal masses: imaging surveillance after radiofrequency ablation. AJR Am J Roentgenol. 2009;192(6):1571–8. https://doi.org/10.2214/AJR.08.1303.
38. Chan YL, Chan KW, Yeung CK, Roebuck DJ, Chu WC, Lee KH, Metreweli C. Potential utility of MRI in the evaluation of children at risk of renal scarring. Pediatr Radiol. 1999;29(11):856–62. https://doi.org/10.1007/s002470050713.
39. Dickerson EC, Dillman JR, Smith EA, DiPietro MA, Lebowitz RL, Darge K. Pediatric MR urography: indications, techniques, and approach to review. Radiographics. 2015;35(4):1208–30. https://doi.org/10.1148/rg.2015140223.
40. Jones RA, Perez-Brayfield MR, Kirsch AJ, Grattan-Smith JD. Renal transit time with MR urography in children. Radiology. 2004;233(1):41–50. https://doi.org/10.1148/radiol.2331031117.
41. Bokacheva L, Rusinek H, Zhang JL, Chen Q, Lee VS. Estimates of glomerular filtration rate from MR renography and tracer kinetic models. J Magn Reson Imaging. 2009;29(2):371–82. https://doi.org/10.1002/jmri.21642.
42. Palmowski M, Schifferdecker I, Zwick S, Macher-Goeppinger S, Laue H, Haferkamp A, Kauczor HU, Kiessling F, Hallscheidt P. Tumor perfusion assessed by dynamic contrast-enhanced MRI correlates to the grading of renal cell carcinoma: initial results. Eur J Radiol. 2010;74(3):e176–80. https://doi.org/10.1016/j.ejrad.2009.05.042.
43. Tofts PS, Parker GJM. DCE-MRI: acquisition and analysis techniques. In: Barker PB, Golay X, Zaharchuk G, editors. Clinical perfusion MRI: techniques and applications. New York: Cambridge University Press; 2013. p. 58–74.
44. Michaely HJ, Schoenberg SO, Oesingmann N, Ittrich C, Buhlig C, Friedrich D, Struwe A, Rieger J, Reininger C, Samtleben W, Weiss M, Reiser MF. Renal artery stenosis: functional assessment with dynamic MR perfusion measurements—feasibility study. Radiology. 2006;238(2):586–96. https://doi.org/10.1148/radiol.2382041553.

5 Motion-Insensitive Contrast-Enhanced Dynamic MR Imaging of the Kidneys

Ramkumar Krishnamurthy and Judd Storrs

Introduction

Renal dysfunction is a growing problem across the world in both pediatrics and adults. Magnetic resonance urography (MRU) is utilized to effectively study the kidney function. MRU provides significant value in the assessment of a variety of disease conditions including obstructive uropathy, reflux nephropathy and renal dysplasia, renovascular disease, Wilms tumor and renal masses, kidney diseases (parenchymal loss, parenchymal infection, dysplasia, and cysts), upper urinary tract assessments (duplex kidney, ureteric course and insertion, narrowing and obstruction), and ureteropelvic junction (UPJ) and mid-ureteral obstruction [1].

Combined with other anatomical imaging sequences, like the heavily T2-weighted acquisition, dynamic contrast-enhanced MRU (DCE-MRU) offers a one-stop comprehensive functional and morphologic imaging [2–5]. MRU provides imaging with no ionizing radiation—making it suitable for children. It also offers optimal spatial and contrast resolution, leading to an improved visualization of small urinary tract structures, obstructed urinary tracts, and subtle renal parenchymal changes [6]. Also, it has high concordance with nuclear scintigraphy to assess kidney function [7].

Dynamic contrast-enhanced imaging has been used to estimate a number of metrics to characterize renal function, including renal transit time, calyceal transit time, and differential renal function. Many studies have looked at estimating glomerular filtration rate (GFR) from functional MRU techniques. Patlak score [8] can also be calculated, which is a surrogate of GFR. Explanation of these metrics is beyond the scope of this chapter, and the readers are encouraged to look at other chapters in this book and published literature [8, 9]. It is imperative that motion artifact-free dynamic images are acquired at a high temporal resolution to both qualitatively and quantitatively assess kidney function.

Dynamic MRI Acquisition Techniques

Dynamic imaging is performed post contrast injection to assess renal and urinary tract anatomy and function [1]. It is performed after the administration of an appropriate diuretic (furosemide). Typically, a gadolinium based contrast agent is slowly injected 10–15 min after furosemide injec-

R. Krishnamurthy (✉)
Medical and Scientific Affairs, ICON Medical Imaging, Philadelphia, PA, USA
e-mail: Ramkumar.Krishnamurthy@iconplc.com

J. Storrs
Nationwide Children's Hospital, Columbus, OH, USA
e-mail: Judd.Storrs@nationwidechildrens.org

S. D. Serai, K. Darge (eds.), *Advanced Clinical MRI of the Kidney*,
https://doi.org/10.1007/978-3-031-40169-5_5

tion, and dynamic imaging is followed for up to 8–10 min to evaluate the combined urinary excretion system [10]. DCE-MRU dynamically assesses signal changes in renal parenchyma after contrast injection and follows the flow of contrast through the entire kidney filtration process, until the bladder is filled. While conventional imaging has been mainly qualitative, in which an expert radiologist visually evaluates the anatomy and the associated function, there can also be quantitative evaluation of function by estimating renal function and differential renal function.

Adequately acquired MRI dynamic images let the radiologist assess renal perfusion, parenchymal enhancement, excretion of contrast material, identification of focal renal parenchymal perfusion defects, and quantitative assessment of renal function.

For a robust qualitative evaluation of dynamic images through 10 minutes of imaging, there are a few essential criteria to be fulfilled:

- Any dynamic imaging technique should be able to image the urinary system at a fast enough temporal resolution between dynamics, so that fast transient function is accurately captured.
- Motion of patients should be limited or compensated. 8–10 min of lying still for a single acquisition is challenging for a non-sedated patient.
  - Breath-hold imaging of dynamics is desired.
  - Image quality in non-sedated patients with poor breath-holding capabilities has to be managed.
- While utilizing automated or semiautomated segmentation programs for quantitative assessment of function, high temporal resolution motion insensitive images will enhance performance [9].

This chapter deals with both a conventional three-dimensional T1 gradient recalled echo (3D-GRE) acquisition technique and a motion-insensitive radial "stack of stars"-based technique. MRI acquisition metrics for each technique is provided, and the relative advantages and disadvantages of each method are provided below.

Conventional Three-Dimensional T1 GRE Dynamic Acquisition

Functional MR urography with dynamic contrast-enhanced imaging has been utilized for many years and has provided valuable information about the excretory system. In earlier days, two-dimensional imaging techniques of excretory system were used [11–14]. Given that motion artifacts were prevalent, and the techniques used were longer for breath-holding, later, respiratory compensation techniques were used for acquisition [15, 16]. These acquisitions were typically longer in duration, prolonging the temporal resolution between dynamics.

Later, three-dimensional D T1-weighted high-resolution GRE acquisitions, which could fit in a single breath-hold or were not too long, started being feasible with hardware improvements that helped with evaluation of functional metrics [17, 18]. For the past decade or so, this Cartesian k-space based three-dimensional T1 GRE acquisition has been the mainstay for dynamic contrast-enhanced evaluation of kidney function [10]. Figures 5.1 (A1-A6) and 5.2a show the methodology of three-dimensional T1 GRE acquisition, as well as sample image acquisition. These acquisitions have a Cartesian filling of k-space, in which multiple slices are acquired. Parallel imaging/acceleration may be used to reduce acquisition duration. The conventional patient images shown in Fig. 5.1 were acquired with a breath-hold time of 20 s.

Typical acquisition parameters for three-dimensional T1 GRE are listed in Table 5.1.

Benefits of the conventional three-dimensional T1 GRE method are the following:

1. Available in all major vendors' MRI machines.
2. Can be easily adopted to MRU requirements.
3. Easy to run the sequence from a technologist's point of view, especially in patients with breath-holding compliance.
4. In sedated patients with shallow breathing, the sequence can be repeated without breath-holding, providing value.
5. Immediate inline reconstruction.

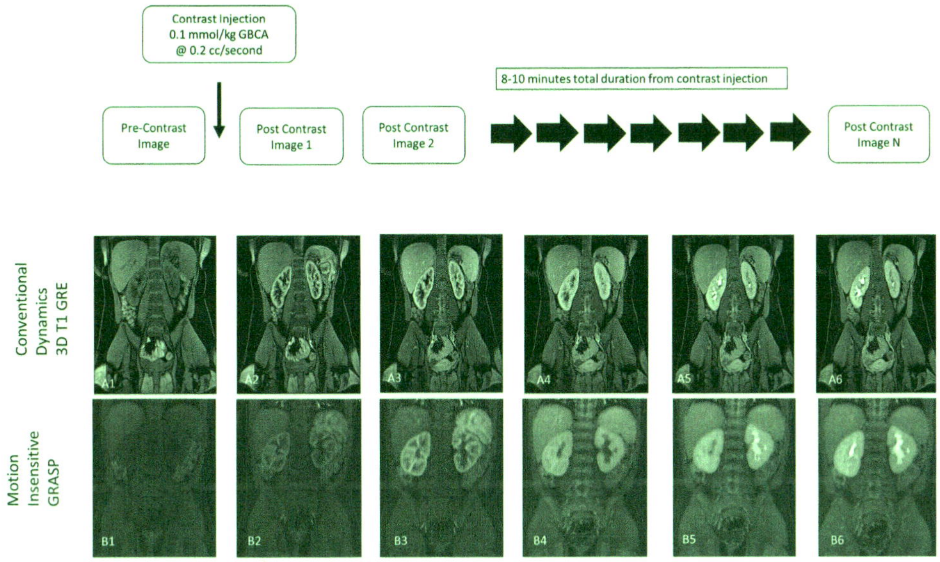

Fig. 5.1 Dynamic imaging with conventional three-dimensional T1 GRE sequence (A1–A6) and a motion-insensitive radial "stack-of-stars"-based GRASP technique (B1–B6) are shown. In a typical MRU acquisition, the contrast-enhanced dynamic acquisition starts around 15 min after furosemide injection. After contrast injection, dynamics are acquired until 8–10 min. Both images were acquired in pediatric patients. The conventional acquisition was made at a temporal resolution of around 40 seconds (including acquisition time and time between dynamics), while the GRASP dynamic was reconstructed at 10 seconds temporal resolution

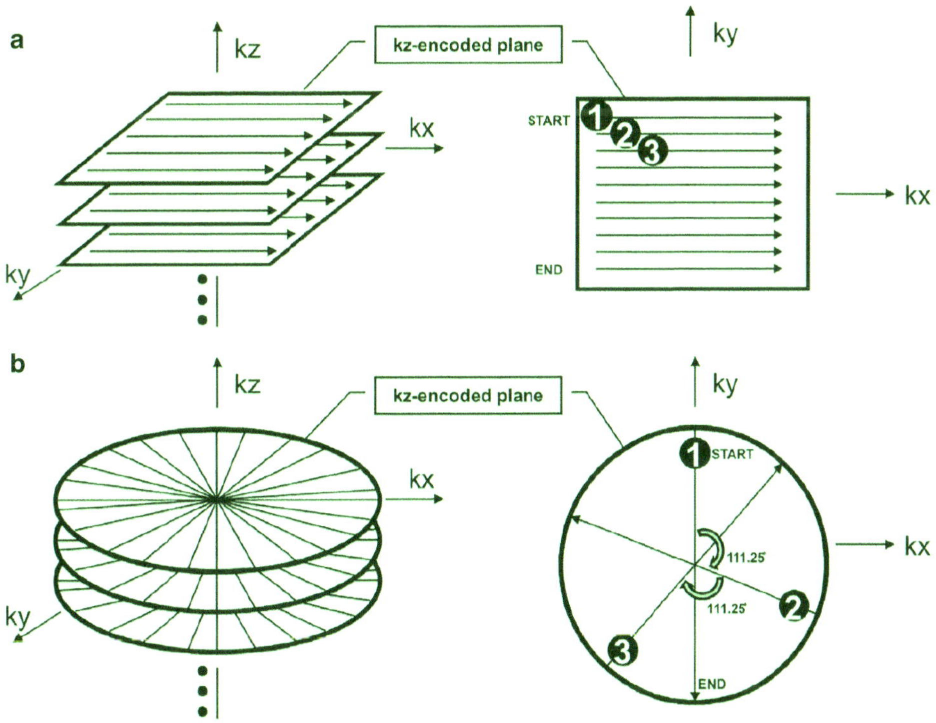

Fig. 5.2 Illustration of three-dimensional k-space comparing conventional (**a**) Cartesian and (**b**) radial "stack-of-stars" acquisition trajectory for radial RAVE/GRASP technique. In Cartesian encoding, all data fall on a rectilinear grid. Typically, consecutive echoes are filled in a sequential pattern. In RAVE, uniform Cartesian grid sampling is maintained along the slice phase encoding direction (kz). However, within each kz-encoded plane, consecutive views are rotated by an angle of 111.25°. For this implementation, a particular spoke is acquired for all kz partitions first before proceeding to the next golden angle spoke

Table 5.1 MRI acquisition metrics for the conventional three-dimensional T1-GRE sequence and the motion-insensitive GRASP acquisition are listed

Parameter	Conventional three-dimensional GRE	Motion-insensitive GRASP
Field strength	1.5 or 3 T	1.5 or 3 T
Sequence	Three-dimensional high-resolution T1 GRE	Radial stack-of-stars
Orientation	Oblique coronal (along kidneys)	Oblique coronal (along kidneys)
Field of view	360 × 340 (depending on patient's body habitus)	360 × 340 (depending on patient's body habitus)
Sequence type	Spoiled GRE	Spoiled GRE
TR	3.2–3.6 ms	3.2–3.6 ms
TE	1.2–1.6 ms	1.2–1.6 ms
Voxel size	2 × 2 × 3 mm^3	1.25 × 1.25 × 3 mm^3
Bandwidth (Hz/pixel)	600	600–1000
Flip angle	~30–40°	10–20°
Parallel imaging	2	NA
Number of slices	32 (depending on patient)	32 (depending on patient)
Temporal Resolution	Acquisition time + wait time between dynamics (~40 s)	Retrospective Reconstruction. Can be as low as 4 s

Some challenges with this acquisition are the following:

1. Each dynamic acquisition may be long (~20 s). Voxel size or acceleration factor can be changed to reduce scan time, with some loss of SNR or resolution.
2. Dynamic temporal resolution may be longer than desired, depending on whether breath-holding is needed.
3. In patients with compromised breath-holding (or suspended respiration in sedated patients), breathing-related motion artifacts may appear.

In certain patient groups, the conventional three-dimensional T1-GRE acquisition might yield sub-optimal images that may not be fully diagnostic. In these cases, having the backup of a motion-insensitive sequence may prove to be useful.

Motion-Insensitive Golden Angle Radial Sparse Parallel (GRASP) Acquisition

Free-breathing three-dimensional golden-angle radial sparse parallel (GRASP) dynamic contrast-enhanced MRI [19] is a dynamic, contrast-enhanced sequence that leverages motion insensitivity of radial acquisition and compressed sensing (acceleration technique) to acquire images that are less afflicted by motion artifacts. It is a continuous, nearly isotropic acquisition that can be reconstructed at a user-selected temporal resolution and reformatted in orthogonal planes. With GRASP, the raw k-space data are acquired in a continuous fashion without predetermined temporal resolution, allowing for retrospective reconstruction at variable temporal resolutions of interest [20].

GRASP k-space data are acquired with consecutive spokes that are rotated by the golden-angle (about 111°) within each kz-slice-encoded plane. This angle ensures the most uniform and nonredundant data sampling scheme. When coupled with compressed sensing and parallel imaging, the data can yield dynamic images across the duration of acquisition. In particular, both high spatial resolution multiphase data sets, analogous to those used for conventional MR urography, as well as high temporal resolution data sets to support robust quantitative perfusion assessment, may be reconstructed from the same continuous GRASP acquisition performed using a single contrast injection.

Figures 5.1 and 5.3 show GRASP images. Patient images in Fig. 5.1 were reconstructed at a 10 s temporal resolution, while the images shown in Fig. 5.3 are reconstructed at a 4 s resolution. The patient in Fig. 5.3 is a four-month-old baby who went through the examination with a swaddle and feed approach, eliminating the need of sedation.

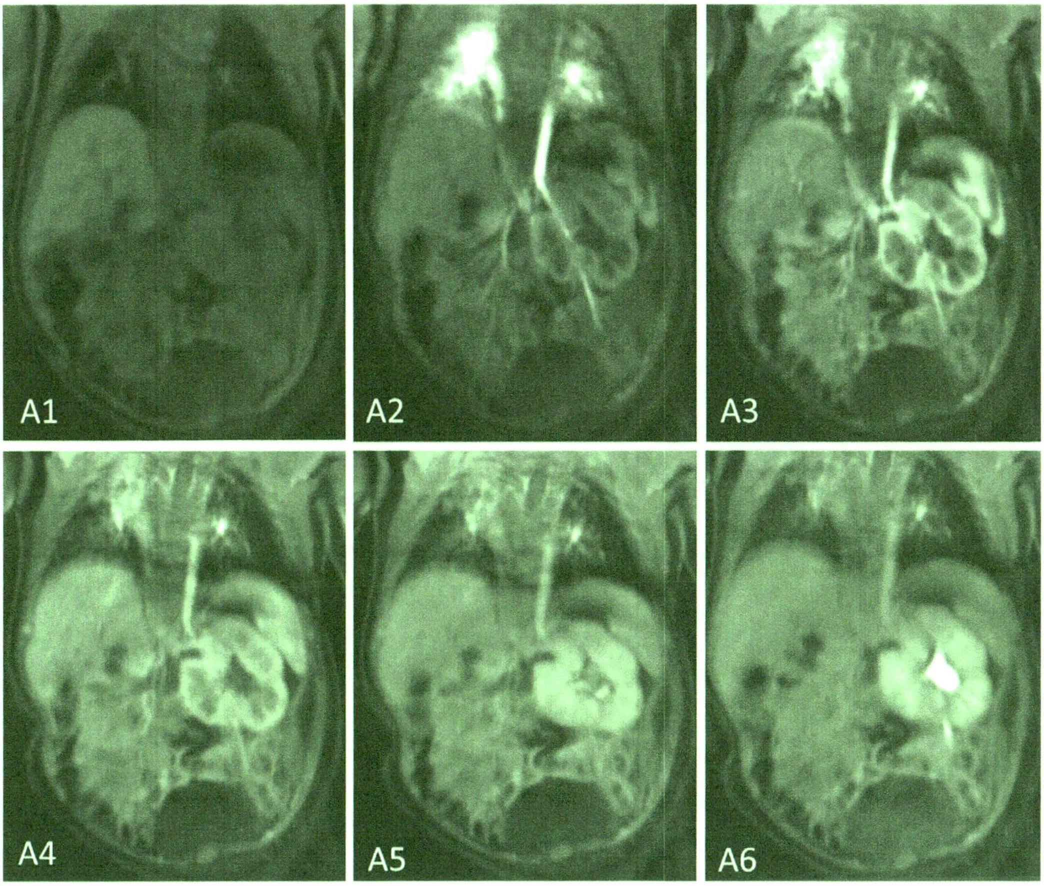

Fig. 5.3 Dynamic enhancement of kidneys using GRASP technique in a non-sedated four-month-old child with a single kidney is shown. The child was immobilized using a feed and swaddle method. The images were reconstructed at a 4 second temporal resolution. All phases of filling of the kidney are seen here

Benefits of GRASP acquisition are the following:

1. Radial acquisitions are naturally motion insensitive, leading to reduced image artifact.
2. Dynamics can be reconstructed at desired temporal resolution retrospectively. It may be feasible to generate both high temporal resolution and low temporal resolution dynamic sets.
3. Higher frame rates (temporal resolution) yield better understanding of kidney function. Figure 5.4 shows data processed using the fMRU program [8]. The high temporal resolution yields better contrast transit timing information, as well as a better fit for kidney function (Patlak score). The explanation of quantitative kidney function using DCE-MRU is explained elsewhere [8, 9].

Some challenges with this methodology are the following:

1. Reconstruction is time consuming currently. It might take a couple of hours to generate a 100 dynamic image set.
2. Availability may be limited. While MRI vendors are starting to provide some variant of the GRASP sequence, it may still need a high-powered post processing machine to reconstruct.

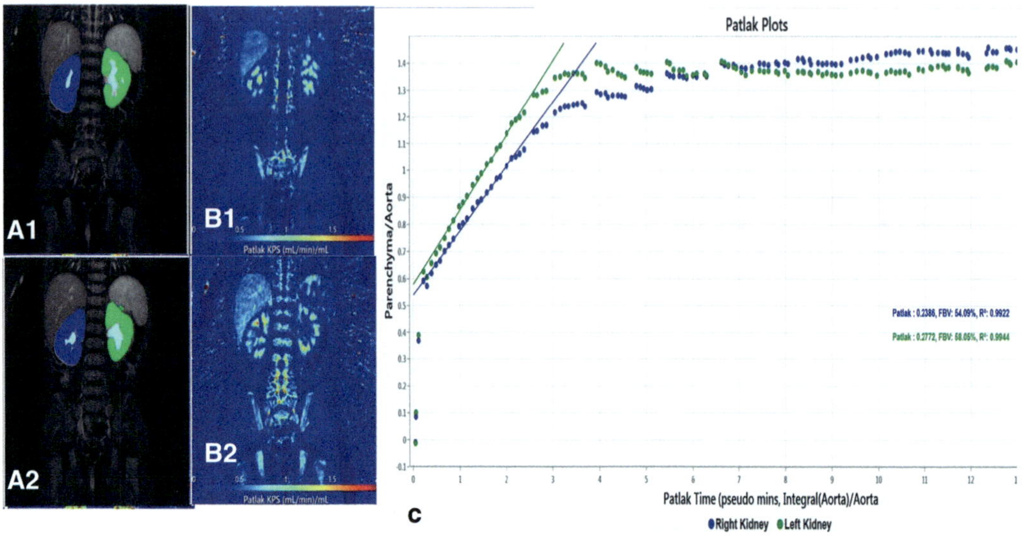

	Right Kidney							Left Kidney						
	vDRF	pDRF	CTT	RTT	TTP	vpDRF	R2 Patlak	vDRF	pDRF	CTT	RTT	TTP	vpDRF	R2 Patlak
#1	NA	NA	NA	NA	NA	NA	NA	100	100	0.340467	1.97475	2.7238	100	0.993106
#2	51.76476	46.57292	0	0	4.97	48.33365	0.99168	48.23524	53.42708	NA	NA	3.313333	51.66635	0.994106

Fig. 5.4 Results from quantitative assessment of kidney function using motion-insensitive MR urography are shown. (**a1**, **a2**) Semiautomated segmentation of kidneys overlaid on magnitude images; (**b1**, **b2**) are the Patlak maps. Results table (**d**) shows the quantitative results from two patients. *CTT* calyceal transit time, *RTT* renal transit time, *TTP* time to peak, *vDRF* volumetric differential renal function, and *pDRF* Patlak DRF. The Patlak plot is shown (**c**) processed with a 5 s dynamic resolution. The Patlak plot shows the data points processed. Increased dynamics from a lower temporal resolution leads to better understanding of kidney function

3. While motion insensitive, this sequence cannot salvage gross motion that may occur during the scanning process.

Conclusion

We have listed acquisition techniques for both a conventional technique and a motion-insensitive radial acquisition scheme. The conventional three-dimensional T1 acquisition technique offers a high spatial resolution imaging at relatively lower temporal resolution that works well with breath-hold compliant patients. It can also be used for quantitative analysis of renal function. In patients with breath-holding difficulty, where shallow breathing is possible, the conventional technique still may offer a viable solution for qualitative analysis.

The radial acquisition scheme offers a motion-insensitive methodology to acquire MRU dynamics. This may also help in acquisition of high temporal resolution that enables better quantitative analysis. While MRI vendors are offering some version of this sequence as a product now, it is not ubiquitously available yet. Also, recent work on automatic segmentation of the kidney [21, 22], with automated estimation of function, renders the ability to analyze kidney function from high temporal dynamic data sets in a relatively simple way.

References

1. Dickerson EC, et al. Pediatric MR urography: indications, techniques, and approach to review. Radiographics. 2015;35(4):1208–30.
2. Avni EF, et al. MR urography in children. Eur J Radiol. 2002;43(2):154–66.

3. Grattan-Smith JD, Little SB, Jones RA. MR urography in children: how we do it. Pediatr Radiol. 2008;38(Suppl 1):S3–S17.
4. Avni F, Riccabona M. The holy grail of anatomic and functional MR urography in children. Pediatr Radiol. 2010;40(5):669.
5. Cerwinka WH, Kirsch AJ. Magnetic resonance urography in pediatric urology. Curr Opin Urol. 2010;20(4):323–9.
6. Dillman JR, Trout AT, Smith EA. MR urography in children and adolescents: techniques and clinical applications. Abdom Radiol (NY). 2016;41(6):1007–19.
7. Boss A, et al. Contrast-enhanced dynamic MR nephrography using the TurboFLASH navigator-gating technique in children. Eur Radiol. 2006;16(7):1509–18.
8. Khrichenko D, Darge K. Functional analysis in MR urography—made simple. Pediatr Radiol. 2010;40(2):182–99.
9. Grattan-Smith JD, et al. Quantitative renal magnetic resonance imaging: magnetic resonance urography. Pediatr Radiol. 2022;52(2):228–48.
10. Jones RA, Grattan-Smith JD, Little S. Pediatric magnetic resonance urography. J Magn Reson Imaging. 2011;33(3):510–26.
11. Rohrschneider WK, et al. Combined static-dynamic MR urography for the simultaneous evaluation of morphology and function in urinary tract obstruction. II. Findings in experimentally induced ureteric stenosis. Pediatr Radiol. 2000;30(8):523–32.
12. Rohrschneider WK, et al. Combined static-dynamic MR urography for the simultaneous evaluation of morphology and function in urinary tract obstruction. I. Evaluation of the normal status in an animal model. Pediatr Radiol. 2000;30(8):511–22.
13. Katzberg RW, et al. Functional, dynamic, and anatomic MR urography: feasibility and preliminary findings. Acad Radiol. 2001;8(11):1083–99.
14. Hackstein N, Heckrodt J, Rau WS. Measurement of single-kidney glomerular filtration rate using a contrast-enhanced dynamic gradient-echo sequence and the Rutland-Patlak plot technique. J Magn Reson Imaging. 2003;18(6):714–25.
15. Borthne A, et al. MR urography in children: current status and future development. Eur Radiol. 2000;10(3):503–11.
16. Staatz G, et al. [Gadolinium-enhanced T(1)-weighted MR urography versus T(2)-weighted (HASTE) MR urography in children]. Rofo. 2001;173(11):991–996.
17. Karabacakoglu A, et al. Diagnostic value of diuretic-enhanced excretory MR urography in patients with obstructive uropathy. Eur J Radiol. 2004;52(3):320–7.
18. Jones RA, et al. Renal transit time with MR urography in children. Radiology. 2004;233(1):41–50.
19. Feng L, et al. Golden-angle radial sparse parallel MRI: combination of compressed sensing, parallel imaging, and golden-angle radial sampling for fast and flexible dynamic volumetric MRI. Magn Reson Med. 2014;72(3):707–17.
20. Parikh N, et al. Performance of simultaneous high temporal resolution quantitative perfusion imaging of bladder tumors and conventional multi-phase urography using a novel free-breathing continuously acquired radial compressed-sensing MRI sequence. Magn Reson Imaging. 2016;34(5):694–8.
21. Yoruk U, Hargreaves BA, Vasanawala SS. Automatic renal segmentation for MR urography using 3D-GrabCut and random forests. Magn Reson Med. 2018;79(3):1696–707.
22. Asaturyan H, et al. Improving automatic renal segmentation in clinically normal and abnormal paediatric DCE-MRI via contrast maximisation and convolutional networks for computing markers of kidney function. Sensors (Basel). 2021;21(23):7942.

6 Clinical Implementation of Image Processing in Kidney MRI

Frank G. Zöllner and Dominik Nörenberg

Renal magnetic resonance imaging nowadays offers multimodal imaging to derive functional imaging parameters. As an example, besides morphological imaging, today diffusion-weighted MRI (DWI) [1], dynamic contrast-enhanced MRI (DCE-MRI) [2] or arterial spin labeling (ASL) [3], blood oxygen level-dependent (BOLD) imaging [4], and relaxometry [5]. Furthermore, x-nuclei imaging like sodium [6] or hyperpolarized approaches [7] is performed. From all these imaging techniques, a large panel of parameters to describe kidney function and disease can be extracted giving information on volume and volume changes, microstructure, perfusion, and permeability and metabolism (Fig. 6.1).

Imaging these parameters with modern scanner hardware comes along with a huge amount of image data ranging from hundreds to several thousands of images per exam and patient. For example, in the paper by Cox et al. [8] and as depicted in Fig. 6.1 compiling a multimodal imaging protocol of 6 imaging techniques, a total of 12 functional renal imaging parameters can be extracted. The shown examples thereby are just one possible combination of the different available imaging techniques in renal MRI. Given this, also the workflow to extract these parameters is highly variable and for the single imaging modality consists of several steps in itself (Fig. 6.2).

Therefore, manual processing of the above-mentioned parameters becomes infeasible and demands for automated image processing. Furthermore, automation of the extraction of renal imaging parameters also removes possible bias due to reader dependencies.

When looking at the different imaging modalities and proposed analysis steps in the literature, three major image processing tasks can be identified: image segmentation, image registration, and modeling.

Image segmentation is an important step in the assessment of total kidney volume (TKV). TKV is the most accessed parameter in patients with autosomal dominant polycystic kidney disease (ADPKD). It has been shown that with disease progression the total volume of the kidney increases while kidney function declines [10]. TKV has been recently qualified as a biomarker by the Federal Drug Association (FDA) [11] for use in drug development in ADPKD. It is also the only MRI-based biomarker so far. Figure 6.3

F. G. Zöllner (✉)
Computer Assisted Clinical Medicine, Mannheim Institute for Intelligent Systems in Medicine, Medical Faculty Mannheim, Heidelberg University, Mannheim, Germany
e-mail: frank.zoellner@medma.uni-heidelberg.de

D. Nörenberg
Department of Radiology and Nuclear Medicine, University Medical Center Mannheim, Heidelberg University, Mannheim, Germany
e-mail: dominik.noerenberg@medma.uni-heidelberg.de

S. D. Serai, K. Darge (eds.), *Advanced Clinical MRI of the Kidney*,
https://doi.org/10.1007/978-3-031-40169-5_6

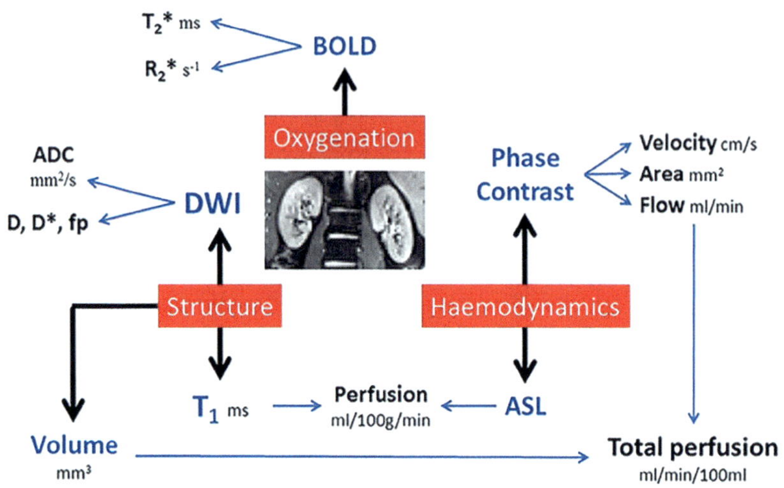

Fig. 6.1 Example of renal imaging techniques, assessment goals, and associated functional imaging parameters that could be derived from the imaging data. (Reproduced with permission from [8])

depicts an example of patients with ADKPD imaged by T1-weighted and T2-wheighted sequences at different disease stages. In green, segmentations of the kidney are shown. An increased load of cysts is obvious.

Volume estimation (not only in ADPKD) is not the only application of renal image segmentation. It also can be used to derive kidney contours and its compartments, that is, the renal cortex and medulla [13, 14] and renal tumors [15] or cysts [16, 17]. This drives further the automation of voxel-based analysis of functional MRI techniques like perfusion, diffusion, or BOLD to help improving diagnosis in kidney diseases like renal hydronephrosis, renal hypoplasia, and chronic kidney disease (CKD) related to diabetes, cardiovascular disease, hypertension, and obesity. Furthermore, assessment of graft function in renal transplantation via volumetry and application in renal artery stenosis (RAS) have been reported. Image segmentation has also been reported in the treatment of renal tumors via cryoablation [18].

Methodologically, image processing techniques applied to renal imaging can be categorized into manual, semiautomated (with limited user intervention), and automated (i.e., fully automated). Zöllner et al. recently analyzed current approaches and found that manual delineation is nowadays mainly used as reference method for the evaluation of new kidney segmentation approaches [12]. Semi- and automatic approaches are, however, still developed to improve segmentation accuracy. These approaches could be divided into image-based and model-based techniques. Regarding the recent literature, most approaches use a combination of algorithms from the abovementioned categories. This is probably because the renal image data (Fig. 6.3) is difficult to process: they suffer from low SNR (signal-to-noise ratio), different amount of cyst or tumor load in adjacent organs like the liver and spleen, and eventually motion artefacts. It seems that a single technique cannot alone sufficiently segment the kidneys. Also, there is a variety of imaging contrasts employed in renal imaging that warrants a robust segmentation approach. Zöllner at el. report that the Dice similarity coefficient, a measure of segmentation accuracy calculating the overlap between ground truth and segmentation by the algorithm at hand, in their reviewed papers ranges between 0.5 and 0.98 depending on the specific application. Furthermore, looking at the volume error, that is, the differences between volumes estimated from the ground truth segmentations and the computed volumes, the mean value and standard deviation are typically a few percent each.

With the rise of deep learning (DL) in medical imaging [19] and subsequent promising results,

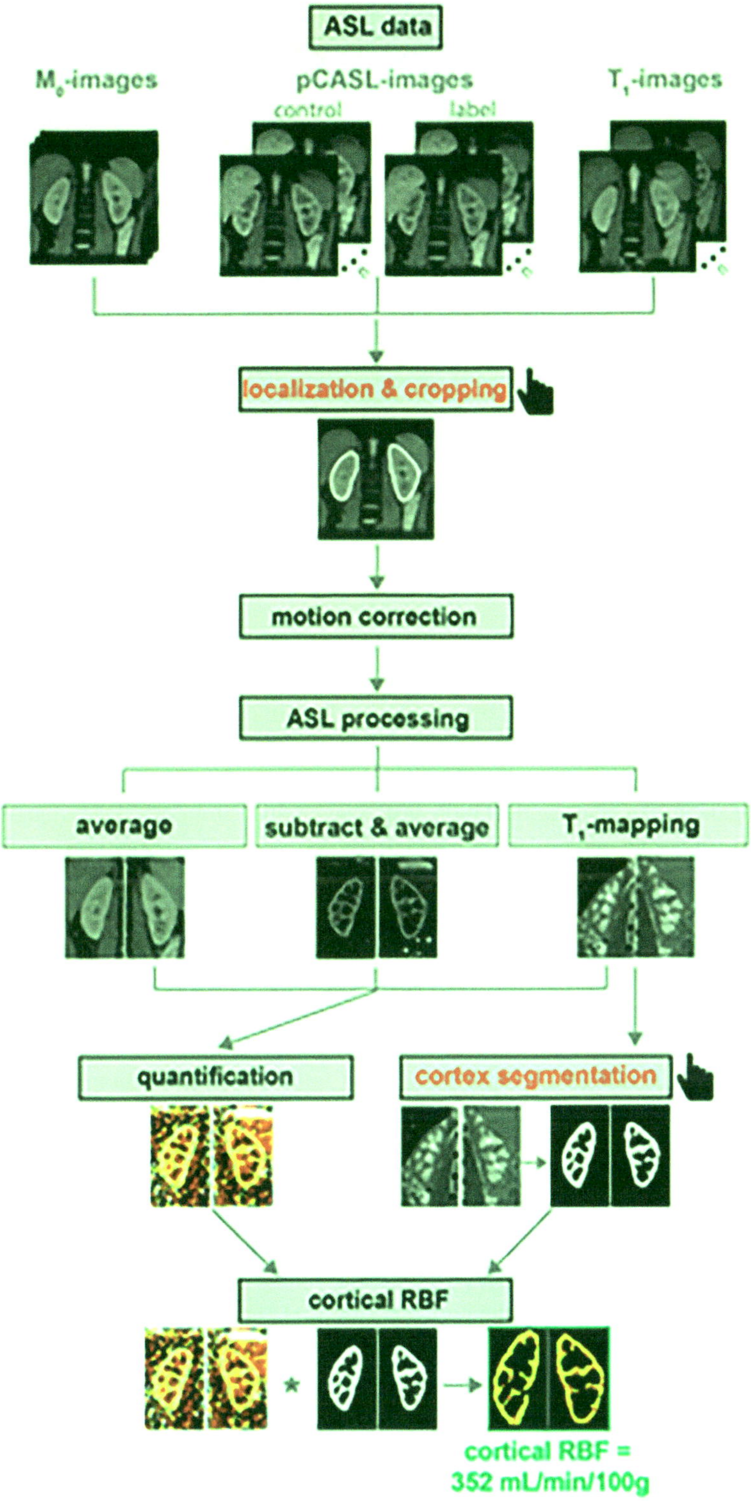

Fig. 6.2 Example of an image processing workflow to estimate cortical perfusion from renal ASL imaging. For the quantification, several image processing steps like segmentation and motion correction are used, but also additional information from T1 mapping is incorporated. (Reproduced with permission from [9])

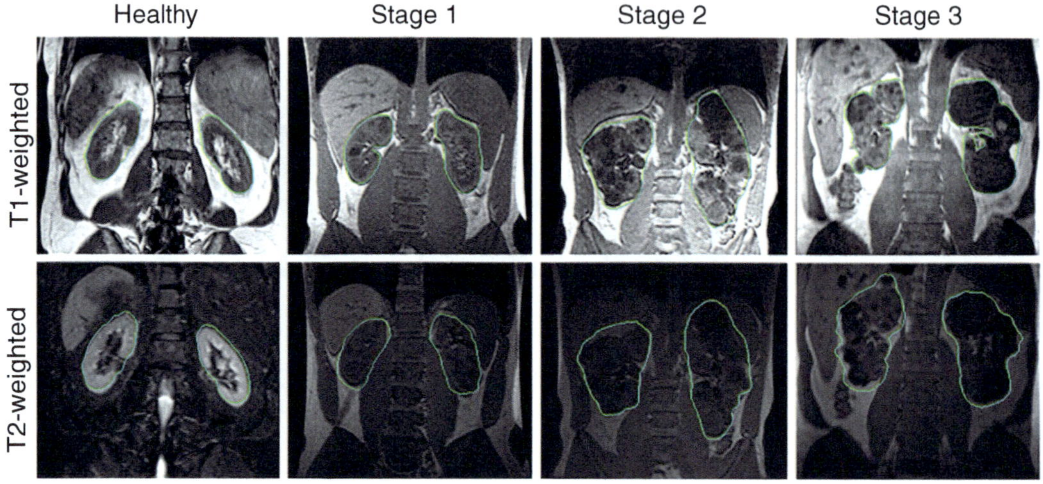

Fig. 6.3 T1-wheighted and T2-wheighted images of patients with different at different disease stages of ADKPD. In green, segmentations of the kidneys are shown. Left, for comparison, an image from a healthy kidney. (Reproduced with permissions from [12])

also these techniques emerge in the field of renal image segmentation. The benefit of deep learning approaches is that they learn their given task, that is, here, segmenting the kidneys. An explicit modeling of the segmentation task like in the image- and model-based approaches is not needed. Recent approaches apply DL to TKV estimation in ADPKD [20, 21]; few started analyzing three-dimensional time-resolved data arising from DCE-MRI [22]. Figure 6.4 depicts an example of a multi-observer convolutional neural network proposed by Kline et al. to segment the kidneys in ADKPD.

Considering results presented in the literature applications of the deep learning methods for fully automated MRI kidney segmentation are encouraging; nevertheless there is a room for further improvement. Current deep learning solutions do not outperform traditional image processing kidney segmentation algorithms [12]. There are several issues that need to be addressed to improve the network performance, such as the lack of the sufficiently large MRI kidney datasets, generalization ability of the network response in case the source of data (data acquisition device) changes, and training with imbalanced data. There are also ideas of combining both deep learning and image processing techniques [23].

Image registration in renal MRI is applied since the image data is hampered by motion, for example, by pulsation, peristaltic, or breathing motion. Such correct for motion is most viable in time-resolved imaging like ASL or DCE-MRI [24, 25]. This motion can hinder subsequent image analysis to estimate hemodynamic parameters like renal blood flow (RBF) or glomerular filtration rate (GFR). A wide range of strategies have been proposed, and renal image registration approaches could be grouped into image acquisition techniques, post-processing methods, or a combination of image acquisition and post-processing approaches. In this chapter, we will focus on post-processing techniques; a review of the others is given in [26].

Image post-processing-based renal MRI registration methods differ according to three key components of image registration techniques, that is, objective function, geometric transformation model, and search method.

The objective function determines the similarity of the registered images, that is, how well the images are aligned. Selection of such an objective function (also known as cost function or loss function) is the most challenging decision at implementation of renal registration algorithms. In dynamic renal MRI, intensity values at the

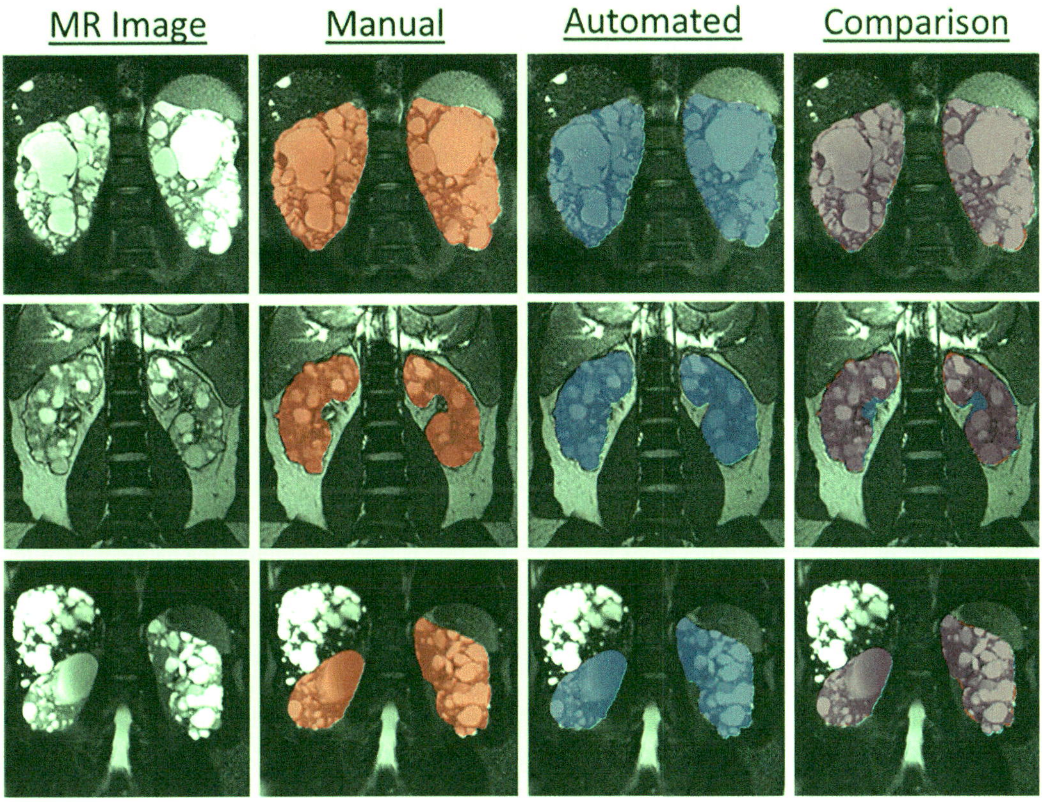

Fig. 6.4 Whole kidney segmentation in ADPKD using a multi-observer DL approach. The first column depicts the input to the networks; the second and third columns show the reference segmentation and the DL segmentation, respectively. The last column is an overlay of the second and third columns, coloring the overlap between ground truth and obtained segmentations in purple, while segmentation errors are given in red and blue. (Reproduced with permission from [20])

same anatomical points may differ considerably for images acquired under different conditions, for example, presence of contrast agent in DCE-MRI or magnetization of the inflowing blood in ASL. Thus, subsequent images do not differ only due to kidney motion that need to be corrected but also due to beneficial information that needs to be preserved. The most common approach to define an objective function is to select an intensity-based similarity metric that best measures alignment of two images. The far most widely selected measures are mutual information (MI) [25, 27] and normalized mutual information (NMI) [28, 29]. Alternatives like point similarity measures that build on top of MI [25, 30], functional intensity dependence [31], or cross-correlation [32] are rarely used. A second group of registration algorithms use gradient information instead of the pure intensity information. Hereby, not only the magnitude but also the direction is used in normalized gradient field (NGF) proposed by Haber and Modersitzki which is applied by several other groups [27, 33]. There are certainly several other possibilities to select the objective function for which the reader is referred to [26].

To register one kidney image to the other, the expected geometric changes of the kidney must be modeled by a geometric transformation model. As outlined before, the geometric changes of kidneys have many causes and are extremely difficult to track or to describe them geometrically [34]. The largest estimate of displacements during normal breathing reported in literature is

7 mm (left–right), 20 mm (head–feet), and 7 mm (anteriori–pasteriori) [35]. In forced deep breathing translations, even up to 86 mm were reported [36]. The deformation component is more difficult to estimate, and the extent of expected deformation is currently not clearly evaluated, although it has been shown that the kidney shape variability can be modeled using an elastic model [37] or an active shape model [38]. In clinical practice, it is considered that the extent of deformation is negligible and a rigid model is sufficient for reaching the correct diagnosis [39, 40]. Nevertheless, some experiments show that visually better results may be obtained using nonrigid approaches, although this may not necessary be due to actual kidney deformation but also due to consideration of other image differences that are not anatomical in nature, for example, movement of the contrast agent. Among nonrigid models, the most commonly used one is a B-spline model [41]. It does not require an additional explicit regularization, because the extent of deformation can be controlled by the density of control points. On the contrary, nonparametric models do need explicit regularization to restrict the amount of deformation and preserve the common shape of the kidney. Regularization can be realized via the physical laws of elasticity [35, 42] or viscosity. Alternatively, smoothness in the spatial and temporal dimension can be applied [43].

Eventually, the above two components have to be connected algorithmically to find the actually best transformation to align the images, that is, an optimization or search methods need to be selected. To increase attraction range, computing efficiency, and reliability of optimization at unavoidable presence of local extrema of criterion functions, the search may hierarchically use images of different resolutions [38] and gradually increase the complexity of transformation model used, from more restrictive rigid ones to more and more detailed deformable ones [41]. It is common that nonrigid registration is preceded by a rigid one [32]. The optimization method is therefore selected depending on the number of transformation parameters.

Similar to (renal) image segmentation, also DL is emerging in the field of image registration. To date, only few approaches employ DL-based image segmentation [19], for renal image registration even less [26]. In general, there are two subtasks of the image registration pipeline that are addressed by deep learning, the objective function and the geometric transformation. The estimated differences are then minimized in a traditional registration procedure, for example, through nonlinear optimization of a geometric transform of image coordinates. The similarity measures are learned straight from the image data to represent complex relationship between local intensity distributions of the images, apparently not captured by traditional handcrafted statistical estimators [44, 45]. The time-consuming iterative optimization is eliminated by employing a neural network predicting the parameters of the voxel coordinate transformation [46]. By this, the registration becomes faster and even can be performed in real time. The work of Cao et al. integrates both approaches [47].

Modeling refers to the part of extracting the functional imaging parameters from images itself after the data has been registered and/or segmented, if necessary. For this, a model reflecting the underlying physics, for example, Brownian motion in DWI, or physiology, for example, compartment models in DCE-MRI, is applied.

Apart from ASL where an analytical solution connecting the (renal) perfusion and the measured magnetization difference exists [3], all other imaging parameters employ a respective model. Commonly, these models are fitted to the obtained data. Thereby, several aspects have to be considered, namely, image data quality and noise, sufficient sampling of the data, fitting parameters especially start values and limits, and eventually that the model reflects the data as best as possible, that is, that overfitting is avoided [48–51].

For instance, in renal DCE-MRI, several compartment models have been proposed ranging from a single-compartment [52] over two-compartment [53] and up to seven-compartment models [54]. Extensive research has been performed to analyze and compare individual models but a consensus has yet not reached [2, 55]. Even more, not only the used model influences the quantification of perfusion and filtration in renal DCE-MRI but also the employed workflow poses potential bias [56].

Recently, new emerging approaches have been proposed to mitigate drawbacks related to the fitting procedure. Magnetic resonance fingerprinting (MRF) converts the typical relaxometry measurements (e.g., via inversion recovery techniques for T1 mapping or multi echo approaches for T2/T2* mapping) and successive model fitting into a database search task [57]. MRF thereby uses the typical MR signal equation to simulate a dictionary of the relaxometry parameters by varying sequence parameters like the flip angle, echo time, or repetition time assigning relaxation times to these signatures that are called fingerprints. In a second step, the same variations in sequence parameters are applied to the real MR acquisition, and the obtained voxel-wise fingerprints are compared to the dictionary and the closest match is selected (Fig. 6.5). Recently, renal MRF has been shown in healthy volunteers (Fig. 6.6) [58] and patients with ADKPD [59].

Besides MRF also machine learning techniques are emerging for enhancing model fitting. Barberie et al. proposed an approach to fit the intravoxel incoherent motion (IVIM) model using a deep learning approach [60]. They use a feed-forward backward propagation deep neural network that is composed of an input layer, three hidden layers, and an output layer. The input layer is made of neurons, which take the normalized diffusion-weighted signal S(b)/S_0 sampled at each b-value as input. The hidden layers are fully

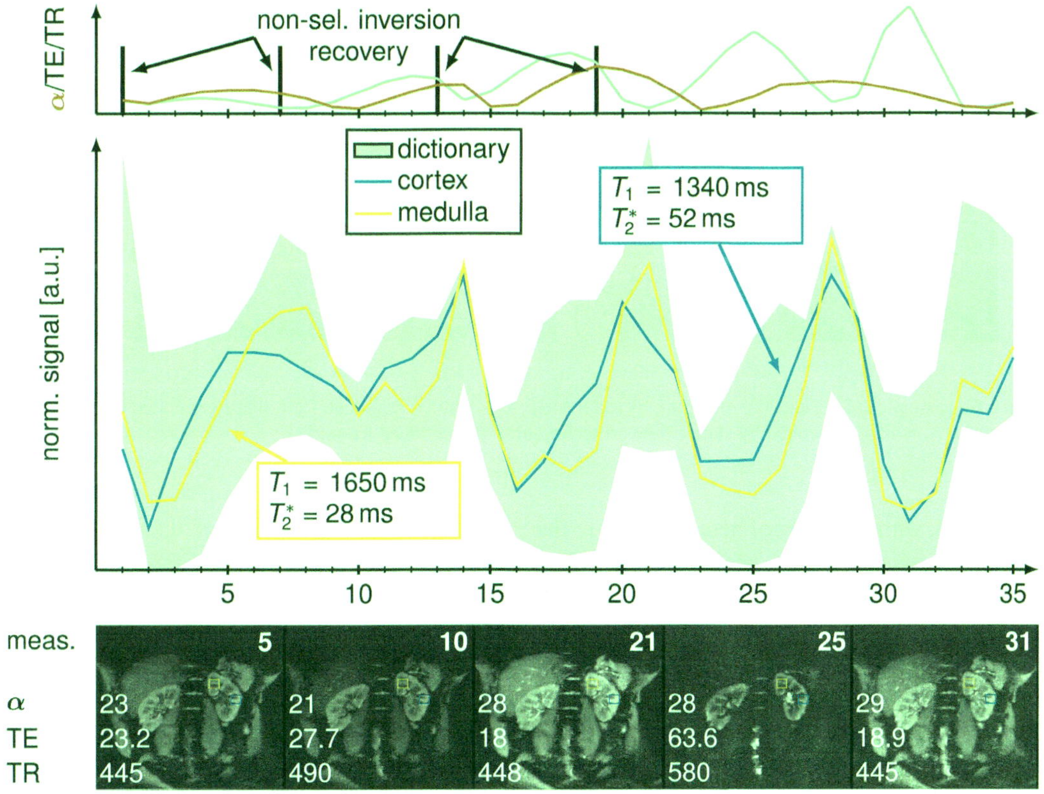

Fig. 6.5 Scheme for renal MRF. In the approach by Hermann et al., a MRF-EPI sequence is used, and dictionary and tissue signal fingerprints are derived by varying flip angle (α), echo time (TE), and repetition time (TR). The evolution curve of the renal cortex (blue) and the renal medulla (yellow) is shown with its corresponding T1 and T2* times for one exemplary measurement. All entries of the full dictionary are depicted as gray area. Baseline images on the bottom show different weightings for several α, TE, and TR along the evolution curve. (Reproduced with permission from [58])

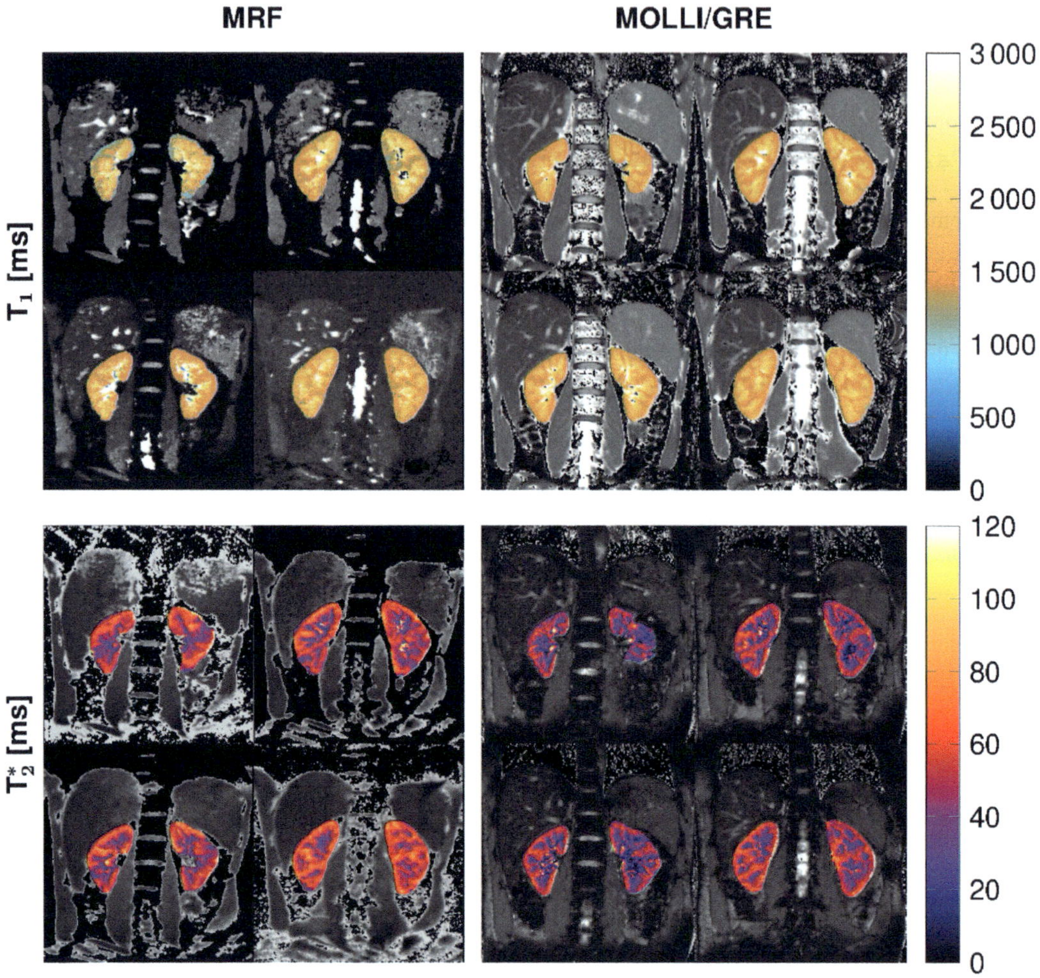

Fig. 6.6 Examples of T1 and T2* mapping by renal MRF in a healthy volunteer. Left, maps generated by MRF, right for comparison maps generated by state-of-the art techniques. (Reproduced from [58])

connected, with a number of neurons equal to the number of b-values of the data of interest and an exponential linear unit activation function (ELU). The output layer is made of three neurons, which hold the estimated IVIM parameters diffusion coefficient D, perfusion fraction f, and pseudo diffusion coefficient D*. A different approach using a CNN to predict IVIM parameters was proposed by Vasylechko et al. [61]. The CNN is coupled to a forward model resembling the IVIM signal model to generate again DWI images. The difference between original input images and predicted images by the forward model is used as loss function.

Despite the assessment of the entire kidney volume and kidney function based on quantitative imaging biomarkers, classical qualitative MRI techniques allow morphologic evaluation of renal cell carcinoma in urooncological imaging. However, qualitative MRI is classically subjective-visual and thus examiner-dependent. In contrast, newer MRI-based methods of quantitative determination of tissue changes show the advantage of an independent and comparable measurement methodology. These quantitative methods include MRI mapping techniques and the entire field of "radiomics" as well as AI-based image analysis. MRI mapping techniques point toward tissue composition via absolute measurements by providing a parametric pixel-by-pixel representation of T1 and T2 relaxation times. This allows direct comparability of tissue signal intensity inter-individually or over time. For example, T1 mapping allows image-based assessment of collagen content. T2 relaxation times reflect tissue composition in terms of water content, among other factors. Adams et al. demonstrated that the quantitative mapping methods were able to detect significant differences in the measured T1 and T2 relaxation times between different tumor grades of clear cell renal cell carcinoma (classified according to WHO/ISUP) [62]. Furthermore, for T1-based mapping methods, there was also a correlation with histologically estimated collagen content. Thus, assuming that higher-grade renal cell carcinomas have a higher degree of fibrosis, T1 mapping of collagen content may provide a noninvasive estimate of tumor grade. In addition, machine learning techniques within the field of "radiomics" and artificial intelligence (AI) have recently contributed to major innovations in the medical software sector. Largely automatic image analysis will play an important role in the future to extract crucial biomarkers for clinical decision-making, especially in urooncological imaging. In addition to image analysis, the methods of AI can also be excellently applied specifically for decision support systems. The selection of a specific minimally invasive therapy or specific surgical therapy procedures (e.g., partial vs. total nephrectomy for renal cancer treatment) in individual patients is composed of many decision criteria, best practices, and guidelines, which are almost impossible to fully overview in everyday life without automated image analysis and processing of data for clinical decision-makers.

In summary, renal image processing is important and needs further investigation to help in automating the processing of multiparametric renal image data and to derive possible biomarker candidates. There are several promising approaches reported in the literature that tackle the three tasks described in this chapter: segmentation, registration, and modeling. A bottleneck toward clinical implementation is often the lack of available open source software, evaluation on large datasets, and consensus on workflows [12, 26].

The COST (European Cooperation in Science and Technology) action PARENCHIMA (Magnetic Resonance Imaging Biomarkers for Chronic Kidney Disease) (http://www.renalmri.org) is working the translation of renal biomarkers into clinical practice [63] and already proposed consensus for a number of renal functional imaging techniques including DWI, ASL, T1/T2 mapping, BOLD, and phase contrast MRI [3, 5, 64–66]. The Working Group II of PARENCHIMA reviewed and investigates renal data analysis algorithms including image segmentation and registration [12, 26] to provide a core software library for a comprehensive and standardized approach to renal data analysis. These efforts might overcome barriers in the development of renal MRI biomarkers.

References

1. Notohamiprodjo M, Reiser MF, Sourbron SP. Diffusion and perfusion of the kidney. Eur J Radiol. 2010;76(3):337–47.
2. Bokacheva L, Rusinek H, Zhang JL, Lee VS. Assessment of renal function with dynamic contrast-enhanced MR imaging. Magn Reson Imaging Clin N Am. 2008;16(4):597–611.
3. Nery F, Buchanan CE, Harteveld AA, Odudu A, Bane O, Cox EF, et al. Consensus-based technical recommendations for clinical translation of renal ASL MRI. MAGMA. 2020;33(1):141–61.
4. Nissen JC, Mie MB, Zöllner FG, Haneder S, Schoenberg SO, Michaely HJ. Blood oxygenation level dependent (BOLD)-Bildgebung der Nieren: Konzepte und Anwendungen. Z Med Phys. 2010;20(2):88–100.
5. Dekkers IA, de Boer A, Sharma K, Cox EF, Lamb HJ, Buckley DL, et al. Consensus-based technical recommendations for clinical translation of renal T1 and T2 mapping MRI. MAGMA. 2020;33(1):163–76.
6. Zöllner FG, Konstandin S, Lommen J, Budjan J, Schoenberg SO, Schad LR, et al. Quantitative sodium MRI of kidney. NMR Biomed. 2016;29(2):197–205.
7. Pedersen M, Ursprung S, Jensen JD, Jespersen B, Gallagher F, Laustsen C. Hyperpolarised 13C-MRI metabolic and functional imaging: an emerging renal MR diagnostic modality. MAGMA. 2020;33(1):23–32.
8. Cox EF, Buchanan CE, Bradley CR, Prestwich B, Mahmoud H, Taal M, et al. Multiparametric renal

magnetic resonance imaging: validation, interventions, and alterations in chronic kidney disease. Front Physiol. 2017;8:696.
9. Bones IK, Bos C, Moonen C, Hendrikse J, Stralen M. Workflow for automatic renal perfusion quantification using ASL-MRI and machine learning. Magn Reson Med. 2022;87:800.
10. Grantham JJ, Torres VE, Chapman AB, Guay-Woodford LM, Bae KT, King BF, et al. Volume progression in polycystic kidney disease. N Engl J Med. 2006;354(20):2122–30.
11. Center for Drug Evaluation and Research. Qualification of biomarker total kidney volume in studies for treatment of autosomal dominant polycystic kidney disease draft guidance for industry [internet]. US Food and Drug Association; 2016. https://www.fda.gov/regulatory-information/search-fda-guidance-documents/qualification-biomarker-total-kidney-volume-studies-treatment-autosomal-dominant-polycystic-kidney.
12. Zöllner FG, Kociński M, Hansen L, Golla A-K, Trbalić AŠ, Lundervold A, et al. Kidney segmentation in renal magnetic resonance imaging—current status and prospects. IEEE Access. 2021;9:71577–605.
13. Gloger O, Tönnies K, Mensel B, Völzke H. Fully automatized renal parenchyma volumetry using a support vector machine based recognition system for subject-specific probability map generation in native MR volume data. Phys Med Biol. 2015;60(22):8675–93.
14. Yang X, Le Minh H, Cheng T, Sung KH, Liu W. Automatic segmentation of renal compartments in DCE-MRI images. In: Navab N, Hornegger J, Wells WM, Frangi A, editors. Medical image computing and computer-assisted intervention—MICCAI 2015. Cham: Springer International Publishing; 2015. p. 3–11.
15. Wake N, Wysock JS, Bjurlin MA, Chandarana H, Huang WC. "Pin the tumor on the kidney:" an evaluation of how surgeons translate CT and MRI data to 3D models. Urology. 2019;131:255–61.
16. Kline TL, Edwards ME, Garg I, Irazabal MV, Korfiatis P, Harris PC, et al. Quantitative MRI of kidneys in renal disease. Abdom Radiol (NY). 2018;43(3):629–38.
17. Bae K, Park B, Sun H, Wang J, Tao C, Chapman AB, et al. Segmentation of individual renal cysts from MR images in patients with autosomal dominant polycystic kidney disease. Clin J Am Soc Nephrol. 2013;8(7):1089–97.
18. Liu X, Tuncali K, Wells WM, Zientara GP. Automatic iceball segmentation with adapted shape priors for MRI-guided cryoablation. J Magn Reson Imaging. 2015;41(2):517–24.
19. Lundervold AS, Lundervold A. An overview of deep learning in medical imaging focusing on MRI. Z Med Phys. 2019;29(2):102–27.
20. Kline TL, Korfiatis P, Edwards ME, Blais JD, Czerwiec FS, Harris PC, et al. Performance of an artificial multi-observer deep neural network for fully automated segmentation of polycystic kidneys. J Digit Imaging. 2017;30(4):442–8.
21. van Gastel MDA, Edwards ME, Torres VE, Erickson BJ, Gansevoort RT, Kline TL. Automatic measurement of kidney and liver volumes from MR images of patients affected by autosomal dominant polycystic kidney disease. J Am Soc Nephrol. 2019;30(8):1514–22.
22. Lundervold AS, Rorvik J, Lundervold A. Fast semi-supervised segmentation of the kidneys in DCE-MRI using convolutional neural networks and transfer learning. In: Berlin, Germany; 2017. (2nd international scientific symposium, functional renal imaging: where physiology, nephrology, radiology and physics meet).
23. Bevilacqua V, Brunetti A, Cascarano GD, Palmieri F, Guerriero A, Moschetta M. A deep learning approach for the automatic detection and segmentation in autosomal dominant polycystic kidney disease based on magnetic resonance images. In: Springer International Publishing; 2018. p. 643–649. http://link.springer.com/10.1007/978-3-319-95933-7{_}73.
24. Workflow for automatic renal perfusion quantification using ASL-MRI and machine learning. [cited 2021 Nov 11]. https://onlinelibrary.wiley.com/doi/10.1002/mrm.29016?af=R.
25. Zöllner FG, Sance R, Rogelj P, Ledesma-Carbayo MJ, Rørvik J, Santos A, et al. Assessment of 3D DCE-MRI of the kidneys using non-rigid image registration and segmentation of voxel time courses. Comput Med Imaging Graph. 2009;33(3):171–81.
26. Zöllner FG, Šerifović-Trbalić A, Kabelitz G, Kociński M, Materka A, Rogelj P. Image registration in dynamic renal MRI—current status and prospects. MAGMA. 2020;33(1):33–48.
27. Hodneland E, Hanson EA, Lundervold A, Modersitzki J, Eikefjord E, Munthe-Kaas AZ. Segmentation-driven image registration—application to 4D DCE-MRI recordings of the moving kidneys. IEEE Trans Image Process. 2014;23(5):2392–404.
28. Fei B, Flask C, Wang H, Pi A, Wilson D, Shillingford J, et al. Image segmentation, registration and visualization of serial MR images for therapeutic assessment of polycystic kidney disease in transgenic mice. Conference proceedings. Annual international conference of the IEEE engineering in medicine and biology society IEEE engineering in medicine and biology society conference. 2005;1:467–469.
29. Melbourne A, Hipwell J, Modat M, Mertzanidou T, Huisman H, Ourselin S, et al. The effect of motion correction on pharmacokinetic parameter estimation in dynamic-contrast-enhanced MRI. Phys Med Biol. 2011;56(24):7693–708.
30. Rogelj P, Zöllner FG, Kovačič S, Lundervold A. Motion correction of contrast-enhanced MRI time series of kidney. In: ERK. Portorož; 2007. p. 191–194.
31. Roche A, Malandain G, Pennec X, Ayache N. The correlation ratio as a new similarity measure for multimodal image registration. In: Wells WM, Colchester A, Delp S, editors. Medical image computing and

computer-assisted intervention—MICCAI'98. Berlin: Springer; 1998. p. 1115–24. (Lecture Notes in Computer Science).
32. Merrem AD, Zöllner FG, Reich M, Lundervold A, Rorvik J, Schad LR. A variational approach to image registration in dynamic contrast-enhanced MRI of the human kidney. Magn Reson Imaging [Internet]. 2012 [cited 2012 Dec 13]. http://www.ncbi.nlm.nih.gov/pubmed/23228308.
33. Hodneland E, Lundervold A, Rørvik J, Munthe-Kaas AZ. Normalized gradient fields for nonlinear motion correction of DCE-MRI time series. Comput Med Imaging Graph. 2014;38(3):202–10.
34. Buonaccorsi GA, Roberts C, Cheung S, Watson Y, O'Connor JPB, Davies K, et al. Comparison of the performance of tracer kinetic model-driven registration for dynamic contrast enhanced MRI using different models of contrast enhancement. Acad Radiol. 2006;13(9):1112–23.
35. Lausch A. Nonrigid registration of dynamic contrast-enhanced MRI data using motion informed intensity corrections. 2011.
36. Siva S, Pham D, Gill S, Bressel M, Dang K, Devereux T, et al. An analysis of respiratory induced kidney motion on four-dimensional computed tomography and its implications for stereotactic kidney radiotherapy. Radiat Oncol. 2013;8(1):248.
37. Hodneland E, Keilegavlen E, Hanson EA, Andersen E, Monssen JA, Rørvik J, et al. In vivo detection of chronic kidney disease using tissue deformation fields from dynamic MR imaging. IEEE Trans Biomed Eng. 2019;66(6):1779–90.
38. Spiegel M, Hahn DA, Daum V, Wasza J, Hornegger J. Segmentation of kidneys using a new active shape model generation technique based on non-rigid image registration. Comput Med Imaging Graph. 2009;33(1):29–39.
39. Positano V, Bernardeschi I, Zampa V, Marinelli M, Landini L, Santarelli MF. Automatic 2D registration of renal perfusion image sequences by mutual information and adaptive prediction. MAGMA. 2013;26(3):325–35.
40. de Senneville BD, Mendichovszky IA, Roujol S, Gordon I, Moonen C, Grenier N. Improvement of MRI-functional measurement with automatic movement correction in native and transplanted kidneys. J Magn Reson Imaging. 2008;28(4):970–8.
41. Sance R, Anderlik A, Roervik J. Towards quantification of kidney function by clustering volumetric MRI perfusion time series. MAGMA. 2006:103–104.
42. Eikefjord E, Andersen E, Hodneland E, Zöllner F, Lundervold A, Svarstad E, et al. Use of 3D DCE-MRI for the estimation of renal perfusion and glomerular filtration rate: an Intrasubject comparison of FLASH and KWIC with a comprehensive framework for evaluation. Am J Roentgenol. 2015;204(3):W273–81.
43. Sun Y, Moura JMF, Yang D, Ye Q, Ho C. Kidney segmentation in MRI sequences using temporal dynamics. In: Biomedical imaging, 2002 proceedings 2002 IEEE international symposium on [internet]. IEEE; 2002 [cited 2011 Dec 20]. p. 98–101. http://ieeexplore.ieee.org/xpls/abs_all.jsp?arnumber=1029202.
44. Simonovsky M, Gutiérrez-Becker B, Mateus D, Navab N, Komodakis N. A deep metric for multimodal registration. In: Ourselin S, Joskowicz L, Sabuncu MR, Unal G, Wells W, editors. Medical image computing and computer-assisted intervention—MICCAI 2016. Cham: Springer International Publishing; 2016. p. 10–8. (Lecture Notes in Computer Science).
45. Wu G, Kim M, Wang Q, Gao Y, Liao S, Shen D. Unsupervised deep feature learning for deformable registration of MR brain images. Med Image Comput Comput Assist Interv. 2013;16(2):649–56.
46. Miao S, Wang ZJ, Liao R. A CNN regression approach for real-time 2D/3D registration. IEEE Trans Med Imaging. 2016;35(5):1352–63.
47. Cao X, Yang J, Zhang J, Wang Q, Yap P-T, Shen D. Deformable image registration using a Cue-aware deep regression network. IEEE Trans Biomed Eng. 2018;65(9):1900–11.
48. Roberts C, Issa B, Stone A, Jackson A, Waterton JC, Parker GJM. Comparative study into the robustness of compartmental modeling and model-free analysis in DCE-MRI studies. J Magn Reson Imaging. 2006;23(4):554–63.
49. Sourbron S. Technical aspects of MR perfusion. Eur J Radiol. 2010;76(3):304–13.
50. Sourbron SP, Buckley DL. On the scope and interpretation of the Tofts models for DCE-MRI. Magn Reson Med. 2011;66(3):735–45.
51. Alhummiany BA, Shelley D, Saysell M, Olaru M-A, Kühn B, Buckley DL, et al. Bias and precision in magnetic resonance imaging-based estimates of renal blood flow: assessment by triangulation. J Magn Reson Imaging [Internet]. [cited 2021 Aug 18];n/a(n/a). https://onlinelibrary.wiley.com/doi/abs/10.1002/jmri.27888.
52. Sourbron SP, Buckley DL. Classic models for dynamic contrast-enhanced MRI. NMR Biomed. 2013;26(8):1004–27.
53. Sourbron SP, Michaely HJ, Reiser MF, Schoenberg SO. MRI-measurement of perfusion and glomerular filtration in the human kidney with a separable compartment model. Invest Radiol. 2008;43(1):40–8.
54. Lee VS, Rusinek H, Bokacheva L, Huang AJ, Oesingmann N, Chen Q, et al. Renal function measurements from MR renography and a simplified multicompartmental model. Am J Physiol Renal Physiol. 2007;292(5):F1548–59.
55. Chandarana H, Lee VS. Renal functional MRI: are we ready for clinical application? AJR Am J Roentgenol. 2009;192(6):1550–7.
56. Hanson E, Eikefjord E, Rørvik J, Andersen E, Lundervold A, Hodneland E. Workflow sensitivity of post-processing methods in renal DCE-MRI. Magn Reson Imaging. 2017;42:60–8.
57. Panda A, Mehta BB, Coppo S, Jiang Y, Ma D, Seiberlich N, et al. Magnetic resonance fingerprinting-an overview. Curr Opin Biomed Eng. 2017;3:56–66.

58. Hermann I, Chacon-Caldera J, Brumer I, Rieger B, Weingärtner S, Schad LR, et al. Magnetic resonance fingerprinting for simultaneous renal T_1 and T_2^* mapping in a single breath-hold. Magn Reson Med. 2020;83(6):1940–8.
59. Rapid B1-insensitive MR fingerprinting for quantitative kidney imaging|Radiology [Internet]. [cited 2021 Nov 23]. https://pubs.rsna.org/doi/pdf/10.1148/radiol.2021202302.
60. Deep learning how to fit an intravoxel incoherent motion model to diffusion-weighted MRI—Barbieri—2020—Magnetic Resonance in Medicine—Wiley Online Library [Internet]. [cited 2021 Nov 23]. https://onlinelibrary.wiley.com/doi/full/10.1002/mrm.27910.
61. Self-supervised IVIM DWI parameter estimation with a physics based forward model—Vasylechko—Magnetic Resonance in Medicine—Wiley Online Library [Internet]. [cited 2021 Nov 23]. https://onlinelibrary.wiley.com/doi/full/10.1002/mrm.28989.
62. Adams LC, Bressem KK, Jurmeister P, Fahlenkamp UL, Ralla B, Engel G, et al. Use of quantitative T2 mapping for the assessment of renal cell carcinomas: first results. Cancer Imaging. 2019; 19(1):35.
63. Mendichovszky I, Pullens P, Dekkers I, Nery F, Bane O, Pohlmann A, et al. Technical recommendations for clinical translation of renal MRI: a consensus project of the cooperation in science and technology action PARENCHIMA. MAGMA. 2020;33:131–40.
64. Bane O, Mendichovszky IA, Milani B, Dekkers IA, Deux J-F, Eckerbom P, et al. Consensus-based technical recommendations for clinical translation of renal BOLD MRI. MAGMA. 2020;33(1):199–215.
65. de Boer A, Villa G, Bane O, Bock M, Cox EF, Dekkers IA, et al. Consensus-based technical recommendations for clinical translation of renal phase contrast MRI. J Magn Reson Imaging. 2020;55:323.
66. Ljimani A, Caroli A, Laustsen C, Francis S, Mendichovszky IA, Bane O, et al. Consensus-based technical recommendations for clinical translation of renal diffusion-weighted MRI. MAGMA. 2020;33(1):177–95.

Part II

MRI Methods, Analysis and Clinical Applications

Quantitative MRI of the Kidneys: Rationale and Challenges

7

Susan Francis

Introduction

Multiparametric MRI provides the potential for a more comprehensive noninvasive assessment of organ structure and function than individual MRI measures. There have been considerable recent advances in multiparametric renal MRI. The combination of highly detailed structural images combined with functional assessment of the kidney is particularly compelling for its potential to provide a comprehensive understanding of pathological changes. This chapter provides an overview of the recent advancements in quantitative renal MRI techniques, outlining their rationale and clinical relevance as well as the challenges in using such measures. Subsequent chapters will describe each method/technique in more detail. This chapter offers an overview of the main renal MRI techniques of morphometric measures to measure total kidney volume (TKV) [1–3], T_1/T_2 relaxometry mapping [4], BOLD (blood oxygen level-dependent) imaging, diffusion-weighted imaging (DWI) [5–12], MR angiography and phase contrast MRI [13], arterial spin labeling (ASL) perfusion [14], and dynamic contrast-enhanced (DCE) MRI, along with other less commonly used methods to measure biophysical tissue properties such as magnetization transfer (MT) [15], T1rho ($T_1\rho$) [16], microstructural methods such as quantitative susceptibility mapping (QSM) [17, 18], diffusion tensor imaging (DTI) [9, 19], and MR elastography (MRE) [20–22] for the study of kidney stiffness. For a detailed description of each renal MRI measure, see Chaps. 8–21.

Comprehensive multiparametric MRI is reproducible and correlates well with available measures of renal function and pathology. In 2018, the COST Action PARENCHIMA initiated a drive toward standardization in renal MRI [23], with a focus on five renal MRI techniques most commonly implemented in multiparametric MRI studies: renal T_1 and T_2 mapping [4], PC MRI [13], ASL [14], diffusion [24], and BOLD [25]. The ultimate goal of the Action was to perform large-scale clinical studies using renal MRI to confirm the value of quantitative renal MRI values as a clinical biomarker. The following section outlines the potential pathological changes which can be studied with quantitative renal MRI measures.

Quantitative Renal Multiparametric MRI

Multiparametric renal MRI offers a range of measures with different pathophysiological origins which provide potential biomarkers, from the assessment of morphology to tissue charac-

S. Francis (✉)
Sir Peter Mansfield Imaging Centre, University of Nottingham, Nottingham, UK
e-mail: susan.francis@nottingham.ac.uk

S. D. Serai, K. Darge (eds.), *Advanced Clinical MRI of the Kidney*,
https://doi.org/10.1007/978-3-031-40169-5_7

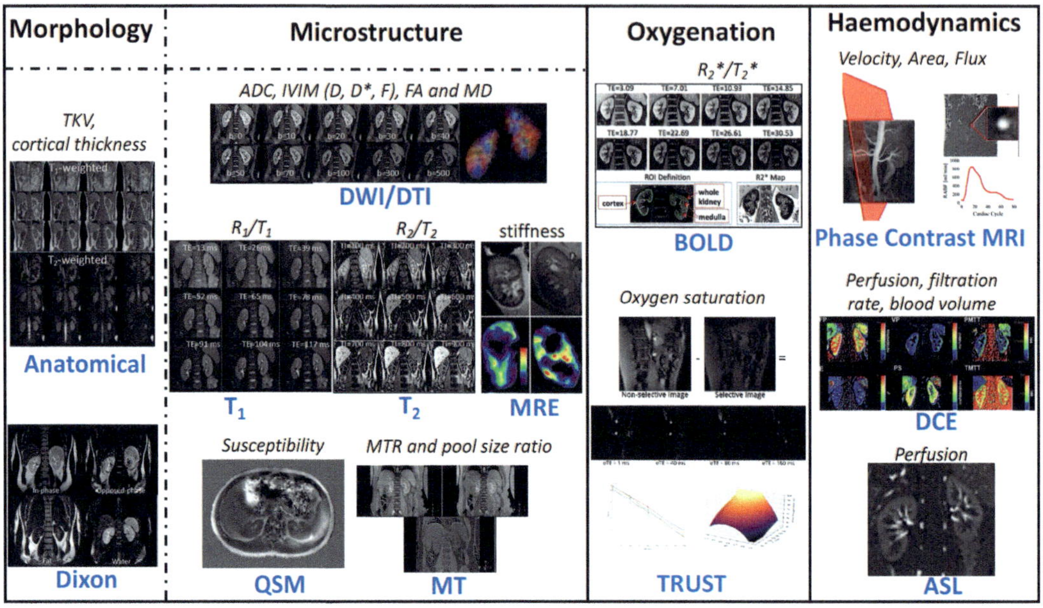

Fig. 7.1 Multiparametric renal functional imaging. Measures characterize kidney morphology, tissue microstructure, hemodynamics, and oxygenation; associated outcome measures are provided in italics. Morphology measures comprise total kidney volume (TKV), cortical thickness, and fat fraction. Microstructural measures can be computed from diffusion-weighted imaging (DWI), apparent diffusion coefficient (ADC), and intravoxel incoherent motion (IVIM) measures (D, D*, and F) and diffusion tensor imaging (DTI), fractional anisotropy (FA), and mean diffusivity (MD), T1 and T2 mapping, quantitative susceptibility mapping (QSM), and magnetization transfer (MT). Oxygenation is measured using blood oxygenation level-dependent (BOLD) contrast and T_2-relaxation under spin tagging (TRUST). Hemodynamic measures are assessed using angiography and phase contrast MRI, dynamic contrast-enhanced (DCE) measures, and arterial spin labeling (ASL) perfusion. Aside from DCE and TRUST, this MRI biomarker panel has been developed and applied in the UKRIN_MAPS and AFIRM protocols

terization, assessment of renal oxygenation, and the study of renal hemodynamics and molecular measures. Combining multiple MRI measures enhances interpretation of MRI measures and allows better understanding of the pathophysiology of the changes as compared with the collection of a single MRI measure alone. This breadth of quantitative renal MRI measures is illustrated in Fig. 7.1 and outlined in Table 7.1.

Studying Renal Morphology

Kidney length and volume and their change over time can be measured with anatomical images, typically using T_2-weighted imaging (T2WI) measures for total kidney volume (TKV) and cyst measures [3, 26], mDIXON for TKV as performed using data from the UK Biobank [27], or T_1-weighted measures for assessment of cortical thickness. Volume measures are key in patients with autosomal dominant polycystic kidney disease (ADPKD) which is characterized by an increase in TKV as a result of cyst formation but may also be important in CKD progression, primary and secondary hyperfiltration in diabetic nephropathy, renal transplants, renal artery stenosis, and vesicoureteric reflux. Cortical thickness may be more variable within a given kidney, limiting reproducibility. Estimated glomerular filtration rate (eGFR) is a measure of how well your kidneys filter blood. It is calculated using blood serum creatinine. The increase in TKV occurs before the decline in eGFR [28, 29], which means that TKV identifies progression at an earlier stage. TKV has been approved by the European Medicines Agency (2015) and the US Food and Drug Administration (FDA, 2016) as a prognos-

Table 7.1 Quantitative renal MRI techniques, a descriptive outline, the pathophysiological process which can be measured, and the associated MRI biomarker

MR technique	Description	Pathophysiological process	Biomarker measured
Morphometry			
Volumetry	Kidney volume measured from T_1- and/or T_2-weighted structural images. Measures have also been assessed from mDIXON scans	Kidney length and volume and their change over time are key measures in patients with ADPKD and may also be important in CKD progression, diabetic nephropathy, renal transplants, renal artery stenosis, and vesicoureteric reflux	Total kidney volume (ml) cortical thickness (mm)
Tissue composition			
Diffusion-weighted imaging (DWI)	Detects Brownian motion of water in tissue by acquiring data at a range of b-values which alters the measured apparent diffusion coefficient (ADC). ADC may be affected by tubular flow and capillary perfusion, so true diffusion (D) can be measured using the IntraVoxel Incoherent Motion (IVIM) model, alongside pseudo-diffusion (tubular/vascular flow, D*) and perfusion fraction (F)	Changes in the renal microstructure, for instance, due to renal fibrosis, cellular infiltration (inflammatory or tumorous), or edema and changes in renal perfusion and in water handling in the tubular compartment	• ADC (mm^2/s) • True diffusion (D) (mm^2/s) • Pseudo-diffusion (D*) (mm^2/s) • Perfusion fraction (F) (%)
Diffusion tensor imaging (DTI) and diffusion kurtosis imaging (DKI)	DTI assesses directionality of diffusion (Brownian motion), which is quantified as a percentage of spatially oriented diffusion signal [fractional anisotropy (FA)]. Allows assessment of the degree of organization in space of oriented tissues DKI measures the deviation from the free diffusion of water molecules	Any changes in the microstructure that lead to a change in the preferred direction of water diffusion, for instance, tubular dilatation, tubular obstruction, or a loss in the organization of medullary tubules	• FA where 0 = isotropic diffusion (equal in all directions) and 1 = complete anisotropy • MD (mean diffusivity) in mm^2/s • Mean kurtosis (MK), axial kurtosis (Ka), and radial kurtosis (Kr) (dimensionless)
T_1 mapping	T_1 is a tissue-specific time variable that can distinguish different tissue compositions. Absolute values of tissue relaxation times differ between 1.5 and 3 T scanners	Changes in the molecular environment, for example, water content, viscosity, temperature, fibrosis (due to the association of collagen with supersaturated hydrogel) and inflammation (interstitial edema, cellular swelling)	T_1 in ms for the whole kidney, cortex, medulla, and corticomedullary difference (CMD)
$T_1\rho$ mapping	$T1\rho$ is the spin-lattice relaxation time constant in the rotating frame, though only a few studies have been performed as outlined in Chap. 9	$T1\rho$ has been shown to be sensitive to low-frequency interactions between water molecules and macromolecules, such as collagen and proteoglycans, fueling interest in the application of $T1\rho$ as a noninvasive marker of microstructure	$T_1\rho$ in ms for the whole kidney, cortex, medulla, and corticomedullary difference (CMD)

(continued)

Table 7.1 (continued)

MR technique	Description	Pathophysiological process	Biomarker measured
T_2 mapping	Provides quantification of T_2 as a tissue-specific time parameter. Changes with tissue water content	Changes in the molecular environment but assumed to be more sensitive to the effects of edema and/or inflammation. Limited experience in human kidney disease to date	T_2 in ms for the whole kidney, cortex, medulla, and corticomedullary difference (CMD)
Magnetization transfer	Dependent on the fraction of large macromolecules or immobilized cell membranes in tissue	The fraction of large macromolecules or immobilized cell membranes in tissue; in the kidney, shown to correlate with fibrosis	MT ratio (%) Bound pool fraction (%)
QSM	Magnetic susceptibility of biological tissue	QSM is sensitive to molecular content, cellular arrangement, and tissue microstructure and has been demonstrated to be sensitive to inflammation and fibrosis	Susceptibility (ppm)
MRE	Magnetic resonance elastography uses external mechanical vibration to quantify organ stiffness on MRI	MRE is sensitive to renal stiffness driven by the replacement of compliant cells with rigid matrix and cross-linking of matrix fibrils	Kidney stiffness (kPa)
Hemodynamics			
Phase contrast (PC) MRI	Measurement of blood flow in renal arteries and veins. Sensitized to flow by using bipolar gradients affecting the phase signal of spins that flow with a uniform velocity in the direction parallel to the gradients. Global perfusion of the kidney can be measured by dividing total blood flow to the kidney by the total kidney volume (TKV)	Increased renal resistance to flow due to downstream microvascular obstruction, large vessel arterial disease, or changes in systemic hemodynamics	• Renal artery blood flow (flux) (mL/s) • Renal artery velocity (cm/s) • Renal artery area (cm) • Global perfusion (mL/100 g/min)
Arterial spin labeling (ASL)	A subtraction technique where arterial blood water is labeled (inverted) prior to imaging. Difference in signals are determined by subtracting imaging data with and without labeling	Cortical perfusion, which can be affected by a number of pathophysiological processes in acute and chronic renal disease	• Cortex and medulla perfusion (mL/100 g/min)
Dynamic contrast-enhanced (DCE)	Uses gadolinium-based contrast agents to change the T_1 relaxation time of water in tissues	Perfusion and filtration per unit tissue, vascularity, and tubular transit times. Allows measurement of perfusion and GFR. Concerns exist when using gadolinium for research in advanced CKD	• Single kidney GFR (mL/min) • Tissue blood flow (mL/100 mL/min) • Tubular flow (mL/100 mL/min) • Filtration fraction (%) • Tubular transit time (s) • Tubular volume fraction (%)

Table 7.1 (continued)

MR technique	Description	Pathophysiological process	Biomarker measured
Blood oxygenation level dependent (BOLD)	Deoxyhemoglobin is paramagnetic and shortens the transverse relaxation constant T_2^* (ms) which is the inverse of the relaxation rate R_2^* (1/s). Besides oxygenation, R_2^* is also influenced by changes in hematocrit and tissue water content	Changes in renal oxygenation or changes in the microstructure of the capillary bed. Other factors such as hydration status, dietary sodium, and susceptibility effects also alter T_2^*	• T_2^* in ms • R_2^* ($1/T_2^*$) As measures of renal oxygenation
T_2 relaxation under spin tagging (TRUST)	Spin tagging of blood, similar to ASL, is used to separate the signals from venous blood from surrounding tissues, and this is collected across a range of T_2-weighted echo times. By acquiring an R_2 signal solely from venous blood, the venous oxygenation (saturation) can be calculated	In contrast to BOLD, TRUST data is not influenced by edema and hematocrit. Renal TRUST is a novel technique with limited previous data and is less explored compared to BOLD. Validation studies are mainly from the central nervous system to study the sagittal sinus	• Global oxygenation • Renal venous saturation (%)

tic enrichment biomarker to identify patients at high risk of disease progression and to identify those who could be included in clinical trials of novel treatments.

Assessing Tissue Microstructure with Quantitative Renal MRI

Renal fibrosis can result from acute or chronic injury to the kidney. The degree of interstitial fibrosis (IF) and tubular atrophy is often the most important determinant of long-term renal outcomes [30]. A number of MRI techniques show promise for the noninvasive characterization of fibrosis on a whole kidney basis including DWI, T_1 and $T_{1}\rho$ mapping, T_2 mapping, and magnetization transfer (MT), as shown in Fig. 7.2.

Diffusion-Weighted Imaging (DWI)

Diffusion-weighted MRI gives information about the motion of water molecules in tissue. In DWI, a strong magnetic gradient field (called the positive diffusion gradient) causes water molecules to accumulate phase. A second gradient field, which is the negative of the first field (called the negative diffusion gradient), undoes this phase accumulation. For water molecules that have not moved in the time between the positive and negative diffusion gradients, the phase accumulation caused by the positive gradient is exactly undone by the negative gradient, and these molecules experience no net change in phase. However, water molecules that are in motion in the short time interval between the two gradients accumulate phase during the positive diffusion gradient, which is not completely undone by the negative gradient. Accumulation of phase causes signal loss. Therefore, moving water molecules give less signal (less intensity on the final image) than water molecules that are stationary. The amount of signal loss increases with increased distance traveled by water molecules in the time between the positive and negative diffusion gradients. Water molecules that diffuse freely experience the greatest signal loss, whereas molecules with motion that is constrained by surrounding structures experience less signal loss. This signal loss can be modeled to give a quantity called the apparent diffusion coefficient (ADC) for each pixel in an image that expresses how freely water is able to diffuse in the tissue. DWI can be performed rapidly with standard MRI equipment, and therefore, technical barriers to clinical implementation are low.

Tissue with higher cellularity generally shows lower ADC, because diffusion of water molecules is impeded by hydrophobic cell

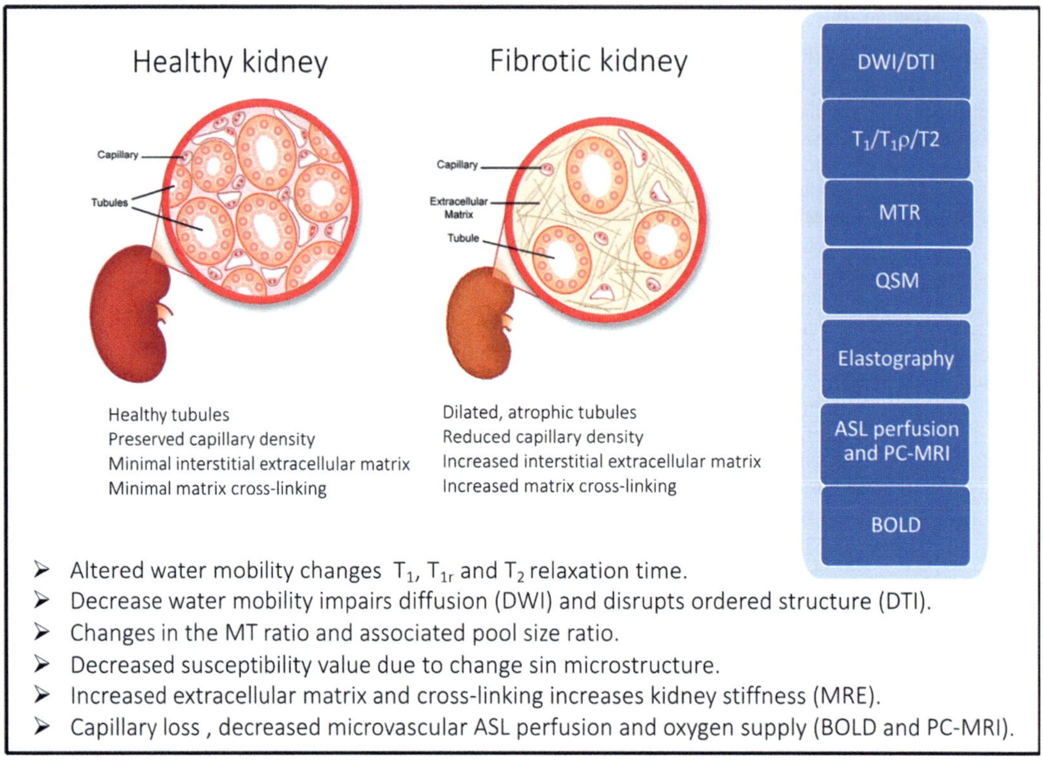

Fig. 7.2 A number of MRI techniques show promise for the noninvasive characterization of fibrosis on a whole kidney basis. The alterations that occur in fibrosis and the associated MRI measures are outlined

membranes. Accumulation of collagen and other matrix components in renal fibrosis would be expected to impair free diffusion of water and thus lower ADC. In the kidney, microstructural barriers that differ depending on tissue composition determine the ADC, but ADC is also affected by microcirculation in the tissue such as tubular flow and capillary perfusion. Intravoxel incoherent motion (IVIM) corrects for the contribution of microperfusion to quantify pure molecular diffusion (D) from perfusion-dependent diffusion (D*) and the perfusion fraction (f). For a full description of DWI methodology, see Chap. 18. A further variant of DWI is diffusion tensor imaging (DTI) which assesses the directionality of diffusion of water molecules by the fractional anisotropy (FA), providing information on the microstructural orientation and homogeneity of tissues. In DTI, diffusion imaging is performed repeatedly with diffusion gradients oriented in different directions. This allows quantification of not only the freedom of water molecules to diffuse (ADC) but also the preferential directions of diffusion. For water in free solution, there is no preferential direction for diffusion; motion is random in all directions. However, in tissues with an organized structure, water may diffuse more freely in one direction than another. For instance, in the tubules of the renal medulla, water may diffuse preferentially along the direction of the tubule. The degree to which diffusion shows a preference for direction is quantified as FA. FA measured by DTI has a range of zero to one and represents the degree of spatial organization of tissue. Non-Gaussian model diffusion kurtosis imaging (DKI) is an extension of DTI; in this model, the deviation from the free diffusion of water molecules can be measured, with the kurtosis index including mean kurtosis (MK), axial kurtosis (K_a), and radial kurtosis (K_r) being obtained [31].

A number of studies have applied DWI in patients with chronic kidney disease (CKD) and in kidney transplants and compared measurements with renal function and renal biopsy, as reviewed in a systematic review and statement paper describing the diffusion-weighted MRI [7]. It has been shown that ADC decreases with increasing fibrosis in chronic kidney disease (CKD) and in kidney transplant patients with acute tubular necrosis, acute rejection, and immunosuppressive toxicity, while FA has been shown to decrease. Further, K_a has been shown to increase with eGFR and interstitial fibrosis [31].

T_1, $T_1\rho$, and T_2 Mapping

The longitudinal (T_1) relaxation time of tissue has been shown to provide an assessment of either fibrosis (due to association of collagen with supersaturated hydrogel) or inflammation (interstitial edema, cellular swelling) [32]. T_1 values have been shown to correlate well with fibrosis and edema in cardiac [33] and liver imaging [34]. The early changes in acute tissue injury such as interstitial edema usually lengthen the T_1 relaxation time. T_1 relaxation values differ between different kidney components (cortex, medulla, urine, etc.); it decreases when paramagnetic contrast agents such as gadolinium chelates or oxygen (O_2) are present, and it may increase or decrease with pathology. In addition, T_1 tends to increase with field strength (B_0). The sensitivity of T_1 to the tissue microenvironment has been employed quite extensively to assess renal structure and function, both in clinical and preclinical studies. In an animal model of acute kidney injury (AKI) induced by ischemia followed by reperfusion, Hueper et al. demonstrated that the T_1 relaxation time of renal tissue increased significantly and was associated with renal inflammation [35]. Breidthardt et al. showed that chronic parenchymal damage, as indicated by prolonged T_1 relaxation, appears to underlie chronic cardiorenal syndrome rather than decreased perfusion [36]. Wu et al. [37] performed T_1 mapping of the renal cortex to determine its utility for assessing renal fibrosis in patients with chronic glomerulonephritis (CGN). They showed that renal cortex T_1 correlated well with CKD stage ($p < 0.05$), except between CKDs 2 and 3 and that T_1 was positively correlated with cystatin C, neutrophil gelatinase-associated lipocalin, and serum creatinine and negatively correlated with hemoglobin, kidney length, estimated glomerular filtration rate, and hematocrit ($p < 0.05$). T_1 values can be affected by a wide variety of changes in the tissue environment, including inflammation and fibrosis. Inflammation can coexist with fibrosis in the kidney tissue, for example, during rejection of transplanted kidneys. T_1 may also be used as baseline measurement for DCE MRI acquisitions. More information on the use of T_1 for quantitative DCE MRI measurements can be found in Chap. 20.

$T1\rho$ is the spin-lattice relaxation time constant in the rotating frame. $T1\rho$ has been shown to be sensitive to low-frequency interactions between water molecules and macromolecules, such as collagen and proteoglycans, fueling interest in the application of $T1\rho$ for the noninvasive marker of microstructure in the kidneys, though only a few have been performed as outlined in Chap. 11. $T1\rho$ may provide a noninvasive indirect measurement of collagen deposition as a result of interstitial fibrosis.

T_2 relaxation time also allows quantification of specific local microstructural composition of the kidney. Tissue T_2 is known to increase in response to inflammation, while it tends to decrease in reaction to severe fibrosis; this characteristic enables discrimination between those conditions. Chapters 8 and 9 review T_1 and T_2 mapping in renal disease. MR fingerprinting (MRF) [38]-based assessments (see Chap. 12) include image synthesis to derive quantification parametric images of multiple tissue parameters such as T_1 and T_2 in a single scan, with the resultant parametric maps being inherently co-registered, allowing the data to be easily combined to enable a more comprehensive evaluation of tissue composition and pathophysiology.

Magnetization Transfer

Magnetization transfer measures the spin exchange between proton pools in different environments and is strongly dependent on the macromolecular content of tissue. To date, semiquantitative measurements of the MT ratio (MTR) [39] have been used to assess renal apoptosis and fibrosis [15, 40]. However, MTR measures can be affected by various factors including relaxation rates and the precise selection of different experimental parameters which reduce the reproducibility and specificity of measurements. Studies [41] suggest that a pool size ratio (PSR) from quantitative MT (qMT) modeling is a more specific and sensitive measure than MTR for detecting changes of macromolecular composition in the cortex in different kidney diseases. For a complete description, see Chap. 13.

Quantitative Susceptibility Mapping

Magnetic susceptibility is a physical property of tissue that varies slightly between different tissue types and has a complex effect on MR images. Sophisticated mathematical analysis of MRI phase images can go beyond susceptibility weighting to yield quantitative maps of estimated tissue susceptibility. Quantitative susceptibility mapping (QSM) provides a method to noninvasively estimate the magnetic susceptibility of biological tissue which is particularly sensitive to molecular content, cellular arrangement, and tissue microstructure [42]. It has been demonstrated in ex vivo mice kidneys that inflammation and fibrosis can be detected, with these pathologies leading to a decreased susceptibility value [43]. QSM in the human kidney is not yet widely used, but the potential diagnostic value QSM possesses in the human has been shown from the susceptibility value between a group of healthy individuals and on a patient with severe kidney fibrosis [44]. This is reviewed in Chap. 16. An extension of susceptibility imaging known as susceptibility tensor imaging has been applied to excised and fixed kidneys and has shown the intriguing potential to provide information about renal tissue microstructure on the scale of the renal tubule that may be relevant to renal fibrosis. However, this method is limited to ex vivo imaging and is not currently feasible for human imaging, because it requires extremely long imaging times and also requires that the tissue be placed in a variety of orientations relative to the main magnetic field of the MRI machine, which is not possible for human subjects positioned in a conventional clinical MRI system.

Magnetic Resonance Elastography

Magnetic resonance elastography (MRE) is a method of quantifying tissue stiffness with MRI. In this method, a mechanical transducer is placed against the body surface and causes mechanical vibration that propagates through the tissue. MRI is performed in synchrony with the mechanical vibration. MRI phase images can detect small displacements of tissue throughout the imaging volume. These displacement maps can then be used to calculate the stiffness of tissue throughout the imaging volume. As a kidney undergoes fibrosis, there is an accompanying increase in renal stiffness driven by the replacement of compliant cells with rigid matrix and cross-linking of matrix fibrils. However, several factors other than fibrosis affect kidney stiffness. Recent data suggest that kidney stiffening is not just a manifestation of the fibrotic process, but fibrosis requires this stiffening to occur. Fibroblasts respond to TGF-b, a profibrotic stimulus, only when grown in a stiff environment, whereas fibroblasts grown on a soft, healthy organ-like surface fail to respond. MRE is particularly suited to renal transplant recipients, given that allografts are placed much closer to the skin surface than native kidneys. There have been some divergent results in the studies so far, with some showing a positive correlation between elastography and fibrosis, while others have found a negative correlation [45]. For a detailed review of the methods and clinical applications of magnetic resonance elastography, see Chap. 17.

Renal Oxygenation

Blood Oxygen Level-Dependent (BOLD) MRI

Hypoxia has been implicated as a key process in the progression and failed recovery of many forms of acute and chronic kidney disease [46, 47]. Renal hypoxia may be a functional rather than anatomic marker for fibrosis. Renal BOLD MRI has evolved over the last two decades with early interest in understanding the acute effects of physiological and pharmacological factors on intrarenal oxygenation. BOLD MRI can provide an indication of tissue oxygenation by utilizing the paramagnetic affect that deoxyhemoglobin exerts to shorten the transverse relaxation time constant (T_2*), which is also expressed as R_2* (1/T2*). Higher R_2* (or lower T_2*) is an indicator of lower tissue oxygenation (pO_2) (Chap. 10). Increased levels of deoxyhemoglobin cause decreased T_2*, and numerous published studies have shown an inverse association of T_2* with renal oxygen levels. Due to their relative positions on the oxygen dissociation curve, BOLD MRI is more sensitive at detecting changes in medullary as compared to cortical pO_2.

Despite the sometimes-demonstrated sensitivity of BOLD MRI in animal models and healthy volunteers, clinical studies have produced inconsistent results. A large number of studies in CKD, diabetic nephropathy, and kidney transplantation, with some animal studies of AKI, are summarized in a comprehensive review by Neugarten and Golestaneh [48]. Whereas some investigators have reported a reduction in oxygenation in CKD, a more recent study by Pruijm et al., which compared healthy controls ($n = 45$), CKD patients ($n = 95$), and treated hypertensives ($n = 58$), found no differences in cortical or medullary R_2* between groups [49]. In part, these inconsistent findings may reflect issues related to both the origin and analysis of BOLD MRI data, combined with a number of clinical factors that may affect BOLD MRI image intensity other than oxygenation, such as hydration status, age, hematocrit, dietary sodium, pH, or even body temperature [48, 50]. At present, additional technical advances to unravel these links are required before the quantitative capabilities of BOLD MRI can be integrated to clinical practice, as evidenced by the failure of BOLD MRI to discriminate between different stages of chronic kidney disease in 280 undifferentiated CKD patients [51]. Historically, manual placement of regions of interest (ROI) in the cortex and medulla has been most frequently used, but other methods to analyze T_2* or R_2* maps have been reported in the literature [52]: the fractional tissue technique, the 12 layer concentric objects (TLCO) technique [53], the compartmental method, and a histogram analysis-based technique that defines masks for the cortex and medulla based on T_1 maps [54]. With the semiautomatic TLCO technique, lower interobserver variability in R_2* across all layers has been reported compared to the ROI technique, improving the detection of differences in R_2* between healthy, mild CKD, and severe CKD groups [55]. Alternative techniques such as quantitative susceptibility mapping (QSM) as described in Chap. 16 may also aid in the interpretation of BOLD. QSM is very sensitive to microstructure and chemical composition and can spatially resolve the source of the signal change in BOLD MRI [18].

T_2-Relaxation-Under-Spin-Tagging (TRUST) MRI

The relationship between the R_2 tissue relaxation rate and oxygen saturation can be used to quantify the oxygen dependence of an organ or tissue. Using a method of T_2-relaxation-under-spin-tagging (TRUST) MRI, it is possible to enhance separation of the blood and tissue signals. In the brain, combining this with measures of blood flow allows the global metabolic rate of oxygen to be calculated [56]. Theoretically, it should be possible to apply the same methods to assess renal oxygen metabolism ($RMRO_2$), providing an alternative to BOLD MRI. Alternatively, recent studies have described the use of two-dimensional multi-echo gradient and spin echo (MEGSE) or triple echo asymmetric spin echo (ASE), combined with arterial spin labeling (ASL) to form spatial maps of $RMRO_2$ [57]. To our knowledge, there are no clinical studies in this area at present.

Measurement of Renal Blood Flow and Perfusion

Changes in large vessel flow as well as changes in tissue perfusion at the capillary level have relevance to a number of different renal diseases but importantly may also provide insights into efficacy of therapies. Measurement of renal perfusion can be separated into those techniques that require exogenous contrast agents (DCE-MRI) and those that do not (ASL).

Phase Contrast MRI

Phase contrast (PC) MRI is the current standard for the measurement of renal blood flow (RBF) in the renal artery and veins. It does not require contrast media and allows noninvasive measurement of RBF in each renal artery in a single two-dimensional slice (2D PC MRI) and recently also in the branches of the vessel of interest (4D flow MRI). PC MRI uses the velocity-induced phase changes of moving blood to quantify blood flow; a consensus paper has been published on renal phase contrast MRI methods [13]. PC MRI has been shown to correlate well with alternative non-MRI measures of renal blood flow [58]. Renal PC MRI is not yet being routinely used in clinical practice, but several studies support its clinical potential. Chapter 15 provides a comprehensive overview of PC MRI and MRA of the renal arteries.

Arterial Spin Labeling

Arterial spin labeling (ASL) uses magnetically labeled water protons in blood that act as a diffusible tracer, providing an alternative to exogenous intravenous contrast. Due to its high physiologic perfusion (both kidneys receive 20% of the cardiac output but their total weight is only ~300 g), the kidney is an ideal candidate for perfusion imaging by ASL. ASL uses the water spins of blood as an endogenous tracer. Tissue perfusion is determined by subtracting control images (no labeling applied to arterial blood) from the labeled image (radiofrequency magnetic labeling). The difference between a labeled image and a non-labeled image can be used to calculate tissue perfusion. While MRI can measure renal perfusion with or without exogenous contrast agents, non-contrast techniques may be preferable due to the risk of nephrogenic systemic fibrosis associated with gadolinium-based contrast agents in patients with renal insufficiency and in the setting of longitudinal monitoring. Animal studies have shown that ASL can detect changes in renal perfusion commensurate with the degree of induced ischemia, which correlate with histological damage and change in renal function [59]. Human renal ASL has been applied in a variety of kidney diseases including CKD, AKI, diabetes, hypertension, lupus nephritis, and renovascular disease [60]. All of the studies have consistently shown that the RBF in the renal cortex is reduced in CKD compared to healthy volunteers [61–63]. Furthermore, the RBF has been shown to decrease with increasing stages of CKD and correlate to eGFR [64]. ASL has also been used in AKI; Dong et al. reported a reduction in both cortical and medullary perfusions in a group of 11 patients with AKI mostly due to intrinsic renal disease [65]. Buchanan et al. [66] also showed a reduction in cortical perfusion in AKI; however, the cross-sectional nature of the study obscured the relationship between ASL measurements and renal recovery.

In renal transplant patients, Heusch et al. employed ASL in a heterogeneous group of 98 renal transplant patients who underwent MRI ASL between 3 days and 11 years after renal transplantation [67]. Despite the wide variation in patient selection, the results demonstrated that renal perfusion was lower in those patients with lower eGFR values. Similar associations between a reduction in perfusion and GFR have been shown in a cross-sectional study of renal transplant patients [68].

It is promising that the clinical studies employing ASL have so far produced relatively consistent results and the technique has great potential. However, there are still technical considerations that need to be addressed before ASL can become more widely utilized [14], including the variation in ASL acquisition schemes that may prevent comparison between different techniques and between different MRI platforms, differences in post processing, and complex analysis requirements. For a detailed review of ASL methods, see Chap. 19.

Dynamic Contrast-Enhanced MRI

Dynamic contrast-enhanced (DCE) MRI monitors the transit of contrast agents, typically gadolinium chelates, through the intrarenal regions, the renal cortex, the medulla, and the collecting system. In this way, DCE MRI reveals the renal uptake and excretion of the contrast agent. By analyzing the enhancement of the renal tissues as a function of time, one can determine indirect measures of clinically important single-kidney parameters as the renal blood flow, glomerular filtration rate, and intrarenal blood volume. Zollner et al. investigated the results of different pharmacokinetic models in a quantitative analysis of renal blood flow (RBF) and GFR in an animal model of AKI using deconvolution analysis and a two-compartment renal filtration model [69]. Significant differences between control and AKI animals were detected by functional parameters (GFR and RBF), suggesting that this technique is useful to determine renal damage as evidenced by spatially resolved abnormal changes in renal tissue. Not only does DCE MRI provide functional information, but it can provide detailed structural information about the kidneys. For example, Woodard et al. used DCE MRI to automatically estimate the volume of cortex, medulla, collecting system, fat, and fibrosis based on the patterns of tissue enhancement following gadolinium administration [70].

Opinion is still divided as to the extent to which these techniques should be utilized in patients with impaired renal function in view of the association of gadolinium and nephrogenic systemic fibrosis, but otherwise DCE MRI is clearly useful for the diagnosis of renal function and for assessing treatment response and post-transplant rejection. Recent studies are therefore limited to those patients with less severe reductions in eGFR and are less numerous as compared to those employing ASL techniques.

Understanding the Biological Specificity of Multiparametric Renal MRI Measures

Renal MRI measures are often equated with a given pathophysiological outcome, such as T_2* with oxygenation and T_1 and ADC with interstitial fibrosis. However, it is important to recognize that a given renal MRI measure is often inherently nonspecific and the relationship between MRI measures is complex due to their sensitivity to many pathophysiological processes. It is important to be aware of this limitation when interpreting results.

The transverse relaxation time T_2* is primarily used in BOLD imaging to indirectly quantify renal oxygenation and hypoxia due to its sensitivity to the oxygenation of blood because of the paramagnetic properties of deoxygenated hemoglobin. However, T_2* is not specific and is also strongly sensitive to renal blood volume, renal blood flow, and tubular function and microstructure [49], and this is likely to play a role in the differences between individuals. BOLD cannot distinguish between renal injuries that affect perfusion from those that affect oxygen consumption. For example, BOLD findings interpreted as confirmation that hypoxia is a driver for CKD progression [71] could also be caused by a reduction of perfusion, and it has been shown that the presence of edema in AKI can compromise the interpretation of BOLD measures [66].

Another example is that of the measurement of fibrosis, which reduces ADC by creating barriers to water mobility in the extracellular space. However, this does not necessarily translate to the kidneys, which under normal conditions have a very small cortical interstitium. While MRE-determined stiffness correlates with the level of fibrosis, it should be recognized that MRE-derived stiffness measurements are not solely dependent on renal fibrosis, and reductions in renal blood flow could mitigate increases in the fibrosis-associated intrinsic stiffness. Garcia et al. [72] used multifrequency MRE (tomoelastography) in patients with lupus nephritis (LN) and found that the MRE-derived stiffness values decreased with increasing CKD stage in the medulla and inner cortex compared to healthy controls. Importantly, the diagnostic accuracy of CKD staging increased when MRE results were coupled with BOLD and DWI compared to MRE alone, highlighting the need for using multiparametric MRI for diagnosis of renal fibrosis.

A priority in renal MRI research must therefore be to improve the specificity to individual biological processes and understanding of how these interact. This will be facilitated by the introduction of other MRI sequences in multiparametric MRI measures which might increase the specificity of MRI as a diagnostic tool, along with associations with histology through biopsy or ex vivo tissue [17, 73, 74].

Combining Information from Multiparametric Renal MRI

Renal MRI can be performed with 1.5 and 3 Tesla (T), although studies have shown the benefits of 3 Tesla for SNR, examination time, and spatial resolution. Most recent studies implementing multiparametric renal MRI comprise a combination of more than one technique of DWI, BOLD, and T_1 and T_2 mapping, volumetric analysis and phase contrast MRI, and less frequently ASL, DTI, MT, and MRE. The choice of MRI biomarkers depends on the clinical question, availability of methods, and scan time allowed. Using the combination of renal MRI techniques to assess changes in perfusion, diffusion, oxygenation, kidney volume, and tissue structure is a promising approach to gain deep insight into the potential of specificity to the individual biological process of each measure and understanding of how the measures interact. For example, it may be possible to build a discrete signature for pathological processes derived such as interstitial fibrosis (IF). Since properties such as cortical perfusion, magnetization transfer, and diffusion tensor imaging are all correlated with IF, they could potentially improve the specificity further.

For quantitative analysis of multiparametric fMRI in the kidneys, organ segmentation is required for the assessment of total kidney volume (TKV). Additionally, definition of the kidney compartments of the cortex and medulla is an essential step to evaluate multiparametric maps. To date, manual segmentation has been the prevalent segmentation technique in renal MRI studies since renal parenchyma is difficult to differentiate from the surrounding organs and structures using signal intensity alone. However, for clinical use of renal fMRI, this time-consuming and laborious method needs to be replaced by more efficient automated segmentation deep learning (DL) techniques to deal with the complex multiparametric datasets. DL has been applied in studies for segmentation of the kidneys to estimate TKV measures [26, 27] or T_1-weighted measures for assessment of cortical thickness. Volume measures are key in patients with autosomal dominant polycystic kidney disease. For the study of spatial variability in multiparametric renal MRI, this poses challenges for data analysis regarding the registration of different MRI measures, which have heterogenous image contrasts. Further motion due to breathing can lead to a considerable variation in the position of the kidneys not only between renal MRI measures but also within measurements. Image registration can perform spatial alignment of kidney images to enable further processing steps. Furthermore, kidneys can vary dramatically in their anatomical position, size, and features, such as cysts. DL seems especially promising to boost further development and the path to the clinical routine. Renal image processing is important and needs further investigation to help in automating the processing of multiparametric renal image data and to derive possible biomarker candidates.

Further, renal multiparametric MRI measures can also be combined with blood- and urine-based biomarkers and clinical information, for example, not only GFR and albuminuria but urine and blood injury markers which may provide an additional way of establishing biological validity (e.g., neutrophil gelatinase-associated lipocalin, kidney injury molecule-1). In summary, combining information across measures will provide deep insight into individual biological process and understanding of how measures interact.

Renal Multiparametric MRI Measures in Clinical Studies

Multiparametric fMRI has recently been applied to examine patients with transplants [75], chronic kidney disease [53, 54, 64, 76–79], acute kidney injury [66], IgA nephropathy [80], autosomal dominant (ADPKD) and autosomal recessive polycystic kidney disease (ARPKD) [81], and interstitial renal fibrosis [82], as well as in patients with coronavirus disease 2019 (COVID-19) [83–85].

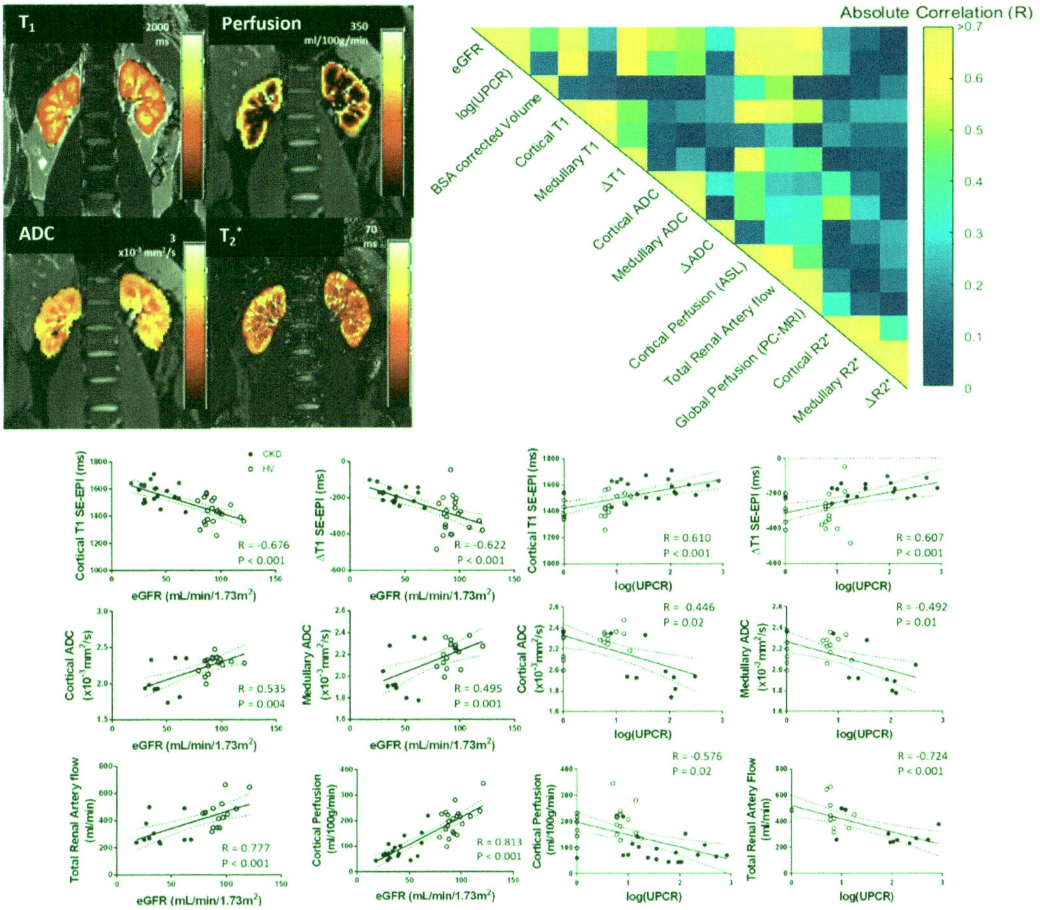

Fig. 7.3 Correlation matrix for combined healthy volunteer (HV) and chronic kidney disease (CKD) groups of biochemical measures [eGFR and log (UPCR)] and multiparametric MRI measures, taken from Buchanan et al. [64]. Significant correlations of MRI measures with biochemical measures are shown. Between the multiparametric MRI measures, significant correlations are observed between cortical T_1 and cortical perfusion ($R = -0.595$, $P < 0.001$), total renal artery blood flow ($R = -0.655$, $P < 0.001$), and global perfusion ($R = -0.435$, $P = 0.001$) and between T_1 CMD ($\Delta T1$) and cortical perfusion ($R = -0.587$, $P < 0.001$), and total renal artery blood flow ($R = -0.397$, $P = 0.05$). Correlations are also seen between cortical ADC and cortical perfusion ($R = 0.452$, $P = 0.02$). Between hemodynamic measures, significant correlations were observed between cortical perfusion and total renal artery flow ($R = 0.596$, $P = 0.002$) and cortical perfusion and global perfusion ($R = 0.44$, $P = 0.04$)

Bane et al. [75] used 1.5 Tesla DWI and DTI, BOLD R_2*, and T_1 to assess renal transplant dysfunction with fibrosis. The combination of cortical ADC and T_1 measurements showed promising results for the noninvasive assessment of renal allograft histology and outcomes. Cortical ADC, D, medullary ADC, and corticomedullary differentiation (CMD) in T_1 were significantly decreased, and cortical T_1 was significantly elevated in fibrotic allografts. The combination of CMD T_1 and cortical ADC had excellent diagnostic performance for detection of chronic dysfunction with fibrosis, while cortical ADC and T_1 had good performance for predicting eGFR decline at 18 months.

In CKD, Buchanan et al. [64] showed using renal MRI at 3 Tesla that ADC, T_1, and cortical perfusion are all associated with IF, as illustrated in Fig. 7.3. Berchtold et al. [5] found that CMD in ADC and T_1 and eGFR were independently correlated with IF. Zhang et al. combined IVIM diffusion-weighted imaging and MRE, and multiple linear regression models were performed to evaluate the correlations between MRI parameters and histology variables [45]. Sugiyama et al. [71] performed a longitudinal study of multiparametric renal MRI measures in CKD, supporting that multiparametric renal MRI can not only improve specificity but also lead to added clinical utility. In a multivariate analysis, baseline eGFR, level of proteinuria, and renal T_2* were independent predictors of the eGFR slope. T_2* was predictive of eGFR decline but did not correlate well with eGFR at baseline, whereas ADC correlated well with eGFR at baseline but was not predictive of eGFR decline. This shows that cross-sectional analyses should evaluate measures that are orthogonal as well as correlated with eGFR. Inoue et al. [86] compared several multiparametric MRI sequences. Using principal component analysis, they showed a similarity between T_1 values and tissue perfusion (ASL) and between FA (DTI) and ADC values (DWI). In multiple regression analysis, only T_2* values, derived from BOLD MRI, were associated with eGFR slope after adjusting for degree of proteinuria, a classic prognostic factor for CKD. Dillman et al. [76] performed quantitative multiparametric MRI in children and young adults with CKD compared to age-matched controls. They showed that renal T_1 relaxation and DWI ADC measurements differ between pediatric healthy controls and CKD patients, correlate with laboratory markers of CKD, and may have histologic correlates. Srivastava et al. [87] assessed ADC and BOLD imaging at baseline and at 12 months in 122 CKD participants in the multicenter, multiparametric trial of CKD Optimal Management with Binders and Nicotinamide (COMBINE) trial [NCT02258074] with results published in *CJASN*. They showed that baseline ADC was associated with change in eGFR over time, but this association was no longer significant after further adjustment for albuminuria. However, these authors found that there was no significant association between baseline R_2* and change in eGFR over time. Li et al. [79] performed DTI to measure FA, and TKV was obtained from DTI and T2WI in CKD. Medullary FA values (m-FA), TKV, and the product of the m-FA values and TKV (m-FA-TKV) were significantly correlated with eGFR ($r = 0.653$, 0.685, and 0.797, respectively, all $P < 0.001$). Receiver operating characteristic curve analysis showed that m-FA-TKV exhibited better diagnostic performance than m-FA values ($P = 0.022$). In Lang et al. [80] multiparametric MRI was used to study advanced stage immunoglobulin A nephropathy (IgAN) using tomoelastography, DWI, and BOLD. Shear wave speed was decreased in IgAN (−21%, $P < 0.0001$), accompanied by lower apparent diffusion coefficient values (−12%, $P = 0.004$), but BOLD imaging was not sensitive to IgAN ($P = 0.12$).

Multiparametric functional renal MRI has not been extensively studied in patients with AKI. The only study of multiparametric renal MRI in AKI is by Buchanan et al. [64]. This study identified significant increases in TKV, T_1 relaxation time, and cortical perfusion that gradually improved during recovery from AKI. Interestingly, by three months serum creatinine had returned to normal in all subjects, but the MRI parameters remained abnormal in some. Coronavirus disease 2019 (COVID-19) caused by a novel coronavirus called severe acute respiratory syndrome coronavirus 2 (SARS-CoV-2) is known to attack the lungs, but other organs such as the kidneys can also be damaged, with proximal acute tubule injury and endothelial cell swelling of the kidneys reported in pathological examinations. AKI is independently associated with increased mortality in hospitalized patients with COVID-19 and may result in higher odds of death than AKI due to other causes, and AKI also increases the risk of impaired kidney function in surviving patients after the acute phase of COVID-19 [88]. A prospective case-control study has investigated differences in renal perfusion, oxygenation, and water diffusion using multiparametric renal MRI in critically ill COVID-19 patients with and without AKI. Total renal blood flow was lower in patients with AKI compared with patients without AKI, and regional perfusion was reduced in both cortex and medulla. Renal venous saturation was similar in both groups, as was regional oxygenation (R_2*). Thus this study concluded that in critically ill COVID-19 patients with AKI, the total, cortical, and medullary renal blood flow are reduced compared with similar patients without AKI, whereas no differences in renal oxygenation were demonstrable in this setting [89]. In studies of recovered COVID-19 participants compared to normal volunteers, increased ADC and f values from both the renal cortex and medulla were observed. Also, renal cortical T_1 and corticomedullary differentiation, markers of renal injury/fibro-inflammation, have been shown to be abnormal in patients, with a significantly higher renal cortical T_1 in 29% of patients [83–85, 90].

Multiparametric renal MRI is now beginning to be used for clinical trials. For example, the TOP-CKD clinical trial [ClinicalTrials.gov Identifier: NCT04258397] is a randomized, double-blind, placebo-controlled interventional study, a phase 2 trial of pirfenidone versus placebo in CKD. One primary outcome is DWI as a measure of kidney fibrosis to evaluate pirfenidone as a potential new treatment for patients with CKD. Renal MRI is also being used to improve understanding of the pathophysiology of the sodium/glucose cotransporter 2 (SGLT2) inhibitor [91] which has been shown to have cardiorenal protective properties through mechanisms beyond glucose control. Zanchi et al. [92] used BOLD to study the cortical and medullary renal oxygenation in response to the acute or chronic administration of empagliflozin [ClinicalTrials.gov Identifier: NCT03093103]. The authors found no acute or sustained changes in renal cortical or medullary tissue oxygenation. A currently ongoing sub-study of the EMPA-KIDNEY trial [ClinicalTrials.gov Identifier: NCT03594110] is performing a full multiparametric protocol (including T_1, DWI, BOLD, and renal perfusion alongside cardiac MRI); results are yet to be published.

Challenges to Clinical Translational Renal MRI

A number of challenges must be resolved before renal MRI techniques can become commonplace in the clinical environment. One key challenge in clinical translation of renal MRI biomarkers is building evidence of clinical utility on scale and with rigor.

The first steps in scaling up the level of evidence are the creation of a more harmonized and standardized approach to data collection across MRI vendors and assessing the repeatability of renal MRI measures as performed in recent studies at 1.5 and 3 Tesla [54, 93]. MRI sequences are complex and depend on many parameters that must be optimized and fine-tuned separately. Many of the newer MRI techniques (such as ASL and T_1 mapping) are not standardized and are currently performed only in dedicated research centers due to the need for a specialized scan. The lack of readily available and generally accepted protocols also creates barriers for new groups and clinical sites, often requiring extensive and costly in-house optimization.

In addition to scan capabilities, methods are needed for data handling, quality assurance, processing, and analysis for the development of multicenter studies. For successful application of multiparametric fMRI protocols in the clinical routine and studies of large patient cohorts in the future, standardized data post-processing and data analysis workflows are needed. This is one of the main limiting factors for use in clinical practice, since it can have a significant impact on data interpretation. Recent advances in deep learning artificial neural networks show great potential for medical imaging technology, data analysis, and diagnostics and might substantially impact the future of healthcare. Patient preparation is an issue, as some parameters are sensitive to external factors; for example, R_2* values are influenced by dietary sodium intake, glycemia, and hydration status. ADC is on the basis of the degree of movement of water molecules in tissues; the latter is not only influenced by tissue fibrosis but also by capillary density or tubular flow (and thus possibly by diuretics). All these factors need to be taken into account when performing functional renal MRI. Further, different magnetic resonance sequences are used by distinctive vendors and centers, and image analysis is not always performed in the same way. The functional renal MRI community is aware of these issues, and the chapters presented in this book are an attempt to help standardize the acquisition and post-processing methods. We have written the book chapters to be a "how-to-do" recipe book on acquisition and data analysis for clinical practice.

The standardization of acquisition and analysis measures is also one of the aims of the UKRIN_MAPS project. The AFiRM (Application of Functional Renal MRI to improve assessment of chronic kidney disease) study [ClinicalTrials.gov Identifier: NCT04238299] is an example of such a clinical study that is underway using the UKRIN_MAPS protocol. This multicenter cohort study is using multiparametric MRI to assess different aspects of kidney structure and function in 450 people with CKD. This comprises structural images, angiography, phase contrast, ASL, BOLD-MRI, DWI and DTI, MTR, and mDIXON measures within a one-hour scan protocol, allowing the relation of MRI results to histology, measured GFR, and progression of CKD over the subsequent 2 years. The overarching aim of the AFiRM study is to determine if multiparametric renal MRI can provide structural and functional assessment of the kidneys in people with CKD that will (1) provide prognostic information and (2) guide treatment options. The prognostic imaging biomarkers for diabetic kidney disease (iBEAt) study of the BEAt-DKD project [94] [ClinicalTrials.gov Identifier: NCT03716401] aims to determine whether renal imaging biomarkers (MRI and ultrasound) provide insight into the pathogenesis and heterogeneity of diabetic kidney disease (DKD) and whether they have potential as prognostic biomarkers in DKD. Finally, in view of the high cost of MRI, the cost-effectiveness of MRI measures and the additional information they provide are key factors in determining their eventual utility in clinical practice. A health economic analysis would be required to evaluate the use of MRI screening to potentially identify those patients at risk of rapid progression.

Conclusion

MRI has been used for many years to depict the anatomy of the kidney. Recent, exciting advances in quantitative multiparametric renal MRI illustrate that complementary measures of kidney structure and function are now possible within a single MR scan session that may provide unparalleled insights into the pathophysiology of renal disease. Ultimately, the aim of developing multiparametric quantitative MRI of the kidneys is not to replace established techniques such as ultrasonography and renal scintigraphy but to broaden and improve renal imaging and help clinicians and patients in the treatment of kidney diseases. The techniques must now be tested in clinical studies; this will be essential prior to translation to clinical practice. Ultimately, multiparametric evaluation could allow for recognition of patterns in MRI parameters characteristic of different pathologies. Future research should focus on improving the characterization of measurement uncertainty, standardization of measurement methods, larger and longitudinal clinical studies in well-defined phenotypes, improving specificity by multiparametric and multimodal signatures, and modeling of potential cost-effectiveness.

References

1. Bae KT, Commean PK, Lee J. Volumetric measurement of renal cysts and parenchyma using MRI: phantoms and patients with polycystic kidney disease. J Comput Assist Tomogr. 2000;24(4):614–9.
2. Christensen RH, Lundgren T, Stenvinkel P, Brismar TB. Renal volumetry with magnetic resonance imaging. Acta Radiol Open. 2017;6(9):2058460117731120.
3. Will S, Martirosian P, Wurslin C, Schick F. Automated segmentation and volumetric analysis of renal cortex, medulla, and pelvis based on non-contrast-enhanced T1- and T2-weighted MR images. MAGMA. 2014;27(5):445–54.
4. Dekkers IA, de Boer A, Sharma K, Cox EF, Lamb HJ, Buckley DL, et al. Consensus-based technical recommendations for clinical translation of renal T1 and T2 mapping MRI. MAGMA. 2020;33(1):163–76.
5. Berchtold L, Friedli I, Crowe LA, Martinez C, Moll S, Hadaya K, et al. Validation of the corticomedullary difference in magnetic resonance imaging-derived apparent diffusion coefficient for kidney fibrosis detection: a cross-sectional study. Nephrol Dial Transplant. 2020;35(6):937–45.
6. Blondin D, Lanzman RS, Mathys C, Grotemeyer D, Voiculescu A, Sandmann W, et al. [Functional MRI of transplanted kidneys using diffusion-weighted imaging]. Rofo. 2009;181(12):1162–1167.
7. Caroli A, Schneider M, Friedli I, Ljimani A, De Seigneux S, Boor P, et al. Diffusion-weighted mag-

netic resonance imaging to assess diffuse renal pathology: a systematic review and statement paper. Nephrol Dial Transplant. 2018;33(suppl_2):ii29–40.
8. Friedli I, Crowe LA, Berchtold L, Moll S, Hadaya K, de Perrot T, et al. New magnetic resonance imaging index for renal fibrosis assessment: a comparison between diffusion-weighted imaging and T1 mapping with histological validation. Sci Rep. 2016;6:30088.
9. Hueper K, Hartung D, Gutberlet M, Gueler F, Sann H, Husen B, et al. Magnetic resonance diffusion tensor imaging for evaluation of histopathological changes in a rat model of diabetic nephropathy. Invest Radiol. 2012;47(7):430–7.
10. Ljimani A, Caroli A, Laustsen C, Francis S, Mendichovszky IA, Bane O, et al. Consensus-based technical recommendations for clinical translation of renal diffusion-weighted MRI. MAGMA. 2020;33(1):177–95.
11. Mao W, Zhou J, Zeng M, Ding Y, Qu L, Chen C, et al. Intravoxel incoherent motion diffusion-weighted imaging for the assessment of renal fibrosis of chronic kidney disease: a preliminary study. Magn Reson Imaging. 2018;47:118–24.
12. Zhao J, Wang ZJ, Liu M, Zhu J, Zhang X, Zhang T, et al. Assessment of renal fibrosis in chronic kidney disease using diffusion-weighted MRI. Clin Radiol. 2014;69(11):1117–22.
13. de Boer A, Villa G, Bane O, Bock M, Cox EF, Dekkers IA, et al. Consensus-based technical recommendations for clinical translation of renal phase contrast MRI. J Magn Reson Imaging. 2022;55(2):323–35.
14. Nery F, Buchanan CE, Harteveld AA, Odudu A, Bane O, Cox EF, et al. Consensus-based technical recommendations for clinical translation of renal ASL MRI. MAGMA. 2020;33(1):141–61.
15. Jiang K, Ferguson CM, Ebrahimi B, Tang H, Kline TL, Burningham TA, et al. Noninvasive assessment of renal fibrosis with magnetization transfer MR imaging: validation and evaluation in murine renal artery stenosis. Radiology. 2017;283(1):77–86.
16. Hectors SJ, Bane O, Kennedy P, El Salem F, Menon M, Segall M, et al. T1rho mapping for assessment of renal allograft fibrosis. J Magn Reson Imaging. 2019;50(4):1085–91.
17. Xie L, Bennett KM, Liu C, Johnson GA, Zhang JL, Lee VS. MRI tools for assessment of microstructure and nephron function of the kidney. Am J Physiol Renal Physiol. 2016;311(6):F1109–F24.
18. Xie L, Lee VS, Wei H, Qi Y, Gurley SB, Johnson GA, et al. Quantitative susceptibility mapping of kidney injury in a model of ischemia reperfusion. ISMRM conference; May 2016; Singapore. 2016.
19. Hueper K, Khalifa AA, Brasen JH, Vo Chieu VD, Gutberlet M, Wintterle S, et al. Diffusion-weighted imaging and diffusion tensor imaging detect delayed graft function and correlate with allograft fibrosis in patients early after kidney transplantation. J Magn Reson Imaging. 2016;44(1):112–21.
20. Kirpalani A, Hashim E, Leung G, Kim JK, Krizova A, Jothy S, et al. Magnetic resonance elastography to assess fibrosis in kidney allografts. Clin J Am Soc Nephrol. 2017;12(10):1671–9.
21. Kim JK, Yuen DA, Leung G, Jothy S, Zaltzman J, Ramesh Prasad GV, et al. Role of magnetic resonance elastography as a noninvasive measurement tool of fibrosis in a renal allograft: a case report. Transplant Proc. 2017;49(7):1555–9.
22. Serai SD, Yin M. MR elastography of the abdomen: basic concepts. Methods Mol Biol. 2021;2216:301–23.
23. Mendichovszky I, Pullens P, Dekkers I, Nery F, Bane O, Pohlmann A, et al. Technical recommendations for clinical translation of renal MRI: a consensus project of the cooperation in science and technology action PARENCHIMA. MAGMA. 2020;33(1):131–40.
24. Ljimani A, Caroli A, Laustsen C, Francis S, Mendichovszky IA, Bane O, et al. Correction to: consensus-based technical recommendations for clinical translation of renal diffusion-weighted MRI. MAGMA. 2020;33(1):197–8.
25. Bane O, Mendichovszky IA, Milani B, Dekkers IA, Deux JF, Eckerbom P, et al. Consensus-based technical recommendations for clinical translation of renal BOLD MRI. MAGMA. 2020;33(1):199–215.
26. Daniel AJ, Buchanan CE, Allcock T, Scerri D, Cox EF, Prestwich BL, et al. Automated renal segmentation in healthy and chronic kidney disease subjects using a convolutional neural network. Magn Reson Med. 2021;86(2):1125–36.
27. Langner T, Ostling A, Maldonis L, Karlsson A, Olmo D, Lindgren D, et al. Kidney segmentation in neck-to-knee body MRI of 40,000 UK biobank participants. Sci Rep. 2020;10(1):20963.
28. Perrone RD, Mouksassi MS, Romero K, Czerwiec FS, Chapman AB, Gitomer BY, et al. Total kidney volume is a prognostic biomarker of renal function decline and progression to end-stage renal disease in patients with autosomal dominant polycystic kidney disease. Kidney Int Rep. 2017;2(3):442–50.
29. Tangri N, Hougen I, Alam A, Perrone R, McFarlane P, Pei Y. Total kidney volume as a biomarker of disease progression in autosomal dominant polycystic kidney disease. Can J Kidney Health Dis. 2017;4:2054358117693355.
30. Fogo AB. Mechanisms of progression of chronic kidney disease. Pediatr Nephrol. 2007;22(12):2011–22.
31. Li A, Yuan G, Hu Y, Shen Y, Hu X, Hu D, et al. Renal functional and interstitial fibrotic assessment with non-Gaussian diffusion kurtosis imaging. Insights Imaging. 2022;13(1):70.
32. Jellis CL, Kwon DH. Myocardial T1 mapping: modalities and clinical applications. Cardiovasc Diagn Ther. 2014;4(2):126–37.
33. Iles L, Pfluger H, Phrommintikul A, Cherayath J, Aksit P, Gupta SN, et al. Evaluation of diffuse myocardial fibrosis in heart failure with cardiac magnetic resonance contrast-enhanced T1 mapping. J Am Coll Cardiol. 2008;52(19):1574–80.
34. Hoad CL, Palaniyappan N, Kaye P, Chernova Y, James MW, Costigan C, et al. A study of T(1) relaxation time as a measure of liver fibrosis and the influence

of confounding histological factors. NMR Biomed. 2015;28(6):706–14.
35. Hueper K, Peperhove M, Rong S, Gerstenberg J, Mengel M, Meier M, et al. T1-mapping for assessment of ischemia-induced acute kidney injury and prediction of chronic kidney disease in mice. Eur Radiol. 2014;24(9):2252–60.
36. Breidthardt T, Cox EF, Squire I, Odudu A, Omar NF, Eldehni MT, et al. The pathophysiology of the chronic cardiorenal syndrome: a magnetic resonance imaging study. Eur Radiol. 2015;25(6):1684–91.
37. Wu J, Shi Z, Zhang Y, Yan J, Shang F, Wang Y, et al. Native T1 mapping in assessing kidney fibrosis for patients with chronic glomerulonephritis. Front Med (Lausanne). 2021;8:772326.
38. European Society of Radiology (ESR). Magnetic resonance fingerprinting—a promising new approach to obtain standardized imaging biomarkers from MRI. Insights Imaging. 2015;6(2):163–5.
39. Wolff SD, Balaban RS. Magnetization transfer contrast (MTC) and tissue water proton relaxation in vivo. Magn Reson Med. 1989;10(1):135–44.
40. Wang F, Jiang R, Takahashi K, Gore J, Harris RC, Takahashi T, et al. Longitudinal assessment of mouse renal injury using high-resolution anatomic and magnetization transfer MR imaging. Magn Reson Imaging. 2014;32(9):1125–32.
41. Wang F, Katagiri D, Li K, Takahashi K, Wang S, Nagasaka S, et al. Assessment of renal fibrosis in murine diabetic nephropathy using quantitative magnetization transfer MRI. Magn Reson Med. 2018;80(6):2655–69.
42. Deistung A, Schweser F, Reichenbach JR. Overview of quantitative susceptibility mapping. NMR Biomed. 2017;30(4):e3569.
43. Xie L, Sparks MA, Li W, Qi Y, Liu C, Coffman TM, et al. Quantitative susceptibility mapping of kidney inflammation and fibrosis in type 1 angiotensin receptor-deficient mice. NMR Biomed. 2013;26(12):1853–63.
44. Bechler E, Stabinska J, Thiel T, Jasse J, Zukovs R, Valentin B, et al. Feasibility of quantitative susceptibility mapping (QSM) of the human kidney. MAGMA. 2021;34(3):389–97.
45. Zhang J, Yu Y, Liu X, Tang X, Xu F, Zhang M, et al. Evaluation of renal fibrosis by mapping histology and magnetic resonance imaging. Kidney Dis (Basel). 2021;7(2):131–42.
46. Fine LOC, Norman JT. Progressive renal disease: the chronic hypoxia hypothesis. Kidney Int Suppl. 1998;65:74–8.
47. Venkatachalam MA, Griffin KA, Lan RP, Geng H, Saikumar P, Bidani AK. Acute kidney injury: a springboard for progression in chronic kidney disease. Am J Physiol Renal Physiol. 2010;298(5):F1078–94.
48. Neugarten J, Golestaneh L. Blood oxygenation level-dependent MRI for assessment of renal oxygenation. Int J Nephrol Renov Dis. 2014;7:421–35.
49. Pruijm M, Hofmann L, Piskunowicz M, Muller ME, Zweiacker C, Bassi I, et al. Determinants of renal tissue oxygenation as measured with BOLD-MRI in chronic kidney disease and hypertension in humans. PLoS One. 2014;9(4):e95895.
50. Zhang JL, Morrell G, Rusinek H, Sigmund EE, Chandarana H, Lerman LO, et al. New magnetic resonance imaging methods in nephrology. Kidney Int. 2014;85(4):768–78.
51. Michaely HJ, Metzger L, Haneder S, Hansmann J, Schoenberg SO, Attenberger UI. Renal BOLD-MRI does not reflect renal function in chronic kidney disease. Kidney Int. 2012;81(7):684–9.
52. Pruijm M, Mendichovszky IA, Liss P, Van der Niepen P, Textor SC, Lerman LO, et al. Renal blood oxygenation level-dependent magnetic resonance imaging to measure renal tissue oxygenation: a statement paper and systematic review. Nephrol Dial Transplant. 2018;33(suppl_2):ii22–8.
53. Li LP, Milani B, Pruijm M, Kohn O, Sprague S, Hack B, et al. Renal BOLD MRI in patients with chronic kidney disease: comparison of the semi-automated twelve layer concentric objects (TLCO) and manual ROI methods. MAGMA. 2020;33(1):113–20.
54. Cox EF, Buchanan CE, Bradley CR, Prestwich B, Mahmoud H, Taal M, et al. Multiparametric renal magnetic resonance imaging: validation, interventions, and alterations in chronic kidney disease. Front Physiol. 2017;8:696.
55. Piskunowicz M, Hofmann L, Zuercher E, Bassi I, Milani B, Stuber M, et al. A new technique with high reproducibility to estimate renal oxygenation using BOLD-MRI in chronic kidney disease. Magn Reson Imaging. 2015;33(3):253–61.
56. Liu P, Xu F, Lu H. Test-retest reproducibility of a rapid method to measure brain oxygen metabolism. Magn Reson Med. 2013;69(3):675–81.
57. Wang C, Zhang R, Jiang L, Wang R, Zhang X, Wang H, et al. MRI-based evaluation of renal oxygenation under the influence of carbogen breathing. ISMRM conference; May 2016; Singapore. 2016.
58. Liss P, Cox EF, Eckerbom P, Francis ST. Imaging of intrarenal haemodynamics and oxygen metabolism. Clin Exp Pharmacol Physiol. 2013;40(2):158–67.
59. Hueper K, Gutberlet M, Rong S, Hartung D, Mengel M, Lu X, et al. Acute kidney injury: arterial spin labeling to monitor renal perfusion impairment in mice-comparison with histopathologic results and renal function. Radiology. 2014;270(1):117–24.
60. Odudu A, Nery F, Harteveld AA, Evans RG, Pendse D, Buchanan CE, et al. Arterial spin labelling MRI to measure renal perfusion: a systematic review and statement paper. Nephrol Dial Transplant. 2018;33(suppl_2):ii15–21.
61. Mora-Gutierrez JM, Garcia-Fernandez N, Slon Roblero MF, Paramo JA, Escalada FJ, Wang DJ, et al. Arterial spin labeling MRI is able to detect early hemodynamic changes in diabetic nephropathy. J Magn Reson Imaging. 2017;46(6):1810–7.
62. Rossi C, Artunc F, Martirosian P, Schlemmer HP, Schick F, Boss A. Histogram analysis of renal arterial spin labeling perfusion data reveals differences

between volunteers and patients with mild chronic kidney disease. Invest Radiol. 2012;47(8):490–6.
63. Tan H, Koktzoglou I, Prasad PV. Renal perfusion imaging with two-dimensional navigator gated arterial spin labeling. Magn Reson Med. 2014;71(2):570–9.
64. Buchanan CE, Mahmoud H, Cox EF, McCulloch T, Prestwich BL, Taal MW, et al. Quantitative assessment of renal structural and functional changes in chronic kidney disease using multi-parametric magnetic resonance imaging. Nephrol Dial Transplant. 2020;35(6):955–64.
65. Dong J, Yang L, Su T, Yang X, Chen B, Zhang J, et al. Quantitative assessment of acute kidney injury by noninvasive arterial spin labeling perfusion MRI: a pilot study. Sci China Life Sci. 2013;56(8):745–50.
66. Buchanan C, Mahmoud H, Cox E, Noble R, Prestwich B, Kasmi I, et al. Multiparametric MRI assessment of renal structure and function in acute kidney injury and renal recovery. Clin Kidney J. 2021;14(8):1969–76.
67. Heusch P, Wittsack HJ, Blondin D, Ljimani A, Nguyen-Quang M, Martirosian P, et al. Functional evaluation of transplanted kidneys using arterial spin labeling MRI. J Magn Reson Imaging. 2014;40(1):84–9.
68. Tao Ren C-LW, Chen L-H, Xie S-S, Cheng Y, Fu Y-X, Oesingmann N, de Oliveira A, Zuo P-L, Yin J-Z, Xia S, Shen W. Evaluation of renal allografts function early after transplantation using intravoxel incoherent motion and arterial spin labeling MRI. Magn Reson Imaging. 2016;34:908–14.
69. Zollner FG, Zimmer F, Klotz S, Hoeger S, Schad LR. Functional imaging of acute kidney injury at 3 tesla: investigating multiple parameters using DCE-MRI and a two-compartment filtration model. Z Med Phys. 2015;25(1):58–65.
70. Woodard T, Sigurdsson S, Gotal JD, Torjesen AA, Inker LA, Aspelund T, et al. Segmental kidney volumes measured by dynamic contrast-enhanced magnetic resonance imaging and their association with CKD in older people. Am J Kidney Dis. 2015;65(1):41–8.
71. Sugiyama K, Inoue T, Kozawa E, Ishikawa M, Shimada A, Kobayashi N, et al. Reduced oxygenation but not fibrosis defined by functional magnetic resonance imaging predicts the long-term progression of chronic kidney disease. Nephrol Dial Transplant. 2020;35(6):964–70.
72. Marticorena Garcia SR, Grossmann M, Bruns A, Durr M, Tzschatzsch H, Hamm B, et al. Tomoelastography paired with T2* magnetic resonance imaging detects lupus nephritis with normal renal function. Invest Radiol. 2019;54(2):89–97.
73. Morozov D, Bar L, Sochen N, Cohen Y. Modeling of the diffusion MR signal in calibrated model systems and nerves. NMR Biomed. 2013;26(12):1787–95.
74. de Boer A, Pieters TT, Harteveld AA, Blankestijn PJ, Bos C, Froeling M, et al. Validation of multiparametric MRI by histopathology after nephrectomy: a case study. MAGMA. 2021;34(3):377–87.
75. Bane O, Hectors SJ, Gordic S, Kennedy P, Wagner M, Weiss A, et al. Multiparametric magnetic resonance imaging shows promising results to assess renal transplant dysfunction with fibrosis. Kidney Int. 2020;97(2):414–20.
76. Dillman JR, Benoit SW, Gandhi DB, Trout AT, Tkach JA, VandenHeuvel K, et al. Multiparametric quantitative renal MRI in children and young adults: comparison between healthy individuals and patients with chronic kidney disease. Abdom Radiol (NY). 2022;47(5):1840–52.
77. Sugiyama S, Yoshida A, Hieshima K, Kurinami N, Jinnouchi K, Tanaka M, et al. Initial acute decline in estimated glomerular filtration rate after sodium-glucose Cotransporter-2 inhibitor in patients with chronic kidney disease. J Clin Med Res. 2020;12(11):724–33.
78. Yu B, Huang C, Fan X, Li F, Zhang J, Song Z, et al. Application of MR imaging features in differentiation of renal changes in patients with stage III type 2 diabetic nephropathy and normal subjects. Front Endocrinol (Lausanne). 2022;13:846407.
79. Li XS, Zhang QJ, Zhu J, Zhou QQ, Yu YS, Hu ZC, et al. Assessment of kidney function in chronic kidney disease by combining diffusion tensor imaging and total kidney volume. Int Urol Nephrol. 2022;54(2):385–93.
80. Lang ST, Guo J, Bruns A, Durr M, Braun J, Hamm B, et al. Multiparametric quantitative MRI for the detection of IgA nephropathy using tomoelastography, DWI, and BOLD imaging. Invest Radiol. 2019;54(10):669–74.
81. MacAskill CJ, Erokwu BO, Markley M, Parsons A, Farr S, Zhang Y, et al. Multi-parametric MRI of kidney disease progression for autosomal recessive polycystic kidney disease: mouse model and initial patient results. Pediatr Res. 2021;89(1):157–62.
82. Zhang J, Zhang LJ. Functional MRI as a tool for evaluating interstitial fibrosis and prognosis in kidney disease. Kidney Dis (Basel). 2020;6(1):7–12.
83. Han Q, Lu Y, Wang D, Zhao Y, Li X, Mei N, et al. Assessment of dynamic hepatic and renal imaging changes in COVID-19 survivors using T1 mapping and IVIM-DWI. Abdom Radiol (NY). 2022;47(5):1817–27.
84. Dennis A, Wamil M, Alberts J, Oben J, Cuthbertson DJ, Wootton D, et al. Multiorgan impairment in low-risk individuals with post-COVID-19 syndrome: a prospective, community-based study. BMJ Open. 2021;11(3):e048391.
85. Raman B, Cassar MP, Tunnicliffe EM, Filippini N, Griffanti L, Alfaro-Almagro F, et al. Medium-term effects of SARS-CoV-2 infection on multiple vital organs, exercise capacity, cognition, quality of life and mental health, post-hospital discharge. EClinicalMedicine. 2021;31:100683.
86. Inoue T, Kozawa E, Ishikawa M, Fukaya D, Amano H, Watanabe Y, et al. Comparison of multiparametric magnetic resonance imaging sequences with labora-

tory parameters for prognosticating renal function in chronic kidney disease. Sci Rep. 2021;11(1):22129.
87. Srivastava A, Cai X, Lee J, Li W, Larive B, Kendrick C, et al. Kidney functional magnetic resonance imaging and change in eGFR in individuals with CKD. Clin J Am Soc Nephrol. 2020;15(6):776–83.
88. Kolhe NV, Fluck RJ, Selby NM, Taal MW. Acute kidney injury associated with COVID-19: a retrospective cohort study. PLoS Med. 2020;17(10):e1003406.
89. Cox E, Luther T, Eckerbom P, Weis J, Palm F, Frithiof R, et al., editors. Inflammation and reduced cortical perfusion in kidneys of critically ill Covid-19 patients. International Society for Magnetic Resonance in Medicine; 2022.
90. Hultström M, Lipcsey M, Wallin E, Larsson IM, Larsson A, Frithiof R. Severe acute kidney injury associated with progression of chronic kidney disease after critical COVID-19. Crit Care. 2021;25(1):37.
91. van der Hoek S, Stevens J. Current use and complementary value of combining in vivo imaging modalities to understand the renoprotective effects of sodium-glucose cotransporter-2 inhibitors at a tissue level. Front Pharmacol. 2022;13:837993.
92. Zanchi A, Burnier M, Muller ME, Ghajarzadeh-Wurzner A, Maillard M, Loncle N, et al. Acute and chronic effects of SGLT2 inhibitor Empagliflozin on renal oxygenation and blood pressure control in nondiabetic normotensive subjects: a randomized, placebo-controlled trial. J Am Heart Assoc. 2020;9(13):e016173.
93. de Boer A, Harteveld AA, Stemkens B, Blankestijn PJ, Bos C, Franklin SL, et al. Multiparametric renal MRI: an intrasubject test-retest repeatability study. J Magn Reson Imaging. 2021;53(3):859–73.
94. Gooding KM, Lienczewski C, Papale M, Koivuviita N, Maziarz M, Dutius Andersson AM, et al. Prognostic imaging biomarkers for diabetic kidney disease (iBEAt): study protocol. BMC Nephrol. 2020;21(1):242.

T_1 Mapping of the Kidney

8

Matthew D. Robson, Carolina C. Fernandes, Rui Teixeira, and Elizabeth M. Tunnicliffe

Introduction

Of all the MRI contrast mechanisms for renal imaging, T_1 was the one that was discovered earliest and has remained in continual use through the use of T_1-weighted images. In the kidney, this contrast mechanism differentiates the perirenal fat, sinus fat, blood vessels, medulla, and cortex. One of the diagnostic criteria for kidney disease is the elevation of the cortical T_1 bringing its value close to that of the medulla, yielding a decrease in cortical medulla differentiation (CMD) in T_1-weighted images.

T_1 mapping of the kidney was reported as early as 1984 [1] when relaxation value measurement was of interest, but subsequently spatial resolution was prioritized, with "weighted" images found to offer diagnostic sensitivity and adopted by the radiology community. In kidney MRI, measurement of the T_1 relaxation time of water molecules may provide a valuable biomarker for a variety of pathological conditions. Due to its sensitivity to the tissue microenvironment, T_1 has gained substantial interest for noninvasive imaging of kidney pathology, including inflammation and fibrosis. More recently, with the clinical availability of rapid T_1 mapping, this approach is enjoying an epiphany. Quantitative mapping has the benefit over T_1 weighting of enabling standardized thresholds to be used, which ensures best practice. Further, quantitative measurement facilitates monitoring of change over time, which is especially valuable in clinical trials.

In this chapter, we focus on the native T_1 (i.e., without additional MRI contrast agents) and describe how to acquire and process standardized T_1 maps of the kidney, the level of precision available, and the pitfalls.

Part I: MRI Physics and Acquisition Protocols

This section explains the source of T_1 image contrast and how to acquire these data.

Origins of T_1

T_1 relaxation time is a fundamental parameter in MRI relating to the interaction and energy exchange between the hydrogen atoms (also known as protons) and their surrounding environment. In this section, we will describe what T_1 is,

M. D. Robson (✉) · C. C. Fernandes · R. Teixeira
Perspectum Ltd., Oxford, Oxfordshire, UK
e-mail: matthew.robson@perspectum.com; carolina.fernandes@perspectum.com

E. M. Tunnicliffe
The University of Oxford Centre for Clinical Magnetic Resonance Research (OCMR), University of Oxford, Oxford, Oxfordshire, UK
e-mail: elizabeth.tunnicliffe@cardiov.ox.ac.uk

S. D. Serai, K. Darge (eds.), *Advanced Clinical MRI of the Kidney*,
https://doi.org/10.1007/978-3-031-40169-5_8

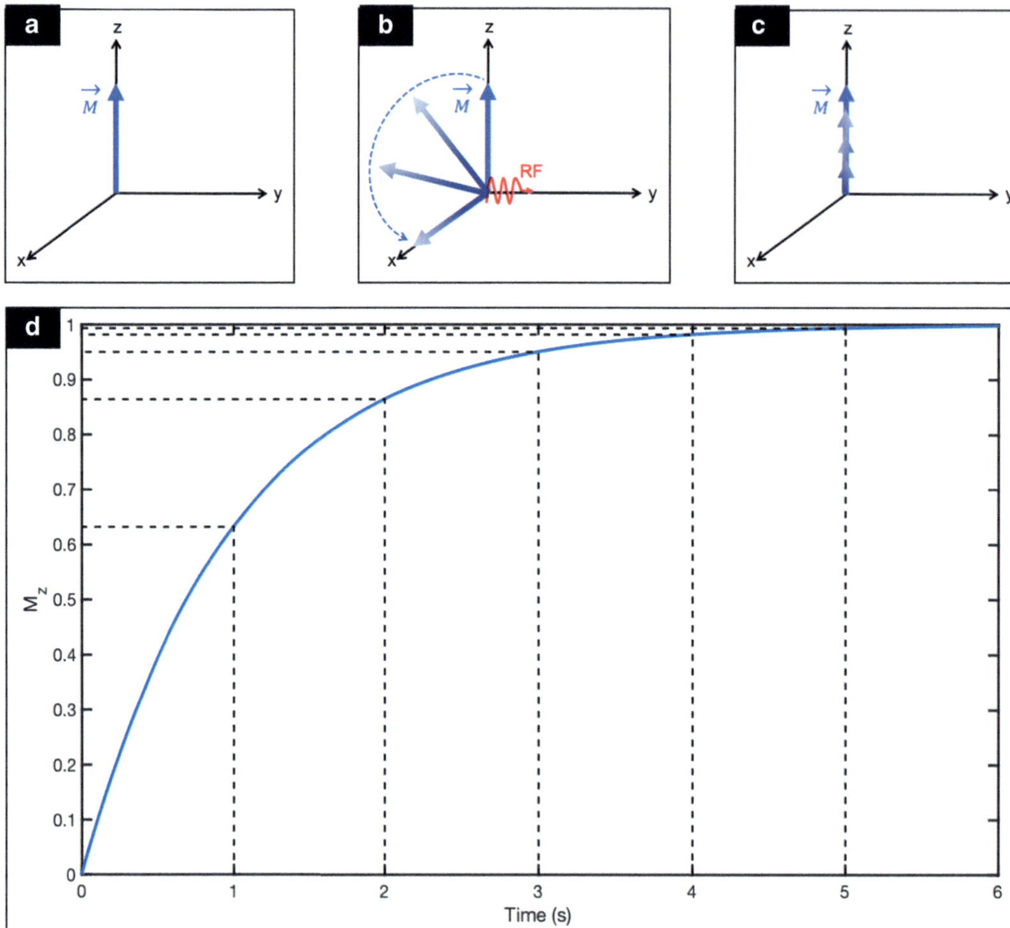

Fig. 8.1 (**a**) Equilibrium magnetization after protons align with main magnetic field B_0. (**b**) RF pulse in red tilts the magnetization away from equilibrium toward the transverse plane. (**c**) Recovery of the magnetization vector toward equilibrium following a 90° RF pulse. (**d**) Plot of the z-component of the magnetization vector as a function of time for a proton system with a T_1 of 1 s. After a time T_1, the magnetization recovers 63% of its equilibrium value; at two and three T_1 times, it recovers 83% and 95%, respectively

what factors might contribute to it, and how to measure it in a clinical setting.

When immersed in an external magnetic field B_0 (typically considered along the z-axis in a three-dimensional coordinate system), protons align with it, originating a small but measurable amount of magnetization (Fig. 8.1a). By applying an external radio frequency (RF) pulse, the magnetization can be perturbed away from equilibrium toward the transverse plane (x-y). The total amount of incurred rotation away from the z-axis is the flip angle; therefore when we say we apply a 90° RF pulse, we are rotating the available magnetization 90° toward the transverse plane (Fig. 8.1b). After rotation, the protons exchange energy with their surroundings and realign with the main magnetic field. The magnetization z-component (M_z) grows with a characteristic time defined as the T_1 relaxation: after one T_1 time, the M_z would have recovered 63% of its initial value, at two T_1 times 86%, and at three T_1 times 95%. Magnetization is approximately back in equilibrium after five T_1 times (Fig. 8.1c and d).

Fundamentally, T_1 is driven by molecular motion and how often the protons interact and exchange energy with their surroundings [2]. Picturing each proton as a tiny magnet, as they vibrate, tumble, and diffuse in a homogenous aqueous solution, they experience varying magnetic fields from nearby protons that, if these happen to be at the Larmor frequency (frequency at which the protons optimally absorb and/or irradiate RF energy), drive the magnetization toward equilibrium. The more often such interactions occur, the more quickly the magnetization recovers. Note that the important factor is not the total amount of interactions but the number of interactions that result in a field variation at the Larmor frequency. This has immediate consequences on which parameters might influence T_1 [2, 3]:

- *Temperature*: At different temperatures, the thermal motion of the protons changes. Hence the T_1 is expected to change because the average time spent on each interaction will be smaller as temperature increases.
- *Tissue composition:* In free fluid (such as CSF), water molecules are free to experience fast molecular motion, making protons less likely to experience field variations at the Larmor frequency and resulting in characteristically long T_1 relaxation times. In soft tissues (such as renal tissues), water molecular motion is restricted, resulting in protons being more likely to experience field variations at the Larmor frequency, and therefore T_1 relaxation is shorter.
- *Field strength:* As the Larmor frequency varies with field strength, T_1 values are expected to vary with it. Hence, T_1 measurements at 1.5 T will typically be shorter than at 3 T.
- *Presence of (para)diamagnetic atoms:* Susceptibility effects (e.g., due to the presence of iron, calcium, etc.) will induce local field variations that alter the Larmor frequency of the protons. Hence for the same temperature/tissue viscosity, a T_1 variation will be observed. MRI gadolinium-based contrast agents utilize this mechanism.

The relationship between T_1 and the environment experienced by the imaged protons explains why some literature might also refer to T_1 as "thermal" or "spin-lattice" relaxation [4]. Furthermore, it demonstrates why the ability to measure T_1 has the potential to be a sensitive tool for predicting clinical outcomes in parenchymal renal disease, since changes in T_1 values can be related to tissue composition such as fibrosis, edema, iron deposition, etc. [5, 6].

Acquisition of Kidney T_1 Maps

Now that we have established a description on the biophysical origins of T_1, we will reflect on how to measure it in a clinical setting. The gold standard approach for measuring T_1 is an inversion recovery pulse sequence [7] where the equilibrium magnetization is inverted, using a 180° RF pulse, left to recover for a specific amount of time (commonly referred to as inversion time TI) after which a spin echo or gradient echo readout image is acquired to sample the magnetization at different values of TI. The sampled data can then be used to compose a voxel-wise estimation of M_0 and T_1 given the expected mono-exponential recovery of Eq. 8.1:

$$M_z = M_0\left(1 - 2e^{-\frac{T_I}{T_1}}\right). \tag{8.1}$$

Although regarded as being accurate, this approach requires long acquisition times because the magnetization is allowed to fully recover before each measurement (repetition times >5 x T_1) making it an inherently slow approach and hindering its clinical applicability. This promoted the development of faster methodologies such as the modified Look-Locker inversion recovery acquisition (MOLLI) [8], saturation-recovery single-shot acquisition (SASHA) [9], variable flip angle (VFA) [7, 10], magnetic resonance fingerprinting (MRF) [11], and IR-EPI [12], among others. Each method has different sensitivities to imperfections such as homogeneity of B_0, the transmit field B_1, imaging timings, and system imperfections. In this chapter, we focus on the MOLLI methodology due to its widespread availability in clinical scanners and wide adoption within the field [13].

MOLLI allows different TI images to be sampled using single-shot balanced steady-state-free precession (bSSFP) acquisitions after a single 180° inversion pulse. With this approach, a single-slice T_1 map can be performed within one breath-hold of around 12 seconds. Because we

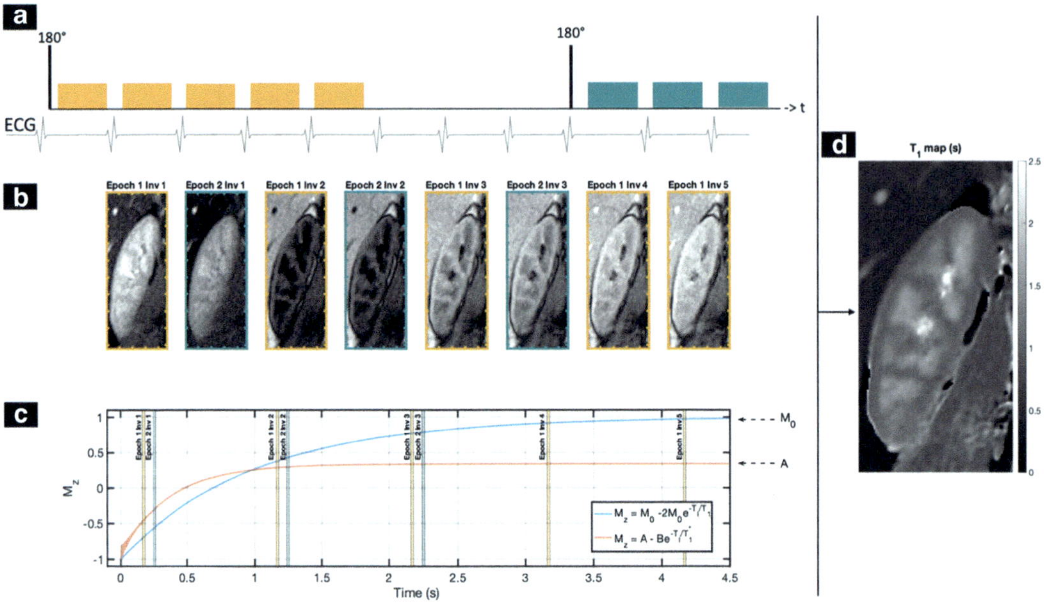

Fig. 8.2 5(3)3 MOLLI renal acquisition scheme. (**a**) Sequence diagram of the 5(3)3 MOLLI scheme. A first inversion pulse is applied followed by five readouts that sample different inversion (Inv) contrasts (yellow) at each heartbeat. This constitutes the first epoch. A recovery period of three heartbeats where no images are acquired is followed by a second inversion pulse and three readout events that sample another three inversion times (green), which constitutes the second epoch. Data are then ordered as a function of TI to estimate T_1*. (**b**) Exemplar images of the different contrasts acquired using diagram of (**a**). (**c**) Exemplar M_z recovery for a T_1 of 1 s when gold standard T_1 recovery is employed (blue) and during the MOLLI assumed recovery of Eq. 8.3 (red). The different timings of the diagrams (**a**) and (**b**) are highlighted. (**d**) Exemplar T_1 map obtained from the methodology summarized in (**a**), (**b**), and (**c**)

are constantly reading the magnetization after the inversion pulse, the influence of the readouts during T_1 recovery must be considered [14]. This is typically done by assuming the magnetization recovers with a mono-exponential recovery of Eq. 8.2:

$$M_z = M_0^* - \left(M_0 + M_0^*\right)e^{-\frac{T_I}{T_1^*}} = A - Be^{-\frac{T_I}{T_1^*}} \quad (8.2)$$

where M_0* and T_1* are the "apparent" equilibrium magnetization and T_1 recovery. Equation 8.3 is used to determine T_1 from T_1*; this equation has dubious validity [15] but is widely used:

$$T_1 = T_1^*\left(\frac{B}{A} - 1\right) \quad (8.3)$$

A comparison between the normal T_1 recovery and T_1* equivalent is shown in Fig. 8.2 for a T_1 value of 1 s. A sequence diagram of a 5(3)3 MOLLI acquisition is also shown where 5 images are acquired after an inversion pulse followed by a 3-heartbeat-pause period, after which a second inversion pulse is employed to prepare the signal for 3 further images.

MOLLI was initially developed for cardiac T_1 mapping, and therefore it is essential to cardiac gate the acquisition of different TI images. In kidney imaging, it is not necessary to synchronize the image acquisition with the cardiac cycle because the kidney pulsation is very minor. Therefore, a heart rate simulator can be used to ensure a fixed interval of 1 s between inversion times. The use of a heart rate simulator thereby producing images at consistent TI times has two benefits: firstly, it may avoid the practical inconvenience of cardiac gating; secondly it removes a bias that can appear in the MOLLI-T_1 value for patients with high heart rate (which shortens the TR). This is a minor confound for cardiac imaging but is more substantial for renal imaging owing to the longer T_1 of the kidney, which results in an incomplete recovery of M_z at the end of the TR, deviating it from the mono-exponential recovery of Eq. 8.2.

Table 8.1 Summary of renal T_1 mapping consensus [5] and authors' notes on how each parameter might affect the image quality

	Consensus [5]	Author's notes
Patient preparation	Normal hydration	
Field strength	1.5 T or 3 T	3 T will allow images with higher SNR at the cost of increased artifacts due to B_0 and B_1 inhomogeneities. Measured T_1 values at 3 T will be longer than at 1.5 T
T_1 mapping method	MOLLI	5(3)3 timing scheme is typically used in the kidney
Orientation	Coronal	Coronal plane allows both kidneys to be simultaneously acquired within a single two-dimensional slice
Number of slices	≥1	Increased number of slices will come at the cost of increased number of breath-holds
Acquired resolution	At least 3 mm in-plane	We note that higher resolutions (smaller voxels) will allow better delineation between the cortex and medulla and mitigate partial volume effects between both structures; SNR decreases with smaller voxel volumes
Slice thickness	≥5 mm	Larger slice thickness will increase the SNR at the cost of increased partial volume effects
Flip angle	35°	Smaller flip angles will reduce the sensitivity of MOLLI to B_0 inhomogeneities at the cost of lowering SNR; T_1 value is also expected to change with flip angle [20]
RR spacing	1 second	Some MR systems provide a physiology simulator that can be used to achieve a fixed RR interval. An external ECG signal simulation box can also be obtained separately
Parallel imaging	2	Parallel imaging values larger than two will result in increased prevalence of imaging artifacts and loss of SNR as a function of the distance between the coils and the kidney
Acquisition duration	1 breath-hold <15 s	Ideally breath-holds should be <10 s for robust, reliable, patient-friendly imaging

Note further that the T_1 as determined by MOLLI is best perhaps called the MOLLI-T_1, owing to the fact that it is biased by several factors as outlined in [13] and so is not an exact measurement of T_1. The great strength of MOLLI-T_1 is in its robustness to B_1^+ variation, its speed of acquisition, demonstrated reproducibility, and high image quality. These have led to its wide adoption in cardiac, liver, and kidney imaging.

Practical Recommendations for Kidney T_1 Mapping

At the time of writing this chapter, several works have been published employing relaxometry to assess kidney health [6, 16–18]; however, different studies employ different methodologies resulting in different cortex and medulla normative ranges [6, 19]. To tackle this, the European Cooperation in Science and Technology (COST) Action Magnetic Resonance Imaging Biomarkers for Chronic Kidney Disease (PARENCHIMA, CA16103, https://renalmri.org) was established and developed the consensus recommendations found in [5]. A precis of these consensus recommendations for T_1 mapping are provided in Table 8.1.

Part II: Post-processing and Data Analysis Methods

In the section below, the reader will become familiar with the methods necessary to generate renal T_1 maps and best practices to report kidney T_1 values, including recommendations for artifact detection and mitigation.

Generation of Kidney T_1 Maps

Following the acquisition of series of images with distinct T_1 weighting (TI series), T_1 maps can be obtained by fitting a model describing the MR signal evolution (as a function of TI) to the acquired data (following Eqs. 8.2 and 8.3). The use of least square methods is the common approach to solving minimization problems. In particular, the Levenberg–Marquardt (gradient-based) and Nelder–Mead (non-gradient-based) [21] algorithms are extensively used to solve the three-parameter (A, B, T_1*) MOLLI T_1 signal recovery curve shown in Eq. 8.2.

The fitting can be performed with input data in either complex or magnitude domains, and different methods will apply depending on the data format. If using magnitude data, the information on the polarity of the signal (positive or negative) is lost. Therefore, the simplest approach is to fit the absolute of the inversion recovery model in Eq. 8.2 to the data. Alternatively, the polarity of the signal could be restored, and Eq. 8.2 is used for model fitting. In this case, the temporal location of the null point will need to be estimated, through iteratively testing whether a given TI data point is closest to the null point by negating (flipping the sign) values up to that point before fitting the data. The approximate location of the zero crossing is given by the solution with the lowest residual error. This multi-fitting inversion recovery method [22] is more robust than fitting the absolute of the inversion recovery model to the magnitude data as the latter is sensitive to local minima in the fit error function.

If fitting complex data, Eq. 8.2 can be fit to the real part of the complex signal. However, extracting exclusively the real component assumes that the data were acquired with a phase of 0°, and thus it might not accurately reflect the polarity of the magnetization. A reliable method for restoring the polarity of the signal in complex images [23] involves estimation of a phase map from the image with the longest TI. The complex data are then phase-corrected and the real part extracted for model fitting.

As with all fitting approaches, good initial estimates of A and B should be provided to avoid convergence to erroneous local minima and shorten processing times. A and B can be set as follows [24]:

$$A_r = S_{\text{longest TI},r} \tag{8.4}$$

and

$$B_r = A - S_{\text{shortest TI},\,r} \tag{8.5}$$

where $S_{\text{longest TI},\,r}$ and $S_{\text{shortest TI},r}$ are the signal intensities of pixel r on the images with the longest and shortest inversion times, respectively. The initial condition for T_1* should be set to a value within the range of biologically relevant T_1 values observed in the kidneys [6] (e.g., a value of 1000 ms would be a valid initial guess) and can be identical for all image pixels.

Evaluation of the quality of the fit can be performed using several statistical measures. A common approach is to compute an R^2 map, which displays the proportion of the variance of the data that can be explained by the fitted model:

$$R^2 = 1 - \frac{\text{SSR}}{\text{SST}} \tag{8.6}$$

where SSR and SST are the sum of squares of residuals and the total sum of squares, respectively.

An alternative approach is to use the residual error of the fitting to calculate the standard deviation of the T_1 estimate, as described in [25], with the advantage that the quality of the fit is depicted on a map calibrated in T_1 units.

If a Look-Locker sequence (or any variant such as MOLLI) is used to acquire the data, a correction is applied to T_1* to yield the true T_1 as shown in Eq. 8.3. The measured T_1 is shortened by the perturbation to M_z caused by the readout pulses; thus $T_1^* < T_1$. Note that the original formulation of the correction assumes a continuous fast low angle shot (FLASH) gradient echo readout [14], while MOLLI uses a noncontinuous bSSFP readout. Despite this inconsistency and potential source of bias in T_1 quantification, the Look-Locker correction is widely used within the scientific community for MOLLI T_1 values.

A correction for the acquired T_1 is not needed if using the IR-EPI or SASHA methods, where $T_1 = T_1^*$. Furthermore, the three-parameter model in Eq. 8.2 can be reduced to a two-parameter model for fitting the data when a perfect inversion is assumed (Eq. 8.1). The fitting methodology used for T_1 mapping with VFA methods is described elsewhere [10]. While this approach is highly appealing, offering rapid acquisition and three-dimensional data, the calculated values depend

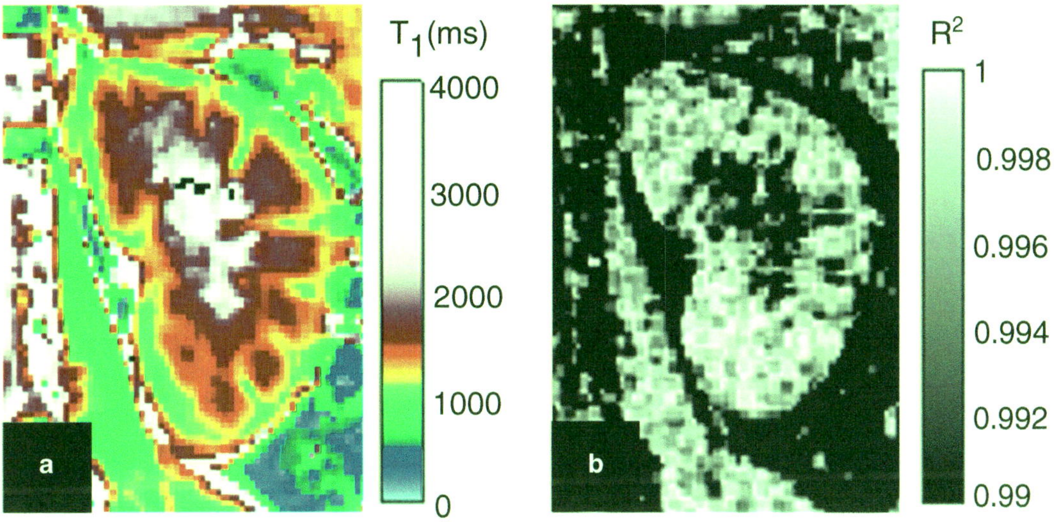

Fig. 8.3 Kidney T_1 map (**a**, in milliseconds) and respective R^2 map obtained from T_1 curve fitting (**b**). Data were acquired on a 1.5 T scanner using the MOLLI scheme

strongly on the transmit field, which should be acquired; consequently VFA methods prove difficult to deploy. More advanced fitting routines can be used that involve the generation of dictionary signals by fully simulating the evolution of the magnetization through any given sequence with the Bloch equations and extracting the parameters (at least T_1, potentially more if the data have sufficient degrees of freedom) that correspond to the simulated signal with maximal similarity to the acquired signal (such as in MRF) [11].

Quality Control

Quality control checks are an essential step to ensure the accuracy of reported kidney measures. There are a number of imaging artifacts that can be visually identified in renal T_1 maps, for which some examples are provided below. The presence of artifacts can also be confirmed using the R^2 map generated from the curve fitting routine (Fig. 8.3). Areas of suspected artifacts may have lower R^2 values when compared to artifact-free regions. It is recommended avoiding ROI placement in regions with R^2 below 0.99 (considering that R^2 values range from 0 to 1) [26]. Similarly, when using standard deviation measures, an increase in the variance of fitted T_1 values might be observed in artifactual regions.

Motion

While the TI series required to generate a T_1 map should be collected in a breath-hold of less than 15 s, superficial breathing and other body movements may still occur. Imaging the kidney in a coronal orientation is advantageous since it allows for an easy identification of respiratory motion, which will appear as a change in the position of the kidneys in the superior-inferior direction throughout the TI series. With breathing, there may also be a slight apparent change in the shape of the kidneys due to motion in the transverse direction (left-right), while through-plane motion should be minimal. Altered T_1 values caused by motion during the acquisition are likely to be most prominent in the periphery of the organ. Careful patient positioning to ensure their comfort and clear instructions on breath-holds may help reduce motion-related artifacts. It is recommended that T_1 maps are reconstructed on the scanner and checked at the time of acquisition to allow reacquisition of data that is affected by motion. If motion artifacts are severe and data reacquisition is not possible, the misalignment of the kidney position across the TI

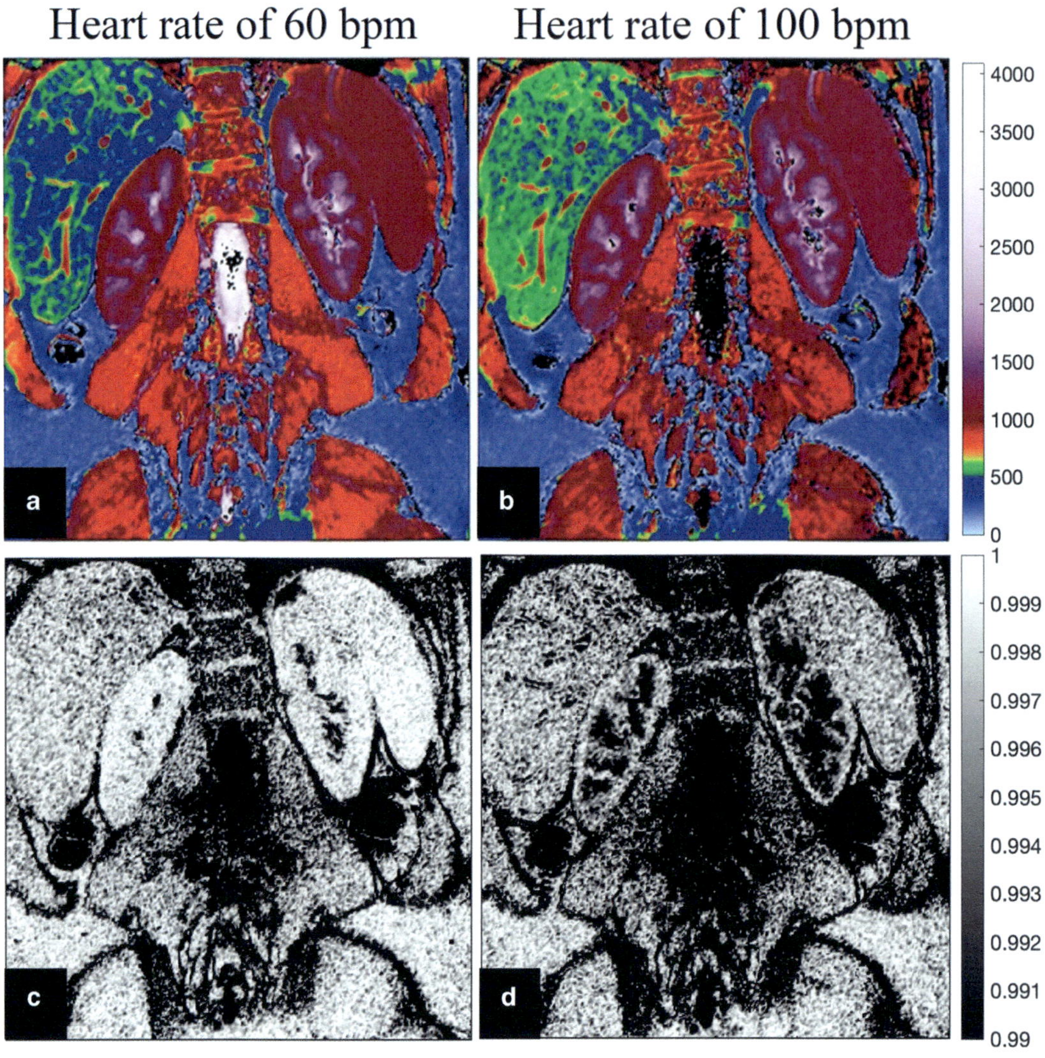

Fig. 8.4 Kidney T_1 maps (in milliseconds) and respective R^2 maps acquired on a healthy volunteer demonstrating the effect of differing heart rates on T_1 quantification. Data were acquired on a 1.5 T Siemens Aera scanner using a 5(3)3 MOLLI scheme. T_1 map acquired with a simulated heart rate of 60 bpm (**a**) shows shorter kidney T_1 values with higher R^2 (**c**), in comparison to the T_1 map acquired with a simulated heart rate of 100 bpm (**b**) and respective R^2 map (**d**). This difference is more noticeable in the renal medulla

series can be corrected through image registration (affine or deformable registration for more severe cases) [5, 18, 27].

Cardiac Gating Issues

It might not always be possible to use the MOLLI sequence in conjunction with a heart rate simulator. In these cases, the sequence is triggered by the patient's heartbeat, which can be measured using a pulse oximeter worn on the patient's finger or with an MRI-compatible ECG. Varying heart rate and misidentification of heartbeats can introduce biases in T_1 quantification [28]. Therefore, kidney T_1 measures may differ significantly between slices acquired with different heart rates if cardiac gating is used (Fig. 8.4).

Reporting of Kidney T_1 Values

Pixel T_1 values can be combined to yield a single value for the cortex and the medulla to provide an

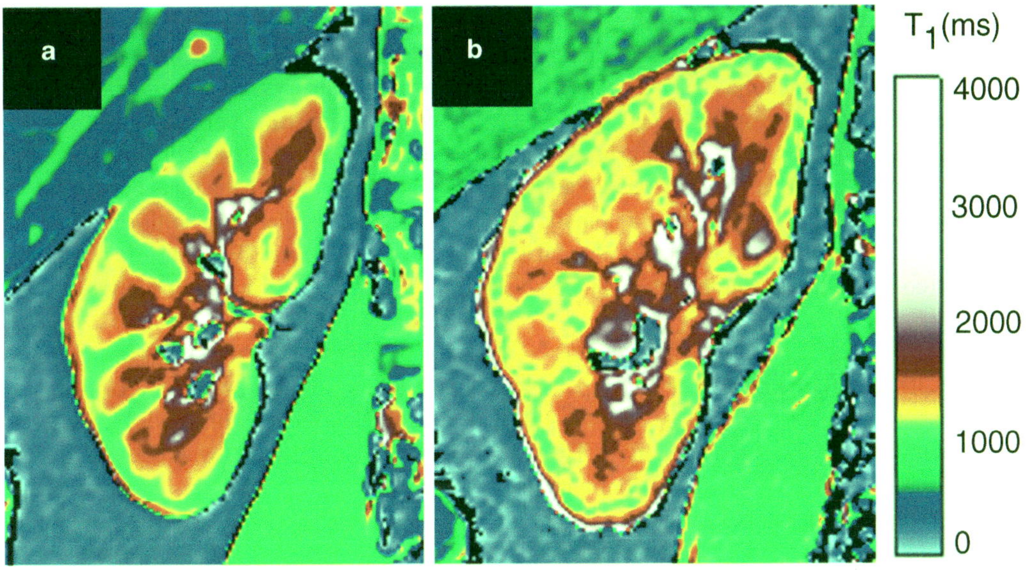

Fig. 8.5 Example of reduced cortico-medullary differentiation in a patient with advanced diabetes. Data were acquired on a 1.5 T scanner using the MOLLI scheme. (**a**) T_1 map of a healthy volunteer shows clear differentiation between the T_1 values in the cortex and the medulla in comparison to the (**b**) T_1 map of a patient with diabetes which shows much reduced difference between the cortex and medulla

overall assessment of kidney health. Several studies have also demonstrated that the degree of kidney impairment observed in patients with chronic kidney disease and renal transplants [6] correlates with an increase in the lack of differentiation between the T_1 values in the cortex and the medulla, also known as corticomedullary differentiation (CMD), as shown in Fig. 8.5. To assess CMD and reduce interindividual variability (see Clinical Applications section below), the cortex–medulla T_1 difference (T_1 medulla–T_1 cortex) [12, 18, 29] and the corticomedullary ratio (T_1 cortex/T_1 medulla) [26] are commonly reported.

A common approach to reporting T_1 in the cortex and the medulla involves manual ROI placement. Consensus on the number, size, and positioning of the ROIs has not been reached [5] with several strategies being suggested: one ROI for each cortex and medulla in a defined region of the kidney [26], three ROIs in different kidney regions (upper, interpolar, and lower poles of renal cortex and medulla) [18], and multiple ROIs placed in multiple slices [29].

A limitation of manual ROIs is the potential increase in intra- and inter-rater variability due to the difficulty in choosing the appropriate location for placement. It is recommended to avoid ROI positioning near tissue interfaces, such as the borders between parenchyma and perirenal fat or renal sinus fat due to partial volume averaging artifacts. Visualization of kidney T_1 maps with color-encoded pixel T_1 values, that is, colormaps, may help distinguish the cortex (usually with shorter T_1) and the medulla (usually with longer T_1) and facilitate ROI selection (Fig. 8.3). Care must be taken in choosing an appropriate colormap; otherwise ROI positioning may be influenced by the creation of artificial boundaries. The cardiac T_1 recommendations encourage the use of a grayscale colormap for ROI placement specifically to avoid bias [13]. Using a T_1 map for segmentation determination of T_1 values has obvious confounds but is a widely used approach. The reduced contrast between the cortex and medulla in advanced kidney disease (decreased CMD) is an additional hindrance to ROI placement. Standardized approaches that include training manuals, blinded analysis, fixed sized ROIs, and rigorous quality control can all improve the inter-rater variability.

The use of semi- or fully automated methods for segmenting the cortex and medulla has been suggested to decrease analysis variability and time. An approach to semiautomated segmentation has been proposed, which involves the computation of a histogram of the T_1 values of the kidney from which the two peaks corresponding to the cortex and the medulla can be identified and used to generate the respective masks [12]. Alternatively, an algorithm based on thresholding and shape detection applied to registered T_1- and T_2-weighted images is able to achieve automatic segmentation of the kidneys and their internal structures (cortex, medulla, and pelvis) [27].

Part III: Clinical Applications

This section will describe the sensitivity of T_1 to kidney disease as well as to additional confounders and how their influence can be minimized to achieve more accurate and precise measurements that can be used for diagnosis.

T_1 as a Biomarker for Kidney Disease

In a T_1-weighted MRI image of a healthy kidney, the anatomical difference between the medulla and the cortex can be visualized owing to the tissue T_1 differences. The medulla has a long T_1 and the value for the cortex is shorter (hence brighter). The contrast seen in these images is known as corticomedullary differentiation (CMD) and is clear in the healthy kidney. Loss of this differentiation is seen in several renal diseases and has generally been found to be due to an increase of the cortex T_1 value, so measurement of cortex T_1 provides a proven metric for kidney disease.

Cortical T_1 has been demonstrated to be influenced both acutely and chronically in animal models of kidney disease [30, 31], which is consistent with the radiological CMD findings. Renal fibrosis is also found to correlate with the cortex T_1 [32]. Note that in these cases changes are also seen in the medulla of the kidney but they are much smaller, may fail to reach statistical significance, and may even move in the opposite direction to the cortical changes. It is accepted that cortical T_1 changes appear to be of most diagnostic relevance. Relative change in T_1 can be beneficial compared to the use of cortex T_1 itself. The use of medulla T_1 difference (T_1 medulla–T_1 cortex) and the corticomedullary ratio may both help mitigate changes that occur in both the medulla and cortex due to acquisition, for example, minor pulse sequence changes, or hydration levels.

An exciting application of kidney T_1 mapping is in the transplanted kidney. In this case, it is hoped that problems with the transplanted kidney can be detected earlier than with conventional blood and urine metrics. Further, it is hoped that MRI may eliminate the need for biopsy (a common theme for MRI-based methods). Routine adoption of kidney T_1 for transplant monitoring is an active area of research with findings that show that cortical T_1 correlates with eGFR [32] and also that renal fibrosis correlates with cortical T_1 [32].

Quantitation and Standardization

One limitation of MRI images is that the pixel intensity values are generally meaningless, so-called arbitrary units that cannot be compared between one patient and another or between one region of the image and another. Thus image contrast (i.e., structure in the image) is all that can be used radiologically. When the measurement means something, such as in CT with the Hounsfield number, then the value can be used directly for analysis that is less user dependent and potentially more robust. Further, this quantitation allows rapid translation of techniques from research into routine clinical usage, accelerating the adoption of best practice.

MRI has already developed several quantitative approaches including phase-contrast flow measurements (cm/s), proton density fat fraction (%), apparent diffusion coefficient (ADC mm/s^2), T_1 mapping in the heart and liver (ms), and T_2* mapping in the heart and liver (ms). In these cases, absolute values can be found to be emerging in diagnostic guidelines.

To get the maximum clinical benefit of quantitative MRI, it helps for the values at one center to be used at another center. This standardization of metrics is expected in science: 1 kg in a New York laboratory is substantially equivalent to 1 kg in a Parisian grocer's shop, and we can trust these measurements. Previous efforts to standardize MRI metrics have struggled and may have been a driver for weighted images (e.g., T_1-weighted and T_2-weighted). Some of the reasons for this variation in values may now have diminished, and there seems to be an opportunity to revisit standardized measurements. Table 8.1 in the review paper from Wolf et al. [6] supports the concept that in 2021 standardization is not complete for kidney T_1 mapping.

Note also that 1.5 T and 3 T scanners will return substantially different T_1 values in the same person owing to the well-known dependence of T_1 on the magnetic field strength. It is also known that changes to the number of phase-encodes, TI, flip angle, TR, TE, MOLLI sampling scheme, inversion pulse, and the fitting methods can all have measurable influence on the MOLLI T_1. Additional variation can be introduced by a particular site's patient preparation (hydration) and the pixels chosen for analysis. Care must therefore be taken when using thresholds and values from the literature when assessing patients. While this remains a problem that has not been solved elegantly, the approach described in the mature T_1 cardiac literature of determining the range for healthy subjects by measuring $N = 20$ [13] cases and evaluating patients relative to that baseline does appear tractable. It should be noted that the changes in T_1 in the kidney are larger than some of the subtle phenomena that cardiac MRI practitioners are attempting to assess; so the precision of the normal T_1 range may require only 20 cases and definitely not the 50 cases specified in the cardiac literature for detecting changes at the ~5% level.

Confounds

Generally, T_1 can be thought of being primarily influenced by the water-to-protein ratio and elevated T_1 relates to increased water content, but there are confounds that warrant consideration.

Fat and Iron

For liver T_1 measurements in the presence of fat and iron, a correction factor is recommended. The kidney, however, does not generally accumulate diffuse fat (unlike the liver) which can bias the MOLLI T_1 measurement. The kidney also typically does not accumulate iron [33]; in the rare circumstances where the kidney does accumulate iron, this would be expected to impact the T_1 of the tissue and also to impact the accuracy of how the T_1 is measured (MOLLI is known to underestimate T_1 when T_2 is short [34], for example).

Hydration

Early heroic experiments by Hricak et al. [16] involved hydration with as much as 4 liters of fluid and observed substantial changes to the T_1 of the kidneys. The authors summarized these changes in healthy subjects: prior to hydration the cortex T_1 ~ 50% of the medulla T_1, with hydration (of the level above) cortex T_1 ~ 80% of medulla T_1. The T_1 of the medulla increases with hydration owing to additional urine, but the cortical increases are larger, which is suggested as being due to increased plasma volume. Note that this work was performed at 3.5 kG (0.35 Tesla), so the values cannot be directly translated to modern MRI at 1.5 T and 3 T, but it is indicative that the impact of hydration may need to be considered as renal problems inevitably can affect hydration.

Liver Cirrhosis

The sensitivity of the kidney's T_1 to water content is seen in patients with liver cirrhosis, where reduced CMD is observed in T_1-weighted images [35, 36]. This phenomenon is independent of renal function (as evaluated by eGFR). Further, it is assumed to be due to shortening of the cortical T_1, but quantitative T_1 measurements were not part of either paper.

Perfusion

MRI relaxation times can be thought of as measures of the tissue. In a general sense, this is true, but other factors can play a part depending on the data acquisition scheme. Kidney perfusion results in a considerable flow of water in and out of the kidney, and this movement of water can impact the measurement of the T_1. Fortunately the MOLLI approach is relatively insensitive to flow effects (e.g., the T_1 of the blood pool of the heart can be measured with reasonable accuracy). However, other methods (perhaps which use slice-selective inversions) could be sensitive to perfusion effects, and perfusion bias might be present in two-dimensional T_1-weighted acquisitions.

Conclusion

Quantification of T_1 in the kidney has emerged as a valuable approach for investigating disease. It has been found to be robust, and the acquisition methods are already available on standard clinical MRI hardware from all the main MRI vendors.

Furthermore, the contrast measured with T_1 mapping has a long history of validity from the mature CMD sign in T_1-weighted images and has been validated against histology as a surrogate for fibrosis. Quantitative measurements of the T_1 may allow this metric of disease to require less skill and experience, potentially making the reporting of CMD more repeatable and reproducible. Care must be taken in the use of this new tool, but T_1 mapping with the MOLLI method appears to be a valuable addition to the medical armamentarium.

References

1. Leung AW, Bydder GM, Steiner RE, Bryant DJ, Young IR. Magnetic resonance imaging of the kidneys. AJR Am J Roentgenol. 1984;143(6):1215–27.
2. Deoni S. Biophysical and physiological principles of T1 and T2 [internet], 1st ed., vol. 1, Quantitative magnetic resonance imaging. Elsevier; 2020. 3–17 p. https://doi.org/10.1016/B978-0-12-817057-1.00003-2.
3. Bloembergen N, Purcell EM, Pound RV. Relaxation effects in nuclear magnetic resonance absorption. Phys Rev. 1948;73(7):679–712.
4. Bloch F. Nuclear induction. Phys Rev. 1946;70(7–8):460–74.
5. Dekkers IA, de Boer A, Sharma K, Cox EF, Lamb HJ, Buckley DL, et al. Consensus-based technical recommendations for clinical translation of renal T1 and T2 mapping MRI. Magn Reson Mater Phys Biol Med. 2020;33(1):163–76.
6. Wolf M, de Boer A, Sharma K, Boor P, Leiner T, Sunder-Plassmann G, et al. Magnetic resonance imaging T1- and T2-mapping to assess renal structure and function: a systematic review and statement paper. Nephrol Dial Transplant. 2018;33(2):ii41–50.
7. Boudreau M, Keenan KE, Stikov N. Quantitative T1 and T1ρ mapping [internet], 1st ed, vol. 1, Quantitative magnetic resonance imaging. Elsevier; 2020. 19–45 p. https://doi.org/10.1016/B978-0-12-817057-1.00004-4.
8. Messroghli DR, Radjenovic A, Kozerke S, Higgins DM, Sivananthan MU, Ridgway JP. Modified look-locker inversion recovery (MOLLI) for high-resolution T 1 mapping of the heart. Magn Reson Med. 2004;52(1):141–6.
9. Chow K, Flewitt JA, Green JD, Pagano JJ, Friedrich MG, Thompson RB. Saturation recovery single-shot acquisition (SASHA) for myocardial T 1 mapping. Magn Reson Med. 2014;71(6):2082–95.
10. Fram EK, Herfkens RJ, Johnson GA, Glover GH, Karis JP, Shimakawa A, et al. Rapid calculation of T1 using variable flip angle gradient refocused imaging. Magn Reson Imaging. 1987;5(3):201–8.
11. Ma D, Gulani V, Seiberlich N, Liu K, Sunshine JL, Duerk JL, et al. Magnetic resonance fingerprinting. Nature. 2013;495(7440):187–92.
12. Cox EF, Buchanan CE, Bradley CR, Prestwich B, Mahmoud H, Taal M, et al. Multiparametric renal magnetic resonance imaging: validation, interventions, and alterations in chronic kidney disease. Front Physiol. 2017;8:696.
13. Messroghli DR, Moon JC, Ferreira VM, Grosse-Wortmann L, He T, Kellman P, et al. Clinical recommendations for cardiovascular magnetic resonance mapping of T1, T2, T2* and extracellular volume: a consensus statement by the Society for Cardiovascular Magnetic Resonance (SCMR) endorsed by the European Association for Cardiovascular Imaging. J Cardiovasc Magn Reson [Internet]. 2017;19(1):75. https://doi.org/10.1186/s12968-017-0389-8.
14. Deichmann R, Haase A. Quantification of T1 values by SNAPSHOT-FLASH NMR imaging. J Magn Reson. 1992;96(3):608–12.
15. Kellman P, Hansen MS. T1-mapping in the heart: accuracy and precision. J Cardiovasc Magn Reson [Internet]. 2014;16(1):2. https://doi.org/10.1186/1532-429X-16-2.
16. Hricak H, Crooks L, Sheldon P, Kaufman L. Nuclear magnetic resonance imaging of the kidney. Radiology [Internet]. 1983;146(2):425–432. https://doi.org/10.1148/radiology.146.2.6849088.
17. Adams LC, Bressem KK, Scheibl S, Nunninger M, Gentsch A, Fahlenkamp UL, et al. Multiparametric assessment of changes in renal tissue after kidney transplantation with quantitative MR Relaxometry and diffusion-tensor imaging at 3 T. J Clin Med. 2020;9(5):1551.
18. Peperhove M, Jang M-S, Gutberlet M, Hartung D, Tewes S, Warnecke G, et al. Assessment of acute kidney injury with T1 mapping MRI following solid organ transplantation. Eur Radiol. 2018;28(1):44–50.
19. Bojorquez JZ, Bricq S, Acquitter C, Brunotte F, Walker PM, Lalande A. What are normal relaxation times of tissues at 3 T? Magn Reson Imaging [Internet]. 2017;35:69–80. https://doi.org/10.1016/j.mri.2016.08.021.

20. Kellman P, Hansen MS. T1-mapping in the heart: accuracy and precision. J Cardiovasc Magn Reson. 2014;16(1):2.
21. Nelder JA, Mead R. A simplex method for function minimization. Comput J. 1965;7(4):308–13.
22. Nekolla S, Gneiting T, Syha J, Deichmann R, Haase A. T1 maps by K-space reduced snapshot-FLASH MRI. J Comput Assist Tomogr. 1992;16(2):327–32.
23. Xue H, Greiser A, Zuehlsdorff S, Jolly M-P, Guehring J, Arai AE, et al. Phase-sensitive inversion recovery for myocardial T1 mapping with motion correction and parametric fitting. Magn Reson Med. 2013;69(5):1408–20.
24. Xue H, Shah S, Greiser A, Guetter C, Littmann A, Jolly M-P, et al. Motion correction for myocardial T1 mapping using image registration with synthetic image estimation. Magn Reson Med. 2012;67(6):1644–55.
25. Kellman P, Arai AE, Xue H. T1 and extracellular volume mapping in the heart: estimation of error maps and the influence of noise on precision. J Cardiovasc Magn Reson. 2013;15(1):1–12.
26. Dekkers IA, Paiman EHM, de Vries APJ, Lamb HJ. Reproducibility of native T1 mapping for renal tissue characterization at 3T. J Magn Reson Imaging. 2019;49(2):588–96.
27. Will S, Martirosian P, Würslin C, Schick F. Automated segmentation and volumetric analysis of renal cortex, medulla, and pelvis based on non-contrast-enhanced T1-and T2-weighted MR images. Magn Reson Mater Phys Biol Med. 2014;27(5):445–54.
28. Piechnik SK, Ferreira VM, Dall'Armellina E, Cochlin LE, Greiser A, Neubauer S, et al. Shortened modified look-locker inversion recovery (ShMOLLI) for clinical myocardial T1-mapping at 1.5 and 3 T within a 9 heartbeat breathhold. J Cardiovasc Magn Reson. 2010;12(1):1–11.
29. Friedli I, Crowe LA, Berchtold L, Moll S, Hadaya K, De Perrot T, et al. New magnetic resonance imaging index for renal fibrosis assessment: a comparison between diffusion-weighted imaging and T1 mapping with histological validation. Sci Rep. 2016;6(1):1–15.
30. Hueper K, Peperhove M, Rong S, Gerstenberg J, Mengel M, Meier M, et al. T1-mapping for assessment of ischemia-induced acute kidney injury and prediction of chronic kidney disease in mice. Eur Radiol. 2014;24(9):2252–60.
31. Hueper K, Hensen B, Gutberlet M, Chen R, Hartung D, Barrmeyer A, et al. Kidney transplantation: multiparametric functional magnetic resonance imaging for assessment of renal allograft pathophysiology in mice. Invest Radiol. 2016;51(1):58–65.
32. Berchtold L, Friedli I, Crowe LA, Martinez C, Moll S, Hadaya K, et al. Validation of the corticomedullary difference in magnetic resonance imaging-derived apparent diffusion coefficient for kidney fibrosis detection: a cross-sectional study. Nephrol Dial Transplant. 2020;35(6):937–45.
33. Schein A, Enriquez C, Coates TD, Wood JC. Magnetic resonance detection of kidney iron deposition in sickle cell disease: a marker of chronic hemolysis. J Magn Reson Imaging [Internet]. 2008;28(3):698–704. https://pubmed.ncbi.nlm.nih.gov/18777554
34. Chow K, Flewitt J, Pagano JJ, Green JD, Friedrich MG, Thompson RB. T(2)-dependent errors in MOLLI T(1) values: simulations, phantoms, and in-vivo studies. J Cardiovasc Magn Reson [Internet]. 2012;14(Suppl 1):P281–P281. https://www.ncbi.nlm.nih.gov/pmc/articles/PMC3304811/
35. Dekkers IA, Lamb HJ. Clinical application and technical considerations of T1 and T2(*) mapping in cardiac, liver, and renal imaging. Br J Radiol. 2018;91(1092):1–13.
36. Yamada F, Amano Y, Hidaka F, Fukushima Y, Kumita S. Pseudonormal corticomedullary differentiation of the kidney assessed on T1-weighted imaging for chronic kidney disease patients with cirrhosis. Magn Reson Med Sci. 2015;14(3):165–71.

T_2 Mapping of the Kidney

9

Marcos Wolf, Diana Bencikova, and Ewald Moser

MRI Physics and Historical Background

Relaxation times are time constants characterizing magnetic interactions between local nuclear spins and the surrounding molecules (lattice). In contrast to spin-lattice relaxation time T_1, which describes an energy exchange based on the interaction between nuclear spins and the lattice, the spin-spin relaxation time T_2 describes changes in entropy due to the dephasing of neighboring spins and local magnetic field fluctuations. Consequently, T_2 relaxation times in heterogeneous tissue are shorter (typically 40–100 ms) than T_1 relaxation times (typically 500–1000 ms), and both may change with physiological or pathological alterations, reflected in local molecular changes. Thus, quantified T_2 changes may be a useful tool for renal tissue characterization and subsequently diagnosis or disease progression analysis.

Historically, and also in terms of practicability, spin-echo experiments described first by Erwin Hahn [1] represent the most simple and robust approach to quantify T_2. He employed two consecutive 90° rf-pulses and described the evolution of spin-echos. The time between those two pulses is called echo-time (TE), and the subsequent signal decay determines how much signal is lost due to dephasing. A T_2 measurement is performed by repeating this experiment several times with varying TE durations. The main problem of that time was the non-homogeneity of the B_1-pulse and, hence, accuracy and reproducibility of spin excitation. These effects were also further pronounced as rf-pulses were only applied on one axis, that is, x-axis, which accumulates phase error from repetitive imperfect pulses and B_1 inhomogeneities. To improve this, Carr and Purcell suggested a more elaborate pulse sequence containing an initial 90° pulse and followed by a train of 180° rf-pulses [2]. This was further improved by Meiboom and Gill [3], who additionally employed refocusing pulses along the ±y-axis to compensate for accumulating errors due to imperfect 180° pulses. Today these methods are summarized in the so-called CPMG (Carr-Purcell-Meiboom-Gill) sequence, and due to its robustness and speed, it is still employed on human MRI scanners.

Modern MRI machines enable local shimming to further improve local magnetic field homogeneity and the application of dedicated rf-pulses to allow for sufficiently homogeneous signal excitation and refocusing despite magnetically heterogeneous settings.

M. Wolf (✉) · E. Moser
High Field MR Center, Center for Medical Physics and Biomedical Engineering, Medical University of Vienna, Vienna, Austria
e-mail: marcos.wolf@meduniwien.ac.at

D. Bencikova
High Field MR Center, Department of Biomedical Imaging and Image-Guided Therapy, Medical University of Vienna, Vienna, Austria

S. D. Serai, K. Darge (eds.), *Advanced Clinical MRI of the Kidney*,
https://doi.org/10.1007/978-3-031-40169-5_9

Acquisition Protocols

Today different acquisition schemes exist to measure the T_2 relaxation time and examples are given in Fig. 9.1. Understanding these principles helps to identify strengths and weaknesses and enables to identify the best practice for specific applications (e.g., phantom measurements and in vivo measurements). The simplest approach to measure T_2 is a single spin-echo (SE) pulse sequence. There is only one initial 90° rf-pulse and a single 180° rf-pulse applied within one time of repetition (TR). This technique acquires one line of k-space per one TR. As previously described, altering the TE on consecutive acquisitions is required to plot the decay of the signal intensity of the echo (also known as TE weightings). However, the associated long acquisition time deems it impractical for in vivo renal measurements, particularly due to motion of the kidney and patient comfort. In contrast, it provides accurate results for phantom measurements. A substantial reduction in measurement time can be achieved by using multi-echo SE (MESE) sequences. After an initial 90° rf-pulse, a train of 180° rf-pulses follow; hence, one line of k-space is acquired for each TE image within one TR. After each refocusing rf-pulse, the signal intensity of the echo decreases. This can be even more accelerated with the turbo SE (TSE) or fast SE (FSE) technique. Similar to MESE acquisitions, a train of refocusing pulses are applied; however, different gradients are set with each refocusing pulse, so that multiple k-space lines are acquired within one TE weighting [4]. This allows to acquire more k-space lines at once but also introduces additional weighting into individual TE images; therefore long echo train

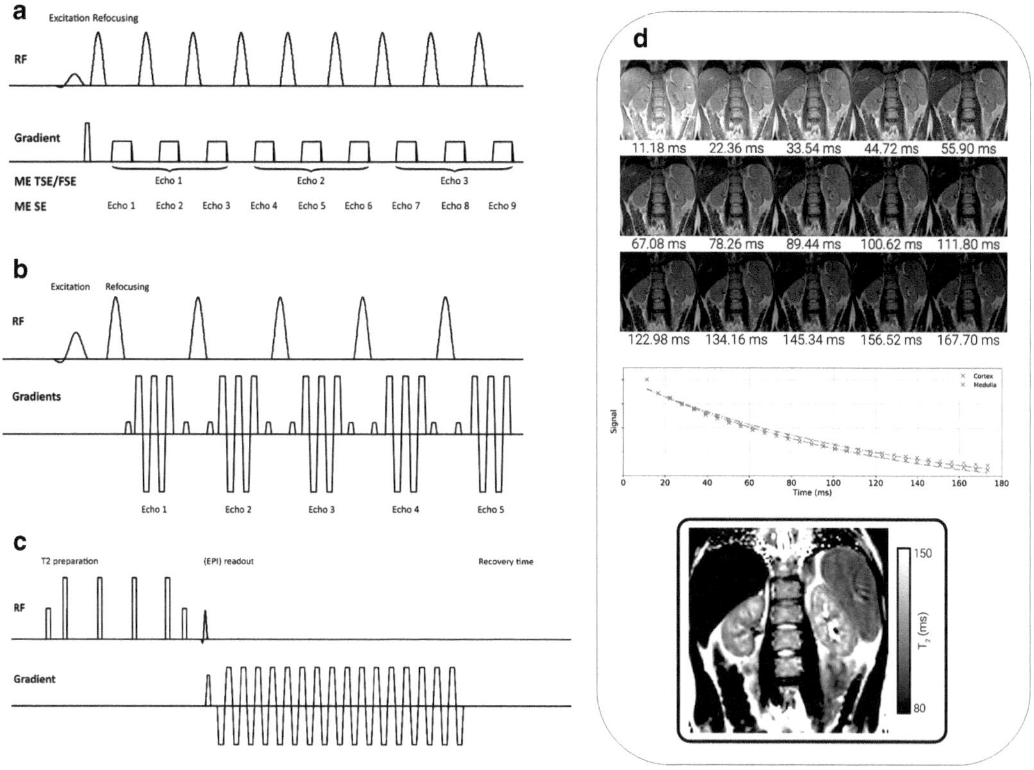

Fig. 9.1 Different excitation and readout schemes for T_2 mapping using MESE (**a**), GRASE (**b**), and T_2 prep (**c**). Example GRASE images (top), signal decay, and post-processing (middle), showing the resulting T_2 map (bottom) (**d**). (Figure reproduced from [12])

lengths (ETL) or high turbo-factors should not be used for T_2 mapping with TSE. Also mixed approaches of gradient-echo and SE sequences, such as GRASE, exist and promise even faster acquisition times [5].

In recent years, novel approaches have been published; however, the concept of an initial excitation (commonly 90° rf-pulse) together with refocusing pulses (commonly 180° rf-pulse) is the common denominator. For example, T_2 preparation pulses (initial 90° rf-pulses and consecutive 180° rf-pulses) can be applied prior to different sequence readouts, such as steady-state-free precession. This approach has been successfully developed for cardiac imaging, where these pulses decrease the influence of imperfect slice selection pulse profiles, diffusion, or flow. They are commonly applied in cardiac MRI where they have shown to improve the diagnostic confidence of edema after myocardial infarction [6, 7]. However, this can lead to slightly higher T_2 values.

Table 9.1 Current technical recommendations for T_2 mapping by a renal imaging expert panel [12]. Some notes regarding these standardizations are shared in the column on the right

	Current consensus extracted from [12]	Author notes
Patient preparation	Normal hydration	Hydration levels could influence T_2 values. A conclusive study is still missing
Field strength and hardware	1.5 T or 3 T with body coil transmitter and multichannel receiver coil	Minor changes of T_2 values with respect to field strength are expected, specifically a decrease in T_2 with increased field strength
Measurement protocol	ME SE, GRASE, and T_2 prep	No final consensus within the community
Orientation	Coronal or coronal oblique	Folding artefacts can be a limiting factor. Hence other orientations could become favorable

Recommendations for Renal T_2 Mapping In Vivo

In general, none of the envisioned acquisition techniques is perfect and there is always a trade-off. At least one of the following aspects may cause a problem: long acquisition times, low spatial resolution, physiologically induced motion artifacts, and inaccurate fittings due to a low number of TE-weighted images with not enough time points to fit reliably [8–10]. Hence, accurate measurement of T_2 in the kidney is not trivial as several aspects have to be taken into account altogether, especially the prohibitive measurement times and the high clinical throughput of patients. Consequently, until today only a limited number of studies exist that focused explicitly on renal T_2 mapping of healthy and diseased kidney (excluding neoplasms and animal studies; [11]), and no detailed consensus was formulated by a group of renal imaging specialists on an optimal renal T_2 mapping approach [12]. Table 9.1 summarizes the current consensus regarding T_2 mapping with notes added.

In addition to Table 9.1, further considerations should be applied in renal T_2 mapping. The correct choice of number of echoes and timing intervals is crucial for a reliable T_2 estimation and should be chosen to span the range of clinically expected T_2 values [11]. The first echo should be as short as technically possible, and there should be as many echos collected as feasible, with ETL up to two to three times the T_2, but without degradation by, for example, motion artifacts or noise. The total number of TEs should be at least five and can be spaced equally or logarithmically. It should be noted that the inter-echo spacing in MESE acquisition influences the resulting T_2 values. Of course the TR has to be set long enough to avoid T_1 effects during the T_2 mapping acquisition.

Post-processing and Data Analysis

In general, the acquired T_2-weighted magnitude images are fitted using a single exponential model [13]:

$$S(\text{TE}) = k \cdot S_0 e^{\frac{-\text{TE}}{T_2}} + \text{offset}, \qquad (9.1)$$

and the first echo, i.e., first T_2-weighted image, is dropped. If the images have a sufficiently high SNR, no offset has to be added (nonzero baseline due to non-convergence toward zero). Another approach is to measure the background signal separately and to subtract it from the images or to stop at echoes with signal equal or lower to the background noise. When comparing T_2 values between scanners, a proportionality constant (k) can be used to correct for specific scanner soft- and hardware influences. S_0 reflects the equilibrium magnetization, that is, proton density. While some scanners provide product licenses for the calculation of T_2 maps inline, these licenses are expensive and not everywhere accessible. In such cases, many simple solutions exist for post-processing. In general, it is recommended to use widely available and open source packages, to enable future comparisons, which are very important due to the limited number of renal T_2 mapping studies. For example, the acquired T_2-weighted images (usually DICOM files) can be converted to the cross platform NifTI format [14]. During this process, the images can be reoriented. If necessary, in vivo data can be co-registered and further segmented [15]. These prepared images can then be processed with various softwares and packages or scripts available, such as Octave and Matlab with the package qMRLab [16]. Also, other solutions exist in Python [17], R [18], 3D Slicer [19], or ImageJ [20]. Besides fitting Eq. 9.1, some software programs speed up the calculation by applying a logarithmic transformation on the data first and then performing linear fit. And other approaches use advanced modeling of the signal to account for the imperfect exponential decay in MESE acquisitions caused by signal contamination of indirect echoes [9, 10].

Study Reports and Quality Assurance

In general, datasets should be checked for artifacts (especially motion artifacts) already on the scanner console during the data acquisition. Subjects should be confident to report breath-hold duration problems.

In order to allow comparability between studies, it is highly recommended to standardize reports. Any hydration protocol should be explained, and any measures to compensate for physiological motion (i.e., breathing and cardiac motion) should be reported. If clinically feasible and possible, the subject's hydration should be controlled. This could shed light on the still unanswered question regarding the influence of hydration on T_2 maps (see Table 9.1).

It comes without saying, the measurement protocol has to be shared and potential impacts on T_2 values have to be discussed. In this context, phantom measurements, that is, data with reference T_2 measurements compared to the applied in vivo protocols, are essential to allow comparability.

Region of interest (ROI) can be placed manually in the cortex and medulla; however, an automated or semiautomated segmentation of the kidney is preferred. If possible renal T_2 reports should distinguish between the cortex and medulla, and the corticomedullary differentiation should be calculated. The associated mean and SD should be reported.

Clinical Applications and Considerations

The T_2 contrast in clinical renal MRI, that is, T_2-weighted imaging, is traditionally used to assess the excretory system, to characterize cysts, intraparenchymal abscesses, hydronephrosis, or to detect solid lesions. However, these weighted images do not contain classical quantification data, and radiologists rather assess anatomical or relative changes. In contrast to the T_1 contrast, the corticomedullary differentiation (CMD) is not so pronounced in T_2-weighted images and

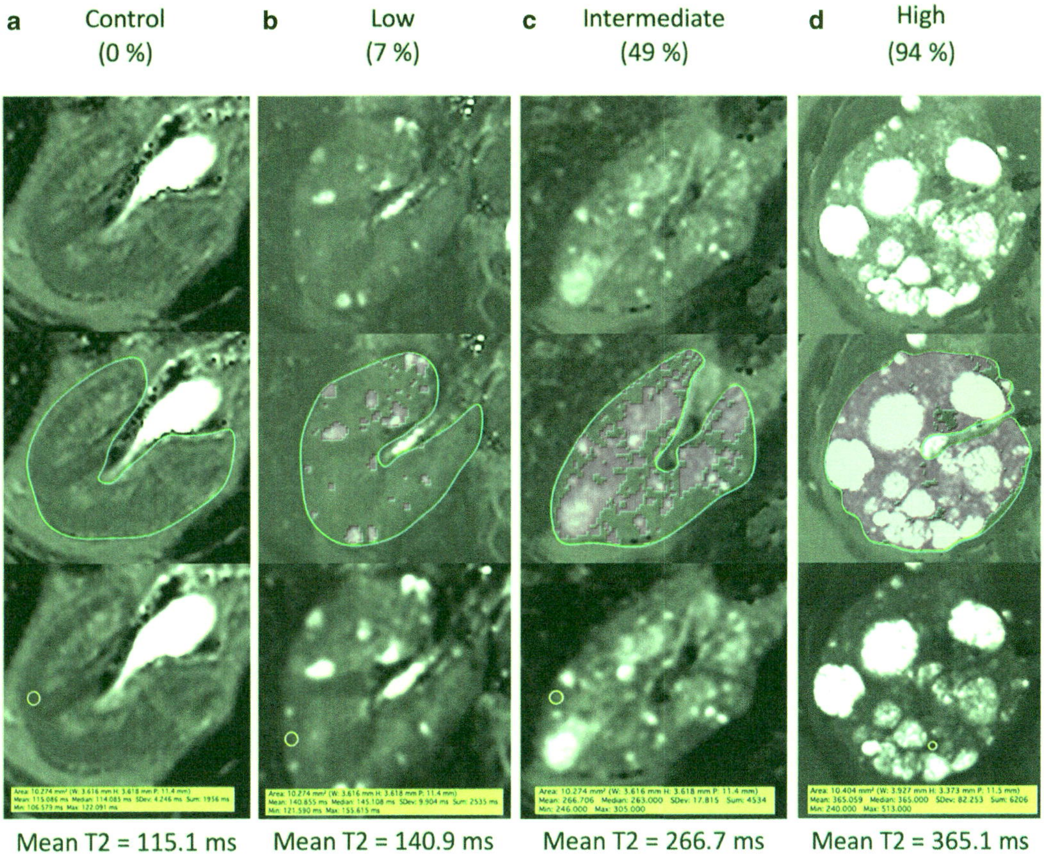

Fig. 9.2 All images are axially oriented T_2 maps with healthy subjects (**a**, a 26-year-old man) and ADPKD patients (**b** a 24-year-old woman with low kidney cyst fraction; **c** a 24-year-old man with intermediate kidney cyst fraction; **d** a 38-year-old woman with high cyst fraction). The calculated cyst fraction is on top of each column. Top row images are before, and middle row images are after segmentation. The purple area on the middle row images (**b**–**d**) reflects the cyst segmentation for the calculation of cyst fraction versus remaining kidney tissue. Bottom row images show ROI in the parenchyma (~0.1 cm^2), with the associated mean T_2 values at the bottom of each column. (Figure reproduced from [24])

thus it is not used for radiodiagnostic assessment of the kidney. T_2 of the renal cortex is shorter than in the renal medulla, and the CMD was reported to decrease during forced diuresis in the early 1980s [21]; however, the latter observation has never been retested so far [11, 12]. First studies regarding T_2 were applied in the 1980s, in particular for renal transplants, where motion or measurement duration do not play a critical role. Increased T_2 was evident in fluid collection in necrotic transplants, perinephric lymphoceles, and hematoma [22]. Increased T_2 in edema or inflammation was indirectly assessed in renal transplants [23]. With regard to the autosomal-dominant polycystic kidney disease (ADPKD; see Fig. 9.2), Siedek et al. could show that T_2 mapping showed a more precise staging and monitoring of ADPKD patients compared to the FDA-approved height-adjusted total kidney volume [24]. While recent studies on renal transplants found no significant change in T_2 relaxation time compared to different fibrosis grades, significant higher T_2 values were found in glomerulitis and patients with antibody-mediated rejection as a sign of increased inflammation. Also, higher T_2 values were associated with proteinuria [25]. The findings of Beck-Tölly et al. were partly reproduced by Adams et al. (Fig. 9.3), a Applied sequence parameters

Spoiled GRE with initial T_2 preparation for T_2 mapping

Scan plane	Oblique coronal
Voxel size (mm)	1.9 x 1.9 x 4
Acquisition time (min)	1:51
Number of slices	7
TR/TE (ms)	766.29/1.44
Averages	1
FoV (mm)	360
Flip angle (°)	12
Matrix	192
Bandwidth (Hz/Px)	1184
Fat saturation	None
Number of preparations (duration in ms)	5 (0, 30, 34, 38, 42)
Trigger delay (ms)	164
Breath-holding procedures	7
Echo spacing (ms)	3.29

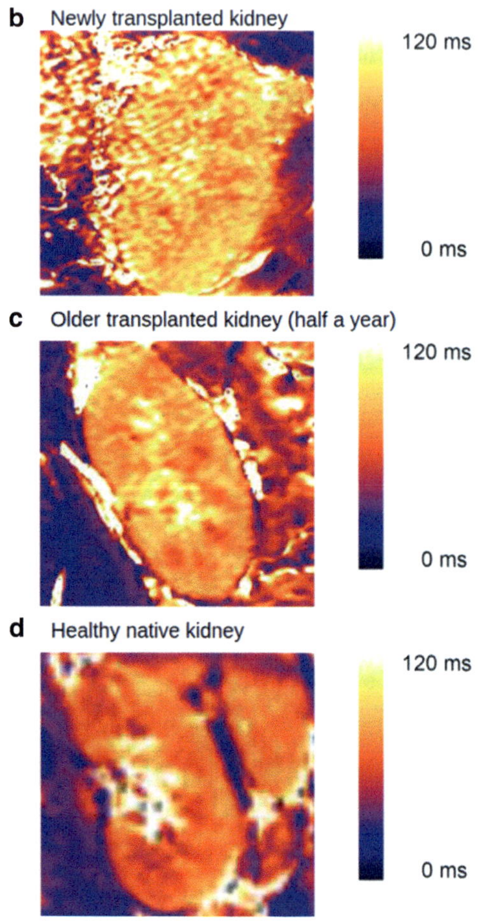

Fig. 9.3 Applied sequence parameters on the left (**a**) and example T_2 maps from transplanted kidneys (**b**, **c**) and healthy subjects (**d**). Highest T_2 values in newly transplanted kidneys (**b**) and lower T_2 values in late transplants (**c**). Lowest T_2 values found in healthy subjects (**d**). This difference was more pronounced in the renal medulla compared to the cortex. The CMD was lowest in newly transplanted patients and healthy subjects showed the highest CMD. Increased T_2 values in early transplants are considered to be linked to inflammation, that is, edema (increased water content). Arguably, this could also explain the higher T_2 values in the surrounding tissue of the newly transplanted kidney, which reduced the delineation of the kidney. Hence, well-segmented renal tissue ROI are needed to reduce the impact of selection-biased ROI. (Figure reproduced from [26])

who found highest cortical T_2 values in early transplants compared to late transplants with generally higher medullary T_2 values. In addition, medullary T_2 values were significantly different between late transplants, early transplants, and control subjects. The CMD being lowered in early transplants compared to late transplants and controls, and the CMD was significantly different between early transplants and controls [26]. These studies are promising results and verify very early observations regarding inflammation, edema, and cyst formation. Further research, especially focusing on standardization of procedures, has the potential to lead to clinical adoption and benefits for patients.

Semiautomated segmentation and associated calculation of T_2 values could reduce the risk of selection-biased T_2 values for the renal parenchyma.

Conclusion

Non-contrast, quantitative renal magnetic resonance relaxometry (MRR), including T_2 relaxation time, is a promising noninvasive modality to quantify specific tissue composition (i.e., local microstructural magneto-chemical environment) of the kidney. Pathophysiological changes in the complex structural and functional organization of the kidney are considered in parts to be quantifiable with T_2, especially regarding inflammation, edema, and cyst formation (water content), which could ultimately lead to a more precise and personalized diagnosis (staging), and enable therapeutic monitoring [27].

While the number of renal T_2 mapping studies is limited [11, 12], evidence for potential clinical adoption of T_2 mapping was introduced by the scientific community [24, 26]. However, more dedicated renal MRR, that is, T_2 mapping studies, have to be conducted with sophisticated and standardized measurement protocols, patient selection and preparations, and quality assurance, that is, comparative phantom measurements.

Acknowledgments Author #1: Financial support via FWF project KLI 736-B30 is acknowledged. This work has been conducted during the COST Action CA16103, PARENCHIMA, renalmri.org.

The funding organizations had no influence whatsoever in terms of scientific content.

Author #2: The financial support by the Christian Doppler Laboratory for Molecular Clinical MR Imaging is gratefully acknowledged.

Author #3: Financial support via FWF project KLI 736-B30 is acknowledged. This work has been conducted during the COST Action CA16103, PARENCHIMA, renalmri.org.

The funding organizations had no influence whatsoever in terms of scientific content.

References

1. Hahn EL. Spin Echoes. Phys Rev. 1950;80:580–94.
2. Carr HY, Purcell EM. Effects of diffusion on free precession in nuclear magnetic resonance experiments. Phys Rev. 1954;94:630–8.
3. Meiboom S, Gill D. Modified spin-echo method for measuring nuclear relaxation times. Rev Sci Instrum. 1958;29:688–91.
4. Kim D, Jensen JH, Wu EX, Sheth SS, Brittenham GM. Breathhold multiecho fast spin-echo pulse sequence for accurate R2 measurement in the heart and liver. Magn Reson Med. 2009;62:300–6.
5. Oshio K, Feinberg DA. GRASE (gradient- and spin-echo) imaging: a novel fast MRI technique. Magn Reson Med. 1991;20:344–9.
6. Giri S, Chung Y-C, Merchant A, Mihai G, Rajagopalan S, Raman SV, Simonetti OP. T2 quantification for improved detection of myocardial edema. J Cardiovasc Magn Reson. 2009;11:56.
7. Kellman P, Aletras AH, Mancini C, McVeigh ER, Arai AE. T2-prepared SSFP improves diagnostic confidence in edema imaging in acute myocardial infarction compared to turbo spin echo. Magn Reson Med. 2007;57:891–7.
8. Oakden W, Stanisz GJ. Effects of diffusion on high-resolution quantitative T2 MRI. NMR Biomed. 2014;27:672–80.
9. McPhee KC, Wilman AH. Transverse relaxation and flip angle mapping: evaluation of simultaneous and independent methods using multiple spin echoes. Magn Reson Med. 2017;77:2057–65.
10. Ben-Eliezer N, Sodickson DK, Block KT. Rapid and accurate T2 mapping from multi-spin-echo data using Bloch-simulation-based reconstruction. Magn Reson Med. 2015;73:809–17.
11. Wolf M, de Boer A, Sharma K, Boor P, Leiner T, Sunder-Plassmann G, Moser E, Caroli A, Jerome NP. Magnetic resonance imaging T1- and T2-mapping to assess renal structure and function: a systematic review and statement paper. Nephrol Dial Transplant. 2018;33:ii41–50.
12. Dekkers IA, de Boer A, Sharma K, et al. Consensus-based technical recommendations for clinical translation of renal T1 and T2 mapping MRI. MAGMA. 2020;33:163–76.
13. Milford D, Rosbach N, Bendszus M, Heiland S. Mono-exponential fitting in T2-relaxometry: relevance of offset and first Echo. PLoS One. 2015;10:e0145255.
14. Li X, Morgan PS, Ashburner J, Smith J, Rorden C. The first step for neuroimaging data analysis: DICOM to NIfTI conversion. J Neurosci Methods. 2016;264:47–56.
15. Zöllner FG, Kociński M, Hansen L, Golla A-K, Trbalić AŠ, Lundervold A, Materka A, Rogelj P. Kidney segmentation in renal magnetic resonance imaging—current status and prospects. IEEE Access. 2021;9:71577–605.
16. Karakuzu A, Boudreau M, Duval T, et al. qMRLab: quantitative MRI analysis, under one umbrella. J Open Source Softw. 2020;5:2343.
17. van Rossum G. Python reference manual. 1995.
18. R Core Team. R: a language and environment for statistical computing. R Foundation for Statistical Computing. 2020.
19. Kikinis R, Pieper SD, Vosburgh KG. 3D slicer: a platform for subject-specific image analysis, visualization, and clinical support. In: Jolesz FA, editor. Intraoperative imaging and image-guided therapy. New York: Springer; 2014. p. 277–89.
20. Schneider CA, Rasband WS, Eliceiri KW. NIH image to ImageJ: 25 years of image analysis. Nat Methods. 2012;9:671–5.
21. Hricak H, Crooks L, Sheldon P, Kaufman L. Nuclear magnetic resonance imaging of the kidney. Radiology. 1983;146:425–32.

22. Geisinger MA, Risius B, Jordan ML, Zelch MG, Novick AC, George CR. Magnetic resonance imaging of renal transplants. Am J Roentgenol. 1984;143:1229–34.
23. Mathys C, Blondin D, Wittsack H-J, Miese FR, Rybacki K, Walther C, Holstein A, Lanzman RS. T2' imaging of native kidneys and renal allografts—a feasibility study. Rofo. 2011;183:112–9.
24. Siedek F, Grundmann F, Weiss K, Pinto Dos Santos D, Arjune S, Haneder S, Persigehl T, Müller R-U, Baessler B. Magnetic resonance kidney parenchyma-T2 as a novel imaging biomarker for autosomal dominant polycystic kidney disease. Invest Radiol. 2020;55:217–25.
25. Beck-Tölly A, Eder M, Beitzke D, et al. Magnetic resonance imaging for evaluation of interstitial fibrosis in kidney allografts. Transplant Direct. 2020;6:e577.
26. Adams LC, Bressem KK, Scheibl S, Nunninger M, Gentsch A, Fahlenkamp UL, Eckardt K-U, Hamm B, Makowski MR. Multiparametric assessment of changes in renal tissue after kidney transplantation with quantitative MR Relaxometry and diffusion-tensor imaging at 3 T. J Clin Med Res. 2020;9(5):1551. https://doi.org/10.3390/jcm9051551.
27. Selby NM, Blankestijn PJ, Boor P, et al. Magnetic resonance imaging biomarkers for chronic kidney disease: a position paper from the European Cooperation in Science and Technology action PARENCHIMA. Nephrol Dial Transplant. 2018;33:ii4–ii14.

10 Probing Renal Oxygenation with T_2*-Sensitized MRI (BOLD-MRI)

Iosif A. Mendichovszky, Bastien Milani, Lu-Ping Li, Thoralf Niendorf, Menno Pruijm, and Pottumarthi V. Prasad

Introduction: The Physiology of Renal Tissue Oxygenation

Human organs and tissues rely on consistent and adequate supplies of oxygen for their normal functioning, existing in a dynamically balanced state between oxygen availability and the demands of cellular energy metabolism. Oxygen delivery to an organ is proportional to tissue delivery of oxygenated blood (perfusion), and it is intrinsically linked to cardiovascular function, resulting in an interdependent relationship between tissue perfusion, blood volume, cellular oxidative energy metabolism, and CO_2 production. In most organs, blood delivery and oxygen consumption are closely related while renal hemodynamics and oxygenation exhibit certain particularities compared to non-renal tissues. One of them relates to an unusually low oxygen extraction fraction (the difference between arterial and venous blood), 10–15% of available oxygen, while most organs extract approximately 45%. This can partly be attributed to the fact that, while receiving 20–25% of cardiac output under resting conditions, the kidneys only consume about 7% of the body's total oxygen, resulting in a whole kidney blood flow being higher than that of most other tissues (on a per gram basis). Renal O_2 consumption is mainly driven by the energy-dependent tubular functions, and it is also limited, in contrast to other organs, by renal perfusion. A raised renal blood flow is, in general, accompanied by increases in glomerular filtration rate and an increase in energy-dependent tubular sodium reabsorption.

Another particularity relates to the kidney's internal architecture that results in highly heterogeneous blood perfusion and oxygenation within the organ. While the renal cortex receives almost all the blood flowing into the kidney, the medulla is perfused only by a small fraction (about 10% of total renal blood flow) of blood that runs

I. A. Mendichovszky (✉)
Department of Radiology, University of Cambridge, Cambridge, UK

Department of Radiology, Addenbrooke's Hospital, Cambridge University Hospitals NHS Foundation Trust, Cambridge, UK
e-mail: im391@cam.ac.uk

B. Milani · M. Pruijm
Department of Medicine, Service of Nephrology and Hypertension, Lausanne University Hospital and University of Lausanne, Lausanne, Switzerland

L.-P. Li · P. V. Prasad
Department of Radiology, NorthShore University HealthSystem, Evanston, IL, USA

T. Niendorf
Berlin Ultrahigh Field Facility (B.U.F.F.), Max-Delbrück Center for Molecular Medicine in the Helmholtz Association, Berlin, Germany

Experimental and Clinical Research Center, A Joint Cooperation Between the Charité Medical Faculty and the Max-Delbrück Center for Molecular Medicine in the Helmholtz Association, Berlin, Germany

S. D. Serai, K. Darge (eds.), *Advanced Clinical MRI of the Kidney*,
https://doi.org/10.1007/978-3-031-40169-5_10

through the cortex (Fig. 10.1). The medulla is essentially perfused by descending vasa recta that depart from post-glomerular arterioles (Fig. 10.2). Due to this, the medullary renal partial pressure of oxygen (pO_2) is very low. The reduced medullary pO_2 is maintained by (1) O_2 shunting from arteries to veins in the cortex as well as from descending to ascending vasa recta in the medulla, (2) "plasma skimming" (the differential distribution of erythrocytes and plasma at certain vessel branches), and (3) the lowering of hematocrit in the long and narrow vasa recta supplying the medulla (Fåhræus–Lindqvist effect). In addition, the higher metabolic rate of the medulla necessary to enable active reabsorption of sodium along medullary thick ascending limbs of Henle's loop places further demands on medullary oxygenation, contributing to a persistently low pO_2 [1].

The crucial role played by renal oxygen availability in kidney metabolism establishes renal tissue ischemia as one of the main mechanisms leading to acute kidney injury and suggests that renal tissue hypoxia is a unifying factor in the development and progression of chronic kidney disease (CKD) [2]. This is discussed in more detail in Sect. 10.4.1. Assessing renal tissue oxygenation in humans is therefore highly relevant to clinical practice. MRI of renal oxygenation using the blood oxygenation level-dependent (BOLD) MR parameter T_2* for image contrast weighting or for parametric mapping has become a widely used method to probe renal tissue oxygenation, although its use remains largely restricted to the research setting.

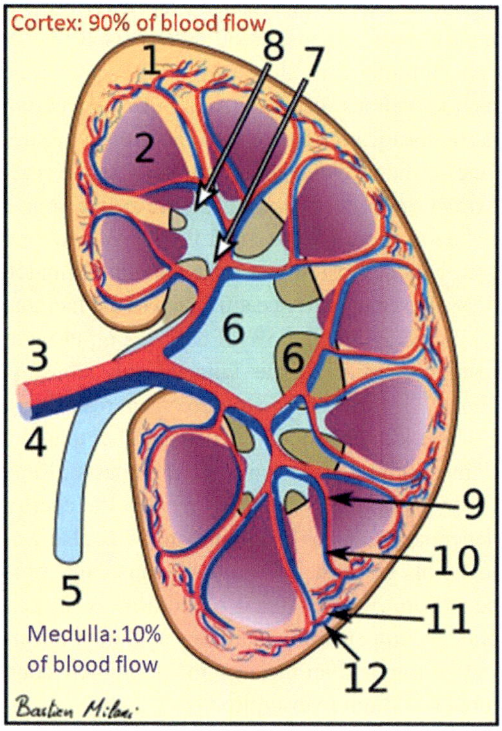

Fig. 10.1 A simplified image of kidney anatomy showing that the outer layers of the kidney parenchyma only contain well-perfused cortex, whereas the deeper layers contain both the cortex and medulla (in the triangular-shaped pyramids). (1) renal cortex, (2) renal medulla, (3) main renal artery, (4) main renal vein, (5) ureter, (6) renal pelvis, (7) major calyx, (8) minor calyx, (9) interlobar artery, (10) interlobar vein, and (11) arcuate artery, (12) arcuate vein

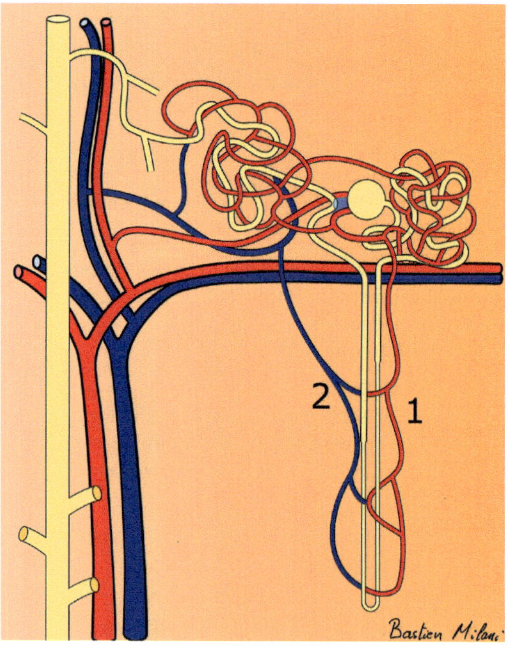

Fig. 10.2 Schematic representation of one nephron, composed of a circle-shaped glomerulus, a tubular system with convoluted and straight parts, and a network of vessels. The descending parts of the vasa recta [1] deliver oxygen to the medulla, but due to shunting between the descending and ascending vasa recta [2], the partial pressure of oxygen in the medulla is low

MRI Physics and Acquisition Protocols

Basic Principles of T_2*-Sensitized MRI (BOLD-MRI)

Hemoglobin in the blood is the primary carrier of oxygen and this oxygenation status determines its magnetic properties. Oxygenated hemoglobin (oxy-Hb) has a zero magnetic moment and is diamagnetic. The four unpaired electrons per Fe atom make deoxygenated hemoglobin (deoxy-Hb) strongly paramagnetic. Since Hb is compartmentalized within the vasculature, the presence of deoxy-Hb causes susceptibility gradients and microscopic magnetic field perturbations around the vessels. The spins in the vicinity of the vessels hence experience spin dephasing. The relaxation parameter T_2* describes the loss of coherence and decay of the MR signal due to spin dephasing. T_2* is governed by $1/T_2^* = 1/T_2 + 1/T_2'$, with T_2 being the transverse relaxation time and T_2' embodying susceptibility-related contributions. T_2*-weighted MRI is sensitive to changes in the amount of deoxygenated Hb (deoxy-Hb) per tissue volume element (voxel). T_2* decreases and a signal attenuation in T_2*-weighted MR images occurs if the volume fraction of deoxy-Hb increases. This effect of the oxygenation status of Hb on T_2* is termed blood oxygenation level-dependent (BOLD) contrast [3]. Although T_2* is widely assumed to provide a surrogate of renal tissue oxygenation, variations in T_2* may only reflect changes in blood oxygenation. This distinction is of relevance since renal blood oxygenation and renal tissue oxygenation can vary independently due to arteriovenous O_2 shunting and plasma skimming. Changes in [vessel volume]/[tissue volume] induced by active vasomotion or passive circular vessel distension/compression also alter the amount of deoxy-Hb per tissue volume and hence T_2*.

T_2* sensitization is given by the echo time (TE). TE is defined by the time between MR signal excitation and MR signal readout. TE governs the loss of phase coherence of the MR signal due to spin dephasing. T_2*-sensitized MRI is most sensitive to blood oxygenation changes when TE is equal to T_2*. Blood oxygenation-induced T_2* changes exhibit a supralinear relationship with the magnetic field strength [4, 5]. T_2*-weighted MRI at higher magnetic field strengths shows enhanced sensitivity to changes in renal blood oxygenation. Clinical applications benefit from renal T_2*-weighted MRI at 3.0 T versus the counterparts at lower magnetic field strengths. The most widely used techniques for T_2*-sensitized renal MRI are gradient echo imaging and echo-planar imaging (EPI). T_2* sensitization can be achieved by a single acquisition using a TE of approximately 20–25 ms that governs T_2* contrast between renal layers, that is, cortex, outer medulla, and inner medulla. Parametric mapping provides quantitative data of the relaxation time T_2*. For this purpose, multiple echo acquisitions are used to estimate either the relaxation time T_2* (s) or the relaxation rate R_2* (s^{-1}). The decay rate constants can be estimated either using a linear fit to Ln(signal intensity(SI)) versus echo time (TE) or by fitting an exponential function to the SI versus TE data. Scanner platforms prefer the use of linear fits because of the less computational burden. When relaxation rates are not known, it may be preferred to use exponential fits. However, when the choice of maximum TE is based on the T_2* or R_2* of the tissue of interest, either method can be used.

Under "perfect" physiological conditions, the pO_2 of capillary blood is in equilibrium with the surrounding tissue, and hence a decrease in R_2* can be thought to represent increased oxygen availability. This is applicable when evaluating acute effects of pharmacological maneuvers such as administration of furosemide. However, when comparing T_2* or R_2* between different individuals or different cohorts such as healthy volunteers versus individuals with CKD, it becomes important to consider other confounding factors that could influence T_2* or R_2* values [6]. For an in-depth discussion, please refer to [7]. This has led to interest in methods to estimate oxygen saturation of Hb (StO_2) [8] or blood pO_2 [9]. However, this would require knowledge of regional fractional blood volume (fBV) and hematocrit. Measurement of fBV requires the use of blood pool contrast agents such as ferumoxytol [8].

Patient Preparation

Patient preparation is important, as several dietary factors may alter kidney parenchyma R_2* and should therefore be taken into account. First of all, hydration status influences the T_2* (BOLD) signal. In one of their first studies, Prasad et al. reported significant decreases up to 30% in medullary R_2* one hour after an acute oral water load of 10 mL/kg in young healthy volunteers [10]. This is probably due to a combination of a reduction in active, oxygen-consuming reabsorption of electrolytes and an increase in the tubular volume fraction. Of note, in more recent studies, oral water loads between 1.5 and 5 mL/kg did not induce changes in R_2* [11]. In a recent consensus paper, most experts advise to restrain from water intake 4 h before the scan [12]. Restraining from water (and food) intake before the scan may also decrease the risk of bowel motion or susceptibility artifacts, but this issue has not been fully resolved. If restraining from water intake before the scan is not feasible, water intake should be standardized, for example, with an hourly intake of water of 1.5 mL/kg. The latter solution has the advantage that similar hydration protocols are used for inulin- or para-amino-hippuric acid clearance studies, thus allowing the combination of clearance studies with BOLD-MRI on the same day.

Dietary salt intake can also influence kidney parenchymal R_2*. This has been demonstrated in a crossover study that included young normotensive and untreated hypertensive male volunteers [13]. After 7 days on a low-salt diet, medullary R_2* were significantly lower than after 7 days on a high-salt diet. The decrease in medullary R_2* (suggesting an increase in oxygenation) was probably due to a reduction in sodium reabsorption in the NKCC2 transporters of Henle's loops. Of note, only men were included in this study, and the differences in salt intake between the two phases were extreme in this study: volunteers consumed on average 19 g/day of salt during high salt and 1.2 g/day on low salt. Therefore, whether smaller variations in dietary salt intake also induce changes in R_2*, in both men and women, remains to be demonstrated. There is no agreement among experts whether salt intake should be standardized before the scan, but when possible, recording salt intake is recommended [12].

In a small cross-over study of ten healthy volunteers, the intake of 1 g/kg of dark chocolate (70% cocoa) reduced medullary R_2* 2 h later, whereas white chocolate did not induce any changes in cortical or medullary R_2* [14]. This difference is possibly explained by cocoa-induced changes in renal perfusion, but as renal perfusion was not measured, this needs further assessment. Clearance studies have demonstrated that high protein foods have the potential to increase renal blood flow and glomerular filtration rate [15]. So far, it is unknown whether high protein meals affect renal BOLD-MRI, from a practical point of view, abstaining from food intake 4–6 h before the scan is recommended. In the abovementioned consensus paper, 8% of experts recommended to abstain from high protein foods 24 h before the scan [12].

Patients suffering from diabetic mellitus (DM) need special attention, as fasting increases their risk of hypoglycemia. Besides, several cross-sectional studies have shown that blood glucose levels at the time of the scan are associated with R_2* levels [11, 16, 17]. For example, in a study by Zheng et al., type 2 DM patients with blood glucose levels >9 mmol/L had higher medullary R_2* levels than those with fasting glucose levels ≤9 mmol/L, despite similar age and eGFR [17]. In a small study of 19 young, overweight but non-diabetic subjects (57.9% women), the intravenous administration of 0.15 g/kg of glucose leads to an acute decrease of R_2* in both the cortex and medulla [16]. Whether this was due to partial volume effects or true changes in oxygenation remained unclear. There was no specific recommendation on blood glucose monitoring in the abovementioned consensus paper, but considering the available data, according to our opinion, glycemia should be measured just before the scan.

The effect of many drugs on R_2* has been studied and is discussed in more detail in Sect. 10.4.5. For several drugs, their potential to alter acutely or chronically renal R_2* has been clearly demonstrated, whereas for many others, this is unknown. Depending on the research question, drugs should be withheld or given when performing T_2*-sensitized MRI. Clearly, when one wishes to study the effects of a particular drug on renal tissue oxygenation as estimated with T_2*-sensitized MRI, other drugs should not be given before the scan, unless withholding them constitutes a risk to the patient. For this reason, it may be preferred to perform the scans in the morning. Of note, Eckerbom and colleagues did not find any circadian rhythm of R_2* in healthy volunteers, despite circadian variations in renal perfusion and GFR [18]. For drugs with longer half-lives, stopping the drug one or several days before the scan may be necessary. In this situation, risks have to be weighed against the benefits.

Many cohort studies have been performed in order to assess the potential of T_2*-sensitized MRI to predict adverse renal outcome. In some of these studies [19], patients were scanned in the early afternoon while taking their usual drugs, arguing that a scan performed under these conditions approaches best the steady state of the patient. In others, RAS blockers and diuretics were withheld one or several days before the MRI [20, 21]. Despite the differences in design, most studies came to the same conclusion, namely, that cortical R_2* is a predictor of consecutive decline of kidney function and adverse outcome. It is therefore difficult to provide recommendations on this subject, and decisions may depend on local ethical and scanning policies. Whatever the decision, recording medication intake is recommended.

Several questions concerning patient preparation remain unanswered. For example, plasma osmolality, pH, and temperature all affect the O_2 dissociation curve, whereas iron status affects the tissue paramagnetic properties. None of the latter factors have been studied for this purpose in humans yet. While awaiting these studies, the authors advise to avoid smoking prior to the MRI examination and to delay the scan at least 2 weeks in case of recent IV iron infusion.

Acquisition Protocol

Initial introductory studies of renal T_2*-sensitized MRI used single-shot echo planar imaging (EPI) [22]. Advantages of EPI include short acquisition time and so it can "freeze motion" when scanning abdominal organs. A series of EPI images acquired with different echo times can be combined to estimate T_2* or R_2*. However, since each echo time-weighted image is acquired during a different breath-hold interval, they may not be perfectly co-registered to each other limiting R_2* mapping. EPI is highly sensitive to bulk magnetic susceptibility artifacts which may result in geometrical distortion and loss of anatomical fidelity of the images, signal loss and signal void, and limited spatial resolution. The image distortion is amplified in regions with poor magnetic field homogeneity such as in the vicinity of bowels filled with gas and at tissue interfaces. There has been one study to investigate the temporal changes following angiotensin II administration using multi-echo EPI acquisition with a 4 s temporal resolution [23].

Most of the studies to date are performed with breath-hold multi-echo gradient echo (mGRE) techniques [24]. mGRE acquisitions provide adequate SNR (signal-to-noise ratio), spatial resolution, and image quality compared to single-shot EPI. mGRE imaging using longer echo times may be constrained by signal losses and signal voids induced by bulk susceptibility artifacts. mGRE can suffer from signal phase and signal amplitude variations between odd and even echoes when both water and fat components are present in renal tissue. These variations are superimposed to the T_2* decay and hence may confound T_2* estimation and T_2* mapping. Choice of echo times cor-

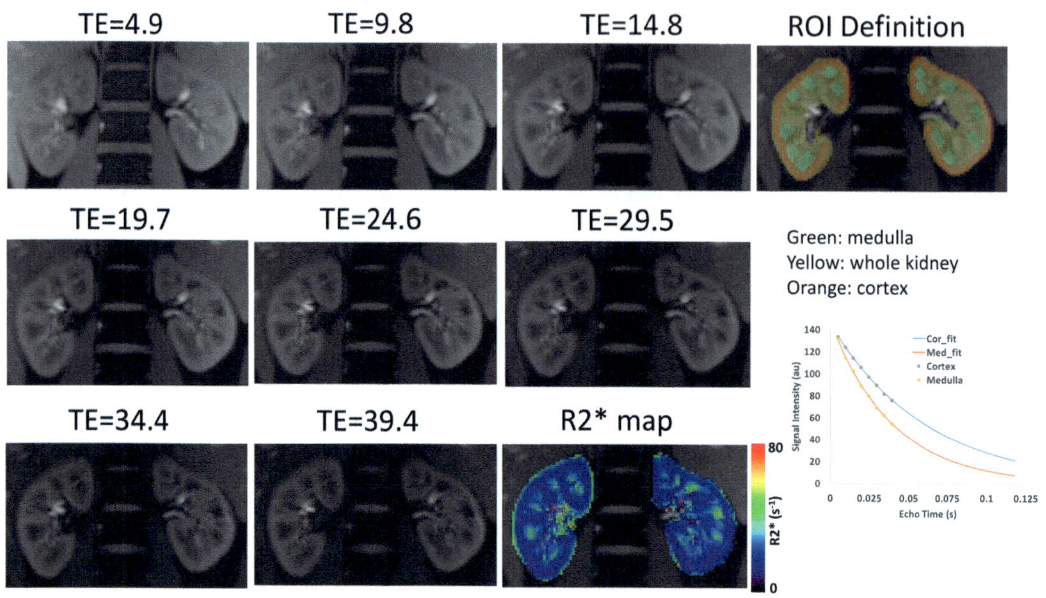

Fig. 10.3 A typical data set acquired with a multiple gradient echo (mGRE) technique showing eight individual images with increasing echo times obtained within a breath-hold interval. Note the increasing T_2* weighting (i.e., darkening of images) with higher echo times. Using the well-defined exponential decay of signal intensity with echo time, an R_2* map can be calculated by performing the exponential fit on a voxel basis. Note the higher R_2* values in the medulla consistent with the lower tissue and hence blood pO_2. For quantitative analysis, regions of interest can be defined in the cortex, medulla, and whole kidney parenchyma

responding to the fat-water in-phase or the fat-water out-of-phase state can minimize or even eliminate such artifacts. In the presence of flow, the use of even echoes may be preferred. Figure 10.3 shows a typical data set with the different echo images acquired in healthy volunteer.

Recently, an international consortium put forward consensus-based technical recommendations for data acquisition protocols for T_2*-sensitized renal MRI [12]. We have adapted the recommendations and drafted Table 10.1 as recommended procedures and parameters for renal T2*/R_2* mapping. For any of the functional renal MRI acquisitions, it was thought to be necessary to normalize the physiological status by either implementing at least a 4-h fasting period before scanning or to follow a controlled fluid intake within 4 h prior to scanning. Because of the known dependence of R_2* on voxel size [25], it is necessary to maintain voxel size between subjects or sites in multicenter studies. It is quite conceivable that technologists would change the field of view based on the body habitus of the subject under investigation.

Common Image Artifacts

Bulk Susceptibility Artifacts (Bowel Gas)

On most occasions, since image artifacts (such as those due to bowel gas) are commonly not appreciated till after the scan is completed, image analysis should not include renal regions affected by artifacts. Alternately, if artifacts are identified during scanning, the acquisitions could be repeated with thinner slices to mitigate the artifacts (Fig. 10.4a and b).

Respiratory Motion Artifacts

mGRE acquisitions can be obtained within a comfortable breath-hold of 10–15 s. However, the participant may not hear the instructions or may fall asleep during the scan. Respiratory motion-induced artifacts can be easily appreciated by playing the multiple echo time images in a cine loop. Alternately, a respiratory triggering belt can be used to monitor the breathing patterns during the scan and alert the participant when not holding their breath.

Table 10.1 Recommendations on renal BOLD-MRI data acquisition, analysis, and interpretation

BOLD-MRI—recommendations on data acquisition, analysis, and interpretation	
Patient preparation	Normal hydration (100 mL water), 4 h fasting from food
Field strength	1.5 T or 3 T (3 T preferred if available)
Sequence	Two-dimensional multi-echo GRE
Slice orientation	Coronal oblique to kidneys
Spatial resolution (in-plane)	2–3 mm
Slice thickness	3–5 mm
Coverage	3–5 slices centered on the kidney hilum
Parallel imaging factor	2
Fat suppression	Yes
TR (msec)	60–75
Number of echoes	8–16
TE (msec)	Minimum to up to 50 with choice of in-phase echoes to account for fat-water
Number of averages	1
Breathing mode	Breath-hold preferred
ROI placement	Manual
Cortical ROI	1 stripe/slice, >3 slices
Medullary ROI	3 samples/slice, >3 slices
Curve fitting	Mono-exponential
Reporting	Cortex and medulla
Reporting metric	R_2* (s−1)
R_2* map format	Color or grayscale quantitative map
Metric statistics reporting	Mean, median, and standard deviation

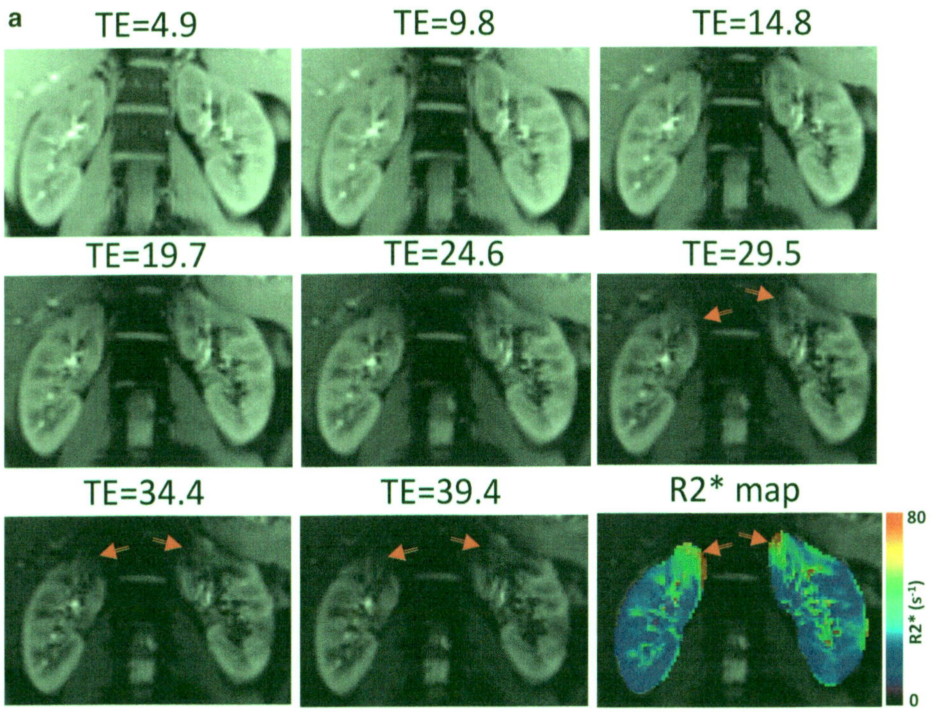

Fig. 10.4 (**a**) mGRE data illustrating bulk susceptibility artifacts (commonly due to presence of air/gas in bowels). These artifacts become apparent at longer echo times and result in artifactually high R_2* values (red arrows). (**b**) mGRE data illustrating bulk susceptibility artifacts at long echo times resulting in artifactually high R_2* values (red arrow bottom left). Note the reduced effects when using thinner slices (red arrow bottom right)

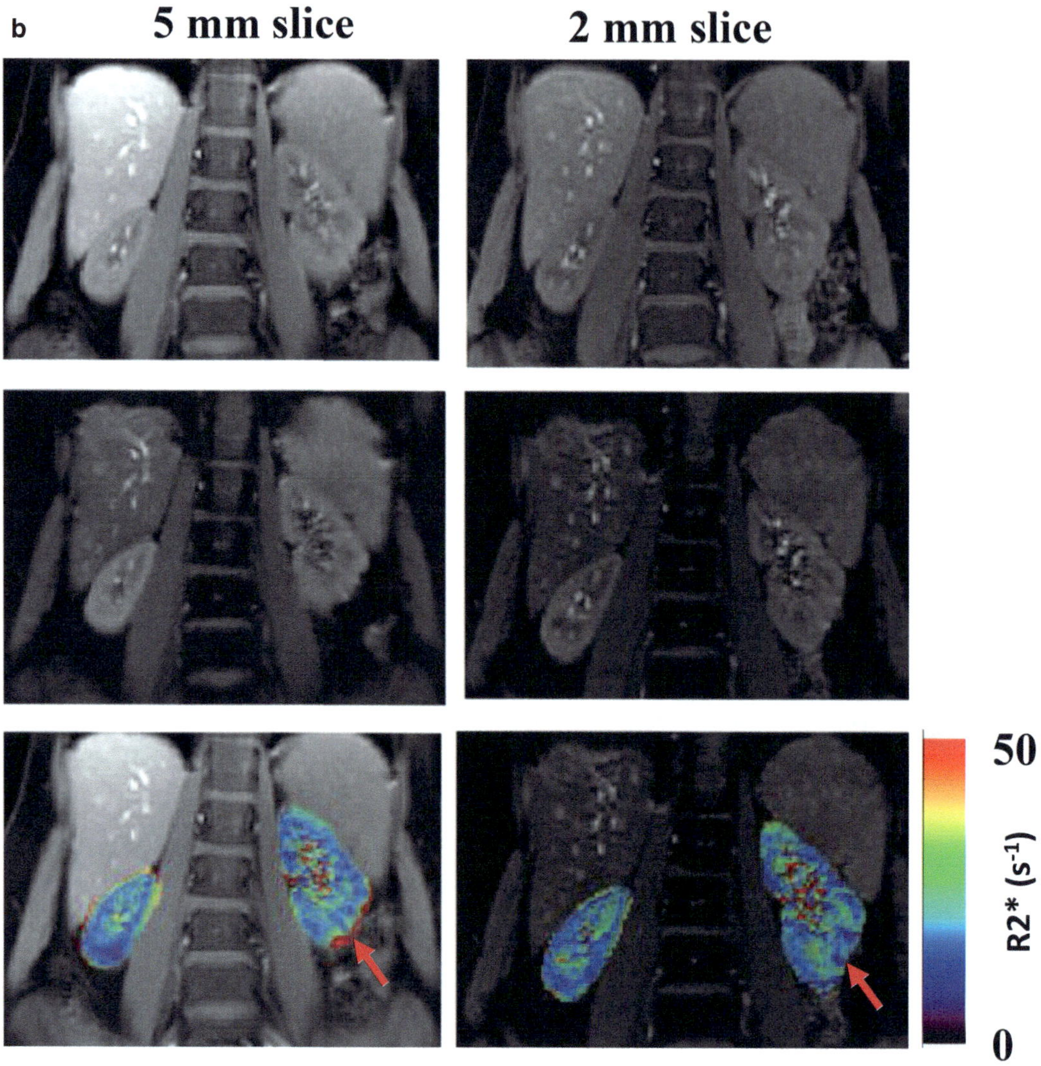

Fig. 10.4 (continued)

Image Post-processing and Data Analysis Methods

Image Post-processing

BOLD-MRI results can be expressed as the T_2* relaxation or R_2* relaxation rate of each voxel. Since 2019, there is a general consensus to report R_2* values. Both exponential and log-linear fitting of the T_2*-signal as a function of the echo time are accepted ways to extract R_2* for each voxel. An R_2* value is a relaxation rate and has the unit 1/s or Hz. An R_2* map is obtained by the voxel-wise fitting of R_2*-weighted values versus echo time. Log-linear fitting can be performed. It can serve, if desired, as the initial step for a more refined exponential fitting with the model:

$$s(t) = As \cdot e^{-t \cdot R_2^*}$$

with parameters A and R_2* and where $s(t)$ is the signal to be fitted. Voxels with outlying values should be excluded, for example, values smaller than 10 Hz and larger than 50 Hz. Another useful exclusion criterium makes use of the root-mean-squared (rms) relative error of the fit given by

$$\sqrt{\sum_{n=1}^{n\mathrm{Echo}} \frac{\left(s\left(t_n\right)-s_{\mathrm{model}}\left(t_n\right)\right)^2}{s_{\mathrm{model}}\left(t_n\right)^2} / n\mathrm{Echo}}$$

where nEcho is the total number of echoes and $s(t)$ is the signal to be fitted. For example, voxels with an rms relative fitting error larger than 0.1 (10%) can be excluded.

The consensus paper provides further guidance on the standardized reporting of quantitative BOLD-MRI values [12]. It outlines that the reported value should be R_2* (rather than T_2*) obtained from exponential or log-linear fit of BOLD signal but cautioned that the results are not comparable between fitting methods and that the log-linear fit increases the influence of noise for later echoes with low SNR [12]. The consensus paper also highlighted that correcting for noise at later echoes may be possible by using a weighted log-linear fit, an exponential fit after identifying the noise floor, or by limiting the maximum TE to the approximate T_2* of tissue of interest.

Data Analysis

Kidneys are structurally heterogeneous organs. The cortex contains both glomeruli, tubuli, and interstitial tissue, whereas the medulla contains tubuli but no glomeruli. The outer layers of the kidneys contain exclusively cortical tissue, whereas the deeper layers contain both cortical and medullary tissues. The medullary tissue is organized in triangular- shaped pyramids. These pyramids can be easily distinguished from the cortex by the human eye in MRI images of healthy volunteers, but this can be difficult in patients with CKD (Fig. 10.5).

As perfusion and oxygenation strongly differ between the cortex and the medulla, distinction of both histological structures is important for a correct interpretation of R_2* maps. Historically, manual placement of regions of interest (ROI) in the cortex and medulla has been most frequently used. With this approach, small ROIs (containing up to 40 voxels) are placed on anatomic images in cortex and medulla and then copied to the R_2* map to obtain the mean R_2* value of each ROI. Some investigators use a slightly different technique and place small ROIs in the pyramids and one large, ring-shaped ROI encompassing the entire cortical tissue for the cortex. Four other methods to analyze T_2* or R_2* maps have been reported in the literature [26]: the fractional tissue technique, the 12 layer concentric objects (TLCO) or multiple layer concentric objects (MLCO) technique, the compartmental method, and a histogram analysis-based technique that defines masks for the cortex and medulla based on T1 maps [27].

Several studies have specifically assessed the interobserver variability (image analysis of the same subject by two or more different observers) of these techniques [28–31]. Piskunowicz et al. reported interobserver coefficients of variation (CV) with the ROI technique of 3.6 and 6.8% of cortical and medullary R_2* values in healthy volunteers, versus 5.7 and 12.5% in CKD [28]. With the semiautomatic TLCO technique, the same research group reported much lower CVs of 2.2, 2.0, and 3.1% in healthy and mild CKD and severe CKD groups [28]. Concerning repeatability (same subject scanned several times), Cox et al. reported a low intra-subject CV of 4.1% in healthy volunteers who underwent 2–3 repeat scans at 3 T on the same or different day [27].

Most authors agree that the ROI technique is reproducible and easy to use in persons with (near) normal renal function (GFR) but less reliable in advanced CKD (stage 3b–5). Li and colleagues showed that the ROI technique performs equally well as the TLCO method in patients with moderate CKD (stage 1–3a) [32]. As the ROI technique is widely available and easy to use, in the consensus paper, most experts recommended the ROI technique for the analysis of BOLD images [12]. However, we recommend the use of semiautomatic methods when locally available, especially when studying patients with advanced CKD.

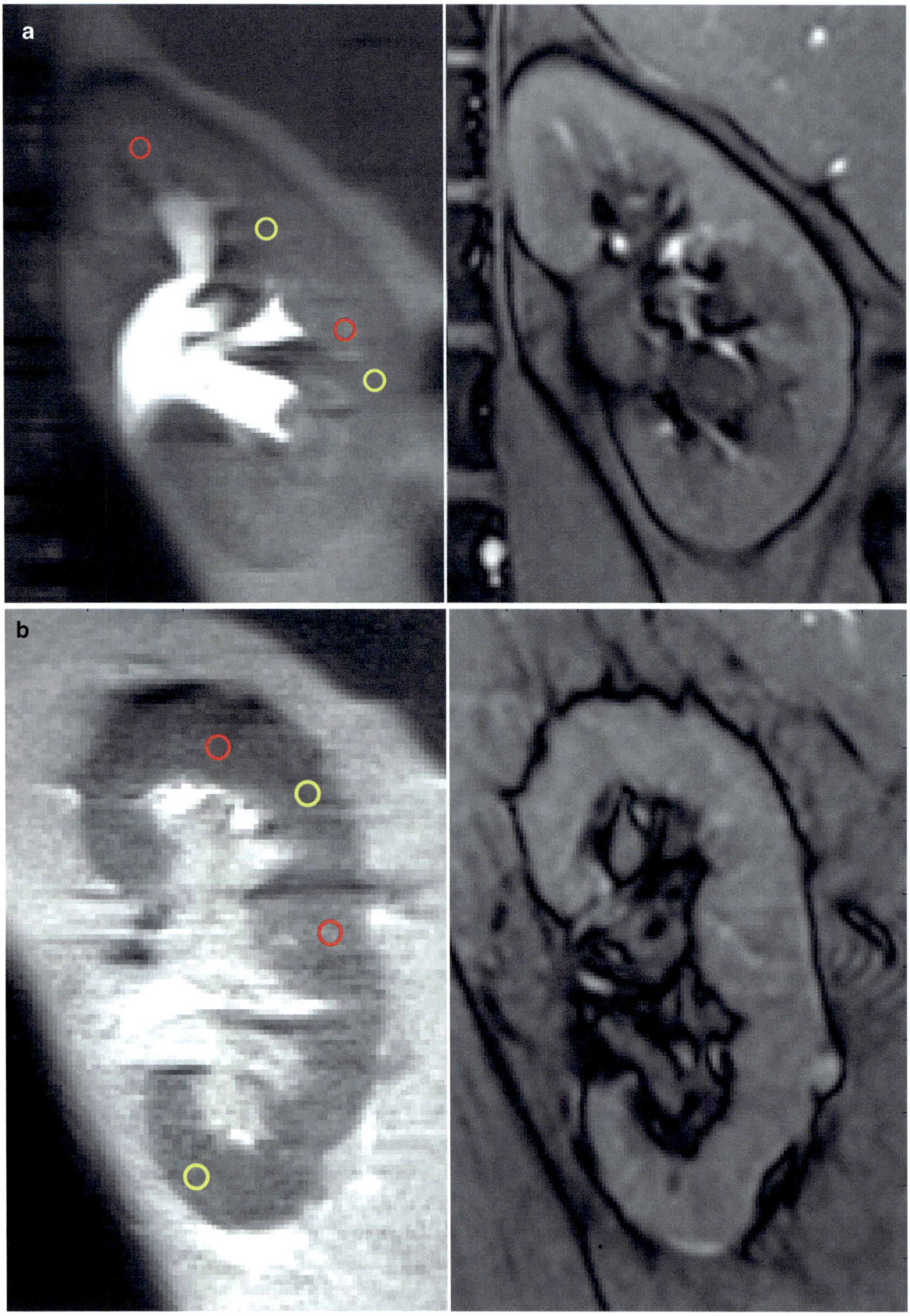

Fig. 10.5 An example of manual placement of ROIs in (**a**) a healthy participant and (**b**) a patient with advanced CKD. Due to the lack of corticomedullary differentiation in the latter, correct placement in the cortex and medulla is challenging

Clinical Studies and Possible Applications

Chronic Kidney Disease

Since the beginning of renal T_2*-sensitized MRI, there has been a specific interest in applying the technique to patients with CKD. The first article on renal BOLD-MRI was published in 1996 [22], whereas the so-called chronic hypoxia hypothesis was formulated around the same time, in 1998 [2]. This hypothesis states that renal tissue hypoxia is a unifying pathway in the development and progression of CKD, irrespective of its cause [2]. According to this hypothesis, primary glomerular injury leads to a simultaneous loss of post-glomerular arterioles and peritubular capillaries, which leads on its term to interstitial hypoxia. The hypoxia will trigger epithelial-mesenchymal transdifferentiation, recruit inflammatory circulating cells and cytokines, and stimulate tubulointerstitial fibrosis. The fibrosis, in turn, leads to the loss of outflow tracts from unaffected capillaries and nephrons and to an ongoing vicious circle of progressive renal injury. Many animal studies have supported this hypothesis, and intrarenal microelectrodes have indeed measured decreased local tissue pO_2 in several experimental models of CKD [33, 34]. However, proof in humans was lacking, as renal tissue oxygenation could not be measured without invasive procedures. The technical development of renal BOLD-MRI overcame this problem and opened a new era of research in humans. However, initially several cross-sectional MRI studies did not find higher R_2* values in CKD patients [11, 35]. This was probably partly due to the lack of standardized patient preparation and the use of low magnetic field strengths (1.5 T). More recent studies—performed under standardized conditions and higher magnetic field strengths (3.0 T)—have systematically reported higher cortical R_2* (corresponding to lower oxygenation) in CKD patients as compared to controls, both in adults and children, irrespective of the cause of CKD [36–38].

Medullary R_2* has shown less consistent results. Some studies reported higher medullary R_2* in patients with CKD [39], whereas others found lower R_2* [30], suggesting higher medullary oxygenation in CKD patients as compared with controls. Heterogenous results have especially been reported in patients suffering from DM [40–42]. As most studies did not measure blood glucose levels just before the scan, differences in glycemia may partly explain this observation. Besides, as oxygenation is the result of the balance between oxygen delivery and consumption, active transport in the tubuli may be reduced more than the medullary perfusion, thus leading to a paradoxical decrease in medullary R_2* in CKD patients. Clearly, it is difficult to interpret the results of these studies, as most BOLD-MRI exams are performed without simultaneous measurement of renal perfusion.

An increasing number of prospective studies have recently assessed whether high baseline R_2* predicts consecutive decline in eGFR. The first reported study was a Swiss cohort of 112 CKD patients and 71 controls. All participants underwent a BOLD-MRI exam at baseline under standardized hydration conditions and regular blood and urine sampling for on average 3 years, in order to assess kidney function decline and proteinuria. CKD patients with high cortical R_2* (>90th percentile) had a faster yearly eGFR decline and needed three times more often renal replacement therapy than those with lower R_2* [19]. Two other studies reported similar results in different populations. In a study by Sugiyama et al. of 91 Asian CKD patients (41.8% with DM), T_2* was, together with the urine protein to creatinine ratio, the only independent predictor of eGFR decline [21]. In another study of 54 individuals (41 with CKD, 32% African-Americans) by Li et al., cortical R_2* values were higher in CKD patients than controls, whereas the furosemide-induced change in R_2* was inversely associated with annual eGFR decline [20]. Taken together, these studies provide evidence for the hypoxia hypothesis in humans and open the road to the implementation of renal BOLD-MRI in the clinical care for CKD patients as a new tool to predict adverse renal outcome. However, the number of patients was fairly small in these studies, and only one study reported data on hard outcomes (the need for renal replacement therapy).

Therefore, these results need confirmation in larger trials. Such trials are actually ongoing: we mention here the European BEAt-DKD study that is recruiting 500 patients with diabetic kidney disease [43] and the Kidney Precision Medicine Project [44] aiming to recruit 1000 CKD patients, of which a subset will undergo renal MRI.

Acute Kidney Injury

Only a small number of studies have evaluated the potential of T_2*-sensitized MRI in patients with acute kidney injury (AKI) with not-so-promising results. BOLD-MRI showed a wide range of R_2* in participants with acute tubular necrosis (ATN) and no statistical differences between these patients and healthy volunteers. Although a study by Bauer et al. did demonstrate R_2* variations in healthy volunteers after the administration of furosemide that did not occur in those with AKI [45], a study by Inoue et al. has shown no consistent trends in R_2* measurements in 23 AKI patients when compared to healthy volunteers and CKD patients, which the authors attributed to interstitial edema and renal hypoxia known to occur in acute renal insults [46]. A more recent study using BOLD-MRI as part of a multiparametric protocol in seven patients, followed up for a year, has shown a nonsignificant trend to R_2* increase over time post-AKI [47]. Overall, the usefulness of BOLD-MRI in acute kidney injury (AKI) warrants further human studies backed up by research in experimental models.

Transplantation

The usefulness of T_2*-sensitized MRI to evaluate acute renal transplant rejection was first proven in 2005 by Sadowski et al. [48]. Their study showed that medullary R_2* was lower in the acute rejection group compared with normally functioning transplants and transplants with acute tubular necrosis (ATN). Cortical R_2* was higher in ATN compared with the other groups. Subsequent findings have confirmed these observations and suggested the medullary-to-cortical R_2* ratio as a potential biomarker [49, 50]. Furthermore, T_2* measured in renal cortex and medulla has proven to be reproducible in subjects with good allograft function, being most useful in differentiating stable well-functioning allografts from acute rejection [51]. Due to fast acquisition times and its reproducibility, BOLD-MRI has often been integrated in more complex MRI protocols, such as perfusion and diffusion-weighted MRI, paving the way to multiparametric renal MRI assessments of the natural evolution of transplanted kidneys, their degree of fibrosis, and the occurrence of episodes of rejection/ATN over time [52, 53]. In a subsequent study integrating T_2* and perfusion MRI, Sadowski et al. showed that allografts with biopsy-proven acute rejection had significantly decreased medullary R_2* and decreased renal perfusion, despite a reduced blood flow, suggesting a decline in oxygen consumption that likely reflects the decrease in filtration and tubular reabsorption during an acute rejection episode [54]. A recent multiparametric renal MRI study by Wang et al. in 103 renal transplant recipients demonstrated a significant correlation between cortical R_2* and biopsy-proven interstitial fibrosis (rho = 0.61; $P < 0.001$), even after adjusting for hemoglobin level (rho = 0.58; $P < 0.001$). This correlation was significantly higher in patients with allograft injury than in normal controls (17.8 s^{-1} versus 15.6 s^{-1}; $P < 0.001$) [53].

Renovascular Disease/Renal Artery Stenosis

Renal artery stenosis (RAS) is characterized by uni- or bilateral reductions in renal blood flow due to reductions in the renal artery lumen. According to the degree of narrowing, RAS is classified as moderate (60–70%) or severe (>70% reduction in the lumen of the renal artery) [55]. RAS is in ~90% of cases caused by atherosclerosis, but fibromuscular dysplasia or inflammatory vascular diseases can also cause RAS. Atherosclerotic RAS is a relatively common disease: it is present in 2–5% of patients suffering from arterial hypertension (AHT) and as such one of the main causes of secondary AHT. Its prevalence increases to 6.8% in elderly patients (>65 years) and reaches 25% in Caucasians with refractory hypertension and 30–40% in persons with peripheral artery disease or abdominal aortic aneurysm [56, 57].

From a physiological viewpoint, reduced renal blood flow (RBF) will diminish oxygen delivery, thereby potentially impacting renal tissue oxygenation. BOLD-MRI seems therefore particularly a suitable surrogate for probing renal oxygenation in patients with RAS, also thanks to its capacity to measure separately R_2* of the stenotic and of the contralateral kidney. Studies in swine models of RAS that used clips around the renal arteries to induce acute [58] or chronic [59] reductions in RBF have indeed demonstrated that BOLD-MRI can detect changes in renal oxygenation, as oxygenation was measured simultaneously with intrarenal oxygen electrodes. Interestingly, studies in humans revealed that cortical and medullary R_2* are preserved in many patients with moderate RAS, despite significant reductions in RBF in stenotic kidneys [60]. This finding underlines the close relationship between oxygen delivery and consumption: significant decreases in RBF lead to simultaneous decreases in GFR, thus attenuating oxygen-consuming solute transport in the tubuli, resulting in a neutral oxygen balance. Besides, adjustments in arteriovenous shunting may also buffer the effects of reduced RBF [61].

However, kidneys distal to severe luminal obstructions (>70–90%) show pronounced increases in R_2* [62], suggesting that there is a threshold above which the adaptability of the kidneys is lost, and ischemia develops [63]. The team from the Mayo Clinic has shown in a series of elegant BOLD-MRI studies that renal tissue hypoxia is directly associated with increased levels of injury biomarkers [neutrophil-gelatinase-associated lipocalin (NGAL) and monocyte-chemoattractant protein-1 (MCP-1)] in the renal vein [64]. Transjugular biopsies have been performed in some patients and showed increases in tissular TGF-β and infiltration of CD-68-positive macrophages in the stenotic, hypoxic kidneys [65]. According to these studies, hypoxia and inflammation quickly develop when the single-kidney GFR falls below 20 mL/min. Taken together, although it was classically believed that RAS is a noninflammatory disease, these data show the opposite. The same paradigm shift has occurred for systemic atherosclerosis that is nowadays considered as a pro-inflammatory disease state. These data show how BOLD-MRI can provide new insights in the pathophysiology of complex disease states.

Moreover, several studies have shown that BOLD-MRI is also an important tool to monitor changes in renal tissue oxygenation after angioplasty of stenotic renal arteries and other therapeutic interventions. In a study of 17 patients with RAS and a clinical indication for angioplasty, fractional kidney hypoxia (defined as the percentage of axial area with R_2* above 30/s) significantly decreased 3 months after angioplasty. However, the level of inflammatory biomarkers did not decrease in the renal vein, and single-kidney GFR only slightly increased [66]. This finding illustrates that restoring RBF alone is probably not enough in RAS patients, as loss of glomeruli is irreversible, and important rarefaction of microvessels probably also occurs in post-stenotic renal tissue. In contrast, patients with RAS receiving adipose-derived autologous mesenchymal stem cells directly injected in the stenotic kidney demonstrate increases in perfusion and oxygenation and reductions in inflammation, even without undergoing angioplasty [67]. This is consistent with an anti-inflammatory effect of mesenchymal stem cells. Similar observations have been made histologically in swine models of RAS using mesenchymal stem cells [68].

It remains an open question whether BOLD-MRI, alone or in combination with other techniques, may predict a positive renal functional response to revascularization, in particular percutaneous transluminal angioplasty (PTA). It is well known that large randomized controlled trials failed to demonstrate a benefit of PTA in patients with atherosclerotic RAS [69, 70]. Nevertheless, PTA can be very beneficial in some patients and lead to significant improvement of blood pressure and stabilization of renal function. Unfortunately, there are actually no noninvasive tools to identify patients who will benefit from PTA. From a physiological viewpoint, RAS patients with renal ischemia but still viable renal tissue are most likely to benefit from PTA. When renal ischemia lasts too long or is too severe, this will lead to renal inflammation, fibrosis, and microvascular rarefaction, resulting in reductions in renal volume and irreversible loss of renal function. In this situation, PTA will probably not improve the clinical condition of the patient.

Some authors have proposed to use BOLD-MRI in combination with GFR assessment of the stenotic kidney (measured by isotope renography) in order to predict the response to PTA. Chrysochou et al. demonstrated that the patients with a favorable response to PTA (>15% increase in GFR, $n = 5$) had a significantly higher R_2*/GFR ratio than those who did not improve ($n = 12$). A high R_2*/GFR ratio may represent metabolically active, suffering tissue yet without irreversible damage. The sensitivity and specificity to predict a favorable response were 66.7 and 85.7% [71]. This study still awaits confirmation in a higher number of patients.

Another interesting marker that may be of help to predict the response to PTA is the furosemide test. This test will be explained in more detail in the next chapter. In brief, furosemide can be administered while the patient is in the scanner, and a lack of change in R_2* after its administration is seen by many as an indirect proof that there is no more viable, metabolically active tissue in the stenotic kidney [72]. Once again, whether the furosemide test can predict a favorable response to PTA remains to be demonstrated.

Drug Research

Furosemide is probably the most extensively studied drug, thanks to its ease of intravenous administration while scanning and the acutely observed decreases in medullary and, to a lesser degree, cortical R_2* occurring within minutes after injection. This decrease in R_2* has been attributed to its effect on oxygen-consuming tubular solute transport. As furosemide blocks sodium reabsorption by the NKCC2 transporters in Henle's loops, its administration leads to an acute decrease in renal tissue oxygen consumption. Studies in rats using Clark-type O_2 microelectrodes inserted into the kidneys have indeed reported increases in medullary pO_2 values after the administration of furosemide [73]. Hence, many have argued that the furosemide-induced decrease in medullary R_2* is an indirect argument for the capacity of BOLD-MRI to capture changes in renal tissue oxygenation. Besides, furosemide-induced changes are smaller in CKD patients and approach zero in atrophic kidneys. The administration of furosemide during scanning is therefore also used as a functional test in CKD patients and patients with renal artery stenosis [11].

A detailed review of other drugs and their effects on R_2* is beyond the scope of this chapter, and we refer to the statement paper published by us and other members of the PARENCHIMA consortium in 2018 [26]. In brief, patients on beta-blockers showed lower R_2* compared to controls without beta-blockers. Inhibitors of the renin-angiotensin system acutely decrease renal R_2*, whereas intravenous angiotensin II perfusion has the opposite effect. Nonsteroidal anti-inflammatory drugs (NSAIDs) have indirect effects and lead to blunted response to water-loading. More recently, the sodium-glucose cotransporter 2-inhibitor (SGLT2i) dapagliflozin acutely decreased cortical R_2* in type 1 DM patients [74]. Such an effect was not observed for the SGLT2i empagliflozin in obese, nondiabetic volunteers [75].

These studies underline the potential of BOLD-MRI to increase our insights in the renal actions of drugs. The possibility to repeat the BOLD-MRI exam minutes or hours later, and to combine it with phase contrast, arterial spin labeling, and other renal MRI techniques without the need of contrast products, makes it a very interesting candidate to demonstrate the metabolic effects of new but also established drugs. For this reason, randomized clinical trials driven by the pharmaceutical industry have started to incorporate multiparametric renal MRI in their study designs. A recently published example is the COMBINE study. In this study, the authors obtained baseline diffusion-weighted and BOLD-MRI in 122 participants to the COMBINE trial, a randomized, double-blind trial of nicotinamide and lanthanum carbonate versus placebo in stage 3b–4 CKD patients [76]. Although no major differences were noted between the placebo and intervention groups, this study paved the way for other trials. An example of such a trial is REMODEL (NCT04865770). This Phase 3 study aims to find out how semaglutide, a GLP-1 agonist used to treat patients with type 2 DM, works by performing multiparametric MRI at baseline, 1 and 12 months after the introduction of semaglutide versus placebo. Results are expected in 2024; many other examples may follow.

Examples of Use in Clinical Practice

As outlined above, BOLD-MRI is thus far essentially used in the research setting. Therefore, the examples that are outlined here come from the personal research experiences of the authors of this chapter.

One of these experiences concerns a 33-year-old male patient with a medical history of Takayasu arteritis. This rare, systemic, inflammatory large-vessel vasculitis had started 5 years before admission and affected most of his major arteries, including the aorta, superior mesenteric artery, both renal arteries, and iliac and femoral arteries. He was treated with low-dose corticosteroids and tocilizumab. He was admitted because of fever, severe left-sided flank pain, and laboratory signs of systemic inflammation (C-reactive protein level of 202 mg/L and sedimentation rate > 110 mm/h). Extended microbiological workup was negative, and conventional imaging, including angio-CT of the abdomen, could not identify an underlying cause for the flank pain. All stenotic lesions of the large vessels were unchanged. As we found no other explanation, left renal ischemia due to activation of Takayasu arteritis was clinically suspected, despite normal LDH values and lack of renal infarction at the CT scan. BOLD-MRI was therefore performed. The left kidney showed higher R_2* values than the right kidney and especially a flatter R_2* curve. This indicated possible ischemia and dysfunction of the left kidney as clinical manifestation of the reactivation of his Takayasu arteritis. Treatment with high-dose corticosteroids was initiated and leads to quick improvement of the patient. The fever and systemic inflammation disappeared, as well as the left-sided flank pain.

Possible Future Developments and Applications

Despite limited examples of direct impact on patient care, the journey of T_2*-sensitized (BOLD) clinical renal MRI is only at its beginning. Major developments in data acquisition, better and faster image reconstructions, and improvements in SNR and (semi-) automated analysis methods, most likely driven by machine learning algorithms [77], promise to address existing obstacles in MRI workflows. A recent report [78] has shown that inclusion of radiomic features of MRI parametric maps facilitates image phenotyping using unsupervised hierarchical clustering analysis and radiomic approaches may provide further insights into the clinical evolution of patients with renal disease. We believe that these technical developments will lead to further standardization and more precise estimations of local tissue oxygenation and potentially facilitate integration into clinical practice.

Among the possible clinical applications for T_2*-sensitized MRI, patients with renal artery stenosis present, to our opinion, the most promising field. In combination with furosemide, T_2*-sensitized MRI can provide information on the functional consequences of the stenosis and assess the viability of the kidney parenchyma. Although randomized clinical studies are lacking thus far, T_2*-sensitized MRI may become an important tool to guide the selection of patients for percutaneous angioplasty. As outlined above, drug research is also a promising area, with the potential to identify some nephrotoxic or nephroprotective properties of drugs at an early stage.

The identification of patients at high risk of future renal function decline is since long considered as a possible clinical application. The technique is, for the moment, too costly to use to this purpose, but the sequences could, for example, be added to CKD patients who undergo an abdominal MRI for another clinical condition. Clearly, post-processing and analysis times have to be drastically shortened and ROI placement further automized.

Even under such favorable conditions, other hurdles must be addressed. As already mentioned, R_2* values depend on many factors, including local scanning conditions. Therefore, it is impossible to provide a universal cutoff value above which renal function will most likely decline. A better understanding of the role of confounding factors such as blood volume and ability to translate T_2*/R_2* in terms of StO_2 [8] OR pO_2 [9] is needed. Nevertheless, some of these confounding factors can be standardized, and others can be measured with other MRI techniques such as phase-contrast MRI, diffusion-weighted MRI, or arterial spin labeling. These multiparametric protocols have quickly gained importance in the research setting and may overcome some of the problems mentioned above. Multiparametric MRI can provide valuable data on many functional parameters and will certainly help to gain further insight in the complex regulation of renal oxygenation.

The results of ongoing and future studies will tell us whether T_2*-sensitized MRI, in combination with other renal MRI techniques, will be able to reliably identify CKD patients at the highest risk and help to identify their underlying diagnosis, without generating excessive additional costs. Only then will T_2*-sensitized MRI lose its connotation "too bold to be true."

References

1. Brezis M, Rosen S. Hypoxia of the renal medulla—its implications for disease. N Engl J Med. 1995;332(10):647–55.
2. Fine LG, Orphanides C, Norman JT. Progressive renal disease: the chronic hypoxia hypothesis. Kidney Int Suppl. 1998;65:S74–8.
3. Ogawa S, Lee TM, Kay AR, Tank DW. Brain magnetic resonance imaging with contrast dependent on blood oxygenation. Proc Natl Acad Sci U S A. 1990;87(24):9868–72.
4. Turner R, Jezzard P, Wen H, Kwong KK, Le Bihan D, Zeffiro T, et al. Functional mapping of the human visual cortex at 4 and 1.5 tesla using deoxygenation contrast EPI. Magn Reson Med. 1993;29(2):277–9.
5. Meloni A, Hezel F, Positano V, Keilberg P, Pepe A, Lombardi M, et al. Detailing magnetic field strength dependence and segmental artifact distribution of myocardial effective transverse relaxation rate at 1.5, 3.0, and 7.0 T. Magn Reson Med. 2014;71(6):2224–30.
6. Prasad PV. Update on renal blood oxygenation level-dependent MRI to assess intrarenal oxygenation in chronic kidney disease. Kidney Int. 2018;93(4):778–80.
7. Niendorf T, Pohlmann A, Arakelyan K, Flemming B, Cantow K, Hentschel J, et al. How bold is blood oxygenation level-dependent (BOLD) magnetic resonance imaging of the kidney? Opportunities, challenges and future directions. Acta Physiol (Oxf). 2015;213(1):19–38.
8. Pohlmann A, Cantow K, Huelnhagen T, Grosenick D, Dos Santos Periquito J, Boehmert L, et al. Experimental MRI monitoring of renal blood volume fraction variations En route to renal magnetic resonance oximetry. Tomography. 2017;3(4):188–200.
9. Zhang JL, Morrell G, Rusinek H, Warner L, Vivier PH, Cheung AK, et al. Measurement of renal tissue oxygenation with blood oxygen level-dependent MRI and oxygen transit modeling. Am J Physiol Renal Physiol. 2014;306(6):F579–87.
10. Prasad PV, Epstein FH. Changes in renal medullary pO2 during water diuresis as evaluated by blood oxygenation level-dependent magnetic resonance imaging: effects of aging and cyclooxygenase inhibition. Kidney Int. 1999;55(1):294–8.
11. Pruijm M, Hofmann L, Piskunowicz M, Muller ME, Zweiacker C, Bassi I, et al. Determinants of renal tissue oxygenation as measured with BOLD-MRI in chronic kidney disease and hypertension in humans. PLoS One. 2014;9(4):e95895.
12. Bane O, Mendichovszky IA, Milani B, Dekkers IA, Deux JF, Eckerbom P, et al. Consensus-based technical recommendations for clinical translation of renal BOLD MRI. MAGMA. 2020;33(1):199–215.
13. Pruijm M, Hofmann L, Maillard M, Tremblay S, Glatz N, Wuerzner G, et al. Effect of sodium loading/depletion on renal oxygenation in young normotensive and hypertensive men. Hypertension. 2010;55(5):1116–22.
14. Pruijm M, Hofmann L, Charollais-Thoenig J, Forni V, Maillard M, Coristine A, et al. Effect of dark chocolate on renal tissue oxygenation as measured by BOLD-MRI in healthy volunteers. Clin Nephrol. 2013;80(3):211–7.
15. Bosch JP, Saccaggi A, Lauer A, Ronco C, Belledonne M, Glabman S. Renal functional reserve in humans.

Effect of protein intake on glomerular filtration rate. Am J Med. 1983;75(6):943–50.
16. Vakilzadeh N, Zanchi A, Milani B, Ledoux JB, Braconnier P, Burnier M, et al. Acute hyperglycemia increases renal tissue oxygenation as measured by BOLD-MRI in healthy overweight volunteers. Diabetes Res Clin Pract. 2019;150:138–43.
17. Zheng SS, He YM, Lu J. Noninvasive evaluation of diabetic patients with high fasting blood glucose using DWI and BOLD MRI. Abdom Radiol (NY). 2021;46(4):1659–69.
18. Eckerbom P, Hansell P, Cox E, Buchanan C, Weis J, Palm F, et al. Circadian variation in renal blood flow and kidney function in healthy volunteers monitored with noninvasive magnetic resonance imaging. Am J Physiol Renal Physiol. 2020;319(6):F966–F78.
19. Pruijm M, Milani B, Pivin E, Podhajska A, Vogt B, Stuber M, et al. Reduced cortical oxygenation predicts a progressive decline of renal function in patients with chronic kidney disease. Kidney Int. 2018;93:932.
20. Li LP, Thacker JM, Li W, Hack B, Wang C, Kohn O, et al. Medullary blood oxygen level-dependent MRI index (R2*) is associated with annual loss of kidney function in moderate CKD. Am J Nephrol. 2020;51(12):966–74.
21. Sugiyama K, Inoue T, Kozawa E, Ishikawa M, Shimada A, Kobayashi N, et al. Reduced oxygenation but not fibrosis defined by functional magnetic resonance imaging predicts the long-term progression of chronic kidney disease. Nephrol Dial Transplant. 2020;35(6):964–70.
22. Prasad PV, Edelman RR, Epstein FH. Noninvasive evaluation of intrarenal oxygenation with BOLD MRI. Circulation. 1996;94(12):3271–5.
23. Schachinger H, Klarhofer M, Linder L, Drewe J, Scheffler K. Angiotensin II decreases the renal MRI blood oxygenation level-dependent signal. Hypertension. 2006;47(6):1062–6.
24. Prasad PV, Chen Q, Goldfarb JW, Epstein FH, Edelman RR. Breath-hold R2* mapping with a multiple gradient-recalled echo sequence: application to the evaluation of intrarenal oxygenation. J Magn Reson Imaging. 1997;7(6):1163–5.
25. Rossi C, Sharma P, Pazahr S, Alkadhi H, Nanz D, Boss A. Blood oxygen level-dependent magnetic resonance imaging of the kidneys: influence of spatial resolution on the apparent R2* transverse relaxation rate of renal tissue. Invest Radiol. 2013;48(9):671–7.
26. Pruijm M, Mendichovszky IA, Liss P, Van der Niepen P, Textor SC, Lerman LO, et al. Renal blood oxygenation level-dependent magnetic resonance imaging to measure renal tissue oxygenation: a statement paper and systematic review. Nephrol Dial Transplant. 2018;33(suppl_2):ii22–i8.
27. Cox EF, Buchanan CE, Bradley CR, Prestwich B, Mahmoud H, Taal M, et al. Multiparametric renal magnetic resonance imaging: validation, interventions, and alterations in chronic kidney disease. Front Physiol. 2017;8:696.
28. Piskunowicz M, Hofmann L, Zuercher E, Bassi I, Milani B, Stuber M, et al. A new technique with high reproducibility to estimate renal oxygenation using BOLD-MRI in chronic kidney disease. Magn Reson Imaging. 2015;33(3):253–61.
29. Ebrahimi B, Gloviczki M, Woollard JR, Crane JA, Textor SC, Lerman LO. Compartmental analysis of renal BOLD MRI data: introduction and validation. Invest Radiol. 2012;47(3):175–82.
30. Milani B, Ansaloni A, Sousa-Guimaraes S, Vakilzadeh N, Piskunowicz M, Vogt B, et al. Reduction of cortical oxygenation in chronic kidney disease: evidence obtained with a new analysis method of blood oxygenation level-dependent magnetic resonance imaging. Nephrol Dial Transplant. 2017;32(12):2097–105.
31. Thacker JM, Li LP, Li W, Zhou Y, Sprague SM, Prasad PV. Renal blood oxygenation level-dependent magnetic resonance imaging: a sensitive and objective analysis. Invest Radiol. 2015;50(12):821–7.
32. Li LP, Milani B, Pruijm M, Kohn O, Sprague S, Hack B, et al. Renal BOLD MRI in patients with chronic kidney disease: comparison of the semi-automated twelve layer concentric objects (TLCO) and manual ROI methods. MAGMA. 2020;33(1):113–20.
33. Manotham K, Tanaka T, Matsumoto M, Ohse T, Miyata T, Inagi R, et al. Evidence of tubular hypoxia in the early phase in the remnant kidney model. J Am Soc Nephrol. 2004;15(5):1277–88.
34. Norman JT, Stidwill R, Singer M, Fine LG. Angiotensin II blockade augments renal cortical microvascular pO2 indicating a novel, potentially renoprotective action. Nephron Physiol. 2003;94(2):39–46.
35. Michaely HJ, Metzger L, Haneder S, Hansmann J, Schoenberg SO, Attenberger UI. Renal BOLD-MRI does not reflect renal function in chronic kidney disease. Kidney Int. 2012;81(7):684–9.
36. Milani B, Ansaloni A, Sousa-Guimaraes S, Piskunowicz M, Vogt B, Stuber M, et al. [Op.4d.06] Reduction of cortical oxygenation in chronic kidney disease: evidence obtained with BOLD-MRI and a new analytic technique. J Hypertens. 2016;34 Suppl 2:e52.
37. Prasad PV, Thacker J, Li LP, Haque M, Li W, Koenigs H, et al. Multi-parametric evaluation of chronic kidney disease by MRI: a preliminary cross-sectional study. PLoS One. 2015;10(10):e0139661.
38. Liang P, Chen Y, Li S, Xu C, Yuan G, Hu D, et al. Noninvasive assessment of kidney dysfunction in children by using blood oxygenation level-dependent MRI and intravoxel incoherent motion diffusion-weighted imaging. Insights Imaging. 2021;12(1):146.
39. Xin-Long P, Jing-Xia X, Jian-Yu L, Song W, Xin-Kui T. A preliminary study of blood-oxygen-level-dependent MRI in patients with chronic kidney disease. Magn Reson Imaging. 2012;30(3):330–5.
40. Wang ZJ, Kumar R, Banerjee S, Hsu CY. Blood oxygen level-dependent (BOLD) MRI of diabetic nephropathy: preliminary experience. J Magn Reson Imaging. 2011;33(3):655–60.

41. Yin WJ, Liu F, Li XM, Yang L, Zhao S, Huang ZX, et al. Noninvasive evaluation of renal oxygenation in diabetic nephropathy by BOLD-MRI. Eur J Radiol. 2011;81:1426.
42. Thelwall PE, Taylor R, Marshall SM. Non-invasive investigation of kidney disease in type 1 diabetes by magnetic resonance imaging. Diabetologia. 2011;54(9):2421–9.
43. BEAt-DKD. https://www.beat-dkd.eu.
44. KPMP. https://www.kpmp.org.
45. Bauer F, Wald J, Bauer FJ, Dahlkamp LM, Seibert FS, Pagonas N, et al. Detection of acute tubular necrosis using blood oxygenation level-dependent (BOLD) MRI. Kidney Blood Press Res. 2017;42(6):1078–89.
46. Inoue T, Kozawa E, Okada H, Inukai K, Watanabe S, Kikuta T, et al. Noninvasive evaluation of kidney hypoxia and fibrosis using magnetic resonance imaging. J Am Soc Nephrol. 2011;22(8):1429–34.
47. Buchanan C, Mahmoud H, Cox E, Noble R, Prestwich B, Kasmi I, et al. Multiparametric MRI assessment of renal structure and function in acute kidney injury and renal recovery. Clin Kidney J. 2021;14(8):1969–76.
48. Sadowski EA, Fain SB, Alford SK, Korosec FR, Fine J, Muehrer R, et al. Assessment of acute renal transplant rejection with blood oxygen level-dependent MR imaging: initial experience. Radiology. 2005;236(3):911–9.
49. Djamali A, Sadowski EA, Samaniego-Picota M, Fain SB, Muehrer RJ, Alford SK, et al. Noninvasive assessment of early kidney allograft dysfunction by blood oxygen level-dependent magnetic resonance imaging. Transplantation. 2006;82(5):621–8.
50. Han F, Xiao W, Xu Y, Wu J, Wang Q, Wang H, et al. The significance of BOLD MRI in differentiation between renal transplant rejection and acute tubular necrosis. Nephrol Dial Transplant. 2008;23(8):2666–72.
51. Xiao W, Xu J, Wang Q, Xu Y, Zhang M. Functional evaluation of transplanted kidneys in normal function and acute rejection using BOLD MR imaging. Eur J Radiol. 2012;81(5):838–45.
52. Vermathen P, Binser T, Boesch C, Eisenberger U, Thoeny HC. Three-year follow-up of human transplanted kidneys by diffusion-weighted MRI and blood oxygenation level-dependent imaging. J Magn Reson Imaging. 2012;35(5):1133–8.
53. Wang W, Yu Y, Wen J, Zhang M, Chen J, Cheng D, et al. Combination of functional magnetic resonance imaging and histopathologic analysis to evaluate interstitial fibrosis in kidney allografts. Clin J Am Soc Nephrol. 2019;14(9):1372–80.
54. Sadowski EA, Djamali A, Wentland AL, Muehrer R, Becker BN, Grist TM, et al. Blood oxygen level-dependent and perfusion magnetic resonance imaging: detecting differences in oxygen bioavailability and blood flow in transplanted kidneys. Magn Reson Imaging. 2010;28(1):56–64.
55. Mishima E, Suzuki T, Ito S. Selection of patients for angioplasty for treatment of atherosclerotic Renovascular disease: predicting responsive patients. Am J Hypertens. 2020;33(5):391–401.
56. Hansen KJ, Edwards MS, Craven TE, Cherr GS, Jackson SA, Appel RG, et al. Prevalence of renovascular disease in the elderly: a population-based study. J Vasc Surg. 2002;36(3):443–51.
57. Olin JW, Melia M, Young JR, Graor RA, Risius B. Prevalence of atherosclerotic renal artery stenosis in patients with atherosclerosis elsewhere. Am J Med. 1990;88(1N):46N–51N.
58. Warner L, Gomez SI, Bolterman R, Haas JA, Bentley MD, Lerman LO, et al. Regional decreases in renal oxygenation during graded acute renal arterial stenosis: a case for renal ischemia. Am J Physiol Regul Integr Comp Physiol. 2009;296(1):R67–71.
59. Warner L, Glockner JF, Woollard J, Textor SC, Romero JC, Lerman LO. Determinations of renal cortical and medullary oxygenation using blood oxygen level-dependent magnetic resonance imaging and selective diuretics. Invest Radiol. 2011;46(1):41–7.
60. Gloviczki ML, Glockner JF, Lerman LO, McKusick MA, Misra S, Grande JP, et al. Preserved oxygenation despite reduced blood flow in poststenotic kidneys in human atherosclerotic renal artery stenosis. Hypertension. 2010;55(4):961–6.
61. Wilcox CS, Palm F, Welch WJ. Renal oxygenation and function of the rat kidney: effects of inspired oxygen and preglomerular oxygen shunting. Adv Exp Med Biol. 2013;765:329–34.
62. Zhao L, Li G, Meng F, Sun Z, Liu J. Cortical and medullary oxygenation evaluation of kidneys with renal artery stenosis by BOLD-MRI. PLoS One. 2022;17(3):e0264630.
63. Gloviczki ML, Glockner JF, Crane JA, McKusick MA, Misra S, Grande JP, et al. Blood oxygen level-dependent magnetic resonance imaging identifies cortical hypoxia in severe renovascular disease. Hypertension. 2011;58(6):1066–72.
64. Abumoawad A, Saad A, Ferguson CM, Eirin A, Woollard JR, Herrmann SM, et al. Tissue hypoxia, inflammation, and loss of glomerular filtration rate in human atherosclerotic renovascular disease. Kidney Int. 2019;95(4):948–57.
65. Gloviczki ML, Keddis MT, Garovic VD, Friedman H, Herrmann S, McKusick MA, et al. TGF expression and macrophage accumulation in atherosclerotic renal artery stenosis. Clin J Am Soc Nephrol. 2013;8(4):546–53.
66. Saad A, Herrmann SM, Crane J, Glockner JF, McKusick MA, Misra S, et al. Stent revascularization restores cortical blood flow and reverses tissue hypoxia in atherosclerotic renal artery stenosis but fails to reverse inflammatory pathways or glomerular filtration rate. Circ Cardiovasc Interv. 2013;6(4):428–35.
67. Saad A, Dietz AB, Herrmann SMS, Hickson LJ, Glockner JF, McKusick MA, et al. Autologous mesenchymal stem cells increase cortical perfusion in renovascular disease. J Am Soc Nephrol. 2017;28(9):2777–85.
68. Eirin A, Zhu XY, Krier JD, Tang H, Jordan KL, Grande JP, et al. Adipose tissue-derived mesenchymal stem cells improve revascularization outcomes to

restore renal function in swine atherosclerotic renal artery stenosis. Stem Cells. 2012;30(5):1030–41.
69. Bax L, Woittiez AJ, Kouwenberg HJ, Mali WP, Buskens E, Beek FJ, et al. Stent placement in patients with atherosclerotic renal artery stenosis and impaired renal function: a randomized trial. Ann Intern Med. 2009;150(12):840–8, W150–1.
70. Cooper CJ, Murphy TP, Cutlip DE, Jamerson K, Henrich W, Reid DM, et al. Stenting and medical therapy for atherosclerotic renal-artery stenosis. N Engl J Med. 2014;370(1):13–22.
71. Chrysochou C, Mendichovszky IA, Buckley DL, Cheung CM, Jackson A, Kalra PA. BOLD imaging: a potential predictive biomarker of renal functional outcome following revascularization in atheromatous renovascular disease. Nephrol Dial Transplant. 2012;27(3):1013–9.
72. Textor SC, Lerman LO. The role of hypoxia in ischemic chronic kidney disease. Semin Nephrol. 2019;39(6):589–98.
73. Brezis M, Agmon Y, Epstein FH. Determinants of intrarenal oxygenation. I. Effects of diuretics. Am J Physiol. 1994;267(6 Pt 2):F1059–62.
74. Laursen JC, Sondergaard-Heinrich N, de Melo JML, Haddock B, Rasmussen IKB, Safavimanesh F, et al. Acute effects of dapagliflozin on renal oxygenation and perfusion in type 1 diabetes with albuminuria: a randomised, double-blind, placebo-controlled crossover trial. EClinicalMedicine. 2021;37:100895.
75. Zanchi A, Burnier M, Muller ME, Ghajarzadeh-Wurzner A, Maillard M, Loncle N, et al. Acute and chronic effects of SGLT2 inhibitor Empagliflozin on renal oxygenation and blood pressure control in nondiabetic normotensive subjects: a randomized, placebo-controlled trial. J Am Heart Assoc. 2020;9(13):e016173.
76. Srivastava A, Cai X, Lee J, Li W, Larive B, Kendrick C, et al. Kidney functional magnetic resonance imaging and change in eGFR in individuals with CKD. Clin J Am Soc Nephrol. 2020;15(6):776–83.
77. Kart T, Fischer M, Kustner T, Hepp T, Bamberg F, Winzeck S, et al. Deep learning-based automated abdominal organ segmentation in the UK biobank and German national cohort magnetic resonance imaging studies. Invest Radiol. 2021;56(6):401–8.
78. Li LP, Leidner AS, Wilt E, Mikheev A, Rusinek H, Sprague SM, et al. Radiomics-based image phenotyping of kidney apparent diffusion coefficient maps: preliminary feasibility & efficacy. J Clin Med. 2022;11(7):1972.

T1ρ Mapping and Its Applications for Assessment of Renal Fibrosis

11

Octavia Bane and Sara Lewis

Part 1: MRI Physics and Acquisition Protocols

Physical Principles and Pulse Sequence Implementation

The longitudinal relaxation of spins in the rotating frame, under the influence of a radio frequency field of low amplitude but long duration, is characterized by the time constant T1ρ (also known as T1rho). T1ρ was first measured by Redfield in 1955 [1] in an NMR spectroscopy spin-locking experiment. Spin-locking experiments were used in the 1960s to investigate low-frequency interactions between macromolecules and bulk water [2, 3]. Starting in the 1980s, spin-locking preparations to measure T1ρ were implemented as part of MRI as a novel way to enhance tissue contrast and differentiate between different types of tissue in the breast [4], the musculoskeletal system [5], liver [6, 7], heart [8], and kidney [9–11].

The timing diagram for the spin-lock pulse cluster used for T1ρ preparation in most T1ρ pulse sequence implementations is shown in Fig. 11.1a. After tipping the magnetization $\vec{M}_0$ of the spin sample to the *x-y* plane by a 90° radio frequency (RF) pulse, a locking RF pulse is applied on resonance, so that $\omega = \omega_0$, for the duration of the spin-lock time (referred to as "TSL"). For the duration of the locking pulse, the magnetization will decay with the time constant $T_1\rho$ and undergoes free induction decay (FID) with time constant T_2^* at the end of the spin-lock interval.

Another 90° pulse rotates the magnetization back to the *z*-axis for data acquisition (ACQ), and a crusher gradient dephases any residual magnetization from the *x-y* plane magnetization. The magnetization stored along the *z*-axis can be read by any 2D or 3D image acquisition methods, such as fast spin-echo (FSE), single-shot fast low-angle shot [6, 9], balanced steady-state free precession (bSSFP) [11], 3D gradient-echo (GRE) [5], 2D spiral imaging [12], or multi-slice spin-lock [13].

As illustrated in Fig. 11.1b, the spins experience an effective spin-locking field B_{eff} during the spin-lock cluster, which is located in the *x-y* plane only if B_1 is on resonance ($\omega = \omega_0$). If this condition is not met, the magnetization will nutate around a B_{eff} pulse not located in the *x-y* plane, and

O. Bane (✉)
Department of Radiology, Icahn School of Medicine at Mount Sinai, New York, NY, USA

BioMedical Engineering and Imaging Institute, Icahn School of Medicine at Mount Sinai, New York, NY, USA
e-mail: octavia.bane@mountsinai.org

S. Lewis
Department of Radiology, Icahn School of Medicine at Mount Sinai, New York, NY, USA
e-mail: Sara.Lewis@mountsinai.org

S. D. Serai, K. Darge (eds.), *Advanced Clinical MRI of the Kidney*,
https://doi.org/10.1007/978-3-031-40169-5_11

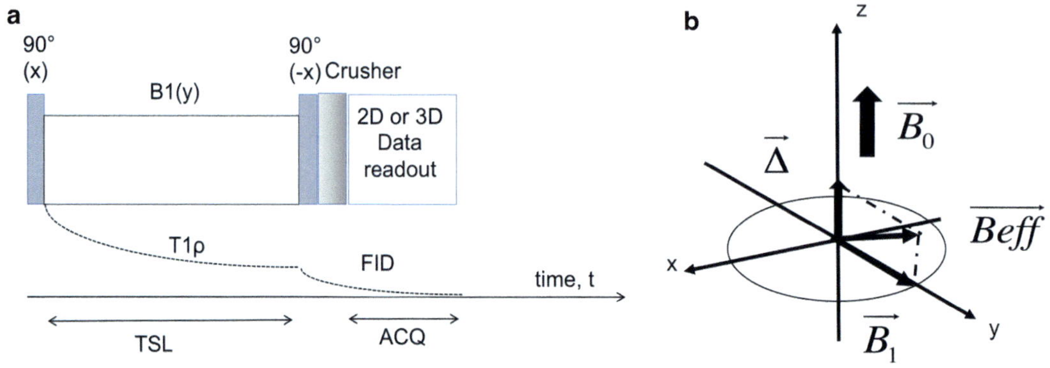

Fig. 11.1 (**a**) Timing diagram for the $T_1\rho$ preparation used in most $T_1\rho$ pulse sequence implementations. After tipping the magnetization $\vec{M_0}$ of the spin sample to the *x-y* plane by a 90° pulse, a locking radio frequency (RF) pulse is applied on resonance, so that $\omega = \omega_0$, for a duration called spin-lock time (TSL). For the duration of the locking pulse, the magnetization will relax with the time constant $T_1\rho$, and undergoes free induction decay (FID) at the end of the spin-lock interval. Another 90° pulse rotates the magnetization back to the *z*-axis for data acquisition (ACQ), and a crusher gradient dephases any residual *x-y* plane magnetization. Data can be acquired with 2D or 3D methods during the FID interval. (**b**) Rotating frame representation of the effective RF field B_{eff} perturbing the magnetization of the spin sample, $\vec{M_0}, \overrightarrow{Beff} = \overrightarrow{B1} + \vec{\Delta}$, where $\vec{\Delta} = \left(B0 - \frac{\omega}{\gamma}\right)\vec{z}$, with ω the frequency of rotation of magnetization $\overrightarrow{M0}$ and γ the gyromagnetic ratio. If the spin-lock field is applied on resonance ($\omega = \omega_0$), $B_{\text{eff}} = B_1$, and the bulk magnetization remains in phase along the direction of B_1 and relaxes with the spin-lattice relaxation time in the rotating frame $T_1\rho$

this off-resonance effect will appear as banding artifacts in the images [5, 14, 15]. To reduce the effects of B_1 inhomogeneities, a "self-compensated" spin-lock pulse is used: the spin-lock pulse is split into two halves of length TSL/2, with alternating phases along *y* and $-y$, so that the pulse halves have a 180° phase difference [16]. However, if there are variations in ω_0 due to a range of chemical shifts in the imaging volume (e.g., change in magnetic susceptibility from bowel gas surrounding the kidneys) or significant B_0 inhomogeneity, a self-compensated spin-lock pulse cannot do away with off-resonance effects. There are several strategies to compensate for both B_1 and B_0 inhomogeneities, such as insertion of a 180° refocusing pulse in the middle of the spin-lock pulse [14, 15] and use of a composite RF pulse in combination with phase cycling [14, 16].

Acquisition Protocols

Typically, $T_1\rho$ mapping is used to investigate the interactions between proton spins and macromolecules such as collagen, which are present in fibrotic renal tissue. For this purpose, a series of $T_1\rho$-weighted images is acquired at the same spin-locking frequency, with varying TSL durations. Sample $T_1\rho$ mapping protocols with a single spin-lock frequency for the kidneys are shown in Table 11.1. The spin-lock frequency is calibrated based on the amplitude (in μT) and length of the B_1 90° pulse. Spin-lock frequency values can vary from 0 to 3000 Hz (Table 11.1), but a spin-lock frequency of 500 Hz is typically used in kidney protocols [9, 11, 12]. The choice of maximum TSL depends on scanner SAR limits and desired SNR [12]. Most $T_1\rho$-weighted sequences developed for kidney and liver imaging have been 2D single-slice; however, 2D multi-slice spin-lock acquisitions [5, 13] have been demonstrated in patellar cartilage, but correction for a $T_2\rho$ factor and compensation for T_1 regrowth is necessary to correctly quantify $T_1\rho$ [13]. He et al. [12] integrated a $T_1\rho$ preparation with single spin-locked frequency into a 2D ASL sequence for measurement of renal perfusion and single-kidney GFR without exogenous contrast agent in healthy volunteers, before and after a protein challenge.

Table 11.1 Sample $T_{1}\rho$ imaging protocols for the kidneys used in human and animal studies

Study	Subjects	Kidney	Clinical question	Field strength (T)	Readout sequence	Respiratory control	Matrix	Voxel size (mm³)	TE/TR (ms)	BW (Hz/Px)	FA (°)	Acquisition time (s)	SL frequency (Hz)	TSL (ms)
Rapacchi et al. (2015)	Human	Native	Diagnosis of renal fibrosis in lupus nephritis	1.5	bSSFP	1 breath-hold	128 × 128	2.7 × 2.7 × 5 (single slice)	1.9/2000	558	70	17	425.8	10, 30, 50, 70
Hectors et al. (2019)	Human	Transplanted	Diagnosis of fibrosis in renal transplant	1.5	FLASH	4 breath-holds	128 × 128	2.8 × 2.8 × 5 (single slice)	3.5/20	260	15	10/TSL	500	4.8, 9. 6, 19. 2, 38.4
He et al. (2014)	Human	Native	Estimation of glomerular filtration rate in healthy volunteers	3	TrueFISP; integrated in FAIR ASL acquisition	7 s breath-hold; timed breathing with ASL acquisition	192 × 144	1.6 × 1.6 × 6 (multi-slice)	1.4/5000	766	70	5/TSL	340.64	20, 40, 60, 80, 100
Hu et al. (2018)	Murine	Native	Assessment of renal fibrosis in a unilateral ureteral obstruction model of fibrosis	3	FSE	NaN	100 × 100	0.6 × 0.6 × 3 (5 slices)	2.4/4.9	NaN	40	NaN	500	0, 27, 54
Wang et al. (2020)	Murine	Native	Assessment of renal fibrosis in a genetic model of fibrosis	7	FSE	NaN	NaN	0.25 × 0.25 × 1	NaN	NaN	NaN	NaN	200, 400, 600, 800, 1000, 1500,2000, 2500,3000	1, 5, 15, 25, 35, 55, and 75

$T_1\rho$ data can be acquired with multiple spin-lock frequencies and multiple spin-lock times to assess the $T_1\rho$ signal dispersion curve; the goal is to select a spin-lock frequency at a smooth and stable point on the dispersion curve [11, 12]. For renal protocols, a spin-lock frequency of 350–500 Hz achieves that goal (Table 11.1). Wang et al. [17] performed dispersion analysis in their murine study (Table 11.1) by acquiring sets of images with different spin-lock field amplitudes (locking frequencies at 200, 400, 600, 800, 1000, 1500, 2000, 2500, and 3000 Hz) and variation in spin-lock times at each spin-lock amplitude (1, 5, 15, 25, 35, 55, and 75 ms). They then mapped $R_1\rho = 1/T_1\rho$ on a pixel-by-pixel basis for each spin-lock frequency and used proton exchange modeling (discussed in the following section) to quantitatively estimate the exchange rates and chemical shifts of exchanging protons between protons in water and in macromolecules (collagen).

Part 2: Post-processing and Data Analysis Methods

Single Locking Frequency

The spin-lock relaxation time $T_1\rho$ is calculated by monoexponential fit of the $T_1\rho$-weighted signal curve at different TSL, according to Eq. 11.1:

$$S(\mathrm{TSL}) = S(0)e^{-\frac{\mathrm{TSL}}{T1\rho}} = S(0)e^{-\mathrm{TSL}*R1\rho} \tag{11.1}$$

where $S(0)$ is the signal at TSL = 0 and TSL is the spin-lock time.

$T_1\rho$ and $S(0)$ are obtained by least-square nonlinear fitting methods, from $T_1\rho$-weighted signal averaged over the region of interest [12], or for each pixel to create pixel-by-pixel maps (Fig. 11.2) [9]. Previous studies have measured $T_1\rho$ in both the cortex and medulla [9, 11, 17], and decreased cortico-medullary differentiation (Fig. 11.3) with fibrosis has been observed by qualitative examination of $T_1\rho$-weighted images and $T_1\rho$ maps [9, 17].

Multiple Locking Frequencies

If $T_1\rho$-weighted data for varying spin-lock times and multiple locking frequencies are available [17], one can obtain a $T_1\rho$ or $R_1\rho$ value for each locking frequency as shown in Eq. 11.1 above. Other parameters reflecting chemical exchange between water protons and macromolecules can be calculated from the dispersion curve of $R_1\rho$ with locking frequency ω_1, according to a model proposed by Chopra et al. and applied by Wang et al. [17, 18] (Eq. 11.2).

$$R1\rho = \frac{R2 + \frac{R1\rho^{\infty}\omega_1^2}{S_\rho^2}}{1 + \frac{\omega_1^2}{S_\rho^2}} \tag{11.2}$$

where R_2 is the transverse relaxation rate, $R_1\rho^{\infty}$ is the spin-lock relaxation rate at infinite spin-lock frequency, and S_ρ is an exchange rate-weighted parameter S_ρ. S_ρ depends on the chemical exchange rate k_{sw} of bound water protons with resonance frequency offset $\Delta\omega_s$ from free water, according to Eq. 11.3:

$$S_\rho^2 \approx k_{sw}^2 + \Delta\omega_s^2 \tag{11.3}$$

One can find the inflection point of the $R_1\rho$ dispersion curve by taking the second derivative of Eq. 11.2 with respect to the locking frequency ω_1, to find the inflection point of the dispersion curve, $\omega_{infl} = \sqrt{\frac{S_\rho^2}{3}}$.

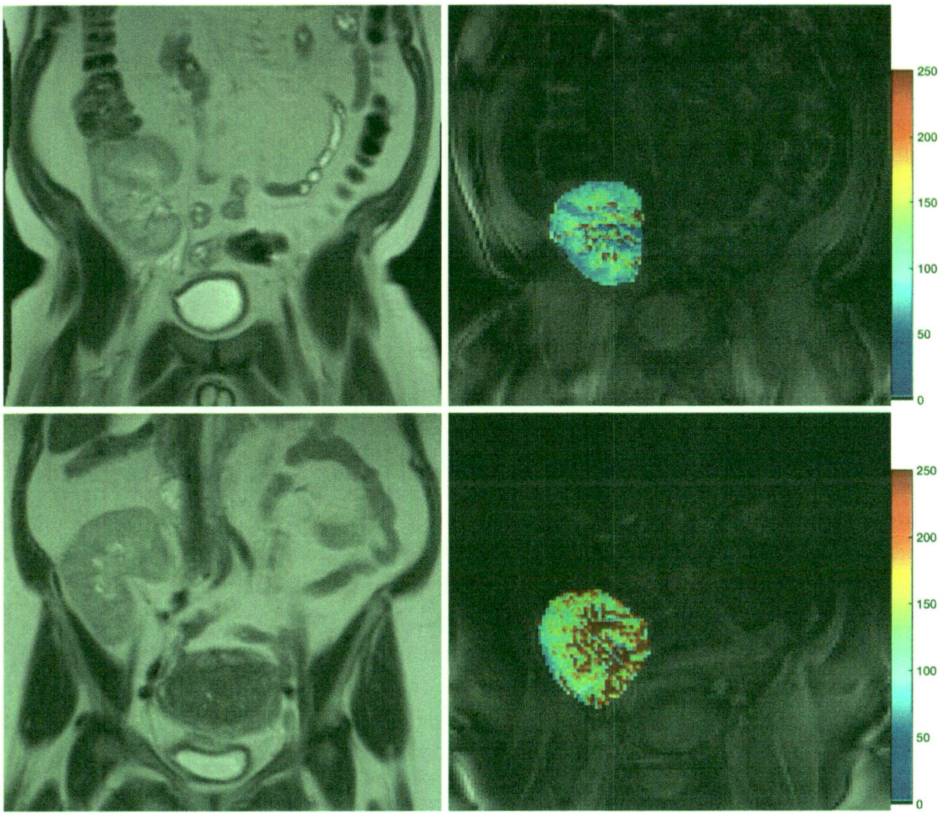

Fig. 11.2 $T_1\rho$ maps in renal allograft (right) with anatomical T_2-weighted coronal image (left) showing location of renal allograft in the pelvis. **Top:** Renal allograft with stable function (GFR = 66.4 mL/min/1.73 m^2) in a 68-year-old male patient; cortical $T_1\rho$ = 78.14 ms; medullary $T_1\rho$ = 115.7 ms. **Bottom:** Renal allograft with dysfunction (GFR = 28.3 mL/min/1.73 m^2) and biopsy-proven moderate fibrosis (B_{anff} interstitial fibrosis ci = 2 of 3, tubular atrophy ct = 2 of 3, inflammation in areas of fibrosis and tubular atrophy iIFTA = 3 of 3) in a 59-year-old female patient; cortical $T_1\rho$ = 131.4 ms; medullary $T_1\rho$ = 131.8 ms. Note the loss of cortico-medullary differentiation and higher $T_1\rho$ values in the fibrotic allograft

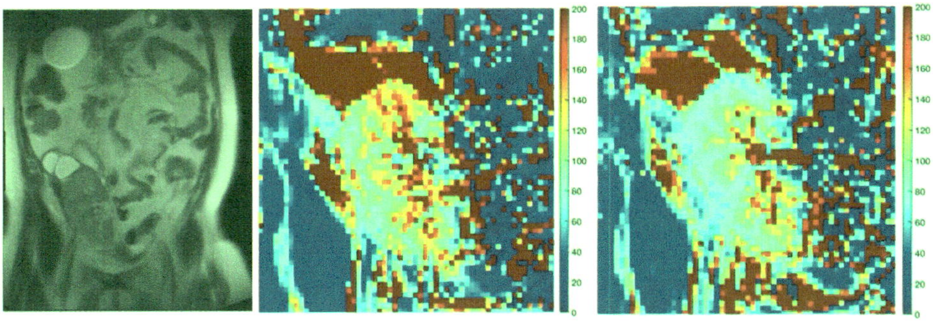

Fig. 11.3 $T_1\rho$ maps in a 30-year-old female patient with a history of two previously failed renal allografts and acute tubular injury (IFTA ci + ct = 0, iIFTA = 0, ti = 0) of her renal allograft. Left: anatomical T_2-weighted coronal image of the renal allograft at hilum, showing its location on the right side of the pelvis, and fluid accumulation around the allograft. Middle: $T_1\rho$ map of the allograft at the hilum (cortex $T_1\rho$: 101 ± 28 ms), acquired at 500 Hz with TSL: 4.8 ms, 9.6 ms, 19.2 ms, 24.9 ms. Right: $T_1\rho$ map of the allograft at the hilum (cortex $T_1\rho$: 89 ± 23 ms), acquired at 350 Hz with TSL = 4.8 ms, 9.6 ms, 19.2 ms, 38.4 ms. Note the fluid accumulation visible on the $T_1\rho$ maps, and the smaller $T_1\rho$ values obtained at 350 Hz

Part 3: Clinical Applications

Background

Renal fibrosis, characterized histologically by interstitial fibrosis/tubular atrophy (IFTA), is the hallmark of chronic kidney diseases (CKD) affecting both native and transplanted kidneys, and is secondary to incremental, sustained, and cumulative damage occurring from virtually any etiology [19]. Fibrosis can affect all the major compartments in the kidney: blood vessels (arteriosclerosis), the glomeruli (glomerulosclerosis), and the tubulointerstitium (interstitial fibrosis) [20]. Renal fibrosis typically progresses silently, often until elevation in serum creatinine (sCr) is identified [21]. Studies with serial allograft biopsies suggest progression of IFTA and a lack of reversibility once developed [22].

The clinical impact of renal fibrosis cannot be overstated. Fibrosis remains the significant cause of kidney disease progression, renal failure, and predictor of outcome for both native and transplanted kidneys [21–23]. For example, CKD/IFTA impacts 15% of the adult population in the US in native kidneys and the reported prevalence of IFTA is approximately 25% in living donor allografts within the first 18 months post-transplant [24, 25]. Early identification and quantification of IFTA is thus essential and may enable direct specific treatments to modulate disease progression (such as administration of antifibrotic agents or alterations of a patient's immunosuppression regimen in the post-transplant setting), thereby aiming to prevent or slow fibrosis progression and the subsequent decline in renal function. Despite the wide variety of causative etiologies, the uniform histopathologic and molecular characteristics of IFTA suggest that this may be an appealing therapeutic target, although few treatment options currently exist [20]. Certain signaling pathway targets, novel antifibrotic agents, and modified immunosuppression regimens are currently being investigated for the treatment of IFTA [26, 27]. Histopathology remains the reference standard for IFTA diagnosis; however, it is plagued by the limitations of biopsy, namely the risk of complications (i.e., hematuria, bleeding, and arteriovenous fistula formation), sampling error (confounded by the fact that IFTA is distributed heterogeneously throughout the kidney), and inter/intra-observer variability in the pathologic assessment [28–30]. A reliable, quantitative, and noninvasive method to diagnose and stage the severity and extent of kidney fibrotic burden is urgently needed and would be highly clinically relevant.

Applications of $T_1\rho$ Imaging in the Kidneys

$T_1\rho$ is the spin-lattice relaxation time constant in the rotating frame, which determines the decay of the transverse magnetization in the presence of a spin-lock radiofrequency field and is the mechanism for deriving tissue contrast [31]. $T_1\rho$ has been previously shown to be sensitive to low-frequency interactions between water molecules and macromolecules, such as collagen and proteoglycans [32]. This has fueled significant interest in the application of $T_1\rho$ as a noninvasive marker of collagen deposition in solid organs, which can potentially overcome the many limitations of biopsy and histopathologic assessment. $T_1\rho$ has been investigated in the myocardium, liver, spleen, and more recently, the kidneys [6–9, 11, 33]. $T_1\rho$ mapping is well suited for renal investigation as both specific region of interest (ROI) measurements in the kidney and its compartments as well as the generation of whole kidney parametric maps, allowing for evaluation of the distribution of disease severity throughout the entire renal parenchyma. Repeated MRI with $T_1\rho$ measurement enables longitudinal monitoring for disease progression or response to therapy.

Only a few published studies have investigated $T_1\rho$ in the kidney. A feasibility study was performed in patients with biopsy-confirmed lupus nephritis ($n = 10$) compared to healthy controls ($n = 10$) demonstrating differences in $T_1\rho$ measurement between the groups, although the $T_1\rho$ measurements were not tested against histopathology given the small sample size [11]. The authors of this study also found good/excellent test–retest measurement repeatability [11]. A prospective study investigated $T_1\rho$ imaging in renal allografts, finding significant differences between cortical $T_1\rho$ values for functional allografts and chronic allograft dysfunction with fibrosis (AUC 0.77, sensitivity 75.0% and specificity 86.7%) [34]. Cortical $T_1\rho$ values correlated with Masson's trichrome-stained fractions at histopathology ($r = 0.515$, $p = 0.044$), as well as after controlling for time since transplant ($r = 0.548$, $p = 0.034$), suggesting that $T_1\rho$ may therefore provide an indirect measurement of collagen deposition due to renal allograft IFTA. Excellent test–retest repeatability was also found in the renal cortex with acceptable repeatability in the renal medulla (CV cortex 7.4 ± 3.5%; CV medulla 13.3 ± 14.4%), similar to values previously reported in the native kidneys and liver [11, 35]. In both studies, $T_1\rho$ was found to be significantly increased in fibrotic compared to healthy kidney parenchyma, which is consistent with increased exchange between free and collagen-bound water protons.

A recent study performed in a murine model of renal fibrosis of different degrees of severity at 7 T, found that spin-lock relaxation rate dispersion, rather than single measurements of relaxation rates, provided more specific information on spatiotemporal changes associated with tubulointerstitial fibrosis [17]. Investigation of the relaxation rate dispersion, which is determined by the variation of relaxation rates $R_1\rho$ ($1/T_1\rho$) with the amplitude of the locking field, provided a method for estimating the exchange rates and chemical shifts of exchanging protons between protons in water and in macromolecules (collagen) [17]. Dispersion analysis was performed by acquiring sets of images with different spin-lock amplitudes (Table 11.1) and variation in spin-lock times at each spin-lock amplitude (Table 11.1). $R_1\rho$ values were then calculated on a pixel-by-pixel basis for each locking field by fitting signals to a single exponential decay with locking time. R1ρ was shown to be sensitive to fibrosis even at an early time point (5–7 weeks) and $R_1\rho$ at the optimal locking frequencies (1000 Hz) was repeatedly found to be significant in detecting differences between normal controls and fibrotic kidneys, as well as for detecting fibrosis at different stages [17]. The exchange rate parameter S_ρ and the inflection frequency ω_{infl} were found to be significantly lower (by a factor of 2) in fibrotic than in healthy murine kidneys and had excellent diagnostic performance (AUC > 0.9) for identifying renal fibrosis at early (5–7 weeks) and late (30–40 weeks) time points after induction of fibrosis [17]. Interestingly, in a separate study in a murine model of fibrosis generated by unilateral ureteral obstruction, which is the standard model of non-immune renal fibrosis, $T_1\rho$ values demonstrated stronger correlations compared to apparent diffusion coefficient (ADC) values for both α-SMA expression ($R^2 = 0.71$ vs. $R^2 = 0.34$, respectively; $p < 0.001$) and Masson's staining at pathology ($R^2 = 0.65$ vs. $R^2 = 0.38$, respectively; $p < 0.001$) [10].

Mechanism

The exact mechanism resulting in $T_1\rho$ elevation in the context of fibrosis has not been firmly established. It is essential to understand whether $T_1\rho$ values are influenced by other physiologic or pathophysiologic processes aside from fibrosis. This is especially important as renal fibrosis needs to be evaluated with other markers of renal injury (i.e., inflammation, endotheliitis, glomerular and vascular damage), as these lesions not only co-exist but also promote IFTA initiation or progression and are independently actionable or prognostic [20, 23, 27, 36]. A previous animal study has demonstrated that the prolongation in liver $T_1\rho$ values is mostly driven by fibrosis and not inflammation [37]. This was further confirmed in a well-controlled study using a rat model of non-alcoholic fatty liver disease induced with a methionine- and choline-deficient diet [38]. The most important findings in this study were the strong correlation between liver collagen content and liver $T_1\rho$ ($r = 0.82$, $p < 0.0001$) and the clear separation of $T_1\rho$ values for healthy controls versus patients with stage 1 fibrosis. There was no significant correlation between $T_1\rho$ value and inflammation ($r = 0.25$, $p = 1.0$) [38].

While $R_1\rho$ measurements were highly correlated with collagen deposition measured at histopathology (picrosirius red) in the fibrotic kidneys in the study by Wang et al., regional differences in $R_1\rho$ among the cortex, outer stripe outer medulla, inner stripe outer medulla, and inner medulla/papilla in healthy control wild type mouse kidneys were found, suggesting that $R_1\rho$ may be sensitive to free water content, capillary density, and tubular density. It is becoming clear that $R_1\rho$ at a single spin-lock frequency is potentially confounded by other factors, and that $R_1\rho$ dispersion may provide a more specific measure of exchange effects by separating relaxation rates, exchange rates, and frequency offsets of exchanging pools as reported by Wang et al. [17]. The authors deliberately selected a renal fibrosis model using hHB-EGF$^{Tg/Tg}$ mice, in which collagen deposition and capillary density reduction were present in the fibrotic regions of kidneys, while confounding tubular dilation or polyuria is absent. This permits attributing decreases of $R_1\rho$ in the areas of histopathologic fibrosis to events specific to fibrosis, such as increase of tubulointerstitial space and matrix deposition of collagen, increased matrix cross-linking, and loss of capillaries [17].

Less Promising Noninvasive MRI Methods for Assessment of Renal Fibrosis

With recent hardware and software advances, several other functional quantitative MRI methods, including magnetic resonance elastography (MRE), diffusion weighted imaging (DWI), T_1 mapping, and blood oxygen level dependent (BOLD) have been explored for the diagnostic assessment of renal fibrosis. ADC values obtained from DWI and T_1 measurements have been shown to be associated with allograft fibrosis, although the measurements also showed significant correlation with inflammation [39]. While MRI enables the quantitative measurement of tissue stiffness by imaging the propagation of mechanical shear waves through the tissue, initial results indicate that MRE-derived stiffness measurements are not solely dependent on renal fibrosis and are confounded by complex renal physiology, anisotropic renal anatomy, and low spatial resolution parametric maps [40–43]. BOLD, which indirectly quantifies renal oxygenation and hypoxia, cannot distinguish between renal injuries that affect perfusion from those affecting oxygen consumption. Furthermore, it is sensitive to other factors than fibrosis that affect renal oxygenation, such as blood volume, medications, and tubular dysfunction [44]. $T_1\rho$ therefore overcomes limitations of other quantitative MRI methods in the measurement of renal fibrosis, especially of MRE.

Future Directions

Published studies have demonstrated a strong association of $T_1\rho$ to renal fibrosis, and further work will need to establish the mechanism while accounting for concomitant physiology and pathologic diagnoses, especially inflammation and changes in capillary density. Measurement of chemical exchange rates obtained through dispersion analysis ought to be explored in both native and transplanted kidneys to validate that differences in collagen quantity result in changes in $T_1\rho$ contrast.

Conclusions

In summary, prior work demonstrates the sensitivity of $T_1\rho$ to collagen deposition in fibrotic native and transplanted kidneys. Further investigation into the exact mechanism can be performed by evaluating the chemical exchange rates from $T_1\rho$ dispersion analysis, which may serve to improve the specificity of $T_1\rho$ metrics to fibrosis. Furthermore, $T_1\rho$ may overcome limitations of other quantitative MRI methods in the measurement of renal fibrosis, since it is potentially less impacted by other concomitant physiologic and pathophysiologic processes, such as inflammation, that may confound assessment. Once validated, $T_1\rho$ may potentially serve a very important role as a quantitative imaging biomarker for the diagnosis and determination of disease severity of fibrosis in native kidneys and allografts, prediction of patient prognosis, and longitudinal disease monitoring for treatment effect or disease progression.

Acknowledgement We gratefully acknowledge the Preclinical PET Imaging Facility and Biomedical Magnetic Resonance Center at Washington University School of Medicine in St. Louis. This work was supported by National Institutes of Health (NIH) Grants R01DK110622, R01DK111861, R01DK129888, and R41DK129138. E. J. Baldelomar also received support by NIH Grant TL1TR002344.

References

1. Redfield AG. Nuclear magnetic resonance saturation and rotary saturation in solids. Phys Rev. 1955;98(6):1787–809.
2. Look DC, Lowe IJ. Nuclear magnetic dipole—dipole relaxation along the static and rotating magnetic fields: application to gypsum. J Chem Phys. 1966;44(8):2995–3000.
3. Hartmann SR, Hahn EL. Nuclear double resonance in the rotating frame. Phys Rev. 1962;128(5):2042–53.
4. Santyr GE, Henkelman RM, Bronskill MJ. Spin locking for magnetic resonance imaging with application to human breast. Magn Reson Med. 1989;12(1):25–37.
5. Wang L, Regatte RR. T1ρ MRI of human musculoskeletal system. J Magn Reson Imaging. 2015;41(3):586–600.
6. Hectors SJ, et al. Splenic T1rho as a noninvasive biomarker for portal hypertension. J Magn Reson Imaging. 2020;52(3):787–94.
7. Rauscher I, et al. Evaluation of T1rho as a potential MR biomarker for liver cirrhosis: comparison of healthy control subjects and patients with liver cirrhosis. Eur J Radiol. 2014;83(6):900–4.
8. van Oorschot JW, et al. Endogenous assessment of diffuse myocardial fibrosis in patients with T1rho -mapping. J Magn Reson Imaging. 2017;45(1):132–8.
9. Hectors SJ, et al. T1rho mapping for assessment of renal allograft fibrosis. J Magn Reson Imaging. 2019;50(4):1085–91.
10. Hu G, et al. Comparison of T1 mapping and T1rho values with conventional diffusion-weighted imaging to assess fibrosis in a rat model of unilateral ureteral obstruction. Acad Radiol. 2019;26(1):22–9.
11. Rapacchi S, et al. Towards the identification of multiparametric quantitative MRI biomarkers in lupus nephritis. Magn Reson Imaging. 2015;33(9):1066–74.
12. He X, et al. Estimation of single-kidney glomerular filtration rate without exogenous contrast agent. Magn Reson Med. 2014;71(1):257–66.
13. Wheaton AJ, et al. In vivo quantification of T1rho using a multislice spin-lock pulse sequence. Magn Reson Med. 2004;52(6):1453–8.
14. Chen W. Errors in quantitative T1rho imaging and the correction methods. Quant Imaging Med Surg. 2015;5(4):583–91.
15. Witschey WR 2nd, et al. Artifacts in T1 rho-weighted imaging: compensation for B(1) and B(0) field imperfections. J Magn Reson. 2007;186(1):75–85.
16. Mitrea BG, et al. Paired self-compensated spin-lock preparation for improved T1ρ quantification. J Magn Reson. 2016;268:49–57.
17. Wang F, et al. Spin-lock relaxation rate dispersion reveals spatiotemporal changes associated with tubulointerstitial fibrosis in murine kidney. Magn Reson Med. 2020;84(4):2074–87.
18. Chopra S, McClung RED, Jordan RB. Rotating-frame relaxation rates of solvent molecules in solutions of paramagnetic ions undergoing solvent exchange. J Magn Reson. 1984;59(3):361–72.
19. Boor P, Ostendorf T, Floege J. Renal fibrosis: novel insights into mechanisms and therapeutic targets. Nat Rev Nephrol. 2010;6(11):643–56.
20. Boor P, Floege J. Renal allograft fibrosis: biology and therapeutic targets. Am J Transplant. 2015;15(4):863–86.
21. Nicholson ML, et al. Early measurement of interstitial fibrosis predicts long-term renal function and graft survival in renal transplantation. Br J Surg. 1996;83(8):1082–5.
22. Nankivell BJ, et al. The natural history of chronic allograft nephropathy. N Engl J Med. 2003;349(24):2326–33.
23. Srivastava A, et al. The prognostic value of histopathologic lesions in native kidney biopsy specimens: results from the Boston kidney biopsy cohort study. J Am Soc Nephrol. 2018;29(8):2213–24.
24. Centers for Disease Control and Prevention. Chronic kidney disease in the United States, 2021. 2021.
25. Khan H, et al. Prevalence and risk factors for early chronic allograft nephropathy in a live related renal transplant program. J Nephropathol. 2014;3(2):69–79.
26. Ishida H, et al. Preventive effect of early introduction of everolimus and reduced-exposure tacrolimus on renal interstitial fibrosis in de novo living-donor renal transplant recipients. Clin Exp Nephrol. 2019;24:288.
27. Lv W, et al. Inflammation and renal fibrosis: recent developments on key signaling molecules as potential therapeutic targets. Eur J Pharmacol. 2018;820:65–76.
28. Korbet SM, Volpini KC, Whittier WL. Percutaneous renal biopsy of native kidneys: a single-center experience of 1,055 biopsies. Am J Nephrol. 2014;39(2):153–62.
29. Furness PN, et al. Protocol biopsy of the stable renal transplant: a multicenter study of methods and complication rates. Transplantation. 2003;76(6):969–73.
30. Elshafie M, Furness PN. Identification of lesions indicating rejection in kidney transplant biopsies: tubulitis is severely under-detected by conventional microscopy. Nephrol Dial Transplant. 2012;27(3):1252–5.
31. Wang YX, et al. T1rho MR imaging is sensitive to evaluate liver fibrosis: an experimental study

in a rat biliary duct ligation model. Radiology. 2011;259(3):712–9.
32. Serai SD. Basics of magnetic resonance imaging and quantitative parameters T1, T2, T2*, T1rho and diffusion-weighted imaging. Pediatr Radiol. 2021;52:217.
33. Allkemper T, et al. Evaluation of fibrotic liver disease with whole-liver T1rho MR imaging: a feasibility study at 1.5 T. Radiology. 2014;271(2):408–15.
34. Hectors SJ, et al. T1rho mapping for assessment of renal allograft fibrosis. J Magn Reson Imaging. 2019;50:1085.
35. Singh A, et al. T1rho MRI of healthy and fibrotic human livers at 1.5 T. J Transl Med. 2015;13:292.
36. Nankivell BJ, et al. The causes, significance and consequences of inflammatory fibrosis in kidney transplantation: the Banff i-IFTA lesion. Am J Transplant. 2018;18(2):364–76.
37. Zhao F, et al. MR T1rho as an imaging biomarker for monitoring liver injury progression and regression: an experimental study in rats with carbon tetrachloride intoxication. Eur Radiol. 2012;22(8):1709–16.
38. Zhao F, et al. Collagen deposition in the liver is strongly and positively associated with T1rho elongation while fat deposition is associated with T1rho shortening: an experimental study of methionine and choline-deficient (MCD) diet rat model. Quant Imaging Med Surg. 2020;10(12):2307–21.
39. Friedli I, et al. New magnetic resonance imaging index for renal fibrosis assessment: a comparison between diffusion-weighted imaging and T1 mapping with histological validation. Sci Rep. 2016;6:30088.
40. Lee CU, et al. MR elastography in renal transplant patients and correlation with renal allograft biopsy: a feasibility study. Acad Radiol. 2012;19(7):834–41.
41. Marticorena Garcia SR, et al. Multifrequency magnetic resonance elastography for the assessment of renal allograft function. Invest Radiol. 2016;51(9):591–5.
42. Streitberger KJ, et al. High-resolution mechanical imaging of the kidney. J Biomech. 2014;47(3):639–44.
43. Gennisson JL, et al. Supersonic shear wave elastography of in vivo pig kidney: influence of blood pressure, urinary pressure and tissue anisotropy. Ultrasound Med Biol. 2012;38(9):1559–67.
44. Leung G, et al. Could MRI be used to image kidney fibrosis? A review of recent advances and remaining barriers. Clin J Am Soc Nephrol. 2017;12(6):1019–28.

12 MR Fingerprinting for Quantitative Kidney Imaging

Yong Chen, Christina J. MacAskill, Sherry Huang, Katherine M. Dell, Sree H. Tirumani, Mark A. Griswold, and Chris A. Flask

Introduction

Magnetic resonance imaging (MRI) plays a critical role in assessment of many kidney diseases due to its ability to depict a wide variety of soft tissue contrasts and its high spatial resolution. However, the current clinical practice using MRI typically relies on qualitative interpretation based on a set of contrast-weighted images instead of actual quantitative tissue properties, which can lead to subjective and even inaccurate image interpretation. Recently, extensive efforts have been devoted to developing novel quantitative imaging biomarkers for kidney imaging [1–6]. Quantification of renal T_1 and T_2 relaxation times has potential usefulness in numerous clinical scenarios, including providing markers to assess the function of transplanted and native kidneys [7], to characterize renal tumors, and to detect and monitor genetic and chronic kidney diseases (CKD) [8, 9] and response to treatment [10, 11]. Another important clinical application of kidney relaxometry assessments is to enable quantitative MRI assessments for both dynamic contrast-enhanced (DCE) MRI (T_1) or blood oxygen level-dependent (BOLD) MRI (T_2/T_2*) [12].

However, quantitative MR imaging can be extremely challenging in the kidney due to patient motion. Our team has recently developed a new quantitative MRI technique named Magnetic Resonance Fingerprinting (MRF). MRF was proposed as a method to deliver simultaneously collected, accurate, and reproducible maps of multiple tissue properties (e.g., T_1 and T_2 relaxation times) in a single scan [13–18]. MRF takes a different approach from conventional MRI for data acquisition and image reconstruction. Conventional MR uses repeated acquisition parameters in a particular sequence until all of k-space is filled, and then this is done serially for other sequences. Image contrast is conventionally

Y. Chen · C. J. MacAskill · M. A. Griswold
Department of Radiology, Case Western Reserve University, Cleveland, OH, USA

S. Huang
Department of Biomedical Engineering, Case Western Reserve University, Cleveland, OH, USA

K. M. Dell
Department of Pediatrics, Case Western Reserve University, Cleveland, OH, USA

Center for Pediatric Nephrology, Cleveland Clinic Children's Hospital, Cleveland, OH, USA

S. H. Tirumani
Department of Radiology, University Hospitals Cleveland Medical Center, Cleveland, OH, USA

C. A. Flask (✉)
Department of Radiology, Case Western Reserve University, Cleveland, OH, USA

Department of Biomedical Engineering, Case Western Reserve University, Cleveland, OH, USA

Department of Pediatrics, Case Western Reserve University, Cleveland, OH, USA
e-mail: caf@case.edu

S. D. Serai, K. Darge (eds.), *Advanced Clinical MRI of the Kidney*,
https://doi.org/10.1007/978-3-031-40169-5_12

created by reconstructing MRI images that weight the images with specific relaxation properties. For example, weighting toward optimization of longitudinal relaxation corresponds to "T_1-weighting," and weighting toward optimization of transverse relaxation corresponds to "T_2-weighting." In contrast, in MRF, the goal is to drive the signal away from a steady state by creating transient variabilities in signal that are highly sensitive to the tissue properties of interest. Because these MRF-based assessments are obtained simultaneously, the resultant parametric maps are inherently co-registered, allowing the data to be easily combined to enable a more comprehensive evaluation of tissue composition and (patho)physiology. Prior human and animal MRF studies have shown that MRF is also inherently resistant to motion artifacts due to the dictionary matching process. Further, our recently developed kidney MRF methodology provides accurate, repeatable, and inherently co-registered kidney T_1 and T_2 maps in 15 seconds or less, providing the opportunity to eliminate respiratory motion by acquiring the MRF data during breath-holds. In this chapter, we will first provide an overview of the MRF method from data acquisition to image post-processing. Next, we will review recent studies related to quantitative kidney imaging using MRF. Finally, we will discuss potential applications of MRF in clinical kidney imaging.

MRF Acquisition Protocols

Conceptual Framework of MRF

The MRF framework is built upon recent developments in parallel imaging, compressed sensing, and non-Cartesian data sampling. The original MRF study, published in *Nature* in 2013, was focused on rapid and accurate determination of quantitative T_1 and T_2 relaxation times for every voxel in an MRF dataset [16]. While the importance of magnetic relaxometry assessments has long been recognized, they are difficult to perform, especially for body imaging applications. Using conventional quantitative MRI methods, several images must be obtained with different acquisition timing parameters (e.g., echo time, repetition time, inversion time) along with least-squared error regression analysis to compute the T_1 and /or T_2 relaxation time maps [19, 20]. This means that multiple full images are needed to map a single relaxometry parameter. This is an inefficient process, and thus quantitative maps are often acquired with suboptimal spatial resolutions or an insufficient number of time points to reduce scan time that can compromise the accuracy and discriminative power in tissue characterization. Most of these prior relaxometric MRI studies are also acquired with a single slice, which does not provide sufficient spatial coverage to fully examine tissues/lesions of interest [21]. For quantitative kidney imaging using conventional methods, long breath-holds or respiratory gating would be required to mitigate motion artifacts for parameter mapping. These processes have been demonstrated to be error-prone and result in image mis-registration, making them impractical in a routine clinical setting.

These difficulties in quantitative MR imaging prompted our team to develop the multi-parametric MRI methodology we termed magnetic resonance fingerprinting. The method was called MR fingerprinting in analogy to traditional fingerprinting, where the match of a fingerprint is utilized to obtain information that is stored in a database and not directly collected. MRF uses a rapid, highly undersampled acquisition with variable acquisition parameters (e.g., flip angle, TR, TE) to generate incoherent magnetization profiles (Fig. 12.1). In this framework, the MRF signal is allowed to evolve dynamically, but in a controlled manner, through a priori acquisition parameter variation. Thus, different tissues or materials have unique resultant signal evolution profiles that depend on the tissue's specific magnetic properties. Using this approach, the MRF signal evolution profiles of all possible tissue types can be pre-calculated using Bloch equation simulations to generate a MRF dictionary. The acquired signal from each voxel of highly accelerated images can then be matched to an entry in this dictionary using an appropriate pattern matching algorithm, which, in turn, yields maps of several MRI parameters simultaneously in a

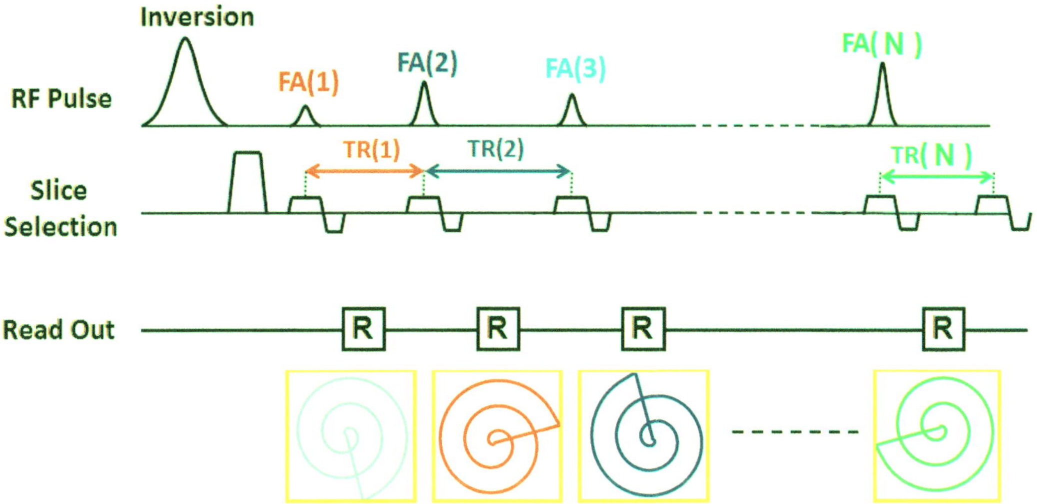

Fig. 12.1 Example sequence diagram for the FISP-MRF sequence. Variable acquisition parameters including flip angles (FA) and repetition times (TR) are used and the data is acquired with an undersampled spiral readout with a high acceleration factor

single, rapid MRI scan [16]. The MRF framework is flexible and can be integrated with different types of MR pulse sequences such as balanced steady-state free precession (bSSFP), fast imaging with steady-state free precession (FISP), and fast low-angle shot (FLASH) sequences, to map out different tissue properties [15, 22, 23]. In addition to relatively stationary brain imaging, MRF has been demonstrated to provide accurate quantification of T_1 and T_2 relaxation times for the abdomen providing rapid, multi-parametric MR analysis in kidney imaging [24]. Compared to conventional approaches, MRF has demonstrated superior performance in tissue quantification with improved accuracy and precision including significantly improved site-to-site and scanner-to-scanner reproducibility [16]. MRF also offers improved motion tolerance, which is advantageous for abdominal imaging [16]. The fact that multiple tissue properties can be acquired simultaneously further enables multi-parametric tissue analysis with improved accuracy for specifically identifying various pathophysiologies by eliminating the need for image co-registration. Next, we will review several recent MRF studies that are focused on quantitative abdominal imaging with a focus on kidney imaging.

MRF Acquisition Methods

MRF for rapid quantitative abdominal imaging [24]. In contrast to stationary brain imaging, one important requirement of an abdominal MRF acquisition is a short acquisition time, preferably within a single breath-hold, to limit respiratory motion artifacts associated with kidney MRI imaging. Inhomogeneities in the B_1 field are another challenge for abdominal imaging assessments as they can result in significant errors in T_1 and T_2 measurements [25]. To overcome these difficulties, we previously developed a B_1-compensated 2D MRF method by combining a 17-s MRF acquisition with a ~2-s Bloch-Siegert acquisition [26] for rapid B_1 mapping [24]. This method has been shown to provide B_1-corrected T_1 and T_2 relaxation time maps of the abdomen (i.e., kidneys or liver) in a single breath-hold. The original MRF acquisition proposed for brain imaging was based on an inversion-recovery bSSFP pulse sequence. The choice of this pulse sequence was based on its high signal-to-noise (SNR) efficiency and its sensitivity to multiple important parameters, including T_1 and T_2 [27]. However, bSSFP sequences are also sensitive to heterogeneities in the main magnetic field (B_0)

which can cause significant banding artifacts in abdominal imaging applications, especially on scanners with higher field strength (e.g., 3.0 T or greater). Therefore, we based our first kidney MRF method on the FISP sequence that has been developed to resolve these challenges [15]. In this first implementation, a total of 2500 MRF time points were obtained in one acquisition, with the repetition times varying between 6.1 and 9.0 ms and the flip angles varying between 0° and 54° (Fig. 12.2). Other imaging parameters included: FOV = 44 × 44 cm; matrix size = 224 × 224 (in-plane resolution = 1.9 mm); echo time (TE) = 1.3 ms; slice thickness = 5 mm; and excitation pulse design = 1 ms sinc pulse with time-bandwidth product = 4. Several simulated signal evolution curves for this kidney MRF design from different abdominal tissues, including the renal cortex and medulla, are plotted in Fig. 12.2c. For the 2-s B_1 mapping scan, a gradient-echo based Bloch-Siegert sequence was implemented with a multi-shot spiral acquisition (24 spiral interleaves for each image; readout duration for each spiral interleaf, 3.0 ms) to improve the imaging speed and to limit the specific absorption rate (SAR). An off-resonance 8-ms Fermi pulse was applied between the excitation pulse and spiral readout to induce a B_1-

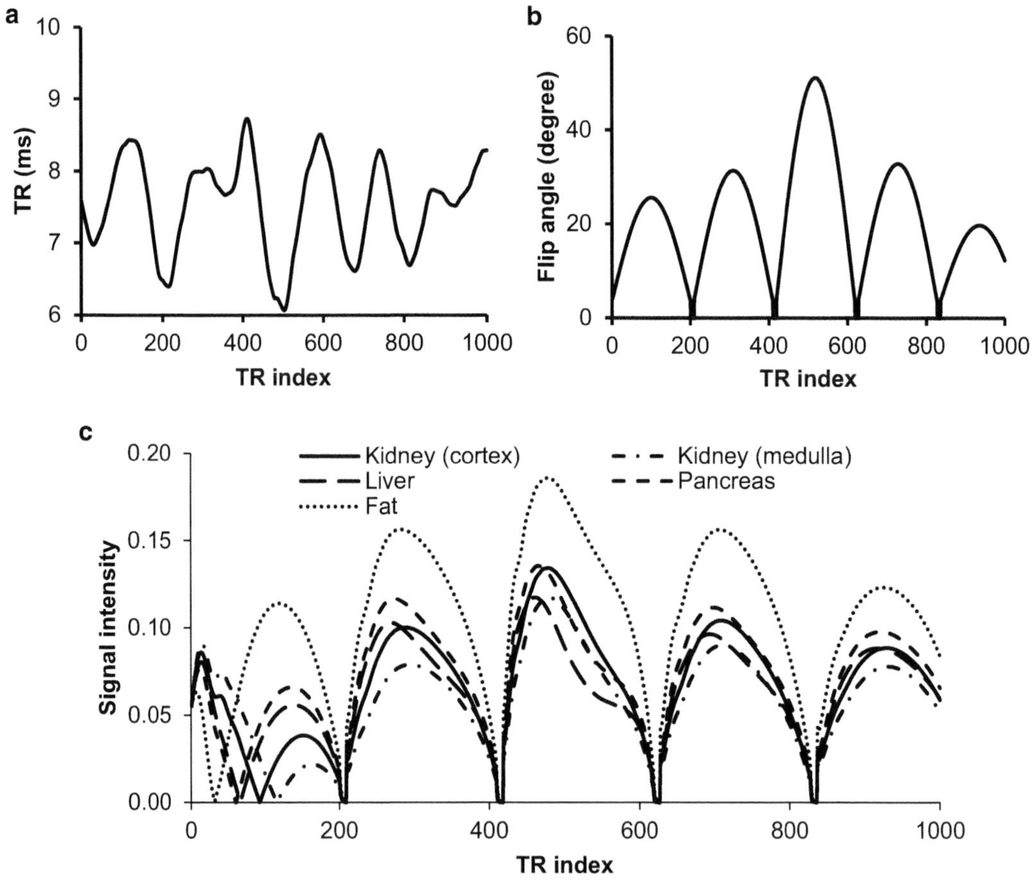

Fig. 12.2 Acquisition parameters and simulation of signal evolutions for abdominal MRF [24]. (**a**) Example of the first 1000 points for repetition time (TR). (**b**) Example of the first 1000 points for flip angle (FA). (**c**) Signal evolution curves for multiple tissues in the abdomen generated using the acquisition patterns shown in (**a**) and (**b**). T_1 and T_2 values, respectively, used to generate the curves included 1140 and 75 ms for the renal cortex, 1540 and 80 ms for the renal medulla, 820 and 35 ms for the liver, 720 and 45 ms for the pancreas, and 400 and 70 ms for fat [28]

dependent phase shift. Additional imaging parameters for the Bloch-Siegert scan were FOV = 44 × 44 cm; matrix size = 128 × 128; slice thickness = 5 mm; repetition time (TR) = 30 ms; and TE = 1.3 ms. Two images were acquired with ±4 KHz frequency off-resonance in an interleaved manner, and the total acquisition time for a B_1 map was 1.8 s. The details of data post-processing including the incorporation of B_1 field map have been described previously. With this method, four tissue property maps including T_1, T_2, proton density (M_0), and B_1 were acquired in one breath-hold. Representative maps obtained from a normal subject are presented in Fig. 12.3.

MRF for simultaneous renal T_1 and T_2 mapping in a single breath-hold* [29]. Besides T_1 and T_2 relaxation times, mapping of T_2* can be utilized to examine the blood oxygenation level-dependent effect, which has been shown to decrease in chronic kidney disease and kidney transplant [30, 31]. Based on the MRF framework, Hermann et al. have recently developed a quantitative imaging method for simultaneous kidney T_1 and T_2* measurement. In this particular study, an MRF protocol based on echo-planar imaging (EPI) was developed to provide quantitative T_1 and T_2* mapping of four slices in one breath-hold of 15 seconds. Compared to the undersampled spiral sampling applied in conventional MRF acquisitions, MRF with EPI readouts provides both high sampling efficiency and images derived from fully-sampled k-space trajectories to generate the MRF signal evolution profiles.

For this MRF implementation, 35 MRF time points were acquired with varying flip angles from 17 to 43°, varying TEs from 16 to 76.5 ms, and varying TR from 363 to 625 ms. Other imaging parameters included FOV = 38 × 38 cm; matrix size 256 × 256 for an effective in-plane resolution of 1.5 mm; slice thickness 5 mm; GRAPPA factor, 3; and Partial Fourier, 5/8. Gaussian smoothing was performed on the baseline EPI images with a kernel size of 5 before

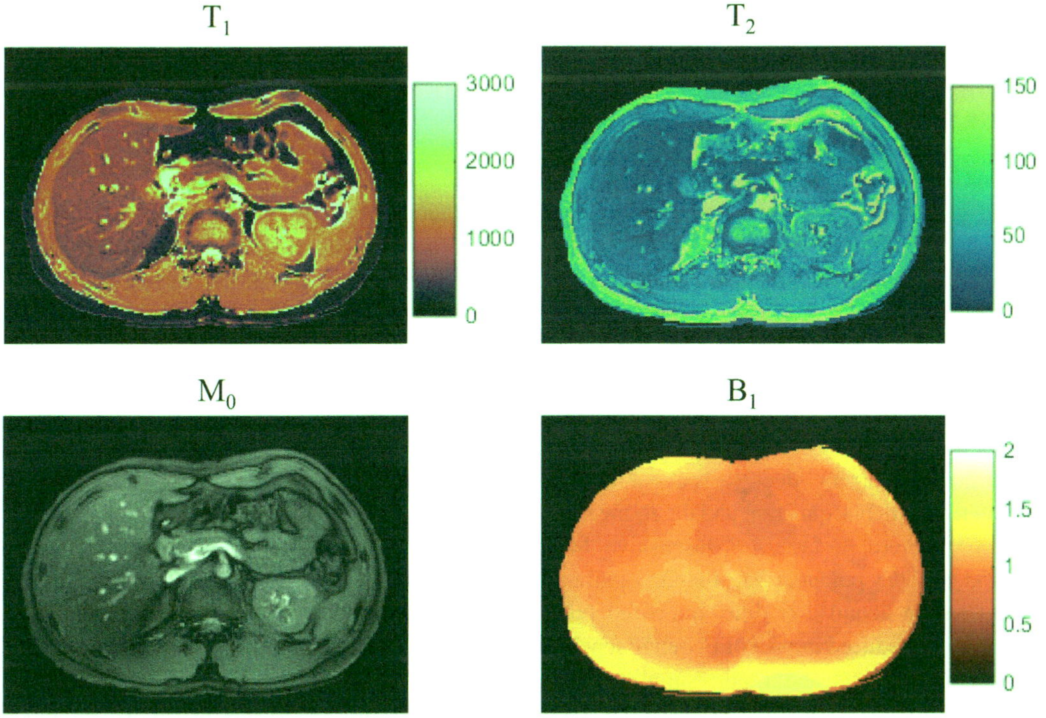

Fig. 12.3 Representative tissue property maps obtained using abdominal MRF from a normal subject [24]. Four quantitative maps, including T_1, T_2, M_0, and B_1, were acquired in one breath-hold of 19 s

the pattern matching process, which improves map quality at a cost of a reduced effective spatial resolution. Representative T_1 and T_2* maps obtained from a healthy volunteer are presented in Fig. 12.4; these results were compared to those obtained using standard approaches (i.e., Modified Look-Locker inversion recovery (MOLLI) for T_1 mapping and a multi-echo gradient-echo sequences for T_2* mapping). Compared to these standard imaging approaches, the developed MRF method demonstrates an improved acquisition speed while also maintaining reasonably accurate quantification of kidney tissues.

In this study, a limited number of MRF evolution time points were implemented to minimize EPI-based ghosting artifacts and overall acquisition time. However, this EPI-based kidney MRF approach has limitations that are common to EPI acquisitions including limited spatial resolution due to a restricted EPI readout length and image distortion from B_0 field inhomogeneities and eddy currents. Therefore, a more flexible MRF implementation was likely needed to meet the needs for the broad set of kidney imaging applications.

Rapid B_1-insensitive MRF for quantitative renal imaging [32]. Based on the abdominal MRF method introduced in Chen et al. [24], our team has recently developed a new B_1-insensitive MRF method for quantitative kidney imaging. While the 19-s breath-hold in the prior study was successful for healthy adult subjects, further reduction in the acquisition time was desired, especially for young pediatric patients or patients with impaired respiratory function. Limiting the need for B_1 correction in the original approach would also reduce the overall scan time/breath-hold duration (~2 s) and would limit the potential quantification errors due to patient motion between the MRF acquisition and the B_1 measurement. Therefore, a faster, B_1-insensitive MRF method has the potential to provide significant reductions in acquisition time, improved precision through reduced impact of B_1 heterogeneities and motion artifacts, and a more simplified post-processing imaging workflow (i.e., no B_1 correction). This B_1-insensitive MRF method also combines multiple features of prior MRF implementations in the brain and heart for improved T_1 and T_2 mapping in the human kidney, including multiple magnetization preparation schema to provide MRF images with both T_1 and T_2 contrast, low flip angles (5°–12°) to limit the impact of B_1 heterogeneities, and a constant TR and TE to minimize the overall scan time. Specifically, this MRF acquisition consists of 12 acquisition segments, each consisting of a different magnetization preparation (i.e., inversion recovery module (n = 3), T_2 preparation (n = 6), or no preparation (n = 3)) followed by a spectrally selective fat suppression pulse to limit the impact of abdominal adipose tissue. After the preparation modules, a total of 144 consecutive MRF readouts were acquired in each acquisition segment. The three inversion recovery modules use non-selective, adiabatic inversion pulses and inversion delays of 21 ms, 100 ms, and 250 ms, respectively. The six T_2 preparations were designed using the Malcom-Levitt algorithm with effective echo times of either 50 ms (n = 3) or 90 ms (n = 3), respectively [33, 34]. The MRF data were acquired using an undersampled spiral readout and FISP kernel with a constant TR (5.74 ms) and TE (1.0 ms). Additional FISP MRF parameters were field-of-view (FOV) = 40 × 40 cm; matrix size = 256 × 256; and slice thickness = 5 mm. A total of 1728 MRF images (12 × 144) were acquired in one breath-hold for a total acquisition time of 15 s.

Figure 12.5 shows T_1 and T_2 maps of a healthy volunteer's kidneys acquired using this approach. For this subject, a ~2-s Bloch-Siegert B_1 mapping sequence [24] was added immediately following the MRF acquisition to measure the B_1 field. The results both with and without incorporation of B_1 correction using the Bloch-Siegert B_1 measurement are presented. Despite visible B_1 differences in the left and right kidneys, the T_1 and T_2 maps obtained with and without B_1 correction were visibly consistent. Note also that the differences between the two versions of the maps resulted in a maximum error of 10 ms in T_1 and 5 ms in T_2, which are single dictionary increments for each value in the MRF dictionary. These results suggest that this new B_1-insensitive MRF method can provide robust tissue property mapping without the need for B_1 correction.

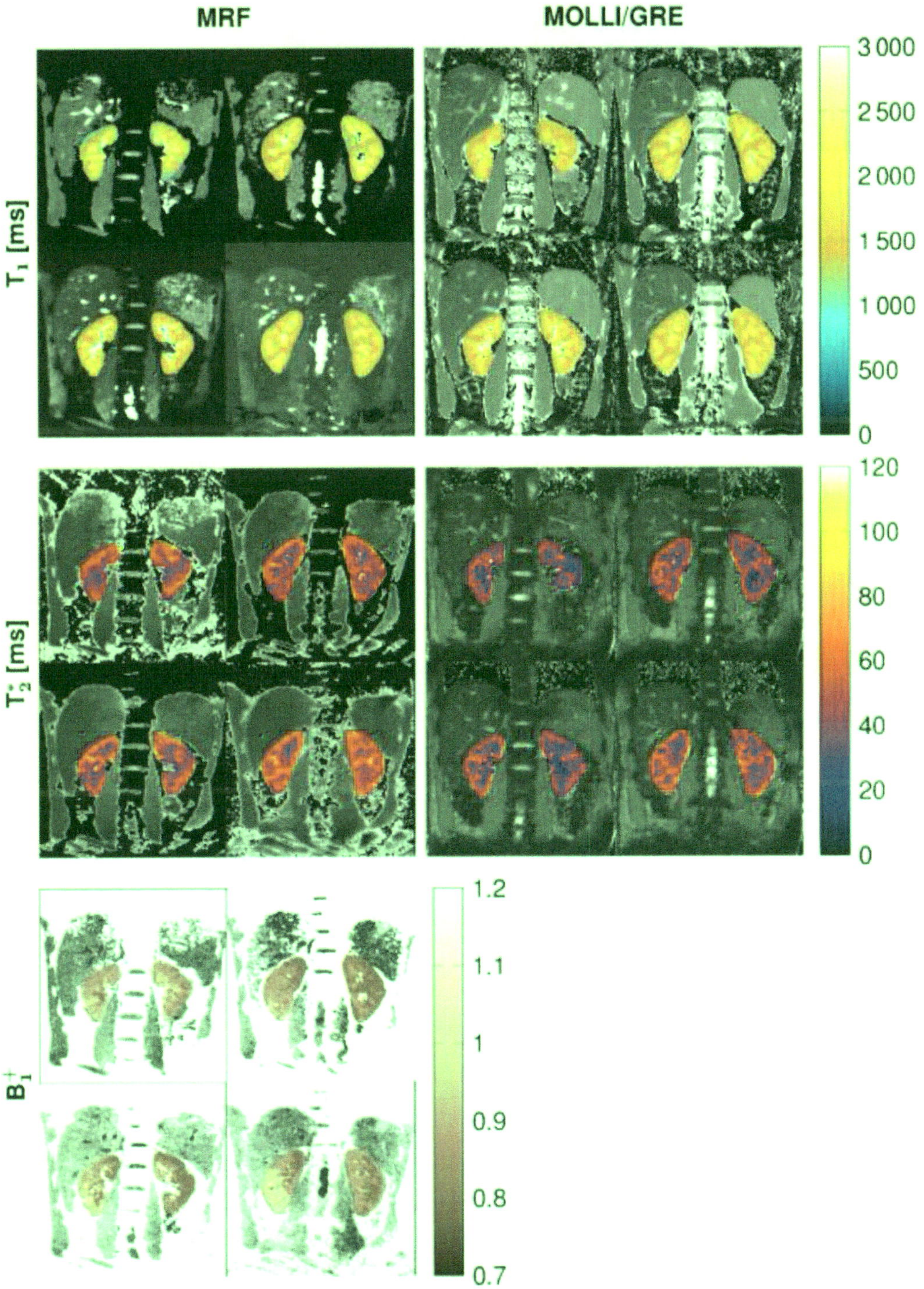

Fig. 12.4 Exemplary baselines image, T_1, T_2*, and B_1 maps for 4 slices of the MRF, MOLLI, and multi-GRE in the kidneys in coronal view (cited from Hermann et al. [29])

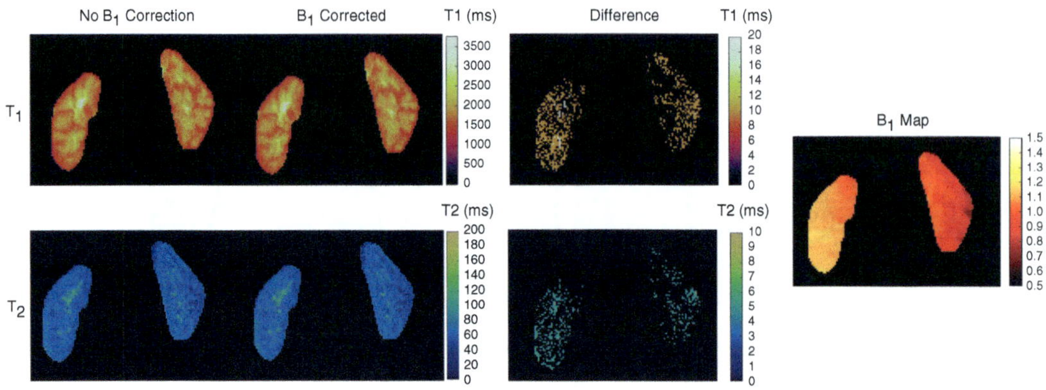

Fig. 12.5 Kidney T_1 and T_2 maps from a healthy volunteer both before and after B_1 correction as well as corresponding difference maps [32]. Corresponding B_1 map acquired using the Bloch-Siegert acquisition is shown on the right

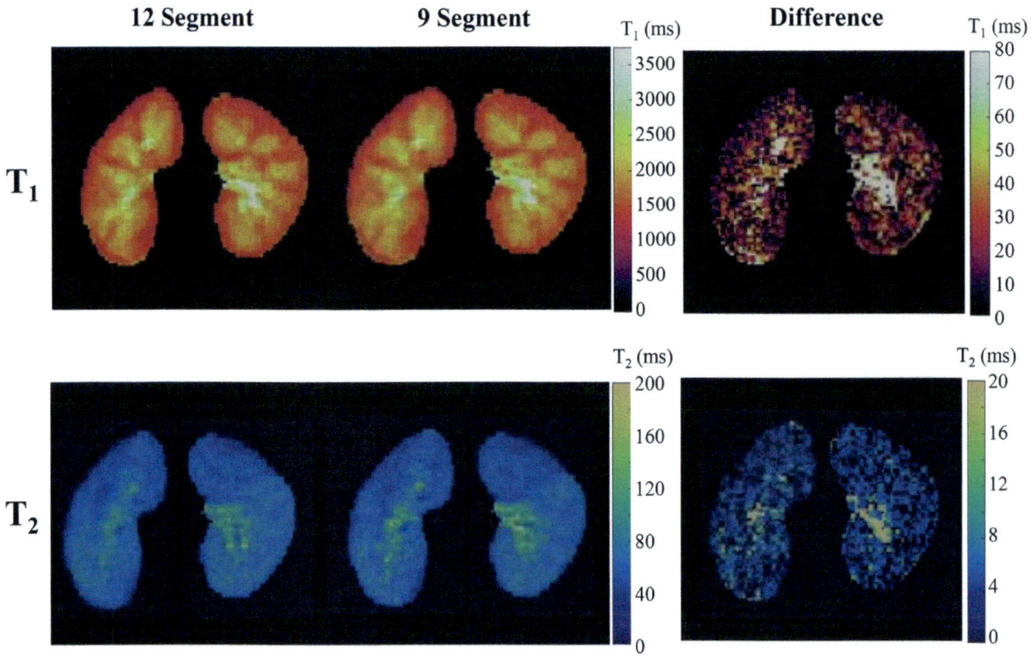

Fig. 12.6 Kidney T_1 and T_2 maps obtained from a healthy volunteer using the B_1-insensitive kidney MRF method [32]. The quantitative maps reconstructed using all 12 segments (15-s scan time) versus 9 segments (11-s scan time) are both presented along with corresponding difference maps

To assess the potential for further reduction in acquisition time, we also generated kidney T_1 and T_2 maps using the same kidney MRF data but with only the first nine MRF segments (1296 MRF time points; scan time, 11 s) instead of all 12 segments. Representative tissue property maps obtained from a healthy volunteer are shown in Fig. 12.6. ROI analysis on a cohort of 10 subjects further demonstrates consistent T_1 and T_2 values for both the renal medulla and cortex as compared to results obtained with conventional methods [28, 35].

Free-breathing abdominal MRF using a pilot tone navigator [36]. All the aforementioned kidney MRF studies were performed with breath-holds, providing quantitative maps of one

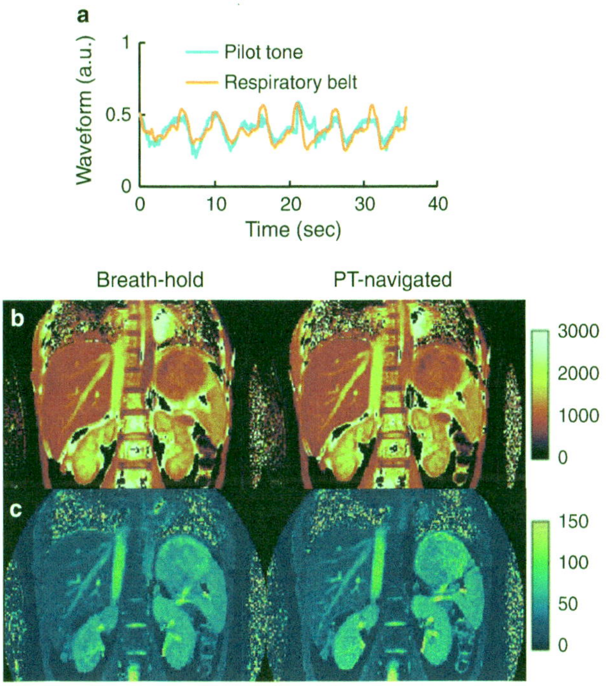

Fig. 12.7 Free-breathing 2D kidney MRF with pilot tone navigator. (**a**) Time courses of respiratory waveform estimated using pilot tone navigator and respiratory belt. Representative T_1 (**b**) and T_2 (**c**) maps obtained using free-breathing 2D MRF with pilot tone navigation. The maps obtained from the same subject using 2D breath-hold MRF are also presented

or a small number of slices in one breath-hold. However, routine clinical kidney imaging using MRF would benefit from volumetric scans for improved coverage and spatial resolution. However, this would be difficult to accomplish with scans obtained in a single breath-hold. Recently, a motion tracking technique called pilot tone (PT) was developed to provide respiratory motion tracking with a high temporal resolution and without additional patient setup or sequence modification [37–40]. The PT signal is a radiofrequency signal that is encoded in the raw MRI data through the receiver coils and directly encodes patient motion (Fig. 12.7a) [40, 41]. We have recently developed free-breathing 2D and 3D MRF that retrospectively analyzes the MRF data using the integrated pilot tone signal [36]. Specifically, principal component analysis was applied to extract respiratory waveform from the pilot tone signal, and the motion information was used to bin the acquired MRF data in respiratory phases. The parameters for the free-breathing 2D MRF acquisition were the same as in the B_1-insensitive kidney MRF method [32]. For each slice, 10 measurements were acquired with a 10-s pause in between for magnetization recovery. Representative 2D T_1 and T_2 maps reconstructed retrospectively from six repeated measurements are shown in Fig. 12.7, and the results demonstrate the effectiveness of the method in motion correction for kidney MRF. A similar approach was also implemented for 3D abdominal MRF and retrospective gating based on four repeated measurements yielded an acquisition speed of ~1 min for each imaging slice. Ongoing work is focused on implementing efficient prospective gating using the pilot tone signal to further reduce the overall MRF acquisition time.

MRF Post-processing

Tissue Property Mapping Using Template Matching

Besides the differences in data acquisition, MRF is also different from most conventional quantitative imaging methods in terms of data post-processing. Since the signal evolution does not follow a certain waveform (for example, the standard exponential recovery or decay for conventional relaxometry mapping methods), a

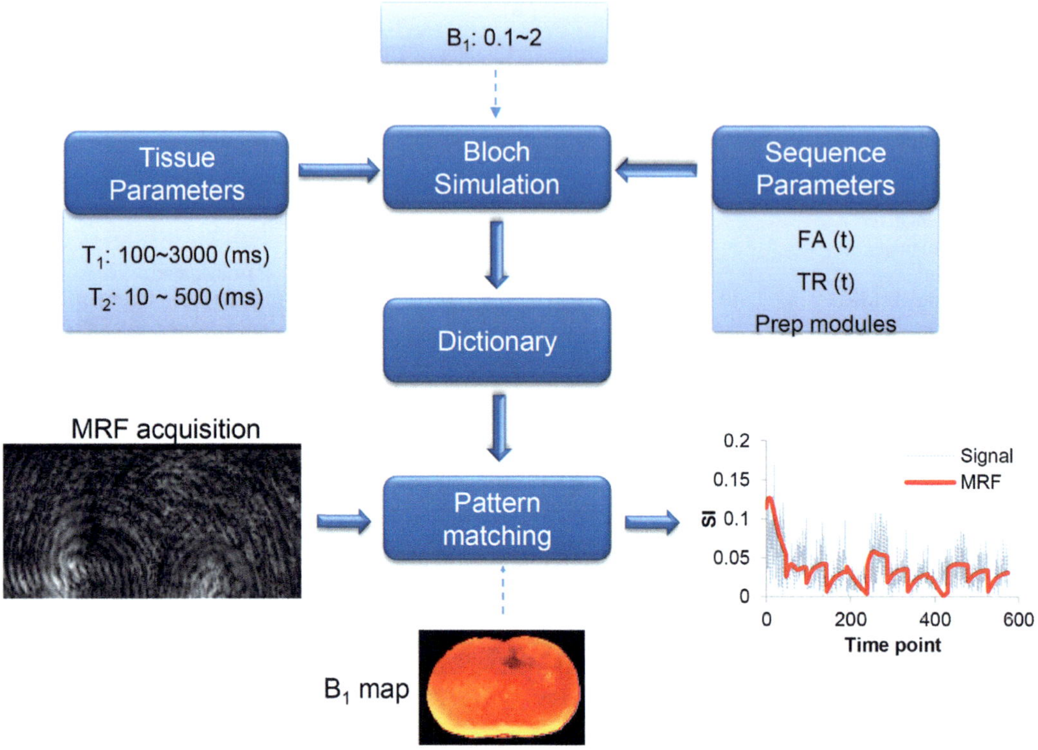

Fig. 12.8 Diagram of the post-processing pipeline for MRF. First, a MRF dictionary is generated using Bloch equation simulations based on tissue property values and acquisition parameters. After MRF image reconstruction, signal evolution of each pixel is compared to the dictionary to identify a best-matched entry, which in turn yields the corresponding tissue properties used to calculate this entry. B_1 information can be integrated in the framework to obtain B_1-corrected tissue properties based on an external measured B_1 map

more sophisticated data analysis algorithm is needed to extract quantitative measurements from the MRF signal evolutions. In the original MRF framework, this was achieved with the template matching approach [16]. The diagram of the MRF post-processing pipeline is illustrated in Fig. 12.8. In brief, an MRF dictionary containing the MRF signal evolutions for all possible combinations of tissue properties (e.g., T_1 and T_2 relaxation times) is first generated. This can be performed with Bloch equation simulations or more efficiently with extended phase graph methods [42, 43]. Besides the information about tissue properties, the MRF acquisition parameters such as flip angles and TRs are also needed to generate the MRF dictionary. Depending on the computational resources and size of the dictionary, the time needed for MRF generation varies from seconds to hours. However, for most applications, including the previously discussed methods for kidney imaging, the MRF dictionary needs to be calculated only once and can be applied to different subjects, scanners, or even field strengths. These dictionaries are also independent of spatial resolution parameters used in the MRF acquisition such as field of view, spatial resolution, and slice thickness.

With the pre-calculated MRF dictionary, template matching or a similar approach is then performed to identify the single entry in the dictionary that most closely matches the acquired MRF signal evolution. This entry, in turn, yields all underlying tissue properties that were used to form the dictionary entry. This process is performed on a voxel-by-voxel basis and repeated over the entire image yielding quantitative maps of the MRI properties of interest. While the raw MRF images are typically aliased due to the high undersampling factor applied in the acquisition, the aliasing artifacts are spatially and temporally incoherent. Thus, they appear as noise in the signal and robust tissue properties can still be extracted using the template matching method. A pair of aliased MRF signal evolution and the matched dictionary entry are plotted in Fig. 12.8 as an example.

Incorporation of B_1 Field Map in Template Matching

One way to minimize the influence of transmit B_1 field inhomogeneities on quantitative tissue properties measured with MRF is to incorporate a B_1 map in the post-processing [24]. As shown in Fig. 12.8, an MRF dictionary was calculated using Bloch simulations and included the signal evolutions from all possible combinations of parameters for a T_1 range of 100–3000 ms, a T_2 range of 5–500 ms, and a B_1 range of 10–200% of the nominal value. A total of 82,914 entries were generated for the dictionary. As previously mentioned, this dictionary only needs to be calculated once and can be applied to MRF measurements obtained from different subjects. For each subject, the acquired signal in each pixel of highly accelerated images was matched to those entries in the dictionary that have the same B_1 values as measured in the Bloch-Siegert sequence. One best entry was identified using the same method in the original MRF implementation.

Accelerated MRF Template Matching with SVD Compression

While the template matching approach can provide accurate tissue quantification in MRF, further improvement in the speed is desired to facilitate clinical workflow. McGivney et al. have proposed an efficient method to accelerate this process by applying singular value decomposition (SVD) along the temporal domain of both the MRF dictionary and acquired signal evolutions [44]. As shown in the study, a FISP-MRF dictionary with 1500 time points can be compressed to only 10 singular vectors with preserved signal-to-noise ratio (SNR) as the template matching with the full-time points. With this SVD compression, the template matching process can be accelerated by a factor of 3.4–4.8 without sacrificing the SNR of the MRF method. This method can be generally applied in most of MRF applications with different pulse sequence designs and tissue property mapping.

Since the invention of MRF, many studies have been conducted to improve its acquisition speed and/or post-processing speed. Readers who are interested in advanced image reconstruction methods for MRF could refer to recent review articles for this topic [45, 46]. In addition, machine learning has developed rapidly in the field, and multiple approaches have been developed to improve MRF from different perspectives. While this is out of the scope of this chapter, readers could refer to this review article by Hamilton et al. for more discussion [47].

Clinical Applications

The quantitative tissue properties obtained using MRF could be applied to various kidney diseases. In this section, we will discuss its potential applications in polycystic kidney disease, kidney cancer, chronic kidney disease, kidney transplant, and sickle cell disease.

Polycystic Kidney Disease (PKD)

Polycystic kidney disease (PKD) is an inherited disorder where renal cysts develop and progressively enlarge over time leading to increased kidney volume and eventually reduced kidney function. There are two common types of PKD: Autosomal Dominant PKD (ADPKD) and Autosomal Recessive PKD (ARPKD). Patients with ADPKD develop distinct renal cysts that progress relatively slowly over a patient's lifetime. In a mouse model with juvenile cystic kidney, kidney T_2 values were found to be highly sensitive to early cystogenesis, yielding better performance in detecting kidney cysts than

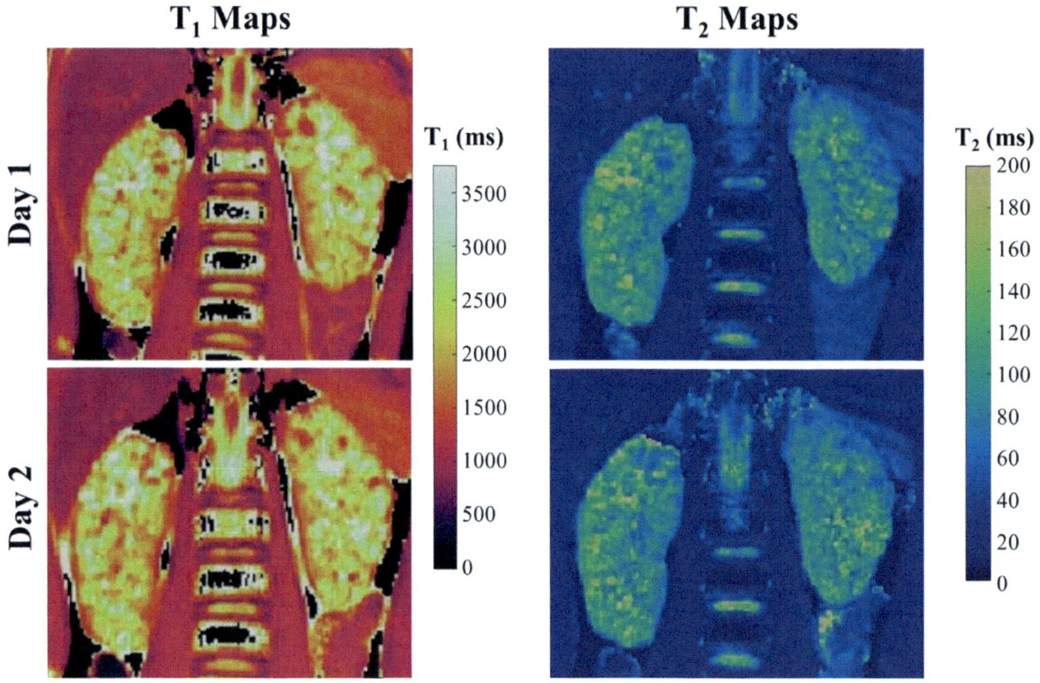

Fig. 12.9 Representative kidney T_1 and T_2 maps of a 13-year-old male patient with ARPKD scanned on successive days. Corticomedullary cysts with high T_1 and T_2 values are clearly visible throughout the kidneys

anatomical-based imaging parameters such as total kidney volume [48]. In another quantitative MRI study, significantly increased renal T_2* was observed in the kidneys of ten ADPKD patients in comparison to age- and gender-matched control subjects (14.9 ± 1.7 vs. $18.1 \pm 1.6\ s^{-1}$, $p < 0.05$), suggesting the potential for detecting and monitoring ADPKD with non-invasive quantitative MRI techniques [5].

ARPKD is another form of PKD that rapidly progresses in children. Even with modern neonatal care, only 70% of ARPKD patients survive beyond the newborn period, and only 80% of those who survive through the neonatal period live beyond 10 years of age [49, 50]. Several novel therapies have shown promise in both ARPKD animal models and adult ADPKD patients. Unfortunately, the major roadblock for implementing clinical trials in ARPKD patients is the absence of sensitive measures of ARPKD kidney disease progression. Conventional measures of kidney disease progression, such as declines in estimated glomerular filtration rate (eGFR), are variable in ARPKD, and eGFR may remain unchanged despite ongoing kidney damage. Therefore, there is an urgent need for alternative markers to stage and monitor ARPKD kidney disease progression. Our group has previously developed an MRI assessment of renal cystic burden for the PCK rat (an ARPKD rodent model) using high resolution, conventional T_2-weighted MRI images to distinguish cystic regions from normal kidney parenchyma [51]. Our results in animal models suggest that T_2-MRI techniques can sensitively detect cystic kidney disease progression and response to therapy.

We have recently applied the B_1-insensitive kidney MRF in three pediatric patients with ARPKD and representative T_1 and T_2 maps are shown in Fig. 12.9. Note the visibly increased renal T_1 and T_2 values consistent with diffuse renal corticomedullary cysts typical of ARPKD kidney disease. Significant differences were seen between the healthy volunteers ($n = 10$) and ARPKD patient populations for both mean kidney T_1 ($P < 0.007$) and T_2 ($P < 0.04$). We further scanned the ARPKD patients on successive days as an initial evaluation of the acquisition's reproducibility in subjects with known pathophysiology. These repeat MRF scans demonstrated very consistent measurements of mean kidney T_1 and T_2 with the largest variation between successive ARPKD patient scans being 2.28% in T_1 and 2.99% T_2.

Kidney Cancer

Kidney cancer is expected to affect 76,080 new patients with 13,780 deaths in the U.S. in the year 2021 [52]. Renal cell carcinoma (RCC) is the most common type of kidney cancer and imposes significant economic burden on the healthcare system [53, 54]. The three major histologic subtypes of RCC are clear cell, papillary, and chromophobe. Clear cell RCC is the most common and aggressive subtype, accounting for 70–80% of RCC with a 5-year survival rate of only 44–69%. Over the last two decades, there has been a global increase in the incidence of RCC due to expanded use of medical imaging, including MRI, as well as improved resolution of imaging techniques. RCC often presents as an incidentally detected, incompletely characterized renal mass [55]. Many of these patients with incidental renal mass either undergo direct surgery or biopsy without further imaging evaluation as accurate histologic diagnosis using modern imaging techniques is not always possible. However, upfront surgery or biopsy is not ideal as nearly 25% incidental renal masses are either benign or low-grade tumors requiring only conservative management with active monitoring. Therefore, accurate characterization of renal masses, especially at the time of diagnosis, has the potential to prevent unnecessary surgery/complications and reduce psychosocial stress and financial toxicity [56].

There is ongoing research to find novel MR imaging biomarkers that are quantitative and reproducible. T_1 and T_2 relaxometry is one such area of increasing interest and can determine quantitative biologic properties in vivo. Use of quantitative T_1, T_2, and T_2* mapping in clear cell RCC has been recently attempted with some success [57–60]. A study with 30 clear cell RCC patients showed significantly lower native T_1 values in low-grade tumors compared to high-grade tumors, resulting in 100% sensitivity, 85% specificity, and 90% accuracy [58]. These changes are likely related to the nucleolar differences between low- and high-grade RCC and are highly correlated with histological collagen volume fraction. This is significant as studies have shown that in RCC upregulation of extracellular matrix proteins like collagen is associated with higher-grade tumors, development of metastases, and overall poor prognosis. In another study, balanced steady-state free precession T_2 mapping sequence showed significant difference between low-grade and high-grade clear cell RCC in 27 patients, with higher T_2 values in low-grade tumors ($T_2 \geq 110$ ms, 83% and 89% sensitivity and specificity, respectively). The lower T_2 values in high-grade RCC may be related to tightly packed cells and irregular tumor vasculature [57]. Similarly, significantly lower T_2* values were also reported for high-grade clear cell RCC in a study of 46 RCC patients. When combined with diffusion, it can provide high accuracy in differentiation of low- and high-grade RCC. These results were in close agreement with pathological findings [60].

We have recently applied the B_1-insensitive 2D kidney MRF in two patients with RCC, one with benign chromophobe RCC (Fig. 12.10) and the other with grade-2 clear cell RCC (Fig. 12.11). Analysis of the T_1 and T_2 maps in the two patients showed that chromophobe RCC had relatively lower T_2 values (66 ± 15 ms) compared to clear cell RCC (89 ± 41 ms). There was some degree of overlap in the T_1 values of the two tumors (1486 ± 137 ms and 1490 ± 225 ms for chromophobe and clear cell types, respectively).

Chronic Kidney Disease

Chronic kidney disease (CKD) is a major health burden approximately affecting 37 million people in the US [61, 62]. It is associated with diabetes, hypertension, and heart disease and is predicted to increase by 5–8% per year [63]. Advanced quantitative MR imaging techniques

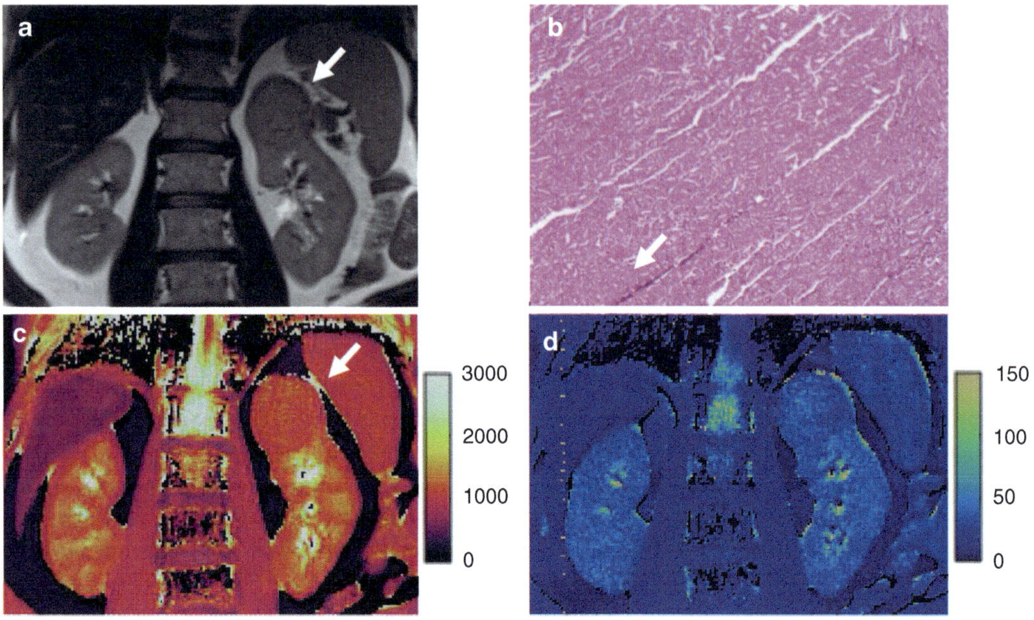

Fig. 12.10 52-year-old man with chromophobe RCC. (**a**) T_2-weighted image shows homogeneously hypointense mass in the upper pole of left kidney. (**b**) Histopathology of the mass shows homogenous sheets of cells with no areas of necrosis. (**c**, **d**) T_1 and T_2 maps obtained with B_1-insensitive kidney MRF and average T_1 and T_2 for the lesion was 1486 ± 137 ms and 66 ± 15 ms, respectively

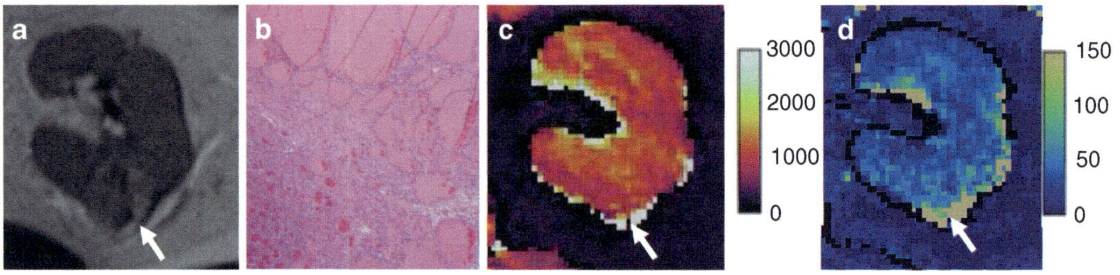

Fig. 12.11 50-year-old man with grade-2 clear cell RCC. (**a**) T2-weighted image shows heterogeneous mass in the left kidney. (**b**) Histopathology of the mass shows intratumoral heterogeneity with few blood vessels (arrowhead). (**c**, **d**) T_1 and T_2 maps obtained with B_1-insensitive kidney MRF and average T_1 and T_2 for the lesion was 1490 ± 225 ms and 89 ± 41 ms, respectively. There was significant difference in standard deviation from slice to slice indicating the intra-tumoral heterogeneity

without the need of gadolinium contrast agents hold great promise in providing non-invasive assessment of kidney structure and function for diagnosis and monitoring of CKD. With a murine CKD model, Schley et al. showed that there were significant differences between the control and diseased kidneys in T_2, T_2*, apparent diffusion coefficient (ADC), and fractional anisotropy in the renal cortex and outer medulla [64]. Among these quantitative measures, T_2 relaxation time presented as the best parameter to distinguish between the two groups. In addition, it correlates well with multiple histological features of CKD, such as the extent of fibrosis, inflammatory infiltrates, and tubular dilation. In another study with 22 CKD patients with matched healthy volunteers, multi-parametric MRI including T_1, ADC, renal artery blood flow, and cortical perfusion shows a good correlation with renal function and pathology [1]. Both studies indicate that multiparametric MR imaging provides complementary information in the assessment of renal function and structure for CKD patients. MRF measurements with T_1, T_2, T_2*, and potentially more quantitative metrics could play a critical role in diagnosing and monitoring the progression of CKD in the future.

Kidney Transplant

Quantitative MR imaging has also been applied to assess function of transplanted and native kidneys. For example, Huang et al. measured T_1 relaxation time from 27 subjects, including 12 with native kidneys and 15 with transplanted kidneys. The T_1 map was acquired using inversion-recovery single-shot fast spin echo sequences [7]. About 7–8 images with the inversion time ranging from 50 to 3500 ms were acquired, each with a separate breath-hold. The results show higher cortical and medulla T_1 in transplanted kidneys versus native kidneys (renal cortex, 1183 ± 136 vs. 1057 ± 94 ms, $P = 0.01$; renal medulla, 1573 ± 132 vs. 1389 ± 48 ms, $P = 0.0001$). Additionally, a correlation between renal T_1 and eGFR was noticed, and subjects with an eGFR less than 60 mL/min/1.73 m^2 showed higher renal T_1 than subjects with an eGFR higher than 60 mL/min/1.73 m^2. Currently, no studies have been reported about MRF applications in kidney transplant. Future studies could attempt to assess the outcome of kidney transplant by simultaneously measuring multiple tissue properties for functional evaluation of kidney tissues.

Sickle Cell Disease

Sickle cell disease (SCD) is an inherited blood disorder affecting nearly 100,000 Americans and millions of people worldwide. An important complication of SCD is CKD, which occurs in approximately one third of SCD patients and contributes to significant morbidity and mortality [65–67]. Like many other forms of CKD, once overt renal impairment is established in SCD, it is not reversible. Multiple factors have been implicated in the pathogenesis of CKD in SCD including focal renal ischemia from "sickling," intravascular hemolysis leading to endothelial activation, renal iron deposition (hemosiderosis), and glomerular "hyperfiltration" [68, 69]. However, current clinical assessments of renal function, such as eGFR and urine albumin excretion, are relatively insensitive to focal renal damage associated with early-stage kidney disease in SCD, a time point when therapies are likely to be most effective [66, 70, 71]. Prior quantitative MRI studies using T_2 relaxation time have shown that renal iron load is associated with the severity of hemolysis for SCD patients [68, 72]. The recent diffusion MRI data also suggests that medullary microstructure is altered in SCD patients in comparison to non-SCD control subjects [73]. Therefore, novel MRF techniques that can provide accurate T_2 and diffusion quantification hold great potential to offer sensitive imaging biomarkers to assess early-stage kidney disease in SCD patients.

To summarize, while multiple MRF methods for quantitative kidney imaging have been developed recently, their usage in clinical applications for various kidney diseases remains to be evaluated. Further technical development in kidney MRF to improve acquisition speed, spatial resolution / coverage, and patient comfort is needed. Its performance—including accuracy, precision, repeatability, and reproducibility—needs to be systematically evaluated in both healthy subjects and patients with different pathologies. All of these developments and their evaluation will directly influence the clinical validation and future adoption in routine clinical applications.

References

1. Buchanan CE, Mahmoud H, Cox EF, McCulloch T, Prestwich BL, Taal MW, Selby NM, Francis ST. Quantitative assessment of renal structural and functional changes in chronic kidney disease using multi-parametric magnetic resonance imaging. Nephrol Dial Transplant. 2020;35:955–64.
2. Caroli A, Pruijm M, Burnier M, Selby NM. Functional magnetic resonance imaging of the kidneys: where do we stand? The perspective of the European COST Action PARENCHIMA. Nephrol Dial Transplant. 2018;33:3–5.

3. Cox EF, Buchanan CE, Bradley CR, Prestwich B, Mahmoud H, Taal M, Selby NM, Francis ST. Multiparametric renal magnetic resonance imaging: validation, interventions, and alterations in chronic kidney disease. Front Physiol. 2017;8: 1–15.
4. Dekkers IA, de Boer A, Sharma K, et al. Consensus-based technical recommendations for clinical translation of renal T1 and T2 mapping MRI. Magn Reson Mater Phys Biol Med. 2020;33:163–76.
5. Kline TL, Edwards ME, Garg I, Irazabal MV, Korfiatis P, Harris PC, King BF, Torres VE, Venkatesh SK, Erickson BJ. Quantitative MRI of kidneys in renal disease. Abdom Radiol (NY). 2018;43:629–38.
6. Ramamurthy NK, Moosavi B, McInnes MDF, Flood TA, Schieda N. Multiparametric MRI of solid renal masses: pearls and pitfalls. Clin Radiol. 2015;70:304–16.
7. Huang Y, Sadowski EA, Artz NS, Seo S, Djamali A, Grist TM, Fain SB. Measurement and comparison of T1 relaxation times in native and transplanted kidney cortex and medulla. J Magn Reson Imaging. 2011;33:1241–7.
8. MacAskill CJ, Erokwu BO, Markley M, et al. Multiparametric MRI of kidney disease progression for autosomal recessive polycystic kidney disease: mouse model and initial patient results. Pediatr Res. 2021;89:157–62.
9. Wolf M, de Boer A, Sharma K, Boor P, Leiner T, Sunder-Plassmann G, Moser E, Caroli A, Jerome NP. Magnetic resonance imaging T1- and T2-mapping to assess renal structure and function: a systematic review and statement paper. Nephrol Dial Transplant. 2018;33:ii41–50.
10. Jamin Y, Tucker ER, Poon E, et al. Evaluation of clinically translatable MR imaging biomarkers of therapeutic response in the TH-MYCN transgenic mouse model of neuroblastoma. Radiology. 2013;266:130–40.
11. Weidensteiner C, Allegrini PR, Sticker-Jantscheff M, Romanet V, Ferretti S, McSheehy PM. Tumour T1 changes in vivo are highly predictive of response to chemotherapy and reflect the number of viable tumour cells—a preclinical MR study in mice. BMC Cancer. 2014;14:88.
12. Nery F, Buchanan CE, Harteveld AA, et al. Consensus-based technical recommendations for clinical translation of renal ASL MRI. Magn Reson Mater Phys Biol Med. 2020;33:141–61.
13. Chen Y, Panda A, Pahwa S, et al. 3D magnetic resonance fingerprinting for quantitative breast imaging. Radiology. 2019;290:33–40.
14. Hamilton JI, Jiang Y, Chen Y, Ma D, Lo WC, Griswold M, Seiberlich N. MR fingerprinting for rapid quantification of myocardial T1, T2, and proton spin density. Magn Reson Med. 2017;77:1446–58.
15. Jiang Y, Ma D, Seiberlich N, Gulani V, Griswold MA. MR fingerprinting using fast imaging with steady state precession (FISP) with spiral readout. Magn Reson Med. 2015;74:1621–31.
16. Ma D, Gulani V, Seiberlich N, Liu K, Sunshine JL, Duerk JL, Griswold MA. Magnetic resonance fingerprinting. Nature. 2013;495:187–92.
17. Ma D, Jiang Y, Chen Y, McGivney D, Mehta B, Gulani V, Griswold M. Fast 3D magnetic resonance fingerprinting for a whole-brain coverage. Magn Reson Med. 2018;79:2190–7.
18. Yu AC, Ponsky LE, Dastmalchian S, Rogers M, McGivney D, Griswold MA. Development of a combined MR fingerprinting and diffusion examination for prostate. Radiology. 2017;283:729–38.
19. Meiboom S, Gill D. Modified spin-echo method for measuring nuclear relaxation times. Rev Sci Instrum. 1958;29:688.
20. Crawley AP, Henkelman RM. A comparison of one-shot and recovery methods in T1 imaging. Magn Reson Med. 1988;7:23–34.
21. Peperhove M, Vo Chieu VD, Jang MS, et al. Assessment of acute kidney injury with T1 mapping MRI following solid organ transplantation. Eur Radiol. 2018;28:44–50.
22. Körzdörfer G, Jiang Y, Speier P, Pang J, Ma D, Pfeuffer J, Hensel B, Gulani V, Griswold M, Nittka M. Magnetic resonance field fingerprinting. Magn Reson Med. 2019;81:2347–59.
23. Wang CY, Coppo S, Mehta BB, Seiberlich N, Yu X, Griswold MA. Magnetic resonance fingerprinting with quadratic RF phase for measurement of T2* simultaneously with δf, T1, and T2. Magn Reson Med. 2018;81:1849–62.
24. Chen Y, Jiang Y, Pahwa S, Ma D, Lu L, Twieg MD, Wright KL, Seiberlich N, Griswold MA, Gulani V. MR fingerprinting for rapid quantitative abdominal imaging. Radiology. 2016;279:278–86.
25. Cloos MA, Assländer J, Abbas B, Fishbaugh J, Babb JS, Gerig G, Lattanzi R. Rapid radial T1 and T2 mapping of the hip articular cartilage with magnetic resonance fingerprinting. J Magn Reson Imaging. 2019;50:810–5.
26. Sacolick LI, Wiesinger F, Hancu I, Vogel MW. B1 mapping by Bloch-Siegert shift. Magn Reson Med. 2010;63:1315–22.
27. Schmitt P, Griswold MA, Gulani V, Haase A, Flentje M, Jakob PM. A simple geometrical description of the TrueFISP ideal transient and steady-state signal. Magn Reson Med. 2006;55:177–86.
28. de Bazelaire CMJ, Duhamel GD, Rofsky NM, Alsop DC. MR imaging relaxation times of abdominal and pelvic tissues measured in vivo at 3.0 T: preliminary results. Radiology. 2004;230:652–9.
29. Hermann I, Chacon-Caldera J, Brumer I, Rieger B, Weingärtner S, Schad LR, Zöllner FG. Magnetic resonance fingerprinting for simultaneous renal T1 and T2* mapping in a single breath-hold. Magn Reson Med. 2020;83:1940–8.
30. Milani B, Ansaloni A, Sousa-Guimaraes S, Vakilzadeh N, Piskunowicz M, Vogt B, Stuber M, Burnier M, Pruijm M. Reduction of cortical oxygenation in chronic kidney disease: evidence obtained with a new analysis method of blood oxygenation level-

dependent magnetic resonance imaging. Nephrol Dial Transplant. 2017;32:2097–105.
31. Pruijm M, Mendichovszky IA, Liss P, Van der Niepen P, Textor SC, Lerman LO, Krediet CTP, Caroli A, Burnier M, Prasad PV. Renal blood oxygenation level-dependent magnetic resonance imaging to measure renal tissue oxygenation: a statement paper and systematic review. Nephrol Dial Transplant. 2018;33:ii22–8.
32. MacAskill CJ, Markley M, Farr S, et al. Rapid B1-insensitive MR fingerprinting for quantitative renal imaging. Radiology. 2021;300:380–7.
33. Weidlich D, Schlaeger S, Kooijman H, Börnert P, Kirschke JS, Rummeny EJ, Haase A, Karampinos DC. T2 mapping with magnetization-prepared 3D TSE based on a modified BIR-4 T2 preparation. NMR Biomed. 2017:e3773.
34. Coolen BF, Simonis FFJ, Geelen T, Moonen RPM, Arslan F, Paulis LEM, Nicolay K, Strijkers GJ. Quantitative T2 mapping of the mouse heart by segmented MLEV phase-cycled T2 preparation. Magn Reson Med. 2014;72:409–17.
35. Dekkers IA, Paiman EHM, de Vries APJ, Lamb HJ. Reproducibility of native T1 mapping for renal tissue characterization at 3T. J Magn Reson Imaging. 2019;49:588–96.
36. Huang S, Boyacioglu R, Bolding R, Chen Y, Griswold MA. Free-breathing abdominal magnetic resonance fingerprinting using a pilot tone navigator. J Magn Reson Imaging. 2021;54:1138–51.
37. Schroeder L. Two-dimensional respiratory-motion characterization for continuous MR measurements using pilot tone navigation. Int Soc Magn Reson Med. 2016;310.
38. Speier S. PT-Nav: a novel respiratory navigation method for continuous acquisition based on modulation of a pilot tone in the MR-receiver. ESMRMB. 2015;129:97–8.
39. Solomon E, Rigie DS, Vahle T, Paška J, Bollenbeck J, Sodickson DK, Boada FE, Block KT, Chandarana H. Free-breathing radial imaging using a pilot-tone radiofrequency transmitter for detection of respiratory motion. Magn Reson Med. 2021;85:2672–85.
40. Vahle T, Bacher M, Rigie D, Fenchel M, Speier P, Bollenbeck J, Schäfers KP, Kiefer B, Boada FE. Respiratory motion detection and correction for MR using the pilot tone: applications for MR and simultaneous PET/MR examinations. Invest Radiol. 2020;55:153–9.
41. Ludwig J, Speier P, Seifert F, Schaeffter T, Kolbitsch C. Pilot tone–based motion correction for prospective respiratory compensated cardiac cine MRI. Magn Reson Med. 2021;85:2403–16.
42. Hennig J. Echoes—how to generate, recognize, use or avoid them in MR-imaging sequences. Part I: fundamental and not so fundamental properties of spin echoes. Concepts Magn Reson. 1991;3:125–43.
43. Hennig J. Multiecho imaging sequences with low refocusing flip angles. J Magn Reson. 1988;78:397–407.
44. McGivney D, Pierre E, Ma D, Jiang Y, Saybasili H, Gulani V, Griswold M. SVD compression for magnetic resonance fingerprinting in the time domain. IEEE Trans Med Imaging. 2014;33:2311–22.
45. McGivney DF, Boyacıoğlu R, Jiang Y, Poorman ME, Seiberlich N, Gulani V, Keenan KE, Griswold MA, Ma D. Magnetic resonance fingerprinting review part 2: technique and directions. J Magn Reson Imaging. 2019;51:993–1007.
46. Poorman ME, Martin MN, Ma D, McGivney DF, Gulani V, Griswold MA, Keenan KE. Magnetic resonance fingerprinting part 1: potential uses, current challenges, and recommendations. J Magn Reson Imaging. 2020;51:675–92.
47. Hamilton JI, Seiberlich N. Machine learning for rapid magnetic resonance fingerprinting tissue property quantification. Proc IEEE. 2020;108:69–85.
48. Franke M, Baeßler B, Vechtel J, et al. Magnetic resonance T2 mapping and diffusion-weighted imaging for early detection of cystogenesis and response to therapy in a mouse model of polycystic kidney disease. Kidney Int. 2017;92:1544–54.
49. Zerres K, Rudnik-Schöneborn S, Deget F, et al. Autosomal recessive polycystic kidney disease in 115 children: clinical presentation, course and influence of gender. Acta Paediatr. 1996;85:437–45.
50. Roy S, Dillon MJ, Trompeter RS, Barratt TM. Autosomal recessive polycystic kidney disease: long-term outcome of neonatal survivors. Pediatr Nephrol. 1997;11:302–6.
51. Erokwu BO, Anderson CE, Flask CA, Dell KM. Quantitative magnetic resonance imaging assessments of autosomal recessive polycystic kidney disease progression and response to therapy in an animal model. Pediatr Res. 2018;83:1067–74.
52. Siegel RL, Miller KD, Fuchs HE, Jemal A. Cancer statistics, 2021. CA Cancer J Clin. 2021;71:7–33.
53. Shih YT, Xu Y, Chien C, Kim B, Shen Y, Li L, Geynisman DM. Rising economic burden of renal cell carcinoma among elderly patients in the United States: part II—an updated analysis of SEER-Medicare data. Pharmacoeconomics. 2019;37:1495–507.
54. Chien C-R, Geynisman DM, Kim B, Xu Y, Shin Y-CT. Economic burden of renal cell carcinoma—part I: an updated review. Pharmacoeconomics. 2019;37:301–31.
55. Silverman SG, Israel GM, Trinh Q-D. Incompletely characterized incidental renal masses: emerging data support conservative management. Radiology. 2015;275:28–42.
56. Sebastià C, Corominas D, Musquera M, Paño B, Ajami T, Nicolau C. Active surveillance of small renal masses. Insights Imaging. 2020;11:63.
57. Adams LC, Bressem KK, Jurmeister P, Fahlenkamp UL, Ralla B, Engel G, Hamm B, Busch J, Makowski MR. Use of quantitative T2 mapping for the assessment of renal cell carcinomas: first results. Cancer Imaging. 2019;19:1–11.
58. Adams LC, Ralla B, Jurmeister P, Bressem KK, Fahlenkamp UL, Hamm B, Busch J, Makowski

MR. Native T1 mapping as an in vivo biomarker for the identification of higher-grade renal cell carcinoma: correlation with histopathological findings. Invest Radiol. 2019;54:118–28.
59. Zhang Y, Udayakumar D, Cai L, et al. Addressing metabolic heterogeneity in clear cell renal cell carcinoma with quantitative Dixon MRI. JCI Insight. 2017;2:e94278.
60. Zhang YD, Wu CJ, Wang Q, Zhang J, Wang XN, Liu XS, Shi HB. Comparison of utility of histogram apparent diffusion coefficient and R2* for differentiation of low-grade from high-grade clear cell renal cell carcinoma. Am J Roentgenol. 2015;205:W193–201.
61. Hill NR, Fatoba ST, Oke JL, Hirst JA, O'Callaghan CA, Lasserson DS, Hobbs FDR. Global prevalence of chronic kidney disease—a systematic review and meta-analysis. PLoS One. 2016;11:e0158765.
62. Eknoyan G, Lameire N, Barsoum R, et al. The burden of kidney disease: improving global outcomes. Kidney Int. 2004;66:1310.
63. Hamer RA, El Nahas AM. The burden of chronic kidney disease. Br Med J. 2006;332:563.
64. Schley G, Jordan J, Ellmann S, Rosen S, Eckardt KU, Uder M, Willam C, Bäuerle T. Multiparametric magnetic resonance imaging of experimental chronic kidney disease: a quantitative correlation study with histology. PLoS One. 2018;13:1–18.
65. Nath KA, Katusic ZS. Vasculature and kidney complications in sickle cell disease. J Am Soc Nephrol. 2012;23:781–4.
66. Guasch A, Navarrete J, Nass K, Zayas CF. Glomerular involvement in adults with sickle cell hemoglobinopathies: prevalence and clinical correlates of progressive renal failure. J Am Soc Nephrol. 2006;17:2228–35.
67. Becker AM. Sickle cell nephropathy: challenging the conventional wisdom. Pediatr Nephrol. 2011;26:2099–109.
68. Vasavda N, Gutiérrez L, House MJ, Drašar E, St Pierre TG, Thein SL. Renal iron load in sickle cell disease is influenced by severity of haemolysis. Br J Haematol. 2012;157:599–605.
69. Davenport A, Buscombe J. Sickle cell kidney. J Nephrol. 2008;21:253–5.
70. Aygun B, Mortier NA, Smeltzer MP, Hankins JS, Ware RE. Glomerular hyperfiltration and albuminuria in children with sickle cell anemia. Pediatr Nephrol. 2011;26:1285–90.
71. Ware HM, Kwiatkowski JL. Evaluation and treatment of transfusional iron overload in children. Pediatr Clin North Am. 2013;60:1393–406.
72. Schein A, Enriquez C, Coates TD, Wood JC. Magnetic resonance detection of kidney iron deposition in sickle cell disease: a marker of chronic hemolysis. J Magn Reson Imaging. 2008;28:698–704.
73. Donnola SB, Piccone CM, Lu L, Batesole J, Little J, Dell KM, Flask CA. Diffusion tensor imaging MRI of sickle cell kidney disease: initial results and comparison with iron deposition. NMR Biomed. 2018;31:1–8.

Magnetization Transfer Imaging 13

Behzad Ebrahimi, Kai Jiang, and Lilach Lerman

Introduction

Magnetic resonance imaging (MRI) is a powerful and versatile imaging modality. It has found many applications in diagnosis and assessment of treatments, due to its ability to acquire images with high temporal and spatial resolution and to provide detailed morphological and functional information, owing to its high contrast in soft tissue. Currently, T1- and T2-weighted sequences (or their derivatives) are commonly used in clinical practice. Many functional MR techniques are also emerging, and we may expect to see them used in the future as standard of care.

Magnetization transfer (MT) MR has been known to the nuclear magnetic resonance (NMR) community for a long time. In fact, early applications of this technique in spectroscopy emerged in the early decades of NMR development. It is worth mentioning the contribution of Adriaan Bax to MT during his work at the National Institute of Diabetes and Digestive and Kidney Diseases in the 1980s [1, 2]. One of the early attempts for implementing quantitative MT by Wolf and Balaban was performed on a mouse kidney and allowed calculation of water exchange between various pools, as will be discussed in detail [3].

Recently, MT MRI has attracted a new wave of interest because of its ability to detect renal fibrosis. New studies have shown promise in using MT in a quantitative framework, which is believed to be more robust in terms of sensitivity to MR parameters and micro-environmental variations. In this chapter, we will briefly discuss the physics of MT, review the mathematical framework, and summarize some of the recent preclinical and clinical studies.

MRI Physics and Acquisition Protocols

MRI Physics

In MR images of biological tissues, water protons are the main source of the signal. Most of these water molecules are unrestricted, meaning that they are free to diffuse and rotate. When small molecules such as water are capable of rotating fast, their impact on the relaxation of surrounding water molecules would be very small. Therefore,

B. Ebrahimi
Department of Radiation and Cellular Oncology, University of Chicago, Chicago, IL, USA
e-mail: behzad.ebrahimi@bsd.uchicago.edu

K. Jiang
Department of Radiation Oncology, University of Maryland School of Medicine, Baltimore, MD, USA
e-mail: KJiang@som.umaryland.edu

L. Lerman (✉)
Division of Nephrology and Hypertension, Mayo Clinic, Rochester, MN, USA
e-mail: Lerman.Lilach@mayo.edu

S. D. Serai, K. Darge (eds.), *Advanced Clinical MRI of the Kidney*,
https://doi.org/10.1007/978-3-031-40169-5_13

a pool of unrestricted water protons has relatively long T1 and T2. This is commonly referred to as a "free water pool," and generally offers the largest contribution to the MR signal. Water protons can also be bound to macromolecules, including proteins, in which case they are referred to as a "bound pool" or "restricted pool" (Fig. 13.1). Such protons would not be able to diffuse or rotate easily (i.e., protons in hydrating water) and typically have very short T2 values. Signals with such short T2 might not be detectable with conventional MRI sequences, making the restricted pool invisible. Some studies have also considered protons from water molecules with loose connection to macromolecules as a third population, which behaves between the free and the restricted protons with T2 values shorter than those in the free pool. In this chapter, we will focus our discussion on two-pool (free-bound) models.

Similar rules regarding the relationship between the mobility and relaxation time apply to macromolecules in tissues as well. However, what limits the motion and rotation are the massive size and links of the macromolecules. Large intracellular proteins and extracellular connective tissues such as collagen are examples of highly restricted macromolecules. Protons on these larger macromolecules typically have very short T2 values, which make them invisible on conventional MR pulse sequences. In contrast, solute protons, which are small enough to rotate within cells, generally have only moderately short T2 values. Such molecules contribute to the MR signal, but they constitute only a small fraction of the total proton pool, and consequently, their contribution to MR signal is very small compared to those of the free water pool. However, using chemical exchange saturation

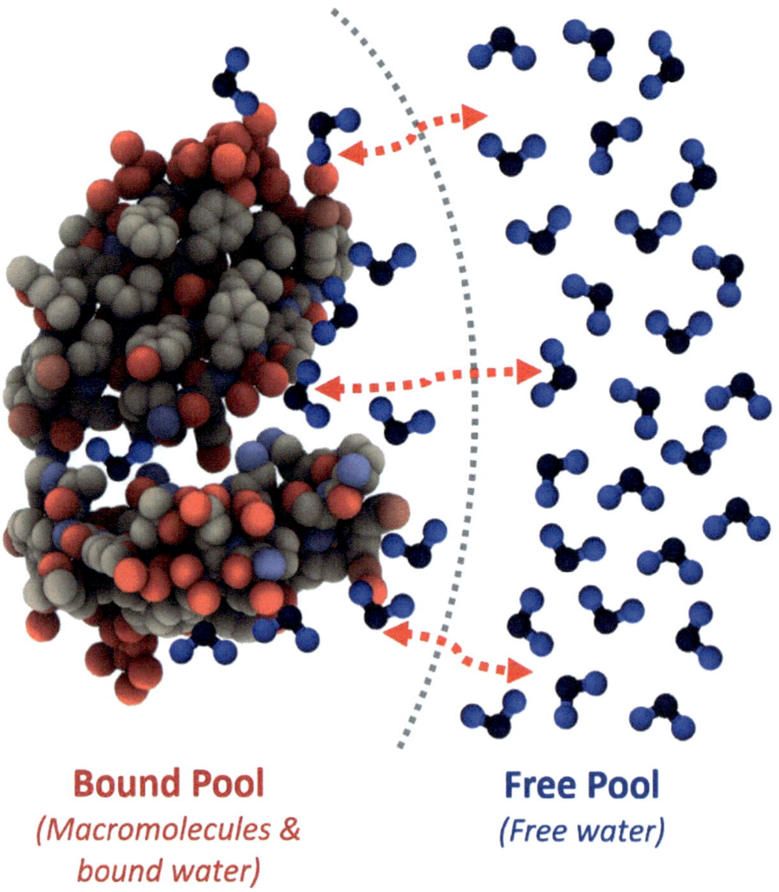

Fig. 13.1 The two water/proton populations in tissues. The "free pool" is composed of free water molecules able to diffuse and freely rotate. The "bound pool" contains protons from macromolecules (such as proteins, lipids, etc.), and the hydrating water molecules bound to macromolecules

transfer (CEST) imaging, valuable functional and metabolic information can be acquired from the MR signal of these solute protons. Interested readers are referred to Chap. 20 of this book titled "Chemical Exchange Saturation Transfer (CEST) MRI for Monitoring Kidney Diseases."

Temporary binding (such as what occurs in hydration) and proton exchange couple the magnetization characteristics of the two pools mentioned above. Macromolecules and water may exchange protons, which means that there might be protons in the free pool that at an earlier stage had been restricted to a macromolecule. Such protons keep some of their spin characteristics for a short time before they relax. Therefore, when the rate of proton exchange is sufficiently fast, exchange allows an accumulation of a great number of such protons in the free pool to be detectable with MR before they lose their initial spin characteristics and adopt those of the free pool. This provides an indirect way to detect the bound pool and study its characteristics. A simple approach to make this MR effect visible uses a radiofrequency (RF) pulse to saturate spins in restricted protons. When protons with saturated spin are exchanged with protons in the free pool with none-zero net magnetization, the signal from the free pool declines. Change in the MR signal provides an indirect way to acquire information from the macromolecules. In other words, MT has the ability to gauge the dynamic relationship between two (or more) nuclei populations. If the exchange is fast enough, such a change in the signal can be detected by subtracting the two images, one acquired with the RF signal and one without it. MT ratio (MTR), a commonly used quantitative marker of MT magnitude, is defined as [4]:

$$\text{MTR} = \frac{S_0 - S_{\text{MT}}}{S_0} \tag{13.1}$$

Clearly, in the absence of MT ($S_0 = S_{\text{MT}}$), this ratio would be equal to zero. For MTR to be equal to one requires an unlikely event, in which the entire free pool participates in the exchange process within a very short time.

MT is a powerful mechanism to create target-specific contrast in MR images (Fig. 13.2). The ability to target the offset frequency at different regions in the NMR spectrum, corresponding to different macromolecules, makes MT a versatile technique. It has been used in many anatomic sites where other contrast mechanisms (T1-weighted, T2-weighted, etc.) might not generate sufficient differentiation [5]. Importantly, compared to other MR techniques such as MR elastography and diffusion-weighted imaging, MT imaging (MTI) has been shown to be less confounded by altered renal hemodynamics and may provide a more reliable tool for fibrosis measurement [6]. However, the feasibility of using MT for any study is not given and requires meeting specific conditions. First, there must be the existence of an offset frequency that allows the targeting of macromolecules of interest with sufficient specificity. In other words, the area with high absorption efficiency in the macromolecules of interest should not overlap with those in any other major molecules. Second, sufficiently fast magnetization exchange between the free and the bound pools should exist so that enough molecules accumulate in order to demonstrate a detectable decline in the signal from the free pool.

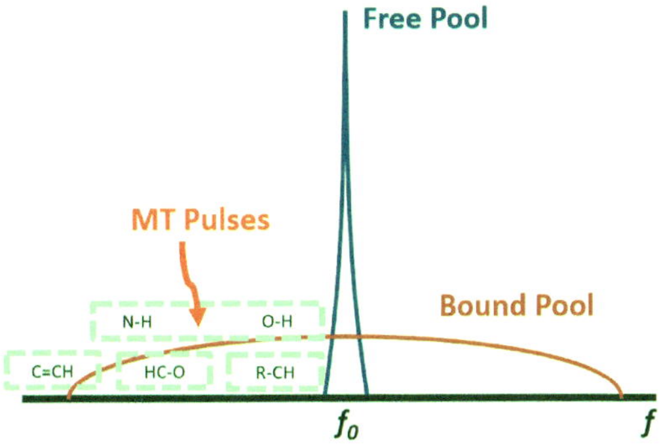

Fig. 13.2 A schematic spectrum of macromolecules and of water protons. The free pool has a narrow bandwidth in the frequency domain, whereas the bound pool has a much broader range. The bound pool is invisible in MRI because of its extremely short T2, and MRI can only detect signal from the free pool. Nevertheless, the bound pool can be indirectly assessed, as it constantly exchanges magnetization with the free pool through cross relaxation and chemical exchange. If the magnetization of the bound pool is saturated at a certain off-resonance frequency away from the Larmor frequency f_0, the measured MR signal from the free pool will also drop because of the magnetization transfer between these two pools

Calculation of MTR is simple and straightforward. However, MTR is not a fully reliable parameter as it may be affected by imaging and tissue NMR characteristics. MT in the two-pool framework could be sensitive to biological changes, such as edema and inflammation, and a complex combination of sequence details and relaxation parameters [7]. This issue becomes more important when MTR is used as a surrogate marker for the fraction of the molecules of interest or the bound pool. Therefore, a quantitative approach is needed to extract fundamental MT parameters. Quantitative MT (qMT) has been proposed to address this issue. The qMT formulation allows identifying and removing the contribution of the factor mentioned above and quantifying the true restricted pool fraction. However, developing such a framework is not straightforward. The model needs to be simple enough to be useful in clinical settings but still sufficiently comprehensive to include the complex biological behavior and pulse sequence characteristics. Moreover, to calculate the unknown parameters in the model, MR imaging-based experiments need to be designed so that they can be implemented in clinical studies [7]. In the following sections, we will discuss the widely applied formulation presented by Henkelman et al. and later expanded by Ramani et al., and review parameter estimations [7, 8].

Off-Resonance MT

To begin, we will use the letters "*A*" and "*B*" to represent the free spin and the restricted spin pools. In tissues, the number of spins in pool *A* is considerably larger than those in pool B. The initial magnetization in either of these two pools is shown by M_{0A} and M_{0B}. Applying an RF pulse at an off-resonance frequency in the absorption domain of the pool *B* will result in significant spin saturation in this pool and a partial direct saturation in the pool *A*. Unfortunately, the direct saturation always exists, but there are methods to account for that in quantitative MT applications. This system can be characterized by three rates, R_A, R_B, and *R*, which represent longitudinal relaxation in pools *A* and *B*, and exchange rate constant between the two pools, respectively (Fig. 13.3). The evolution of magnetization over time can be expressed by Bloch equation [8]:

$$\frac{dM_{zA}}{dt} = R_A\left(M_{0A} - M_{zA}\right) - RM_{0B}M_{zA} + RM_{0A}M_{zB} + \omega_1 M_{yA} \tag{13.2}$$

$$\frac{dM_{zB}}{dt} = R_B\left(M_{0B} - M_{zB}\right) - RM_{0A}M_{zB} + RM_{0B}M_{zA} + \omega_1 M_{yB} \tag{13.3}$$

$$\frac{dM_{xi}}{dt} = -\frac{M_{xi}}{T_{2i}} - 2\pi\Delta M_{yi} \tag{13.4}$$

$$\frac{dM_{yi}}{dt} = -\frac{M_{yi}}{T_{2i}} + 2\pi\Delta M_{xi} - \omega_1 M_{zi} \tag{13.5}$$

where in Eqs. 13.4 and 13.5, *i* represents either of the pools *A* and *B*. ω_1 is the angular frequency of the precision by saturating RF pulse, and Δ is the offset frequency. Solving for M_{zA} gives:

$$M_{zA} = \frac{R_B RM_{0B} + R_{rfB}R_B + R_B R_A + R_A R}{\left(R_A + R_{rfA} + RM_{0B}\right)\left(R_B + R_{rfB} + R\right) - RRM_{0B}} \tag{13.6}$$

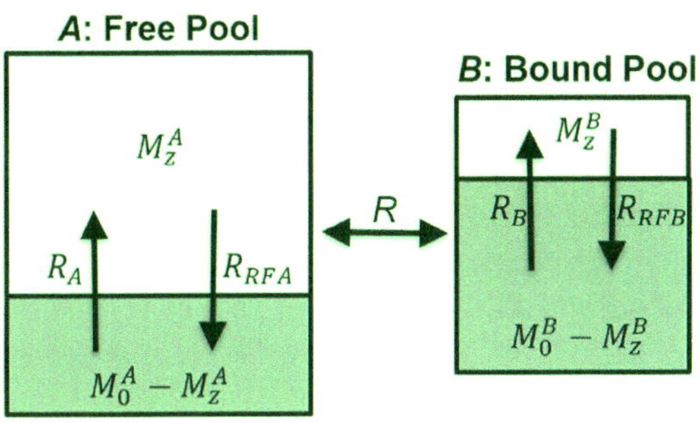

Fig. 13.3 A two-pool model to delineate the magnetization transfer between the free and bond pools. M_0^A and M_0^B are the full magnetization of the free and bound pools, respectively; M_Z^A and M_Z^B indicate the loss of magnetization due to the magnetization saturation; R_A and R_B the longitudinal relaxation rates; R the magnetization exchange rate between the two pools; R_{RFA} *and* R_{RFB} the free and bound pool RF absorption rates dictated by a super-Lorentzian line shape. The bound pool fraction f is quantified as $M_0^B / \left(M_0^A + M_0^B\right)$

Where:

$$R_{rfA} = \frac{\omega_1^2 T_{2A}}{1+\left(2\pi\Delta T_{2A}\right)} \tag{13.7}$$

$$R_{rfB} = \frac{\omega_1^2 T_{2A}}{1+\left(2\pi\Delta T_{2B}\right)^2} \tag{13.8}$$

Equation 13.3 could be problematic because attempts to find the unknown parameters through fitting to experimental data generally does not give unique values for R_A, T_{2A}, R_B, T_{2B}, R, or M_{0B}. An alternative approach based on the assumption that $(2\pi\Delta T_{2A})^2 \gg 1$ allows us to simplify Eq. 13.6 and keep five independent parameters, R_B, T_{2B}, R, $[RM_{0B}/R_0]$, and $1/R_AT_{2A}$, which can be uniquely quantified by fitting to the experimental data:

$$M_{Az} = \frac{R_B\left(\dfrac{RM_{0B}}{R_A}\right) + R_{rfB} + R_B + R}{\left(\dfrac{RM_{0B}}{R_A}\right)\left(R_B + R_{rfB}\right) + \left(1 + \left(\dfrac{\omega_1}{2\pi\Delta}\right)^2\left(\dfrac{1}{R_AT_{2A}}\right)\right)\left(R_B + R_{rfB} + R\right)} \tag{13.9}$$

While the formulation above incorporates the key parameters of MT, it is not formulated in the most suitable format for in vivo studies. Further modifications are needed to bring Eq. 13.9 into the same framework of clinical sequences. The first step of this reformulation involves determination of an equivalent to continuous wave power (CW) for pulsed MT. Ramani et al. defined such a CW pulse as:

$$\omega_{1CWPE} = \gamma\sqrt{P_{SAT}} = \gamma B_{1CWPE} \tag{13.10}$$

where P_{SAT} is the mean square saturating field averaged over repetition time (TR) and is unknown. This parameter can be calculated if B_{SAT}, the maximum amplitude, is known or if Θ_{SAT}, the effective flip angle, is known. The relationship between these two parameters is given by:

$$P_{SAT} = p_2 B_{SAT}^2 \frac{\tau_{SAT}}{TR} \tag{13.11}$$

$$\theta_{SAT} = \frac{180}{\pi}\gamma p_1 B_{SAT}\tau_{SAT} \tag{13.12}$$

where p_2 is the ratio of the square of the mean amplitude of the saturation pulse to that of a rectangular pulse of the same height. p_1 is the ratio of the mean amplitude of the saturation pulse to that of a rectangular pulse of the same amplitude. τ_{SAT} is the duration of the pulse.

Incorporating ω_{1CWPE} and the fraction of restricted pool, f, into Eq. 13.9 gives:

$$M_{Az} = \frac{R_B\left(\dfrac{RM_{0A}f}{R_A(1-f)}\right) + R_{rfB} + R_B + R}{\left(\dfrac{RM_{0A}f}{R_A(1-f)}\right)\left(R_B + R_{rfB}\right) + \left(1 + \left(\dfrac{\omega_{CWPE}}{2\pi\Delta f}\right)^2\left(\dfrac{1}{R_AT_{2A}}\right)\right)\left(R_B + R_{rfB} + R\right)} \tag{13.13}$$

where:

$$f = \frac{M_{0B}}{M_{0B} + M_{0A}} \quad (13.14)$$

To estimate f requires knowing R_A. The relationship between this parameter and the measured R_{Aobs} can be calculated as:

$$R_A = \frac{R_{Aobs}}{\frac{\frac{RM_{A0}f}{(1-f)R_A}(R_B - R_{Aobs})}{(R_B - R_{Aobs}) + RM_{A0}}} \quad (13.15)$$

Using parameters from Eq. 13.13, R_A can be calculated. Knowing that and $f/R_A(1 - f)$ from Eq. 13.13, f can be calculated.

On-Resonance MT

An alternative approach to quantifying the restricted fraction uses an on-resonance RF pulse. The underlying assumption here is that in ideal balanced steady-state free precession (bSSFP), the restricted pool would be fully saturated. This decouples Eqs. 13.2 and 13.3. They can be rewritten as:

$$\frac{dM_{xA}}{dt} = R_{2A} M_{xA} \quad (13.16)$$

$$\frac{dM_{yA}}{dt} = -R_{2A} M_{yA} + \omega_1(t) M_{zA} \quad (13.17)$$

$$\frac{dM_{zA}}{dt} = (R_A + RM_{0B})\left(\frac{R_A}{R_A + RM_{0B}} M_{0A} - M_{zA}\right) - RM_{0B} M_{zA} + \omega_1 M_{yA} \quad (13.18)$$

This equation, with the following modifications, resembles the equation that describes bSSFP for single pool [9]:

$$R_A \to R_A + RM_{0B} \quad \text{and}\; M_{0A} \to \frac{R_A}{R_A + RM_{0B}} M_{0A} \quad (13.19)$$

Solving the differential Equations 13.16–13.18 for M_y gives a solution that in general format resembles the equation that describes the y component of magnetization in bSSFP with single pool:

$$M_y = M_{0A} \sin(\alpha) \frac{(1 - E_{1A})B + C}{A - BE_{1A}E_{2A} - (BE_{1A} - AE_{2A})\cos(\alpha)} \quad (13.20)$$

where

$$A = 1 + F - f_w E_{1B}(F + f) \quad (13.21)$$

$$B = 1 + f_k\left(F - f_w E_{1B}(F + 1)\right) \quad (13.22)$$

$$C = F(1 - E_{1B})(1 - f_k) \quad (13.23)$$

$$f_k = \exp\left(-(k_A + k_B)TR\right) \quad (13.24)$$

$$f_w = \exp\left(-\langle W(\Delta \to 0)\rangle TR\right); M_{0f} = 1 \quad (13.25)$$

$$E_{ij} = \exp\left(-R_{ij} TR\right), \quad i = 1\, or\, 2\, and\; j = A\, or\, B \quad (13.26)$$

Fitting Eq. 13.20 to the data acquired for various repetition time (TR) values and flip angles allows extraction of F, k_r, and k_f.

Acquisition Protocols

MT Protocols

Currently, no consensus exists regarding the best MT protocol for the kidney. Considering broad potential applications for MT in the kidney, developing various application-specific protocols is perhaps more feasible. In this section, we will discuss several MT MRI acquisition protocols used in previous studies, but the main focus will be on those developed for fibrosis imaging. This will also include sequences used to define regions of interest (ROI) and perform segmentation. The accuracy of quantitative MT requires post-acquisition corrections. Sequences used to obtain the information needed for such corrections (i.e., B_0 and B_1 field corrections) will also be reviewed in this section. The implementation of the parameters and post-processing will be discussed in the following sections.

In previous studies, MT scans have been carried out over a broad range of scanners, from clinical MR units with conventional fields (1.5 and 3 T) to small bore high field animal scanners. Various factors are involved in selecting MR parameters, including magnetic field strength, desired matrix size, imaging time, and available sequences and coils. In the following section, we will begin with reviewing protocols of studies performed on clinical scanners, then briefly discuss MT protocols for high field scanners.

Higher fields are generally preferred for MT imaging as they allow better signal-to-noise ratio (SNR) and enhance chemical shift dispersion, which results in higher spectral resolution. However, in kidney imaging, this may come at the cost of more artifacts due to the kidneys' vicinity to the bowel. Phased-array coils are commonly used as they permit faster imaging and SNR. Imaging can be performed under different initial magnetization conditions such as steady-state or spoiled magnetization and shorter TR, and echo time (TE) is generally beneficial. The choice of spatial resolution and slice thickness strongly depends on the type of application and target. For instance, in MT imaging, to assess fibrosis, higher spatial resolution and thinner slices may reduce the partial volume effect and enhance sensitivity. Smaller voxel size comes at the cost of lower SNR, often requiring multiple repetitions for noise reduction through image averaging. For the acquisition, various fast sequences are available; however, most commonly, gradient echo imaging is used (Fig. 13.4). A key element of MT imaging is the RF pulse used for magnetization saturation. Pulsed and continuous wave (CW) are the two modes of off-resonance RF irradiations. However, pulsed RF is the one commonly used in imaging studies due to its availability on clinical scanners. The shape of the RF pulse may have no significant impact as long as its Fourier transform has no component near the Larmor frequency of the free water pool [4].

In a human study by Ito et al., 44 patients underwent MT MR scans using a spoiled gradient echo sequence on a 3 T scanner [10]. Scans were performed using phased-array torso coils. MT images were acquired in the coronal plane, with TR = 80 ms, TE = 2.67 ms, matrix size 320 × 160, flip angle 25°, field of view (FOV) 35 × 35 cm^2, and slice thickness = 6 mm. Scans were carried out over a single breath-hold (21 s). A Gaussian-shaped MT pulse with flip angle = 500° was used for saturation at 1500 Hz offset frequency. A similar sequence with slightly longer TE (3.2 ms) was used by Kline et al. for MT imaging in patients with autosomal dominant polycystic kidney disease (ADPKD) [11].

Using a 3 T clinical scanner, we performed MT MR scans on porcine kidneys with distal to renal artery stenosis, as well as during recovery after revascularization of renal artery stenosis [12, 13]. MTR was measured using a gradient echo sequence. Images were acquired in the coronal plane with TR = 300 ms, TE = 3.4 ms in the first study and 5.3 ms in the second, flip angle = 30°, slice thickness = 4 mm, FOVs were from 15 × 15 to 35 × 35 cm^2, and matrix size at 192 × 128 or 128 × 128. The saturating RF pulse was a Fermi pulse before the gradient echo image acquisition, with flip angle = 800°, pulse width = 16 ms, and offset frequencies at 600 and 1000 Hz.

MT studies on small animals have been carried out mostly on high field scanners. Here, we will briefly review the sequences and parameters for some of these studies. High field scanners deliver greater SNR and allow higher spatial resolutions. However, in contrast to clinical scanners (1.5 vs. 3 T), the protocols for high field small animal scanners' imaging parameters may drastically differ due to greater variations in their magnetic field strengths (i.e., 4.7 vs. 16.4 T).

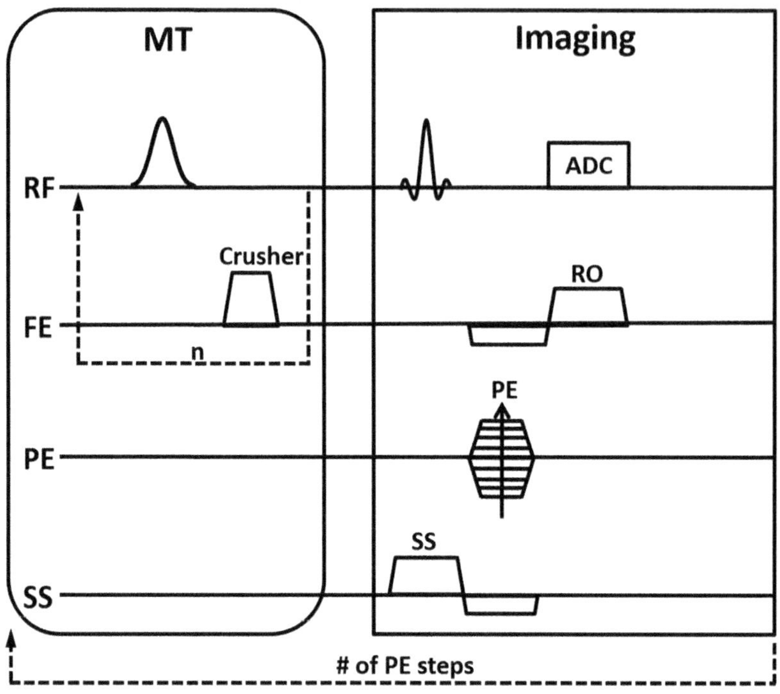

Fig. 13.4 Magnetization transfer-prepared gradient echo sequence diagram. This sequence contains an MT-preparation module followed by imaging using the gradient echo technique. In the MT module, a magnetization saturation pulse is applied at a certain off-resonance frequency to saturate the magnetization of the bound pool, and then a spoiler gradient is applied to eliminate the transverse magnetization. Such an MT module can be applied multiple times to increase saturation power before the imaging module is applied. *MT* magnetization transfer, *RF* radiofrequency, *FE*, frequency encoding, *PE* phase encoding, *SS* slice selection, *RO* readout, *ADC* analog-to-digital converter

In an investigation of renal fibrosis using MTR as the marker, we performed MT imaging using a 16.4 T Bruker scanner with an inner diameter of 38 mm equipped with a birdcage coil. The MT parameters were initially optimized with the help of phantom experiments (Fig. 13.5). Images were acquired with MR parameters as TR = 400 ms, TE = 2.9 ms, flip angle = 20°, section thickness = 1 mm, field of view = 30 × 30 mm, and matrix size = 128 × 128, w/wo Gaussian MT pulses with offset frequencies from −6 k to 6 kHz (14). Then an optimal offset frequency at 1500 Hz was selected to achieve a satisfactory MT contrast as well as low direct saturation of the free water pool.

When using the MTR as an index of the macromolecule content in tissues, there are several factors that need to be considered with regard to MR parameter selection. First, sequences with rapid acquisition times such as gradient echo with short TR are preferred because they provide fast imaging while maintaining sufficient MT saturation. Moreover, if imaging is performed under breath-hold, temporal resolution should allow acquisition under a single breath-hold, since the variation in breathing cycle will cause inconsistent MT saturation and thus incomparable MTR values between subjects, even with implementation of respiratory gating. Second, the off-resonance MT pulse parameters, including the offset frequency, the pulse flip angle, TR, and the number of pulses per repetition, are paramount in achieving satisfactory MT contrast. A pilot study exploiting an optimal combination of the sequence parameters is recommended on either a phantom or an isolated kidney. Finally,

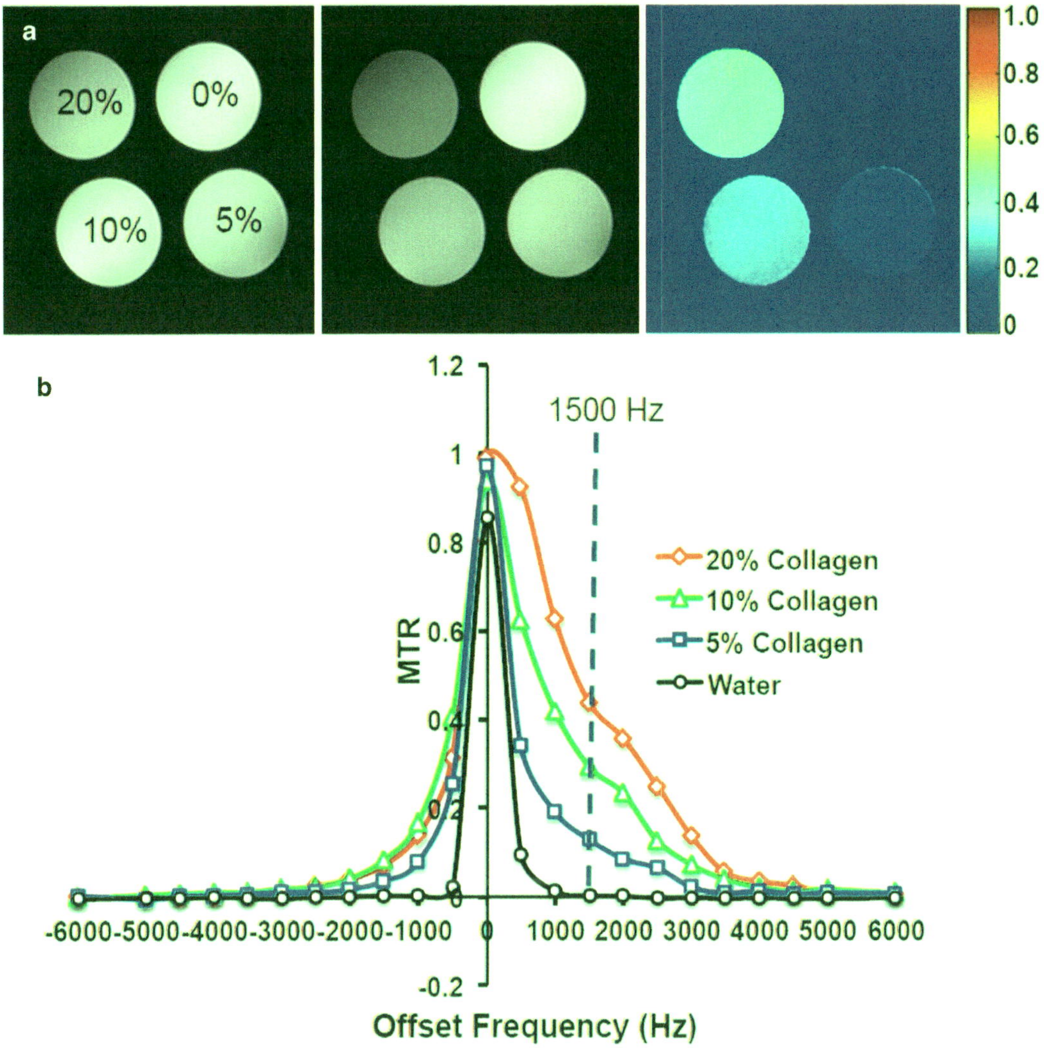

Fig. 13.5 Phantom study to find optimal offset frequency for collagen detection at 16.4 T. (**a**) From left to right are the images without and with magnetization saturation and the calculated magnetization transfer ratio (MTR) map for different concentrations of collagen, with offset frequency at 1500 Hz and bandwidth at 300 Hz. (**b**) Changes in MTR with offset frequency. The optimal offset frequency for collagen detection is selected to be 1500 Hz, which offers a satisfactory MT contrast without inducing a significant amount of direct saturation on the water pool. (Figure reproduced with permission from Jiang et al. Radiology. 2017; 283:77–86)

3D (or at least multi-slice) acquisitions are recommended to cover a larger portion of the kidney for more comprehensive sampling.

For the qMT, we used an MT-prepared fast-low-angle-shot (FLASH) sequence with TR = 120 ms, TE = 2.7 ms, flip angle = 20°, and number of averages = 4. A Gaussian pulse with a pulse width = 9.3 ms was used for magnetization saturation at eight offset frequencies (1, 2, 5, 8, 10, 20, 30, 50 kHz), with two flip angles at 450° and 900°, providing two different degrees of MT saturation [14].

In contrast, using a 16 cm horizontal bore, 7 T Bruker, Wang et al. pursued a different strategy that involved considerably shorter TR and a smaller flip angle, with a large number of repetitions to compensate for SNR (spoiled gradient echo sequence with TR = 24 ms and flip angle = 7°). The matrix size = 256 × 256 and number of acquisitions = 24. They used Gaussian-shaped saturation pulses with flip angles = 220° and 820° (pulse width = 10 ms) and acquired images at 12 RF offsets frequencies between 1 and 80 kHz [15].

Since qMT relies on curve fitting of the MT contrast with different offset frequencies, a large dynamic range of the MT contrast is deemed necessary for reliable quantification of the qMT parameters. Thus, qMT protocol should encompass a wide range of offset frequencies and sufficient MT contrast at the smallest offset frequency (e.g., <30–40% of that without off-resonance magnetization saturation). Similar to the MTR, an appropriate combination of the MT pulse parameters and sequence repetition time is necessary for a robust qMT study.

On-Resonance MT

A protocol for on-resonance MT consists of several sequences. Initially, data is collected using multiple flip angles for calculation of a T1, which would be used later for extraction of *f*. Two spoiled gradient echo (SPGR) sequences (TR = 9.8 ms, TE = 4.77 ms) and bandwidth = 140 Hz/Pixel with flip angles = 4° and 15° were acquired. Additionally, multiple bSSFP samples were acquired with various RF pulse time widths with flip angle = 35°, bandwidth = 790 Hz/Pixel, and varying RF pulse durations ($TR1/T_{RF1}$ = 2.92 ms/0.23 ms, $TR2/T_{RF2}$ = 2.99 ms/0.3 ms, $TR3/T_{RF3}$ = 3.09 ms/0.4 ms, $TR4/T_{RF4}$ = 3.26 ms/0.58 ms, $TR5/T_{RF5}$ = 3.53 ms/0.84 ms, $TR6/T_{RF6}$ = 3.88 ms/1.2 ms, $TR7/T_{RF7}$ = 4.28 ms/1.6 ms, $TR8/T_{RF8}$ = 4.78 ms/2.1 ms). Eight bSSFP sequences are acquired with TR/TRF = 2.99 ms/0.27 ms (bandwidth = 790 Hz/Pixel) and varying flip angles (5°, 10°, 15°, 20°, 25°, 30°, 35°, 40°).

Segmentation

Generally, high resolution MR images with high contrast, particularly for corticomedullary differentiation, are used to delineate renal regions. Segmentation of and defining the ROI depend on the regions involved and the pathology of interest. Some studies have reported drawing ROIs directly on MT images with RF pulse on or off [10, 15]. Using T1 and T2-weighted images for this purpose has been reported as well [16]. T1-weighted sequences, such as MPRAGE, might have low contrast for applications that require differentiation of the cortex and medulla. T2-weighted images may particularly be useful when differentiation of the medulla from the cortex is required.

Field Mapping and Corrections

Two types of field corrections may be applied to improve the accuracy, particularly in qMT assessments. The necessity of such corrections becomes more important in studies performed at high field strengths. B_0 mapping and correction are applied to reduce the impact of inhomogeneity in the static magnetic field. B_1 correction is important in MT because the MTR value is dependent on the amplitude MT RF pulse [17].

We performed B_0 mapping using a dual-echo gradient echo sequence with TR = 120 ms, TE1 = 2.04 and TE2 = 4.08 ms, flip angle = 20°, and number of averages = 4 [14]. In this approach, B_0 is estimated through an additional phase component it produces, as will be discussed later in the post-processing section of this chapter. More detailed discussion about this method is available in [18].

We acquired B_1 maps using the method proposed by Yarnykh with two different repetition times: TR1 = 40 and TR2 = 200 ms, TE = 2.4 ms, flip angle = 60°, and number of averages = 8 [14, 19]. An alternative approach was used by Wang et al. where B_1 maps were obtained based on two flip angles of 40° and 80°, using the method presented earlier by Smith et al. [20].

Post-Processing and Data Analysis Methods

Bound Pool Fraction Calculation

The quantitative off- and on-resonance mathematical frameworks for assessment of bound pool fraction were discussed earlier. In an off-resonance-based model of qMT, MR data acquired from a set of offset frequencies is fitted to Eq. 13.13. This allows estimation of five independent quantities, one of which is $f/R_A(1-f)$. To find the bound pool fraction f, R_A is calculated using Eq. 13.15 and the R_{Aobs}, which is determined from T1 measurements.

In the on-resonance framework, a collection of images is acquired for various TR/TE and flip angles. Then the model in Eq. 13.20 is fitted to this data to extract the variable from Eqs. 13.21–13.26. Other parameters, including F, k_r, and k_f, can be calculated through simultaneously solving the equations.

B_0 Field Correction

B_0 maps are calculated from the two images, acquired with respective phase shifts of 0 and π. If the systematic phase is removed from the two images, then the signal corresponding to images can be written as:

$$S_0 = \rho_1 + \rho_2 \tag{13.27}$$

$$S_\pi = \left|\rho_1 + \rho_2\right| e^{i\phi} \tag{13.28}$$

Where ρ_1 and ρ_2 are the water and fat signals and ϕ is the phase component corresponding to the B_0 inhomogeneity.

B_1 Field Correction

In fact, in this correction, the actual flip angle (as opposed to the implemented flip angle) is determined using an approach that requires two spoiled SSFP images with short but different TR values. The actual flip angle can be measured from:

$$\alpha \approx \arccos\frac{rn-1}{n-r} \tag{13.29}$$

Where $n = TR_2/TR_1$, α' is the implemented flip angle in the sequence, and

$$r \approx \frac{1+n\cos(\alpha')}{n+\cos(\alpha')} \tag{13.30}$$

Clinical Applications

In this section, we will review some of the applications of MT in renal imaging. At this point, a limited number of MT studies have been performed in patients and most novel applications are in the preclinical stage. However, if successful, due to the non-invasive nature of MT, which does not require any intervention or injection of an exogenous contrast agent, translation to the clinical side is believed to be rather straightforward.

Contrast Enhancement

An early study by Kajander et al. in patients with end-stage kidney disease showed superiority of MT images over T2 in differentiating kidney remnants and their fatty surroundings at a very low field (0.1 T) [21]. The study was performed in a cohort of patients with a transplanted kidney but was aimed at investigation of the shrunken right native kidney, which was difficult to differentiate from the surrounded tissue. They applied an RF pulse, at 4 kHz offset frequency, and reported a contrast index (signal intensity of renal parenchyma/signal intensity of surrounding tissue) of 0.82 and 0.46, for pulse widths of 50 and 800 ms, respectively, compared to that in the T2-weighted image that was close to 1.0, indicating the two tissues were not differentiable. Considerable MT effect in these tissues can potentially be explained based on excessive fibrosis in native kidneys and its contribution to renal MT.

Kidney Function

Ito et al. investigated the correlation between MT and estimated glomerular filtration rate (eGFR) on a 3 T scanner [10]. They investigated 44 subjects (22 healthy controls and 22 with declined GFR) and found significant inverse correlation between GFR and MTR in the cortex ($r = -0.645$) but not in the medulla. They also reported higher MTR in patients compared to controls (30.7% vs.

25.3%). The offset frequency was 1500 Hz (~10 ppm), which is relatively close to those previously reported for fibrosis detection [22, 23].

In a different study, Afarideh et al. showed that MTR may serve as a predictor of the outcome of revascularization in renal artery stenosis (RAS) [13]. They found significant correlations between pre-revascularization cortical MTR and post-vascularization perfusion and renal blood flow, at an offset frequency of 600 Hz. Moreover, they reported strong and significant correlation between the change in perfusion and GFR before and after revascularization, and changes in cortical MTR.

Kidney Histology—Fibrosis

As mentioned earlier, feasibility of detecting renal fibrosis is perhaps the most important quest of studies on MT in kidney [24]. In recent years, several studies have been performed to examine this possibility. In the MT-based approach, collagen deposited in fibrotic tissues serves as the direct marker of fibrosis. In the two-pool system, water molecules hydrating collagen molecules act as the restricted pool [25].

We used on-resonance MT in a mouse model of unilateral RAS [23]. Our results showed significant correlation between the fibrosis fraction and the exchange rate constants, k_f. Moreover, we found that the bound pool tended to be larger in the stenotic compared to the contralateral kidney. Using the off-resonance framework, we showed close correlation between MTR and histological markers of fibrosis. Additionally, the results indicated progressive increases in MTR, 2, 4, and 6 weeks after induction of RAS (Fig. 13.6). Similar findings were observed when MT was used to study the swine model of RAS using a 3 T clinical scanner, and a saturation RF pulse at 600 and 1000 Hz offset frequency [12].

Using the qMT framework, Wang et al. observed a significantly larger bound pool in animals with a mild-to-moderate level of fibrosis when using threshold-based small ROIs, such as in the db/db mice model of diabetic nephropathy. Moreover, they reported that the threshold-based quantification of bound pool had higher sensitivity and specificity than other relaxation- and MT-driven markers [16]. We have also reported bound pool fraction in RAS and shown strong correlation between this parameter and fibrosis quantified from histology (Fig. 13.7) [26].

Feasibility of using MTR as a surrogate marker for ADPKD progression has also been explored in an animal study [27]. This study investigated MTR in a mouse model of ADPKD, at 9, 12, and 15 months of age. The assumption was that MTR sensitivity to microscopic tissue remodeling may allow higher sensitivity and precision compared to total kidney volume, a clinically accepted marker of ADPKD progression. The study showed a close correlation between MTR and both histology-derived cystic and fibrotic burden.

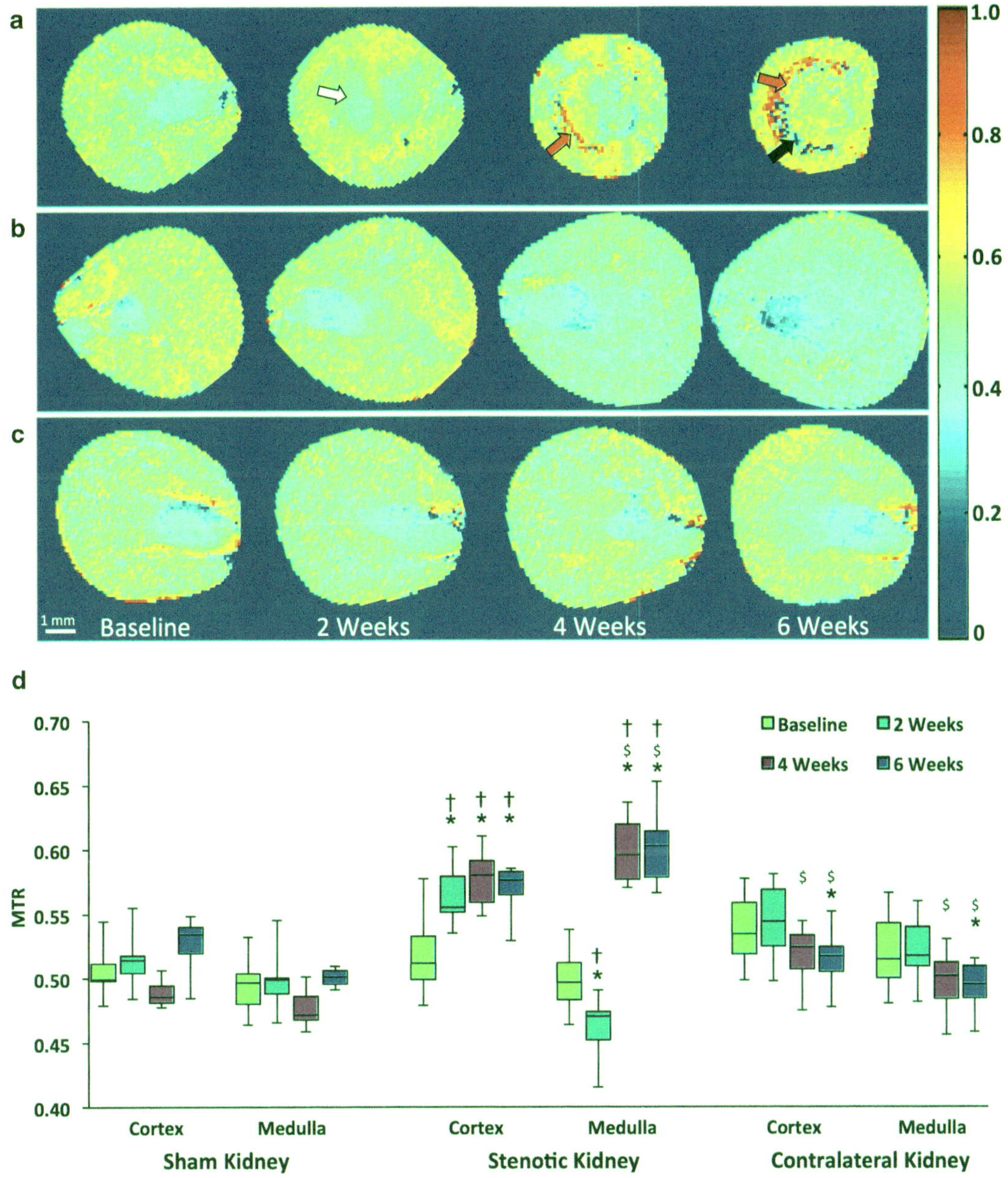

Fig. 13.6 Longitudinal assessment of murine renal fibrosis using magnetization transfer ratio (MTR) maps. With the development of renal fibrosis, the kidney MTR also increased progressively over 6 weeks after induction of renal artery stenosis (**a**), but remained unchanged in the contralateral (**b**) and control (**c**) kidneys. The red, white, and black arrows indicate renal fibrosis, edema, and necrosis, respectively. The MTR values at baseline, 2-, 4-, and 6-weeks post RAS induction are shown below (**d**). $^{*}P < 0.05$ compared to baseline; $^{\$}P < 0.05$ compared to 2 weeks; $^{\dagger}P < 0.05$ compared to sham. (Figure reproduced with permission from Jiang et al. Radiology. 2017; 283:77–86)

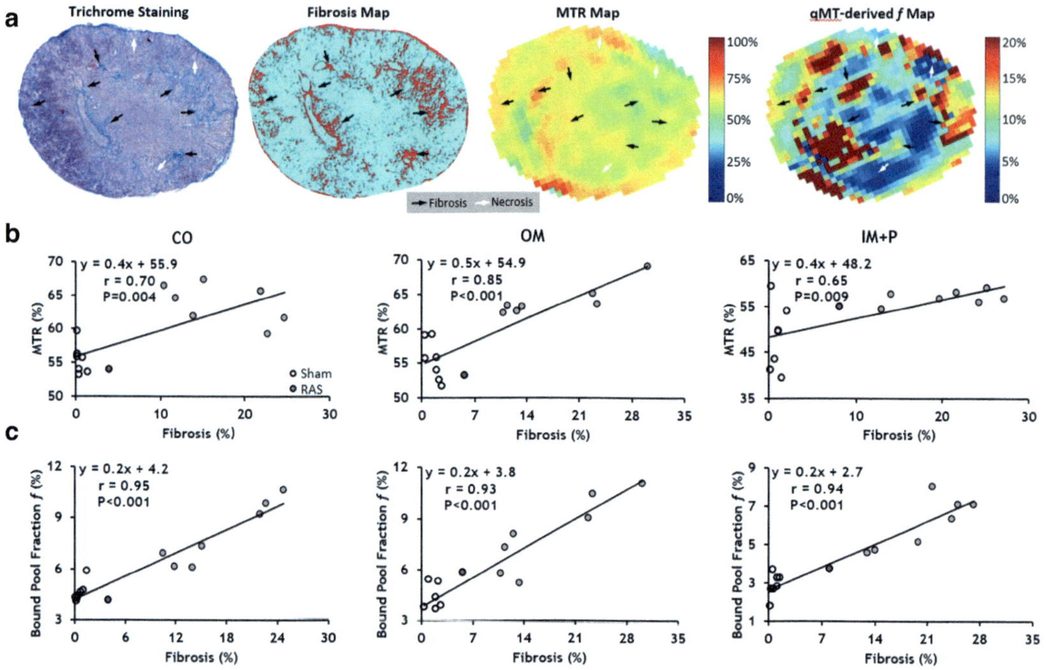

Fig. 13.7 Association between renal fibrosis and the MTR and bound pool fraction *f* in mouse kidneys. (**a**) Masson's trichrome-stained kidney section of a RAS kidney with fibrosis appearing blue and marked by the black arrowheads, whereas kidney regions with edema are marked by the white arrowheads. A thresholding technique generated renal fibrosis map shows fibrosis in red on an aqua background. The MTR map at 1500 Hz and the corresponding qMT-derived *f* map of the same kidney are also shown. (**b**) Correlation between the measured MTR and renal fibrosis in the CO (left), OM (middle), and IM + P (right). (**c**) Correlation between the qMT-derived *f* and renal fibrosis in the CO (left), OM (middle), and IM + P (right). *qMT* quantitative magnetization transfer, *MTR* magnetization transfer ratio, *RAS* renal artery stenosis, *CO* cortex, *OM* outer medulla, *IM + P* inner medulla plus papilla. (Figure reproduced with permission from Jiang et al. JMRI. 2020)

Conclusion

In recent years, there has been a new surge in MTI studies in kidneys, mainly motivated by assessing this technique's ability to noninvasively detect renal fibrosis. The two major quantitative indices, the MTR and bound pool fraction, are sensitive to macromolecule content in kidneys, such as excessive collagen deposited in fibrotic tissue. In fact, with careful selection of imaging parameters and image processing, the quantified MTR and bound pool fraction have been demonstrated to be reliable biomarkers of renal fibrosis. Compared to the bound pool fraction by qMT, the measurement of MTR is easy to implement with only two sets of images required. Nevertheless, the MTR is inherently semi-quantitative and may be affected by factors other than the macromolecule content, such as the MR sequence parameters and field inhomogeneities. The bound pool fraction by qMT, on the other hand, decouples the macromolecule content from all these perturbing factors but requires more intricate image acquisition and post-processing. So far, the ability of renal MTI in measuring fibrosis has only been demonstrated in animal models of kidney diseases; however, the promising results warrant further studies to test its utility in patients.

References

1. Bax A, Hawkins BL, Maciel GE. Off resonance cross-polarization: A technique to reduce rf power requirements for magnetization transfer experiments in solids. J Magn Reson (1969). 1984;59(3):530–5.
2. Bax A, Davis DG. MLEV-17-based two-dimensional homonuclear magnetization transfer spectroscopy. J Magn Reson (1969). 1985;65(2):355–60.
3. Wolff SD, Balaban RS. Magnetization transfer contrast (MTC) and tissue water proton relaxation in vivo. Magn Reson Med. 1989;10(1):135–44.
4. Henkelman R, Stanisz G, Graham S. Magnetization transfer in MRI: a review. NMR Biomed. 2001;14(2):57–64.
5. Wolff SD, Balaban RS. Magnetization transfer imaging: practical aspects and clinical applications. Radiology. 1994;192(3):593–9.
6. Jiang K, Ferguson CM, Woollard JR, Landes VL, Krier JD, Zhu X, et al. Magnetization transfer imaging is unaffected by decreases in renal perfusion in swine. Investig Radiol. 2019;54(11):681–8.
7. Ramani A, Dalton C, Miller D, Tofts P, Barker G. Precise estimate of fundamental in-vivo MT parameters in human brain in clinically feasible times. Magn Reson Imaging. 2002;20(10):721–31.
8. Henkelman RM, Huang X, Xiang QS, Stanisz G, Swanson SD, Bronskill MJ. Quantitative interpretation of magnetization transfer. Magn Reson Med. 1993;29(6):759–66.
9. Gloor M, Scheffler K, Bieri O. Quantitative magnetization transfer imaging using balanced SSFP. Magn Reson Med. 2008;60(3):691–700.
10. Ito K, Hayashida M, Izumitani S, Fujimine T, Onishi T, Genba K. Magnetisation transfer MR imaging of the kidney: evaluation at 3.0 T in association with renal function. Eur Radiol. 2013;23(8):2315–9.
11. Kline TL, Edwards ME, Garg I, Irazabal MV, Korfiatis P, Harris PC, et al. Quantitative MRI of kidneys in renal disease. Abdom Radiol (NY). 2018;43(3):629–38.
12. Jiang K, Ferguson CM, Woollard JR, Zhu X, Lerman LO. Magnetization transfer MRI noninvasively detects renal fibrosis in swine atherosclerotic renal artery stenosis at 3.0 T. Investig Radiol. 2017;52(11):686.
13. Afarideh M, Jiang K, Ferguson CM, Woollard JR, Glockner JF, Lerman LO. Magnetization transfer imaging predicts porcine kidney recovery after revascularization of renal artery stenosis. Investig Radiol. 2021;56(2):86–93.
14. Jiang K, Fang Y, Ferguson CM, Tang H, Mishra PK, Macura SI, et al. Quantitative magnetization transfer detects renal fibrosis in murine kidneys with renal artery stenosis. J Magn Reson Imaging. 2020;53(3):884–93.
15. Wang F, Katagiri D, Li K, Takahashi K, Wang S, Nagasaka S, et al. Assessment of renal fibrosis in murine diabetic nephropathy using quantitative magnetization transfer MRI. Magn Reson Med. 2018;80(6):2655–69.
16. Wang F, Wang S, Zhang Y, Li K, Harris RC, Gore JC, et al. Noninvasive quantitative magnetization transfer MRI reveals tubulointerstitial fibrosis in murine kidney. NMR Biomed. 2019;32(11):e4128.
17. Samson RS, Wheeler-Kingshott CA, Symms MR, Tozer DJ, Tofts PS. A simple correction for B1 field errors in magnetization transfer ratio measurements. Magn Reson Imaging. 2006;24(3):255–63.
18. Skinner TE, Glover GH. An extended two-point Dixon algorithm for calculating separate water, fat, and B0 images. Magn Reson Med. 1997;37(4):628–30.
19. Yarnykh VL. Actual flip-angle imaging in the pulsed steady state: a method for rapid three-dimensional mapping of the transmitted radiofrequency field. Magn Reson Med. 2007;57(1):192–200.
20. Smith SA, Edden RA, Farrell JA, Barker PB, Van Zijl PC. Measurement of T1 and T2 in the cervical spinal cord at 3 tesla. Magn Reson Med. 2008;60(1):213–9.
21. Kajander S, Kallio T, Alanen A, Komu M, Forsström J. Imaging end-stage kidney disease in adults: Low-field MR imaging with magnetization transfer vs. ultrasonography. Acta Radiol. 2000;41(4):357–60.
22. Jiang K, Ferguson CM, Ebrahimi B, Tang H, Kline TL, Burningham TA, et al. Noninvasive assessment of renal fibrosis with magnetization transfer MR imaging: validation and evaluation in murine renal artery stenosis. Radiology. 2017;283(1):77–86.
23. Ebrahimi B, Macura SI, Knudsen BE, Grande JP, Lerman LO, editors. Fibrosis detection in renal artery stenosis mouse model using magnetization transfer MRI. Medical imaging 2013: biomedical applications in molecular, structural, and functional imaging; 2013: International Society for Optics and Photonics.
24. Ebrahimi B, editor. Quantitative magnetization transfer detects renal fibrosis in murine kidneys with renal artery stenosis. Wiley Online Library; 2021.
25. Edzes HT, Samulski ET. The measurement of cross-relaxation effects in the proton NMR spin-lattice relaxation of water in biological systems: hydrated collagen and muscle. J Magn Reson (1969). 1978;31(2):207–29.
26. Jiang K, Fang Y, Ferguson CM, Tang H, Mishra PK, Macura SI, et al. Quantitative magnetization transfer detects renal fibrosis in murine kidneys with renal artery stenosis. J Magn Reson Imaging. 2021;53(3):884–93.
27. Kline TL, Irazabal MV, Ebrahimi B, Hopp K, Udoji KN, Warner JD, et al. Utilizing magnetization transfer imaging to investigate tissue remodeling in a murine model of autosomal dominant polycystic kidney disease. Magn Reson Med. 2016;75(4):1466–73.

Metabolic Imaging: Measuring Fat in the Kidney

14

Ilona A. Dekkers and Hildo J. Lamb

Introduction

Chronic kidney disease (CKD) affects over 10% of the general population [1] and is paralleled by an increased prevalence of obesity and type 2 diabetes [2, 3]. Obesity is not only directly associated with renovascular risk factors, but is also an independent risk factor for CKD progression [4]. Obese individuals have a weight-dependent two-to-seven-fold increased risk of progressive CKD [5]. Current methods to assess CKD (e.g., serum creatinine, albuminuria, and ultrasound) are insensitive to early kidney damage, unspecific to underlying etiology, and unreliable for individual patient stratification. These limitations indicate the need for novel approaches to assess CKD, such as multiparametric renal MRI biomarkers [6] that aid in early recognition of obesity-related kidney damage. One promising biomarker for obesity-related renal disease is intrarenal triglyceride content [7] (e.g., fat accumulating inside the renal parenchyma). Intrarenal triglyceride content relates to postulated concept of dysfunctional adipose tissue expandability [8], in which the accumulation of the excess of fat is presumed to cause ectopic lipid accumulation in non-adipose tissue such as the kidney parenchyma (similar to steatosis occurring in the liver, heart, and skeletal muscle) [9]. Translational studies in humans on obesity-related kidney damage are scarce because it is considered unethical to perform biopsies in obese individuals without overt renal disease. Technical advances of MR spectroscopy over the last decade have opened a window of opportunity to explore physiologic processes in the kidney and have shown that it is feasible to measure intrarenal triglyceride content of human kidney in vivo using ^{1}H-MRS on 1.5 Tesla (T) [10] and at 3 T [11]. In this chapter, we will focus on the use of ^{1}H-MRS for measuring fat in the kidney parenchyma at 3 T in humans and discuss potential clinical applications.

Part 1: MRI Physics and Acquisition Protocols

Magnetic resonance spectroscopy is a technique that allows for the measurement of metabolites or particular chemical compounds that are involved in metabolic processes in living organisms. The involved molecules or metabolites often contain hydrogen and can thus be resonated using ^{1}H-MRS. The use of non-hydrogen nuclei for MRS is not discussed in this chapter.

Field Strength

^{1}H-MRS is a unique imaging modality to study obesity-related kidney disease because of its abil-

I. A. Dekkers (✉) · H. J. Lamb
Department of Radiology, Cardiovascular Imaging Group (CVIG), Leiden University Medical Center, Leiden, The Netherlands
e-mail: i.a.dekkers@lumc.nl; h.j.lamb@lumc.nl

S. D. Serai, K. Darge (eds.), *Advanced Clinical MRI of the Kidney*,
https://doi.org/10.1007/978-3-031-40169-5_14

ity to non-invasively quantify triglycerides based on tissue-specific metabolite spectra. ^{1}H-MRS has evolved over recent years as a valid non-invasive technique to study lipid content in tissue such as liver parenchyma, skeletal muscle, and myocardium. Renal triglyceride content (RTGC) measured using ^{1}H-MRS in humans in vivo was initially explored at 1.5 T and demonstrated feasibility and reproducibility [10]. However, the substantially lower lipid content in the kidney compared to other organs such as the liver makes the acquisition of ^{1}H-MRS particularly challenging. Since increasing field strength results in better resolution and spectral peak quantification, adjustment of the scan protocol to higher field strengths has been explored. Translating ^{1}H-MRS to higher field scanners is challenging. These difficulties are related to the increase in inhomogeneities in the transmit field (B_1^+) and static field (B_0), and artifacts caused by respiratory motion and susceptibility effects. The benefits of scanning at higher field strengths are increased signal-to-noise ratio (SNR) and improved metabolite separation, resulting in better quantification (Fig. 14.1). It should be noted that B_0 shimming (e.g., experimental minimization of B_0 variation) needs to be improved at higher field strengths in order to address broadening of the line widths, which could otherwise result in lower SNR gain than the theoretically expected gain of doubled field strength.

Acquisition

With regard to subject preparation, little is known about physiological influences such as hydration state and fasting state on renal lipids. A standardized preparation of subjects is therefore advised; common practice is to scan after overnight or ≥4 h fasting. To improve voxel planning, 3D fat images from a water-fat acquisition can be used (such as the modified DIXON sequence) because on these fat images, the extrarenal fat in the renal sinus and around the kidney is clearly visible (Fig. 14.2a). To improve the homogeneity of the B_0 field, first-order pencil beam shimming can be used at the voxel location. By applying multiple projections (e.g., 9), this method measures multiple beams through the voxel of interest and reconstructs the B_0 distribution within the voxel. The main advantage of this method is that it is performed in the preparation of the spectroscopy measurement and does not require user input. The shim volumes need to be centered around the ^{1}H-MRS voxel, where the shim volumes need to exceed the sizes of the spectroscopy voxel, e.g., $50 \times 20 \times 20$ mm^3 and $40 \times 10 \times 10$ mm^3, respectively. In renal spectroscopy, the Single voxel Point Resolved Spectroscopy (PRESS) spectra are mainly used and will be the focus in this chapter. PRESS spectra for renal lipids are preferably acquired

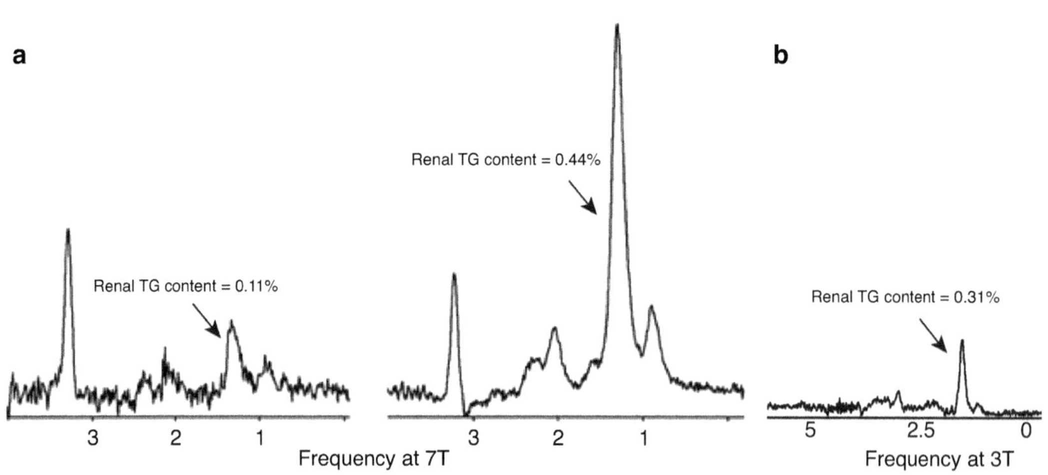

Fig. 14.1 Differences in spectral resolution between field strengths. (**a**) On the *left*, two renal spectra obtained at 7 T showing the triglyceride peak, and (**b**) on the *right*, a renal spectrum obtained at 3 T

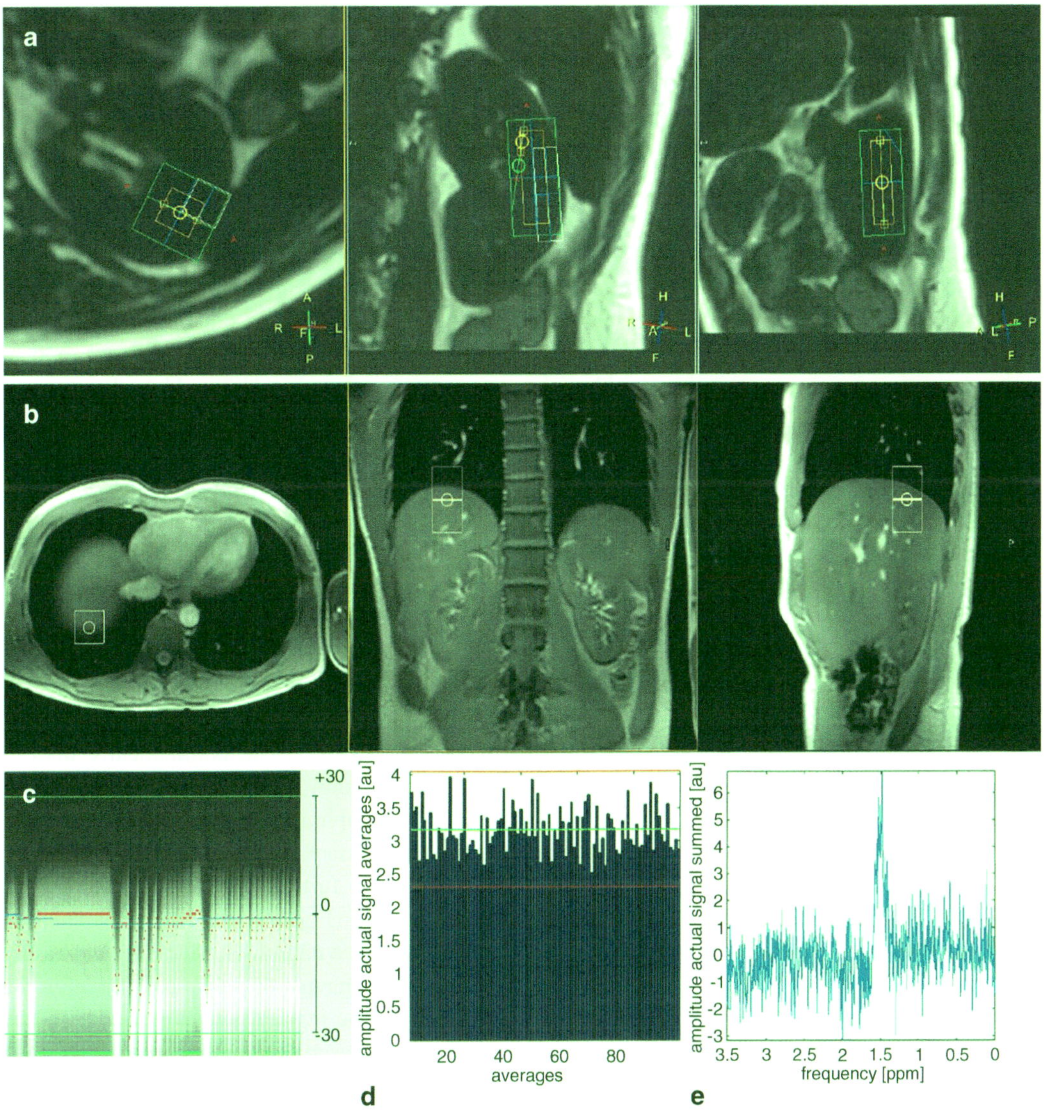

Fig. 14.2 Planning and acquisition of renal ^{1}H-MRS. (**a**) Planning of single voxel ^{1}H-MRS (*orange*) and shim box (*green*) in renal parenchyma on different planes on the Dixon fat only sequences, (**b**) placement of the breathing navigator at liver–lung interface in different planes. (**c**) Navigator profile during acquisition (bottom white part accounts for the liver and the dark upper part represent the lungs). (**d**) Distribution of amplitudes of lipid resonances for all water-suppressed signal averages (dotted *green* line indicates mean amplitude and ±2.5 standard deviations (SDs) are visualized in *red*). Signal averages outside this range can be considered outliers. I Raw spectrum of the summed averages of the actual signal

with a TE of 40 ms and TR of 3 s for the water-suppressed acquisition (e.g., 64 signal averages) and 8 s for the unsuppressed acquisition (e.g., 8 averages), ensuring full relaxation of the water and lipid signals [12, 13]. The number of signal averages can vary; however, it should be noted that the choice of the number of averages is a compromise between scan duration and quality of the obtained spectra. Spectral bandwidth can be set at 1700 Hz, and 1024 samples should be taken for a spectral resolution of 1.66 Hz/sample.

Water Suppression and Local Power Optimization

Considering the fact that the water signal is much larger than the lipid signal in the kidney, adequate suppression of the water signal is needed to minimize baseline distortions and spurious signals that could otherwise complicate renal lipid quantification. Previous research in cardiac ^{1}H-MRS showed that Multiply Optimized Insensitive Suppression Train (MOIST) performed best when the water signal was suppressed, although excitation pulse water suppression should be avoided since this introduces bias in the baseline of the spectra [14]. The water-suppressed spectra can be acquired using MOIST with a bandwidth of 150 Hz.

Power optimization is another important parameter that needs to be addressed in renal spectroscopy. Inadequate estimation of the power of the excitation will lead to a suboptimal choice of the flip angle and result in signal loss. Due to the use of multiple refocusing pulses, this signal loss plays a larger role in single voxel spectroscopy than in most imaging sequences. In particular, for the PRESS sequence, the signal dependence on the flip angle is even greater due to the two 180 degree refocusing pulses that are being used [12]. Local power optimization within the spectroscopic VOI has shown to result in a significant increase in SNR, in contrast to global power optimization where power optimization is performed by integrating the signal intensity throughout the entire slice [14]. The following steps to apply local power optimization can be performed on the scanner and do not require changes to the software of the MR system. First, monitor the intensity of the water peak. Second, incrementally increase the tip angles of the excitation pulse and the two refocusing pulses in the PRESS sequence in steps of 5% (range, 90–150% of the global power optimization result). Finally, select the power setting that produced the highest signal intensity.

Motion Correction

Adequate motion correction is of particular relevance in renal spectroscopy as the kidneys move substantially during breathing. For respiratory triggering, the pencil beam navigator technique is recommended [15]. Breath holding is not recommended as the amount of air in the lungs is known to have significant variation and could thus substantially affect the reproducibility. Moreover, breath holding is not preferred in clinical applications since patients have limited breathing capacity. The pencil beam navigator triggers the spectroscopy acquisition to occur in the same respiratory state. However, it should be noted that to apply the pencil beam navigator, the scanner software needs to be adapted. Moreover, the pencil beam navigator tracks the lung–liver interface in only the feet-to-head direction. The navigator volume needs to be placed at the right diaphragm liver–lung interface (Fig. 14.2b). Triggering of the spectroscopy measurement will start when the diaphragm passes in the automatically defined acceptance window; for example, a window could be the 5 mm diaphragm displacement in end-expiration. Motion tracking of the lung–liver interface can be used to further minimize the respiratory motion effects (Fig. 14.2c). Navigator stability and performance can be improved by increasing the size of the navigator preparation voxel to the same size of the regular navigator voxel, and by using the surface coil rather than the built-in body coil for signal reception. To improve approximation of the navigator voxel location, use of the surface coil is preferred as it increases the respiratory navigator signal. It should be noted that subject repositioning during the scan is not taken into account by the motion correction steps described above; nevertheless, it could be an important source of spectral contamination of non-parenchyma tissue introduced by fat outside the renal parenchyma, such as sinus fat and perirenal fat. If possible, if repositioning during the acquisition is noted, a post-spectroscopy plan scan can be made to check whether the location of the planned single voxel has changed. Moreover, in the post-processing, the separate average of the spectroscopy data can be evaluated, as discussed in Part 2.1 of this chapter.

Part 2: Post-Processing and Data Analysis Methods

Quantification of Renal Triglyceride Content

As on-scanner reconstruction and post-processing methods for spectroscopy data are limited, additional steps using offline post-processing and analysis of the spectral data are needed. Here we describe steps for post-processing and data analysis. After phase correction of the raw data, the weighted sum of the channel signals can be calculated for every average. Eddy current correction can be taken into account by calculating the phase variation over time. Lipid signal amplitude variation between the signal averages is visualized in Fig. 14.2d and in Fig. 14.2e the distribution across parts per million is visualized. Despite the use of motion correction during acquisition of the data, renal spectra can be affected by residual motion, resulting in contamination of the renal lipid spectra with lipids originating from fat in the close proximity of the kidney. Analyzing the averages separately and reconstructing the signal averages over time can allow evaluation of whether sudden changes in the amplitudes have occurred. Such changes would be indicative of contamination of the averages by perirenal or sinus fat. These steps of separate analysis and reconstruction can also serve to exclude outlier signal averages outside the 95% confidence interval. As a final step in the reconstruction process of the spectral data, the included averages can be summed. In order to achieve estimates of RTGC content, the peak areas of the reconstructed spectral data need to be estimated. This estimation requires a mathematical approach that can be done using dedicated software packages, which often require additional physical correction factors that must be taken into account. Existing packages that enable fitting to estimate peak area are Magnetic Resonance User Interface (MRUI). With regard to renal ^{1}H-MRS, the existing literature has been based on the java-based MRUI (Magnetic Resonance User Interface) software [16, 17], and thus will be discussed here. The MRUI software is freely available software that provides fitting in the time domain with eddy current correction and fitting by both linear and non-linear procedures. In addition, MRUI offers the ability to remove the residual water signal using the Hankel-Lanczos filter, which is a singular-value decomposition-based method (Fig. 14.3). This is particularly relevant in renal spectroscopy, as the concentrations of renal lipids are extremely low compared to the water signal, and even after water suppression residual water signal will be present. Non-linear fit in MRUI can be done using the Advanced Method for Accurate, Robust and Efficient Spectral fitting (AMARES) algorithm [18]. Fitting the water-suppressed spectra can be done by using a Gaussian line shape and starting values for renal lipids based on known frequency (ppm) and line width (Hz) estimates: triglyceride methyl (CH_3) 0.9 ppm, 10.0 Hz; triglyceride methylene $(CH_2)_n$ 1.3 ppm, 13.6 Hz; COO-CH_2 2.1 ppm, 10.0 Hz; trimethylamines (TMA) 3.25 ppm, 8.0 Hz (Fig. 14.3b) [11]. In addition, MRUI offers the ability to add prior information on relative resonance frequencies, resonance amplitudes, and line width of the resonances. For RTGC, the relative resonance frequencies and resonance amplitudes can be kept unconstrained, while soft constraints can be applied on the line width of the resonances: CH_3 0–30 Hz; $(CH_2)_n$ 0–30 Hz; COO-CH_2 0–30 Hz; TMA 0–21 Hz (Fig. 14.3b) [11]. In a separate step, the unsuppressed spectra for the water signal can be analyzed using a starting value of 4.7 ppm. In the final step, renal triglyceride content can be calculated as a percentage of the (unsuppressed) water peak using the following equation [11]:

$$\text{Renal TG\%} = \frac{\text{Triglyceride methyl}(CH_3) + \text{Triglyceride methylene}(CH_2)_n}{\text{Water} + \text{Triglyceride methyl}(CH_3) + \text{Triglyceride methylene}(CH_2)_n} \times 100\%$$

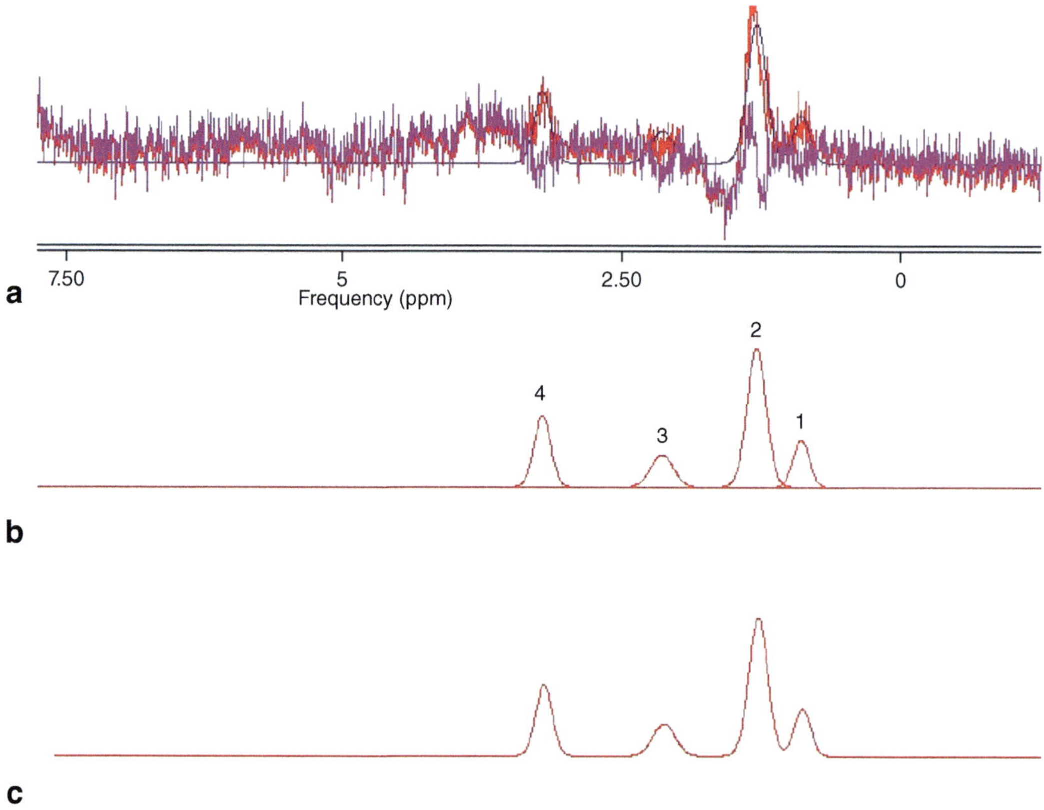

Fig. 14.3 Spectral post-processing of renal 1H-MRS. (**a**) Single voxel renal ^{1}H-MRS spectra with water suppression. (**b**) Resonances from protons of water (peak at 4.7 ppm, H_2O), methylene (peak at 1.3 ppm, $[CH_2]_n$), and methyl (peak at 0.9 ppm, CH_3) are highlighted. Spectral fitting of renal signal amplitudes using estimates for resonances from protons of renal lipids (prior knowledge). Peak number, peak name, frequency, line width: 1. CH_3, 0.9 ppm, 10.0 Hz; 2. $(CH_2)_n$ 1.3 ppm, 13.6 Hz; 3. COO–CH_2, 2.1 ppm, 10.0 Hz; 4. TMA 3.25 ppm, 8.0 Hz. (**c**) AMARES result of individual components of renal lipid signal amplitudes based on original signal and estimated signal using prior knowledge

The concentrations of triglycerides are substantially lower in the kidneys than in other organs such as the liver; this fact is known to negatively affect SNR. For these reasons, several quality criteria have been defined that could be helpful in the evaluation of unreliable renal spectra [19]. These quality criteria are the following:

- Variation in lipid signal amplitudes between the signal averages should be analyzed to exclude potential contamination of the RTGC signal with triglyceride signal originating from renal sinus fat or perirenal fat.
- The Cramér–Rao lower bound divided by the triglyceride amplitude of <20% should be taken into account to discriminate well-fitted metabolites from more poorly fitted metabolites.
- Line width of triglyceride peaks should be <100 Hz.
- Spectra and residuals with artifacts or strongly asymmetric line shapes after eddy correction should be discarded.

Reproducibility and Validation of Renal Triglyceride Content

The intrinsically low renal triglyceride (TG) concentration and voxel size are important limiting factors of the SNR at 3 T despite the theoretical gains due to higher field strength compared to 1.5 T. Local variation of acquired spectra may be introduced unintentionally by differences in voxel planning and subject repositioning during the examination. These variations could cause spectral contamination of non-renal parenchyma tissue such as renal sinus fat and peri-renal fat, which could substantially influence the acquired spectra. Since renal ^{1}H-MRS involves metabolites with extremely low concentrations, adequate water suppression and shimming are of great importance for sufficient spectral quality, in addition to other general factors such as chemical shift displacement and phasing errors. All of these factors contribute to the inter-subject, intra-examination, and inter-examination variability of RTGC measured by ^{1}H-MRS [20]. Intra-examination differences, which represent the unchanged position of the single volume and the receive coils, mainly reflect physiologic motion rather than SNR-related variance. Positioning of the surface coil and planning of sensitive volumes are aspects of ^{1}H-MRS measurements that are reflected in inter-examination differences. In the reproducibility study calibrations, data acquisition parameters and data post-processing were kept identical for both the first and the second measurements, and the differences between inter-examination renal TG percentages reflect measurement variation [11]. Inter-subject differences (SDs or inter-quartile ranges [IQRs]) are a combination of technical factors (spectral noise and partial volume effects) and biological variability (low intrinsic concentrations of renal lipids, total kidney volume, and cortical thickness). The inter-subject difference of RTGC of 0.14% IQR reported in healthy subjects is relatively large [11], which limits the statistical sensitivity to detect significant differences when a single patient or a small group of patients is compared to healthy controls.

In humans, it has been estimated that the kidney consists of 79.5% water, and overall lipid content has been estimated to comprise 0.6% and 1.64% of mean wet kidney weight in the cortex and the medulla, respectively [21]. Moreover, these pathology studies have estimated that overall lipid content in the normal human kidney is composed of approximately one-fifth triglycerides, one-tenth free fatty acids (non-esterified fatty acids), and one-twentieth or less intracellular cholesterol concentration [22]. The large peaks between 1.2 and 1.4 ppm at 3 T originate mainly from the proton resonances of methylene (CH_2) groups of triglyceride. Cholesterol, although it too contains methylene groups, is likely not represented in the spectra with the current resolution due to its more restricted movement, which results in spectral broadening and resonance loss in the background. Renal triglyceride content measurements using ^{1}H-MRS have been validated at 7 T against post mortem samples of porcine kidneys (similar size to human kidneys) to demonstrate proof-of-concept [23]. Good correlation was found for lipid content measured by ^{1}H-MRS and enzymatic assay ($r = 0.86$, $P < 0.0001$) (Fig. 14.4). It should be noted that renal ^{1}H-MRS measures primarily triglycerides while the enzymatic essay measures all lipids, and this may contribute partly to the variance in this study. Using single voxel ^{1}H-MRS, it is not possible to discriminate resonances originating from the cortex or medulla, or from the renal glomeruli or tubuli. Oil Red O staining of the histological porcine specimens in the 7 T validation study showed that renal tubuli exhibited the highest concentrations of renal lipids and that the glomeruli did to a lesser extent [23], which is in accordance with previous findings in human nephrectomies [7]. The tubular uptake of

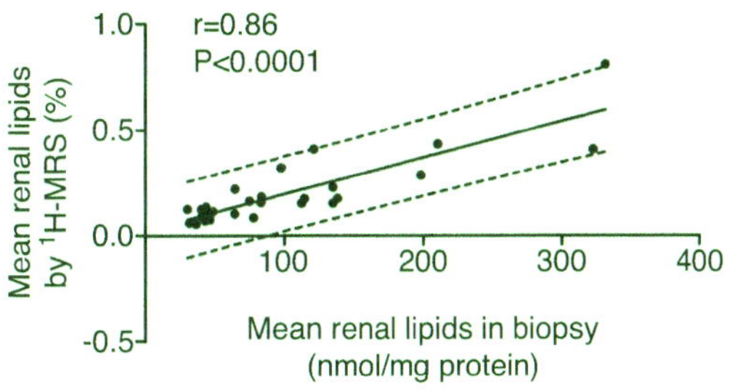

Fig. 14.4 Correlation between mean lipid content measured by ^{1}H-MRS at 7 T and enzymatic assay using post mortem samples of porcine kidneys ($r = 0.86$, $P < 0.0001$). Regression equation: lipids measured by ^{1}H-MRS = 0.02 + 1.7e−3 * lipids measured by enzymatic assay [23]

non-esterified fatty acids depends on plasma levels of non-esterified fatty acids and the luminal concentration of reabsorbed albumin, which is the major carrier of circulatory non-esterified fatty acids [4]. It remains unclear whether increased tubular lipid accumulation directly contributes to tubular atrophy and interstitial fibrosis (e.g., lipid toxicity) or whether decreased fatty acid oxygenation is primarily involved [24].

Part 3: Clinical Applications

Renal Triglyceride Content and Obesity-Related Kidney Disease

The accumulation of lipids in renal parenchyma, referred to as fatty kidney, occurs in obesity, and has been hypothesized to contribute to obesity-related kidney disease [4]. This emerging concept has been supported by the finding of a positive association between BMI and triglycerides in human kidney cortex samples from nephrectomy samples [7]. Translational studies in humans on ectopic lipid accumulation in obesity-related CKD are scarce as biopsies are considered unethical to perform in obese individuals without overt renal disease. In particular, the combination of obesity and type 2 diabetes mellitus (T2DM) has been linked to ectopic lipid accumulation, which in turn has been linked to structural changes such as glomerular hypertrophy [25], and maladaptive functional responses such as hyperfiltration and albuminuria [26]. Renal steatosis has been associated with renal gluconeogenesis in experimental models [4]; however, it is unknown whether glycemic control is conversely linked to ectopic lipid accumulation in the kidney. The application of ^{1}H-MRS for measuring renal triglyceride content in the kidney is a unique and novel way to measure fat metabolism of the kidney non-invasively. This method provides new possibilities to study the pathophysiology of fatty kidney in humans and evaluate potential treatment strategies. Studies performed thus far in diabetic and obese patients and T2DM patients indicate elevated levels of renal lipids compared to healthy controls scanned under similar conditions [11, 27]. Reported medians of triglyceride content in obese T2DM patients at 3 T range between 0.20% and 0.75%, and between 0.12% and 0.21% in healthy controls [11, 19, 27]. It should be noted however that results between studies are hard to compare due to differences in scan protocols and scanning conditions. These factors warrant seeking local normative data in controls that are scanned under the same conditions and scan parameters, rather relying on values from healthy volunteers reported in the literature.

Dietary Effects on Ectopic Fat Storage in the Kidney

One of the landmark studies in obesity-induced hypertension by Hall et al. in dogs showed that obesity induced by a beef fat supplement is associated with hypertension and increased glomerular filtration rate (GFR) and filtration fraction (FF) even under conditions of standardized salt intake [28]. Studies on short-term caloric reduction in severely obese type-2 diabetics with stage two CKD and advanced diabetic nephropathy showed that caloric restriction also influenced GFR [29, 30], but it remains unknown whether these changes relate to ectopic lipid accumulation in the kidney. Previous ^{1}H-MRS studies showed that myocardial triglyceride content and hepatic triglyceride content show a differential response to caloric restriction [31] and to a high-fat high-energy diet [32], indicating that redistribution of endogenous triglyceride stores is likely highly tissue-specific. Additionally, this study found that high fat intake results in increased intracellular fat in the liver but not in the heart, and the effects for the kidney are unknown. No studies thus far have evaluated the physiological variation of intrarenal triglyceride content following dietary intervention in humans. However, the dietary effects on intrarenal lipids have been studied in Göttingen mini-pigs using ^{1}H-MRS at 7 T [23]. In this study, the mini-pigs were used to investigate the effects of a 6-month fast food cafeteria diet and standard diet, as well as T2DM induced by low-dose streptozotocin (STZ). STZ causes beta cell damage and overt hyperglycemiain the presence of normal insulin concentrations and can be used to induce T2DM in animals such as the Göttingen mini-pig [33]. This study found a close correlation between ectopic lipid assessed by ¹H-MRS in the liver parenchyma and in the kidney, supporting the notion that non-alcoholic fatty liver disease might constitute a proxy of fatty kidney [23]. Histological examination of the specimens showed that the mini-pigs with induced type-2 diabetes had significantly higher levels of renal cortex TG quantity compared to the mini-pigs that had only a fast food diet and standard diet [23] (Fig. 14.5). This pre-clinical study using ¹H-MRS supports the pathophysiological role of high caloric intake, obesity, and type-2 diabetes in the context of fatty kidney.

Effects of Glycemic Control on Renal Triglyceride Content

Leading studies such as the UKPDS [34] and ADVANCE [35] studies have demonstrated that improved glycemic control reduces microvascular disease and end-stage kidney disease (ESKD). Moreover, antihypertensive treatment and treatment of proteinuria, in particular using RAAS inhibitors, resulted in a 30% reduction of risk for ESKD [36, 37]; however, the incidence of ESKD due to diabetic nephropathy continues to rise despite the presence of these cornerstone therapies. This indicates that other (non-proteinuric) pathways are possibly related to metabolic regulation and hyperfiltration [38] that remain unaddressed in the current treatment strategies. Novel

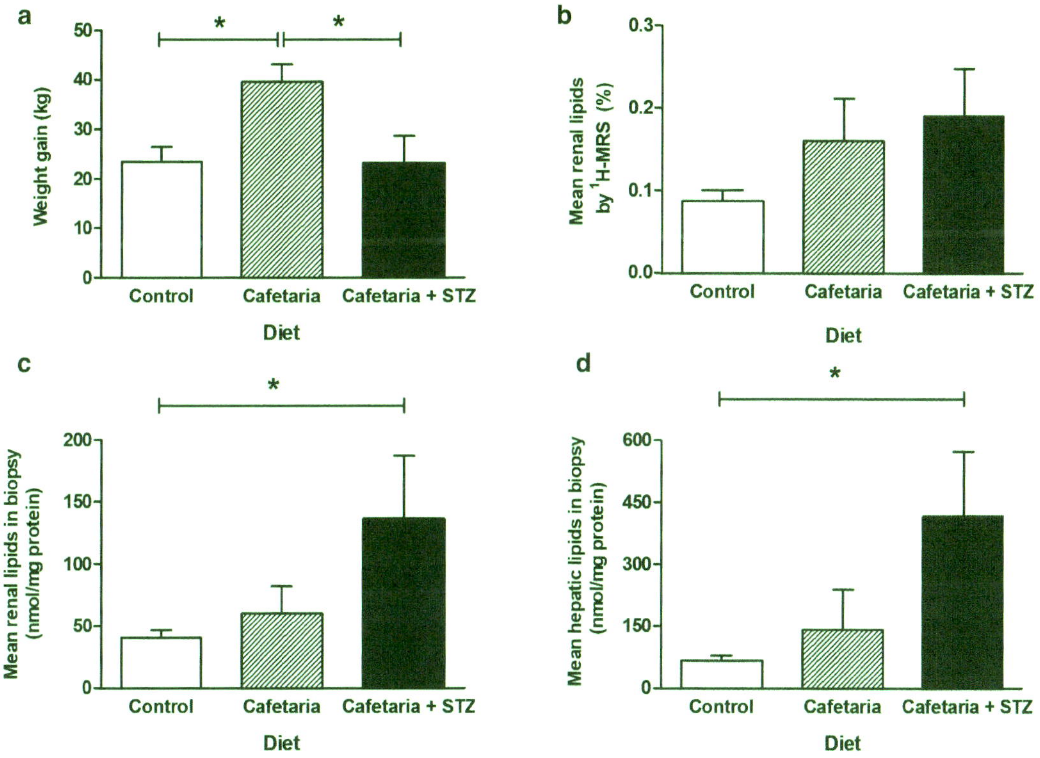

Fig. 14.5 Resultsof the clinical trial to study the dietary effects of 9 months of control diet (*left*), cafeteria diet (*middle*), or cafeteria diet with streptozocin (STZ) (*right*) in Göttingen mini-pigs. (**a**) Weight gain in kilograms for the different treatment arms. (**b**) Renal lipid content measured by proton magnetic resonance spectroscopy (¹H-MRS). (**c**) Renal lipid content from kidney biopsy by enzymatic assay. (**d**) Hepatic lipid content from liver biopsy by enzymatic assay. Data are represented as mean ± SEM. $N = 15$ for renal lipids, $n = 14$ for hepatic lipids. *$P < 0.05$ [23]

antihypertensive medications such as glucagon-like peptide 1 (GLP1) agonists and sodium–glucose transporter 2 inhibitors have created new possibilities for treating diabetic kidney disease, as evidenced by recent trials where they demonstrated beneficial effects on major reno-cardiovascular endpoints [39–42]. With regard to the GLP1 agonist liraglutide, the beneficial effects for the kidney as shown in the LEADER trial [41] are possibly related to improved glycemia, amended blood pressure regulation, and reduction of weight and/or ectopic fat depots such as liver fat [43, 44]. However, direct actions of GLP1 agonists have also been proposed [45], and experimental studies have suggested that liraglutide might have a reno-protective effect in restoring renal metabolism via the inhibition of fat accumulation in the kidney parenchyma [46, 47]. In a recent secondary end-point study of the MAGNA VICTORIA study, T2DM patients were randomized to liraglutide or placebo added to standard glycemic care; this was the first study to assess change in RTGC after 26 weeks of glycemic control measured by proton-spectroscopy and difference in RTGC between treatment groups [19]. Seventeen T2DM patients were included with a baseline mean HbA1c of 61.6 ± 8.4 mmol/mol and log-RTGC of −0.68 ± 0.30%. After 26 weeks of glycemic control, mean HbA1c changed to 56.3 ± 9.5 mmol/mol ($P = 0.046$) and log-RTGC to −0.83 ± 0.32% ($P = 0.049$) irrespective of treatment group (Fig. 14.6). In addition, this study showed that 26-weeks-to-baseline RTGC ratio (95% CI) was significantly different between liraglutide (−0.30 [−0.50,-0.09]) and placebo added to standard care (−0.003 [−0.34,0.34]) ($P = 0.04$) (Fig. 14.7). This exploratory study supports the hypothesis that renal steatosis is a potential driver of diabetic kidney disease, and that tight glycemic control might reduce the risk of diabetic nephropathy, particularly when combined with novel antihyperglycemic agents such as liraglutide. It should be noted, however, that larger clinical studies are needed to assess whether these changes reflect a true effect of glycemic control on renal steatosis, and pre-clinical studies are needed to investigate the underlying biological mechanism. Moreover, it remains uninvestigated whether concomitant useof medications such as statins and antihypertensives also influences RTGC levels.

Future Outlook

Renal spectroscopy is a novel technique that enables the quantification of metabolites in the kidney in humans in vivo. Thus far, this application has mainly been explored for the quantification of renal triglyceride content, which is of particular interest in the evaluation of obesity-related kidney disease and diabetic influences on the kidney. Pioneering work has shown that renal spectroscopy is reproducible and can be used in clinical trials to assess treatment effects. The complexity of the acquisition and required post-processing makes renal spectroscopy a technique that is currently only used by research centers that have a long-standing tradition in body MR spectroscopy. Technical innovations such as multi-voxel spectroscopy, a 3D navigator, and fast scanning solutions could further improve renal ^{1}H-MRS. Ultimately, renal spectroscopy could be used in a personalized medicine-based approach in the management of obesity-related kidney disease and could be combined with other relevant quantitative renal MRI sequences.

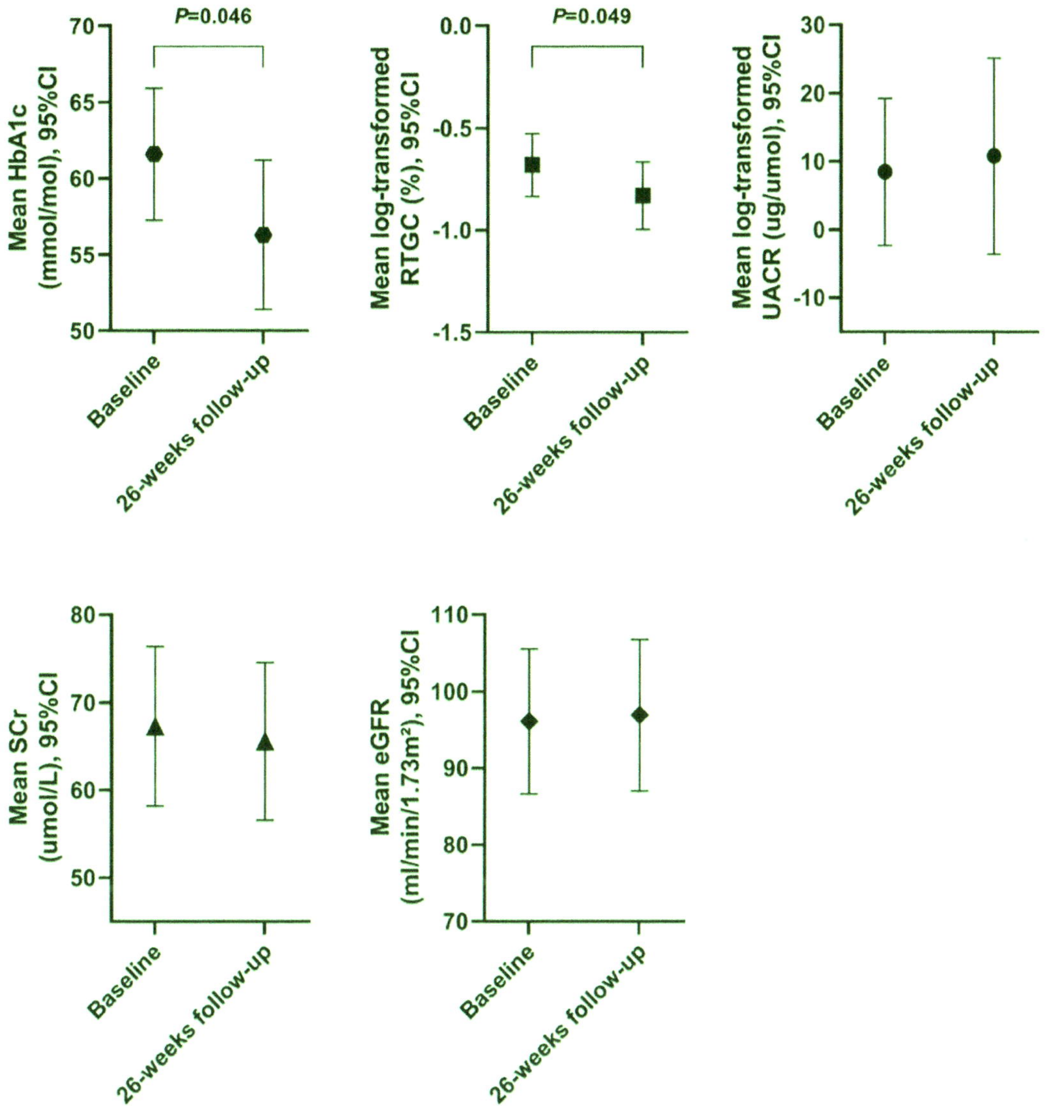

Fig. 14.6 Treatment effect of glycemic control on glycated hemoglobin A1c (HbA1c), renal triglyceride content (RTGC), urine-albumin-creatinine ratio (UACR), serum creatinine (SCr), and estimated glomerular filtration rate (eGFR) irrespective of randomized treatment group ($n = 17$) [19]

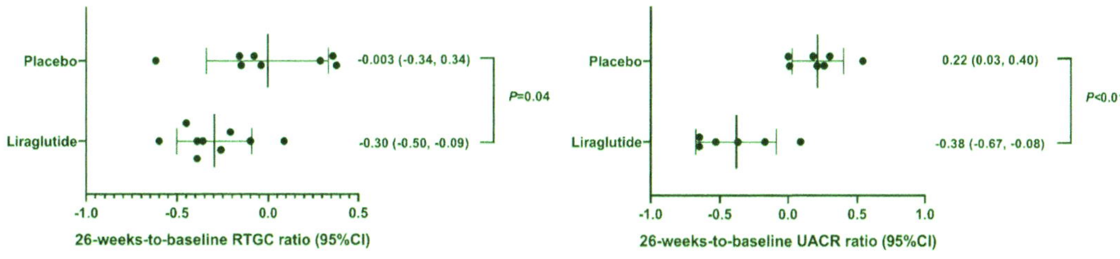

Fig. 14.7 Treatment effectof liraglutide ($n = 9$) versus placebo ($n = 8$) on renal triglyceride content (RTGC) and urinary albumin-creatinine ratio (UACR) [19]

References

1. Webster AC, Nagler EV, Morton RL, Masson P. Chronic Kidney Disease. Lancet. 2017;389(10075):1238–52.
2. Bentham J, Di Cesare M, Bilano V, Bixby H, Zhou B, Stevens GA, et al. Worldwide trends in body-mass index, underweight, overweight, and obesity from 1975 to 2016: a pooled analysis of 2416 population-based measurement studies in 128·9 million children, adolescents, and adults. Lancet. 2017;390(10113):2627–42.
3. Kovesdy CP, Furth S, Zoccali C. Obesity and kidney disease: hidden consequences of the epidemic. Clin Kidney J. 2017;10(1):1–8.
4. de Vries APJ, Ruggenenti P, Ruan XZ, Praga M, Cruzado JM, Bajema IM, et al. Fatty kidney: emerging role of ectopic lipid in obesity-related renal disease. Lancet Diabetes Endocrinol. 2014;2(5):417–26.
5. Ejerblad E, Fored CM, Lindblad P, Fryzek J, McLaughlin JK, Nyrén O. Obesity and risk for chronic renal failure. J Am Soc Nephrol. 2006;17(6):1695–702.
6. Selby NM, Blankestijn PJ, Boor P, Combe C, Eckardt KU, Eikefjord E, et al. Magnetic resonance imaging biomarkers for chronic kidney disease: a position paper from the European Cooperation in Science and Technology Action PARENCHIMA. Nephrol Dial Transplant. 2018;33(suppl_2):ii4–ii14.
7. Bobulescu IA, Lotan Y, Zhang J, Rosenthal TR, Rogers JT, Adams-Huet B, et al. Triglycerides in the human kidney cortex: relationship with body size. PLoS One. 2014;9(8):101285.
8. Hammarstedt A, Gogg S, Hedjazifar S, Nerstedt A, Smith U. Impaired adipogenesis and dysfunctional adipose tissue in human hypertrophic obesity. Physiol Rev. 2018;98(4):1911–41.
9. Neeland IJ, Ross R, Després J-P, Matsuzawa Y, Yamashita S, Shai I, et al. Visceral and ectopic fat, atherosclerosis, and cardiometabolic disease: a position statement. Lancet Diabetes Endocrinol. 2019;7(9):715–25.
10. Hammer S, de Vries APJ, de Heer P, Bizino MB, Wolterbeek R, Rabelink TJ, et al. Metabolic imaging of human kidney triglyceride content: reproducibility of proton magnetic resonance spectroscopy. PLoS One. 2013;8(4):e62209.
11. Dekkers IA, de Heer P, Bizino MB, de Vries APJ, Lamb HJ. 1 H-MRS for the assessment of renal triglyceride content in humans at 3T: a primer and reproducibility study. J Magn Reson Imaging. 2018;48(2):507–13.
12. Bottomley PA. Spatial localization in NMR spectroscopy in vivo. Ann N Y Acad Sci. 1987;508(1):333–48.
13. Klose U. Measurement sequences for single voxel proton MR spectroscopy. Eur J Radiol. 2008;67(2):194–201.
14. de Heer P, Bizino MB, Lamb HJ, Webb AG. Parameter optimization for reproducible cardiac 1H-MR spectroscopy at 3 tesla. J Magn Reson Imaging. 2016;44(5):1151–8.
15. Schär M, Kozerke S, Boesiger P. Navigator gating and volume tracking for double-triggered cardiac proton spectroscopy at 3 tesla. Magn Reson Med. 2004;51(6):1091–5.
16. Naressi A, Couturier C, Devos JM, Janssen M, Mangeat C, de Beer R, et al. Java-based graphical user interface for the MRUI quantitation package. MAGMA. 2001;12(2–3):141–52.
17. Stefan D, Di CF, Andrasescu A, Popa E, Lazariev A, Vescovo E, et al. Quantitation of magnetic resonance spectroscopy signals: the jMRUI software package. Meas Sci Technol. 2009;20(10):104035.
18. Vanhamme L, Van Den Boogaart A, Van Huffel S. Improved method for accurate and efficient quantification of MRS data with use of prior knowledge. J Magn Reson. 1997;129(1):35–43.
19. Dekkers IA, Bizino MB, Paiman EHM, Smit JW, Jazet IM, de Vries APJ, et al. The effect of glycemic control on renal triglyceride content assessed by proton spectroscopy in patients with type 2 diabetes mellitus: a single-center parallel-group trial. J Ren Nutr. 2021;31(6):611–9.
20. Dekkers IA, de Heer P, Bizino MB, de Vries AP, Lamb HJ. ^{1}H-MRS for the assessment of renal triglyceride content in humans at 3T: a primer and reproducibility study. J Magn Reson Imaging. 2018;48(2):507–13.
21. Druilhet RE, Overturf ML, Kirkendall WM. Cortical and medullary lipids of normal and nephrosclerotic human kidney. Int J BioChem. 1978;9(10):729–34.
22. Druilhet RE, Overturf ML, Kirkendall WM. Structure of neutral glycerides and phosphoglycerides of human kidney. Int J BioChem. 1975;6(12):893–901.
23. Jonker JT, de Heer P, Engelse MA, van Rossenberg EH, Klessens CQF, Baelde HJ, et al. Metabolic imaging of fatty kidney in diabesity: validation and dietary intervention. Nephrol Dial Transplant. 2018;33(2):224–30.
24. Kang HM, Ahn SH, Choi P, Ko YA, Han SH, Chinga F, et al. Defective fatty acid oxidation in renal tubular epithelial cells has a key role in kidney fibrosis development. Nat Med. 2015;21(1):37–46.
25. Li L, Zhao Z, Xia J, Xin L, Chen Y, Yang S, et al. A long-term high-fat/high-sucrose diet promotes kidney lipid deposition and causes apoptosis and glomerular hypertrophy in Bama Minipigs. PLoS One. 2015;10(11):e0142884.
26. D'Agati VD, Chagnac A, De Vries APJ, Levi M, Porrini E, Herman-Edelstein M, et al. Obesity-related glomerulopathy: Clinical and pathologic characteristics and pathogenesis. Nat Rev Nephrol. 2016;12(8):453–71.
27. Diserens G, Valenzuela W, Seif M, Mani L, Fuster D, Stettler C, et al. Are renal lipids increased in overweight diabetic patients? A MR spectroscopy and dixon fat/water imaging study. Proc Intl Soc Mag Reson Med 24. 2016.

28. Hall JE, Brands MW, Dixon WN, Smith MJ. Obesity-induced hypertension: renal function and systemic hemodynamics. Hypertension. 1993;22(3):292–9.
29. Ruggenenti P, Abbate M, Ruggiero B, Rota S, Trillini M, Aparicio C, et al. Renal and systemic effects of calorie restriction in patients with type 2 diabetes with abdominal obesity: a randomized controlled trial. Diabetes. 2017;66(1):75–86.
30. Friedman AN, Chambers M, Kamendulis LM, Temmerman J. Short-term changes after a weight reduction intervention in advanced diabetic nephropathy. Clin J Am Soc Nephrol. 2013;8(11):1892–8.
31. Hammer S, Van Der Meer RW, Lamb HJ, Schär M, De Roos A, Smit JWA, et al. Progressive caloric restriction induces dose-dependent changes in myocardial triglyceride content and diastolic function in healthy men. J Clin Endocrinol Metab. 2008;93(2):497–503.
32. Van Der Meer RW, Hammer S, Lamb HJ, Frölich M, Diamant M, Rijzewijk LJ, et al. Effects of short-term high-fat, high-energy diet on hepatic and myocardial triglyceride content in healthy men. J Clin Endocrinol Metab. 2008;93(7):2702–8.
33. Marshall M, Sprandel U, Zöllner N. Streptozotocindiabetes beim Miniaturschwein. Res Exp Med. 1975;165(1):61–5.
34. Holman RR, Paul SK, Bethel MA, Matthews DR, Neil HAW. 10-year follow-up of intensive glucose control in type 2 diabetes. N Engl J Med. 2008;359(15):1577–89.
35. Perkovic V, Heerspink HL, Chalmers J, Woodward M, Jun M, Li Q, et al. Intensive glucose control improves kidney outcomes in patients with type 2 diabetes. Kidney Int. 2013;83(3):517–23.
36. Brenner BM, Cooper ME, de Zeeuw D, Keane WF, Mitch WE, Parving H-H, et al. Effects of losartan on renal and cardiovascular outcomes in patients with type 2 diabetes and nephropathy. N Engl J Med. 2001;345(12):861–9.
37. Lewis EJ, Hunsicker LG, Clarke WR, Berl T, Pohl MA, Lewis JB, et al. Renoprotective effect of the angiotensin-receptor antagonist Irbesartan in patients with nephropathy due to type 2 diabetes. N Engl J Med. 2001;345(12):851–60.
38. Porrini E, Ruggenenti P, Mogensen CE, Barlovic DP, Praga M, Cruzado JM, et al. Non-proteinuric pathways in loss of renal function in patients with type 2 diabetes. Lancet Diabetes Endocrinol. 2015;3(5):382–91.
39. Neal B, Perkovic V, Mahaffey KW, de Zeeuw D, Fulcher G, Erondu N, et al. Canagliflozin and cardiovascular and renal events in type 2 diabetes. N Engl J Med. 2017;377(7):644–57.
40. Heerspink HJL, Stefánsson BV, Correa-Rotter R, Chertow GM, Greene T, Hou F-F, et al. Dapagliflozin in patients with chronic kidney disease. N Engl J Med. 2020;383(15):1436–46.
41. Mann JFE, Ørsted DD, Brown-Frandsen K, Marso SP, Poulter NR, Rasmussen S, et al. Liraglutide and renal outcomes in type 2 diabetes. N Engl J Med. 2017;377(9):839–48.
42. Packer M, Anker SD, Butler J, Filippatos G, Pocock SJ, Carson P, et al. Cardiovascular and renal outcomes with Empagliflozin in heart failure. N Engl J Med. 2020;383(15):1413–24.
43. Bizino MB, Jazet IM, Westenberg JJM, Van Eyk HJ, Paiman EHM, Smit JWA, et al. Effect of liraglutide on cardiac function in patients with type 2 diabetes mellitus: randomized placebo-controlled trial. Cardiovasc Diabetol. 2019;18(1):55.
44. Bizino MB, Jazet IM, de Heer P, van Eyk HJ, Dekkers IA, Rensen PCN, et al. Placebo-controlled randomised trial with liraglutide on magnetic resonance endpoints in individuals with type 2 diabetes: a pre-specified secondary study on ectopic fat accumulation. Diabetologia. 2020;63(1):65–74.
45. Muskiet MHA, Tonneijck L, Smits MM, Van Baar MJB, Kramer MHH, Hoorn EJ, et al. GLP-1 and the kidney: from physiology to pharmacology and outcomes in diabetes. Nat Rev Nephrol. 2017;13(10):605–28.
46. Wang C, Li L, Liu S, Liao G, Li L, Chen Y, et al. GLP-1 receptor agonist ameliorates obesity-induced chronic kidney injury via restoring renal metabolism homeostasis. PLoS One. 2018;13(3):e0193473.
47. Guo H, Wang B, Li H, Ling L, Niu J, Gu Y. Glucagon-like peptide-1 analog prevents obesity-related glomerulopathy by inhibiting excessive autophagy in podocytes. Am J Physiol Ren Physiol. 2018;314(2):F181–9.

15 MR Angiography and Phase-Contrast MRI: Measuring Blood Flow in the Kidney

Anneloes de Boer, Giulia Villa, and Anna Caroli

Introduction

As part of the wide spectrum of kidney magnetic resonance imaging (MRI) sequences, phase-contrast (PC) MRI allows the assessment of blood flow velocity and volume in the renal arteries, while MRA allows assessment of renal vasculature.

The assessment of renal blood flow (RBF) is important for the diagnosis and monitoring of a range of renal diseases in which RBF decreases from the earliest stages. PC-MRI, requiring no contrast media and thus involving no risks for patients with renal disease, provides a non-invasive alternative to traditional and more cumbersome RBF measurements such as para-aminohippurate (PAH) renal clearance, and allows the differentiation of single kidney blood flow. Despite renal PC-MRI not yet being routinely used in clinical practice, several clinical studies support its potential in the diagnosis and monitoring of renal diseases [1].

Unlike PC-MRI, MRA is routinely used in clinical practice to establish the diagnosis of renal artery stenosis in hypertensive patients. Compared to digital subtraction angiography, it has the advantage of being non-invasive and does not depend on iodinated contrast administration, which carries a small risk of inducing acute kidney injury in patients with impaired renal function [2]. Although MRA also requires administration of a contrast agent, promising contrast-free angiography sequences have been developed. While their diagnostic performance still needs to be confirmed in larger clinical studies, those sequences can be used in patients in whom administration of any contrast agent is contra-indicated. Furthermore, the relatively new agent Ferumoxytol provides excellent depiction of both arterial and venous vasculature and is especially promising in patients with renal dysfunction as it is clinically used as an iron supplement in patients with renal failure.

This chapter provides a comprehensive overview of PC-MRI and MRA of the renal arteries, including patient preparation, physics and acquisition protocols, post-processing and data analysis methods, common issues and artifacts, and clinical applications, with the aim of fostering their wider adoption first in clinical research and ultimately in clinical practice.

A. de Boer
Department of Radiology, University Medical Center Utrecht, Utrecht University, Utrecht, The Netherlands
e-mail: a.deboer-13@umcutrecht.nl

G. Villa · A. Caroli (✉)
Bioengineering Department, Istituto di Ricerche Farmacologiche Mario Negri IRCCS, Bergamo, Italy
e-mail: giulia.villa@marionegri.it; acaroli@marionegri.it

S. D. Serai, K. Darge (eds.), *Advanced Clinical MRI of the Kidney*,
https://doi.org/10.1007/978-3-031-40169-5_15

Phase-Contrast MRI

Patient Preparation

In preparation for PC-MRI acquisition, there is no need for patients to maintain strict control of diet and hydration [3]. However, patients should be scanned in a normal state of hydration and asked to avoid salt- and protein-rich meals, since hydration state, salt, and protein intake may influence renal blood flow. To gather as much information as possible from PC-MRI acquisition, it is recommended to concurrently measure a few clinical (blood pressure), blood (hematocrit), and functional parameters (measured or estimated GFR), which allow computation of derivative hemodynamic parameters.

PC-MRI Physics and Acquisition Protocol

PC-MRI acquisition can be performed by established two-dimensional (2D) sequences as well as by more recent four-dimensional (4D) techniques.

2D PC-MRI

The physical principle behind any phase contrast sequence (2D and 4D) is to encode velocity in the phase of a moving proton. This is achieved by sequentially applying magnetic gradients with equal magnitude but opposite polarity (also called bipolar gradients) (Fig. 15.1). A stationary proton will subsequently experience a magnetic field of equal magnitude, but opposite direction, and will therefore gain no net phase shift ($\Delta\phi = 0$). It can

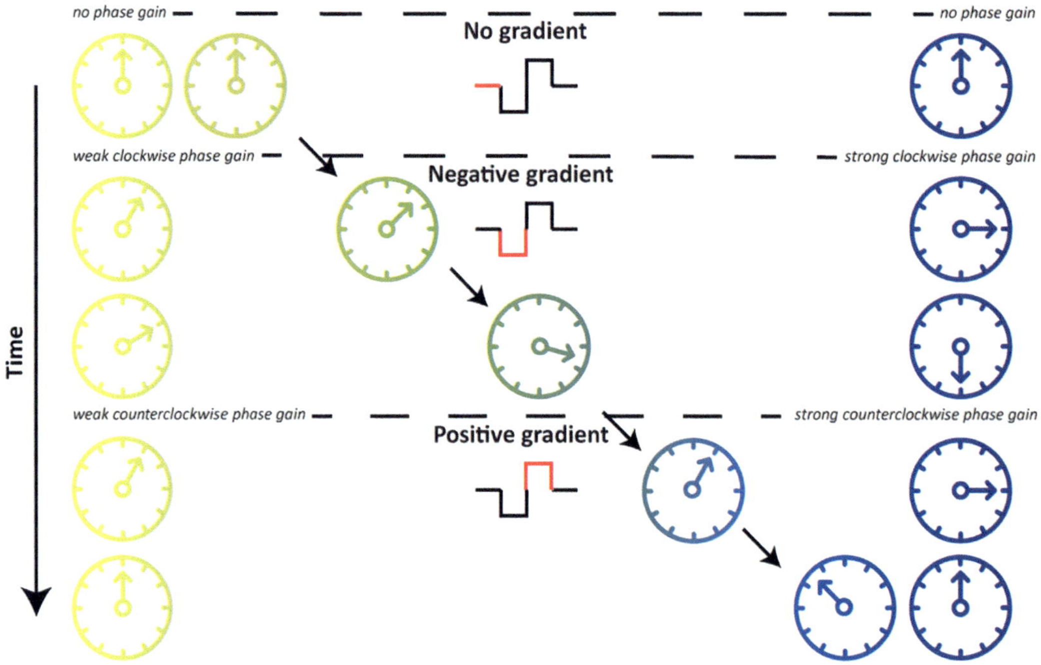

Fig. 15.1 Schematic representation of phase-contrast MRI physical principles. If spins move through a changing magnetic field, the speed at which they precess changes. The top spins all experience the same magnetic field and therefore remain in phase. When the negative gradient lobe is applied, the yellow spins gain phase slower than the blue spins. When a spin moves from the left to the right, the speed at which it gains phase increases, so it will gain phase compared to the yellow spins, while it still lags behind the blue spins. When the magnetic field gradient is inverted, the blue and yellow spins return to their original phase, but the moving spin does not return completely to its initial position: it gains a phase shift which is proportional to its velocity

be mathematically derived that a proton moving with constant velocity v will acquire a phase shift proportional to its velocity. If we assume a bipolar gradient of magnitude -G between $0 < t < T$; G for $T < t < 2T$ and zero otherwise, and if we assume all motion to be in the direction of G, we can state that for $t > 2T$ (after application of the gradients):

$$\Delta\varphi(t > 2T) = \gamma \int_0^t \boldsymbol{G}(\tau) \cdot \boldsymbol{r}(\tau) d\tau$$

$$= \gamma \left(\int_0^T -G(x_0 + v\tau) d\tau + \int_T^{2T} G(x_0 + v\tau) d\tau \right)$$

Here, $\Delta\gamma$ equals the gyromagnetic ratio, $\boldsymbol{G}$ the gradient vector, and $\boldsymbol{r}$ the vector location of the proton, and x_0 the initial position of the proton along the gradient direction. For stationary spins, this cancels out, but for moving spins, the phase shift equals:

$$\Delta\phi = \gamma G v T^2$$

Note that we made some important assumptions here. First, we assumed all flow to be in the direction of the gradient. Practically, this means that we must ensure that our imaging plane is orthogonal to the vessel, since in that case, the scanner will apply a gradient in the direction of the vessel. Second, we ignored all higher-order terms: we only considered stationary spins and spins moving with constant velocity. The equation therefore is not valid if blood is accelerating (or decelerating). In case of turbulent flow, as may occur close to vessel stenosis, both conditions are violated. Therefore, 2D phase contrast MRI always has to be applied in a straight part of the vessel, avoiding any vessel wall irregularities.

Any spin moving at a velocity resulting in a phase shift of more than $\pm\pi$ radians will cause aliasing or phase wrapping on the resulting phase image. This can be avoided by choosing a gradient strength (G) that is small enough to ensure that the phase shift will be below $\pm\pi$ even for the fastest moving spins. On the scanner, this can be achieved by choosing the encoding velocity v_{enc} slightly higher than the highest velocity expected. The encoding velocity may be computed using the following equation:

$$v_{enc} = \frac{\pi}{\gamma G T^2}$$

In terms of venc, the velocity map can be calculated from the phase image as follows:

$$v = \frac{\Delta\phi}{\gamma G T^2} = \frac{v_{enc}}{\pi} \Delta\phi$$

Note that image signal-to-noise ratio (SNR) depends on venc as well, and in terms of SNR, it is preferable to keep venc as low as possible.

To account for local changes in magnetic field strength, the entire acquisition is repeated in the opposite order (first applying G and subsequently $-G$). By subtracting the obtained phase maps, susceptibility-induced phase shifts cancel out.

Since the application of a bipolar gradient does not delete the local susceptibility contribution, it is necessary to repeat the process and apply an inverted bipolar gradient, which causes the phase shift to switch in the opposite direction. By subtracting the two signal values from each other, no signal is detected in stationary tissue and at the same time motion-related signal enhances. Because susceptibility changes are in the same direction for both bipolar gradients, the contribution of susceptibility to the phase shift is also removed [4].

Since arterial flow is pulsatile, ECG triggering is typically used. Cardiac-gated flow measurement produces a set of *frames* that offer the anatomy and velocity information at different points of time in the cardiac cycle. The most widely used technique to acquire data in all time frames is k-space segmentation: within each heartbeat, a number of k-space lines, called views per segment (VPS), are sampled for each frame. The time resolution T_{res} is defined as the product of TR and VPS and represents the number of times that each k-space line is sampled. In some systems, it is possible to increase the number of frames by linear interpolation of data from adjacent frames. This technique, named *view sharing*, can improve the temporal resolution and allows the more efficient collection of data [5]. The user can set the VPS only if the sequence provides the option of modifying the number of cardiac frames to be reconstructed from the acquired data. At least 20 flow-encoded 2D images are typically

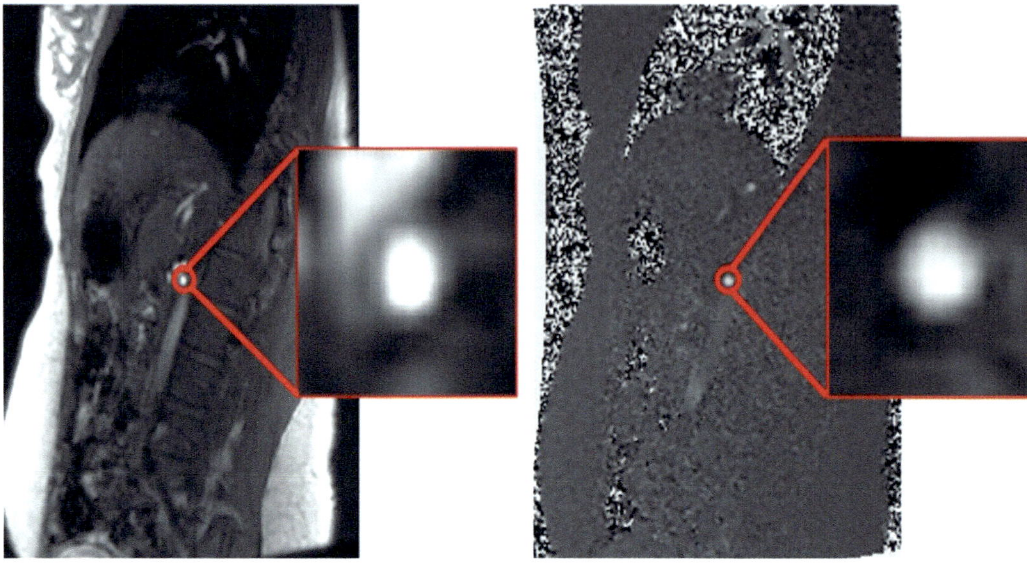

Fig. 15.2 Representative magnitude (left) and velocity images (right) obtained by 2D phase-contrast MRI of the renal artery. The Figure was modified from Villa G. et al. MAGMA 2020 [1] under the terms of Creative Commons Attribution 4.0 (CC-BY-4.0) International license

acquired within the cardiac cycle, and 10–20 cardiac cycles are needed to completely fill the k-space. After reconstruction, PC-MRI acquisition finally provides two sets of images: the magnitude images that depict the anatomy and the velocity maps, also called phase images (Fig. 15.2).

Recently, the renal MRI network "Magnetic Resonance Imaging Biomarkers for Chronic Kidney Disease" (PARENCHIMA) has published a set of technical recommendations for renal 2D PC-MRI acquisition based on consensus by an international panel of experts in the field [Table 15.1] [3].

2D PC-MRI of the renal arteries is generally based on a 2D spoiled gradient echo pulse sequence.

Repetition time (TR) and echo time (TE) should be as short as possible to allow fast imaging and avoid artifacts. The flip angle (usually between 10° and 30°) should be low enough to allow rapid imaging but higher than the minimum flip angle to increase inflow enhancement. One breath-hold acquisition per renal artery should be acquired, preferably within 20 s [3].

The spatial resolution should be high enough to obtain multiple voxels in the renal artery (and thus obtain reasonably accurate RBF values) and low enough to maintain a sufficient SNR. An in-plane resolution below 1.5 mm and a through-plane resolution of 3–6 mm are recommended.

The orientation of the measurement slice should be perpendicular to the vessel direction, as only the through-plane velocity component is acquired. To provide PC-MRI data of sufficient quality, a high-quality vascular survey is recommended (such as time-of-flight (TOF) MR angiography or inflow-dependent inversion recovery (IFDIR) scan, see section Non-Contrast-Enhanced MRA), reconstructed in all three orthogonal views. This will allow accurate planning of the acquisition plane, ensuring its orthogonality to the vessel direction and positioning prior to any artery bifurcation (Fig. 15.3a). Acquisition should be performed in a single breath-hold, preferably in expiration to improve reproducibility, using either cardiac triggering or, if the patient is uncooperative, respiratory triggering [3].

Measuring RBF directly on the renal arteries is generally recommended. If the tortuosity or small size of the renal arteries hinders the posi-

Table 15.1 2D PC-MRI acquisition recommendations

1. Preparation of acquisition
1.1 A vascular survey should be performed at least in the coronal and transverse directions to ensure perpendicular planning. Optimal vascular survey depends on experience and availability in the center, with IFDIR or TOF MRA being recommended
2. Planning of acquisition
2.1 2D PC-MRI should be scanned perpendicular to the vessel of interest, preferably on the renal arteries
2.2 If planning on the renal arteries is not possible due to limited size or tortuosity of the vessels, blood flow can be measured through the aorta above and below the branches of the renal arteries.
2.3 2D phase contrast MRI should be planned on a linear part of the renal artery without apparent vascular abnormalities (stenoses, string-of-beads), preferably not too close to the aorta (roughly >1 cm)
2.4 In case of planning on the aorta, the upper acquisition plane should be placed below the superior mesenteric artery and above the renal arteries, while the lower acquisition plane should be planned below the main renal arteries, below any accessory renal arteries and above the ovarian/testicular arteries
3.Acquisition
A slice thickness of 3–6 mm is recommended
3.1 The acquired in-plane voxel size is recommended to be below 1.5 mm
3.2 The shortest possible TE should be used, with a max value of 4 ms
3.3 The shortest possible TR (Siemens and GE: Echospacing) should be used, with a max value of 10 ms
3.4 A flip angle between 10 and 30° is recommended for non-contrast acquisitions.
3.5 Parallel imaging is recommended when there is need to shorten breath-hold duration.
4. Choice of venc
4.1 It is recommended to choose a fixed venc throughout the study but check the examination for phase wrapping and repeat with higher venc if necessary
4.2 For the renal arteries, a venc of 100–120 cm/s is recommended for healthy volunteers, while for populations with suspected vascular disease, a higher venc of 150 cm/s can be indicated
4.3 For the aorta, a venc of 150 cm/s is recommended for healthy volunteers, while for populations with suspected vascular disease, a venc of 200 cm/s is recommended
5. Motion correction
5.1 Cardiac synchronization should be performed either using retrospective or prospective triggering
5.2 Cardiac triggering should preferably be performed with ECG
5.3 The number of time points acquired should be maximized within reasonable scan time, with at least 20 time points per cardiac cycle
5.4 Breath-holding is preferred for respiratory compensation. If impossible, respiratory triggering can be used
5.5 The max breath-hold time should preferably be below 20s
5.6 If breathholding is used, preferably one breathhold per artery should be used

tioning of the acquisition plane, blood flow can be measured in the aorta just above and below renal arteries' branching, and total RBF can be computed as the difference between the two aortic flows [6], since inflow should equal outflow. Main advantages of measuring blood flow in the aorta are: easier vessel detection, easier planning of the acquisition plane, and limited respiratory motion that minimizes blurring of the vessel contour [6]. Conversely, the main disadvantage is accidental inclusion of other arteries (i.e., mesenterical or gonadal arteries) and consequently incorrect estimation of RBF (Fig. 15.3b) [3]. There is no single optimal venc value for the acquisition of renal 2D PC-MRI. A venc of 100–120 cm/s is recommended to acquire RBF in healthy volunteers, while a venc of 150 cm/s is recommended in subjects with suspected vascular disease, to reflect the higher peak velocities reached in (atherosclerotic) vascular disease. Due to higher peak flow in the aorta, a higher venc is recommended for the aorta [3].

4D Flow MRI

Recent developments allow the investigation of blood flow dynamics with full volumetric cover-

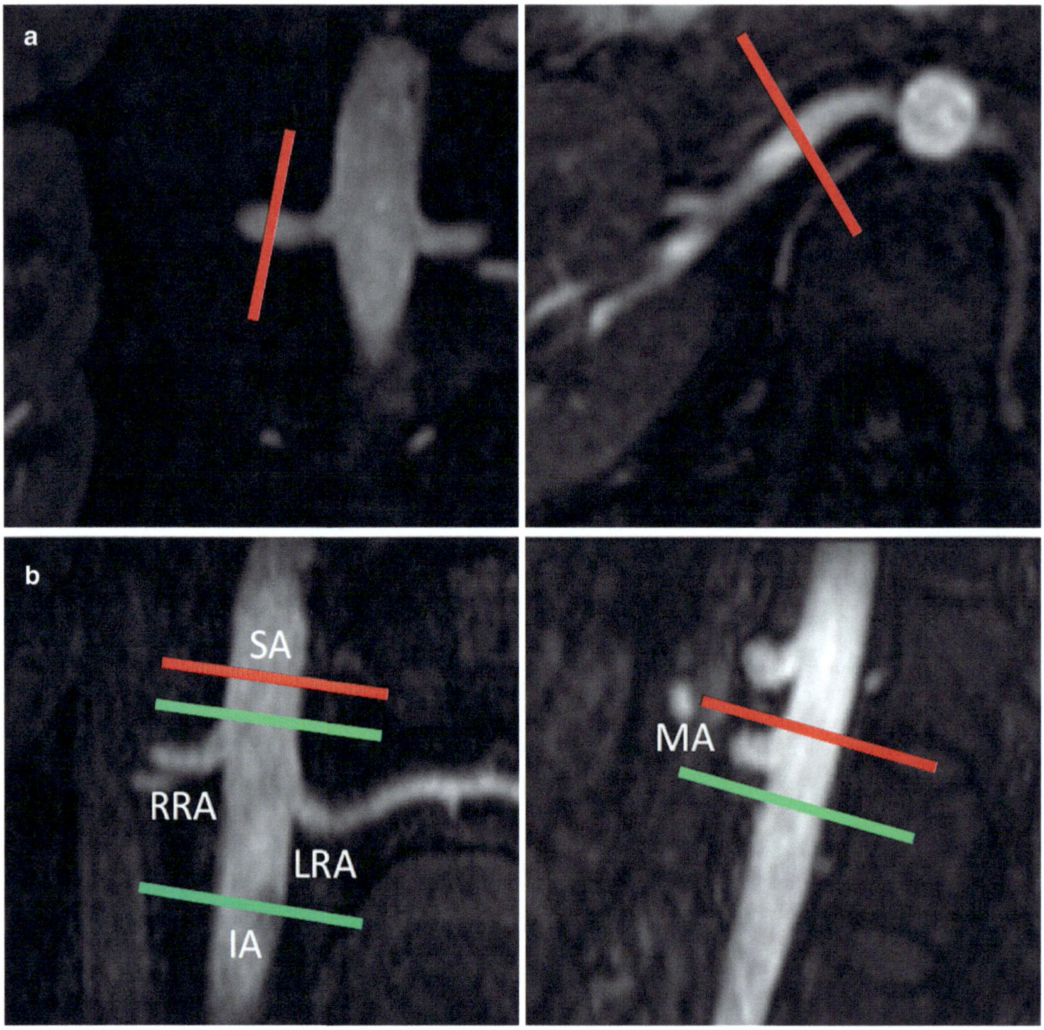

Fig. 15.3 2D phase-contrast MRI acquisition plane setting. (**a**) While acquiring 2D-PC MRI of the renal arteries, the acquisition plane should be placed orthogonally to the direction of the vessel of interest, prior to any bifurcation, taking a survey image as reference (in this case, a non-contrast-enhanced MR angiography, reconstructed in both coronal (left) and axial views (right)). (**b**) While acquiring 2D-PC MRI of the aorta, to compute renal blood flow as the difference between aortic flows, special care should be taken not to include between superior and inferior aorta planes any unwanted arteries, such as the superior mesenteric artery (as in the case of the red plane) or the testicular/ovarian arteries. Abbreviations: SA (Superior Aorta), IA (Inferior Aorta), RRA (Right Renal Artery), LRA (Left Renal Artery), MA (Mesenteric Artery)

age of the anatomical area of interest. The term "4D flow MRI" (or 3D-CINE PC-MRI) refers to three-dimensional (3D) data acquisition in time, with three-directional velocity encoding. 4D flow MRI data can be obtained by standard Cartesian or radial image acquisition [7]. As in 2D PC-MRI, cardiac synchronization is used to obtain a velocity map for each point in the cardiac cycle and segmented k-space acquisition is used to distribute data acquisition over as many cardiac cycles as needed.

Similar to 2D PC-MRI sequence acquisition, originally the six-point method was used to acquire 4D flow MRI: for each direction (x, y, and z), a pair of measurements was obtained (to correct for susceptibility errors). Essentially, the

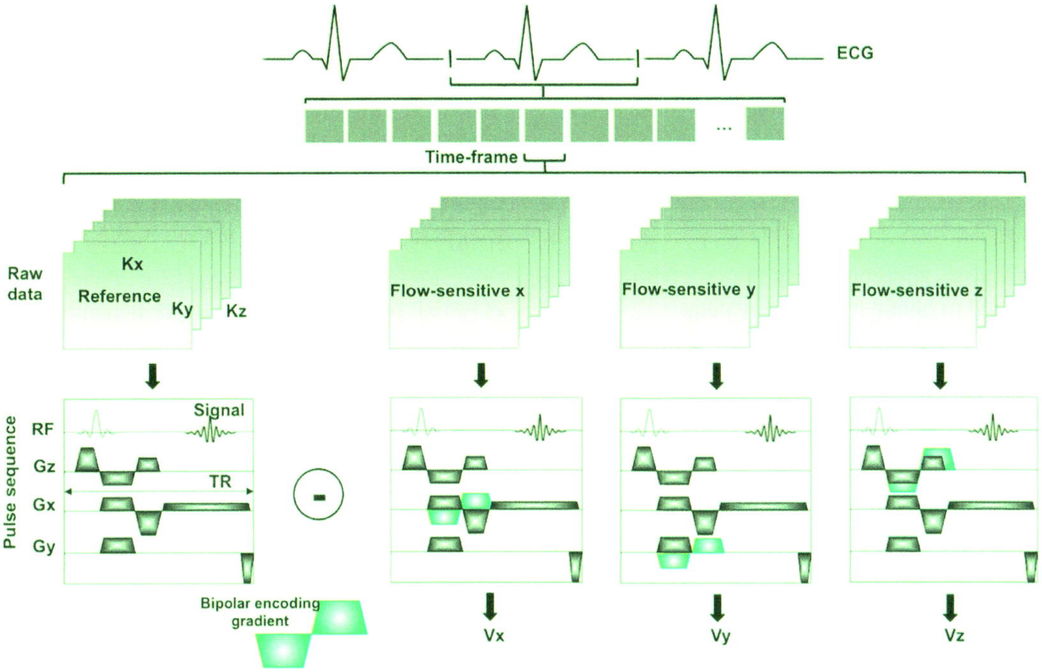

Fig. 15.4 Schematic overview of 4D flow MRI. For each time frame acquired within the cardiac cycle, a reference and three flow-sensitive scans are collected. Velocity encoding gradients are applied in all three directions, and subtraction of phase images provides phase difference images that contain quantitative blood flow velocities

velocity maps for each direction were acquired sequentially, applying velocity encoding in only one direction at a time. However, it is possible to obtain all necessary information in only four scans. For each scan, velocity encoding gradients in all three directions are applied simultaneously. A clever combination of the four resulting images yields velocity maps in all three directions and a magnitude image. This is called the four-point method (Fig. 15.4) [7].

Despite the one-third reduction in scan time achieved by the four-point method compared to the traditional six-point approach, acquisition time in 4D flow MRI remains extremely long: a 3D volume has to be sampled at around 15 points in the cardiac cycle, and this has to be repeated four times to obtain data in all three directions. Therefore, advanced techniques for scan-time reduction have been employed to comply with the need for high spatial resolution or large volumetric coverage while keeping the scan time to clinically feasible durations. Examples include parallel imaging, which yields a reduction in scan time up to a factor of 3 [8] and alternative sampling strategies employing correlations in the spatiotemporal domain, for example k-t BLAST (Broad-use Linear Acquisition Speed-up Technique) or combinations of both (k-t SENSitivity Encoding, k-t SENSE). Another approach makes use of radial undersampling [7]: PC VIPR (vastly undersampled isotropic projection reconstruction) offers large imaging volume coverage with high and isotropic spatial resolution, allowing for lossless reformatting in oblique planes. Furthermore, partial voluming artifacts and intravoxel dephasing are minimized. This comes at a cost in SNR, as streak artifacts and sometimes image degradation (blurring and signal loss) can result from mistakes in implementation. The latter can be overcome by k-space trajectory corrections and off-resonance corrections [7]. It is possible to save additional scan time for cardiac-gated acquisitions by using temporal filtering, which provides a greater flexibility for "view sharing" of radial data when compared with Cartesian datasets [7].

Since 4D flow MRI requires considerably longer scan time than the traditional 2D-CINE PC-MRI sequence, it cannot be performed in a single breath-hold, hence the need for respiratory control (usually performed by respiratory bellows reading or navigator gating) to attenuate motion artifacts. Radial imaging is relatively insensitive to motion and is therefore preferred. However, additional respiratory control is still needed to obtain high-quality data.

However, if data is acquired with a breathing position outside the predefined range, respiratory gating results in data loss and becomes less effective. Adaptive k-space reordering prevents the formation of ghosting artifacts when the acceptable range of breathing positions is extended, instead of generating diffuse noise along the phase-encoding direction. This is achieved by grouping the k-space lines according to their respiratory position, rather than acquiring them incrementally, thus removing the periodicity in k-space in the phase-encoding direction. For example, all lower lines might be acquired in inspiration and all higher k-space lines in expiration [7]. Navigator gating, despite being widely adopted for 4D flow measurements, has the disadvantage of permitting only one or two navigators per cardiac cycle, often hampering prediction of respiratory motion for the cardiac phases acquired long after the navigator signal. Furthermore, the incorporation of the navigator within the scan naturally causes an increase in acquisition time. To overcome this, self-gating methods have been developed, based on the fact that every point in k-space carries information of the entire excited volume and therefore contains information on motion (both respiratory and cardiac) as well. Hence, motion can be estimated by repetitive sampling of a single predefined k-space profile during image acquisition. In radial sequences, this self-navigator can be implemented without an additional increase in acquisition time and can be used both for respiratory and cardiac gating [7].

Lastly, instead of rejecting any data that happened to be acquired outside of the motion window, retrospective motion correction algorithms have been developed. Based on an estimate of the underlying motion, which can be obtained by respiratory belts, navigators, or self-gating signals, the data is motion-corrected and can be used for image formation [7].

PC-MRI Post-Processing and Data Analysis Methods

PC-MRI postprocessing changes depending on the acquisition sequence.

2D PC-MRI

Before processing the velocity images, a careful visual inspection is needed to rule out the presence of possible issues and artifacts. If artifacts occur in a single time frame, the affected frame should be removed; if artifacts occur in multiple time frames, the entire examination should be discarded [1].

Post-hoc motion correction can be performed by either rigid or affine image registration to deal with possible misalignments due to artery motion during the cardiac cycle and/or those misalignments that occur despite breath-holding [3].

Circular and elliptical regions of interest (ROIs) are commonly drawn either on magnitude or velocity images, covering the lumen but not the wall of the vessel of interest (Fig. 15.5) using manual, semi-automatic, or automatic methods (such as adaptive thresholding [9], graph searching [10], active contour [11, 12], paraboloid velocity profiles [13], and k-means clustering) [14].

The mean blood velocity (expressed in cm/s) is computed as the average of the signal in the velocity images over all segmented pixels of all time frames [6, 15]. Then, the mean blood flow (Q, expressed in mL/min) is computed by multiplying the mean velocity (v_{mean}, in cm/sec) by the ROI area (A) and the conversion factor from seconds to minutes (Fig. 15.6):

$$Q = 60 \cdot A \cdot v_{\text{mean}}$$

Making use of clinical (arterial pressure), blood (hematocrit), and functional parameters (measured or estimated GFR), a number of derivative hemodynamic parameters can be computed in addition to RBF, the main ones being: 1) renal

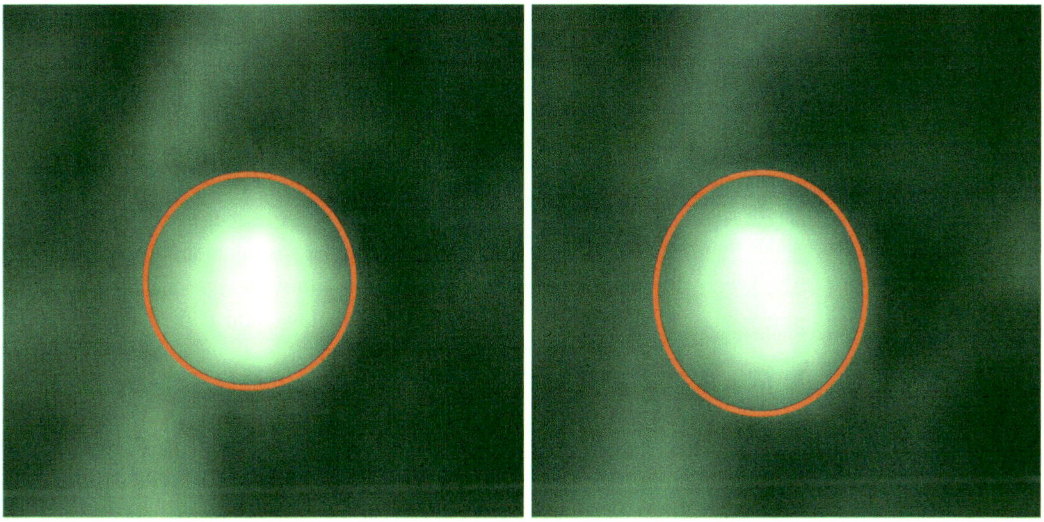

Fig. 15.5 Example of circular (left) and elliptical renal artery regions of interest (right)

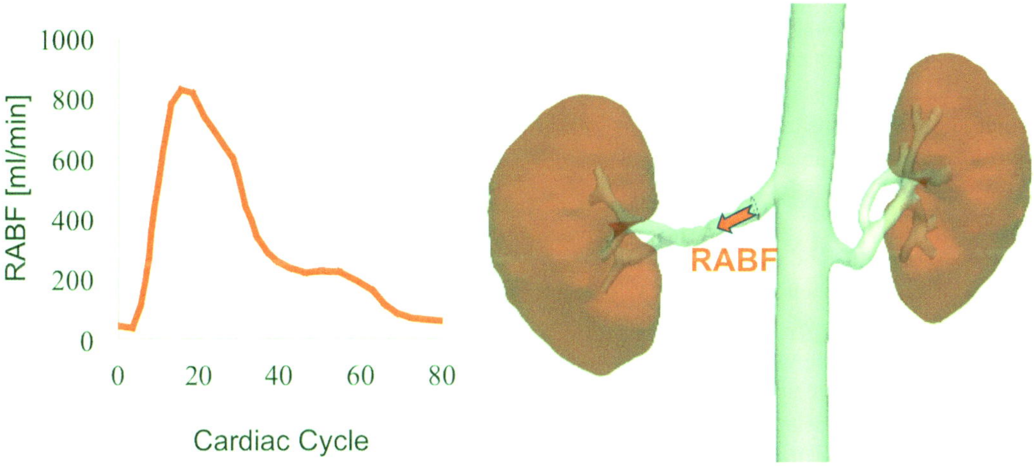

Fig. 15.6 Renal artery blood flow computation. Renal artery blood flow (RABF) is computed in each time frame of the cardiac cycle as blood flow velocity by renal artery area, resulting in a RABF plot (left). Mean RABF, visually shown on the 3D reconstruction (right), is computed as the average over the cardiac cycle. The Figure was modified from Villa G. et al. MAGMA 2020 [1] under the terms of Creative Commons Attribution 4.0 (CC-BY-4.0) International license

plasma flow (RPF), computed as product of RBF times (1-hematocrit) and representing the volume of plasma that reaches the kidneys per unit time; 2) renal vascular resistance, obtained as the ratio of RBF to mean arterial pressure (MAP) [16–19], which measures the degree to which the blood vessels of the kidneys impede the flow of blood through them; and 3) filtration fraction, obtained as the ratio of the GFR to the renal plasma flow, and measuring the proportion of fluid reaching the kidneys that passes into the renal tubules [17, 20, 21].

Consensus recommendations for 2D PC-MRI processing include, beyond post-hoc motion correction, the use of (semi-)automated approaches to select ROIs, either based on thresholding of magnitude or phase images or based on the flow profile. If the use of a (semi-)automated approach

Table 15.2 2D PC-MRI postprocessing recommendations

1. Post-hoc motion correction (ie. Image registration, either rigid or affine) is recommended
2. A (semi-)automated approach for ROI selection is recommended; however, if that is not available, manual ROI selection can be used
3. If ROIs are drawn manually, it is recommended to draw them on each magnitude frame
4. In case of manual ROI selection, it is recommended to draw a circular ROI
5. In case of artifacts in a single time frame, the affected frame should be removed
6. In case of artifacts in multiple time frames, the entire examination should be discarded
7. Phase unwrapping should be performed if necessary

The Table was adapted from de Boer et al. J Magn Reson Imaging 2020 [3] under the terms of Creative Commons Attribution 4.0 (CC-BY-4.0) International license.

is not possible, circular ROIs should be drawn manually on each magnitude image. In the latter case, post-hoc motion correction is not necessary but special attention should be paid to cover the whole lumen to ensure capturing the whole velocity spectrum [Table 15.2] [3].

4D Flow MRI

Prior to 4D flow MRI data processing or visualization, it is recommended to address possible issues and artifacts that could affect the 3D visualization and blood flow quantification, such as background phase contributions from eddy-currents, velocity aliasing and noise, or Maxwell terms or gradient field distortions [7]. Appropriate correction strategies have been proposed and validated in the literature [22–24].

For optimal 4D flow MRI analysis and 3D hemodynamic visualization, it is recommended to combine anatomical information with 3D blood flow data. 4D flow MRI can generate 3D MR angiograms (PC MRAs), obtained by projection reconstruction, depicting vascular morphology of the kidney. As previously mentioned, the choice of venc value strongly influences the quality of the vessel depiction: small venc values allows accurate depiction of small vessels characterized by slow flow, but not larger vessels due to aliasing of higher flow velocities. An increment in venc can improve the visualization of large arterial vessels but increases noise in the venous signal [7].

The most widely used method for visualizing 4D flow MRI data is the vector graph display. Intuitively, the vector graph shows the magnitude and direction of blood velocity within a specific voxel based on three-directional velocity data. Streamlines can be visualized, showing the path that a particle without mass would take in a temporally constant flow field (Fig. 15.7) [25]. For nonstationary pulsatile flow, a visualization of the current path over time is obtained using time-resolved 3D particle tracing or pathlines, showing massless particles that are delivered at user-defined points (regions, planes, or volumes) within the acquired data volume and follow the flow field over time. This is an intuitive method to visualize the temporal evolution of the blood flow velocity data over one or multiple heartbeats [7].

In 4D flow MRI, the selection of the volume of interest and the quantification of blood flow velocities can be performed post hoc, and therefore, errors due to misalignment of the analysis plane are reduced compared to traditional 2D PC-MRI. Moreover, planning of the scan volume is simpler, requiring the positioning of a single 3D volume rather than a series of double oblique scan planes orthogonal to the vessels of interest. Recent studies have demonstrated excellent correlation between standard 2D CINE PC-MRI and 4D flow MRI for quantitative blood flow measurements [26]. As for standard 2D CINE PC-MRI, 4D flow MRI also allows the calculation of regional flow parameters such as peak velocity, time-to-peak flow, total flow, and retrograde flow. In addition, 4D flow MRI makes it possible to determine other hemodynamic parameters such as wall shear stress, pulse wave velocity, pressure difference, or turbulent kinetic energy [7].

PC-MRI Clinical Applications

Despite renal PC-MRI being not yet routinely used in clinical practice, there are several clinical studies showing potential for clinical application in renal disease.

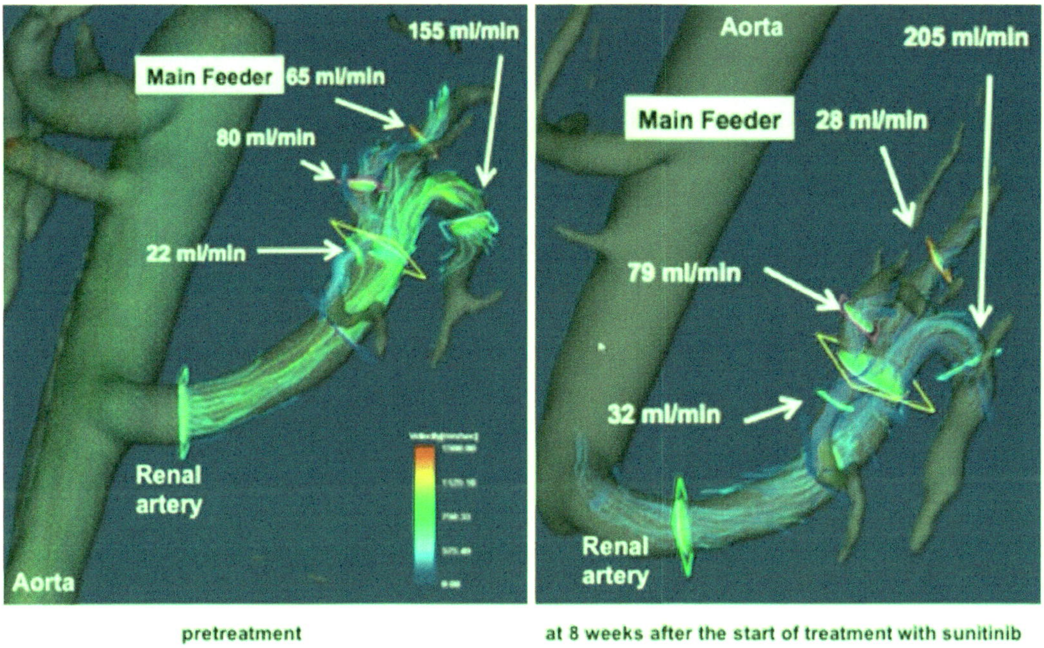

Fig. 15.7 Example of 4D flow MRI data visualization. Renal artery flows were measured by 4D flow MRI in a renal cell carcinoma patient treated with sunitinib and visualized as streamlines. The regions of branches where flows were measured are shown. Blood flow in the main feeder to the tumor decreased after treatment (right), while flow rates in the other branches increased simultaneously, possibly indicating flow redistribution from the tumor to other kidney segments. Figure reprinted from Takayama T et al. BMC Res Notes 2014 [25] under the terms of the Creative Commons Attribution 2.0 (CC-BY-2.0) International license

Chronic Kidney Disease

Hemodynamic and metabolic factors play an important role in the development of chronic kidney disease (CKD). Reduced renal blood flow accompanied by intrarenal ischemia may contribute to the formation of fibrosis in the renal parenchyma. In healthy subjects, the kidneys can regulate blood flow over a wide range of blood pressures, maintaining glomerular pressure and filtration rate. But in CKD patients, the kidneys lose this capability, and renal function declines with RBF decrease. Furthermore, in CKD patients, renal hemodynamics can be influenced by a wide range of drugs, including diuretics and renin-angiotensin-system inhibitors.

Despite PC-MRI not being routinely used in clinical practice to assess RBF in CKD patients, it has been used in a few clinical studies with promising findings. Khatir et al. have demonstrated a good reproducibility of respiratory-gated PC-MRI in CKD patients and healthy volunteers (HVs), examined 1–2 weeks apart [16]. RBF measured by PC-MRI was significantly lower in CKD patients compared to HVs [16, 27, 28], even in patients with mild-to-moderate CKD, although the HVs were 8 years younger [29]. Thanks to the combination of PC-MRI and arterial spin labeling (ASL), it was possible to differentiate healthy kidneys from kidneys with vascular, parenchymal, or combined disease [30]. In CKD patients, measured GFR decreased more than RBF, causing a reduction in filtration fraction that may reflect an adaptation to maintain intra-renal oxygenation within normal range [28]. Lastly, Khatir et al. used PC-MRI to measure RBF and calculate renal vascular resistance for evaluating and comparing vasodilatory and non-vasodilatory antihypertensive treatment in CKD patients. After 18 months, RBF had significantly increased in both groups, although the change was not different between groups [31].

Acute Kidney Injury

The increase or decrease in RBF is considered critical to the etiology of acute kidney injury (AKI). However, PC-MRI has been used rarely in AKI patients, perhaps due to the logistical difficulties of scanning acutely unwell patients. PC-MRI has been successfully performed in a pilot study in 10 patients with sepsis-associated AKI (eight mechanically ventilated, nine on continuous hemofiltration, and five requiring vasopressors). RBF and cardiac output (CO) were measured and compared with 11 HVs, showing a significantly reduced RBF in AKI patients as compared with HVs (482 vs. 1260 mL/min), a considerable inter-individual variability in RBF measures in the AKI group (ranging 335–1137 mL/min), and a reduction in the renal fraction of cardiac output [32].

Renovascular Disease/Renal Artery Stenosis

Renal artery stenosis (RAS) occurs in 1–5% of people with hypertension, often in combination with peripheral arterial or coronary artery disease. Beyond hypertension, RAS may result in ischemic nephropathy and multiple long-term complications. Among the elderly, RAS prevalence may increase up to 7%.

Few studies have investigated PC-MRI clinical utility in the context of renovascular disease [30, 33–36]. 2D Cine PC-MRI demonstrated a dampened but longer systolic wave in RAS [35–37] and showed that blood flow velocity curves had 100% sensitivity and 93% specificity to anatomical stenosis in 23 patients with 48 areas of RAS [38]. Renal hilar velocity waveforms, measured using non-breath-hold PC-MRI with or without an ACE inhibitor, were insufficiently accurate to predict renal artery stenosis [33]. In a pilot study, interleaved gradient echo-planar technique (IGEPI) and conventional Cine PC-MRI techniques were compared, and IGEPI was able to detect 5/5 high-grade stenosis versus 3/5 (66%) detected with conventional Cine PC-MRI [39]. Later, Schoenberg et al. studied the combination of morphologic (3D gadolinium MRA) and functional MR examination (cine phase-contrast flow measurement) demonstrating that this significantly reduced inter-observer variability across seven readers evaluating 43 renal arteries, offering reliable and reproducible grading of RAS if compared with X-ray digital subtraction angiography (DSA) [36–40]. In another study, RBF and renal volume were combined to determine functional significance of RAS lesions [35]. Eighteen out of 31 RAS kidneys had significantly reduced volume and significantly reduced blood flow (91.56 vs 279.15 mL/min without RAS). The Renal Flow Index (RFI, computed as the ratio of blood flow to renal volume) had only minimal overlap between kidneys with and without RAS, showing promise to predict RAS hemodynamic significance. Later, the same group investigated whether positive clinical outcomes (defined as a fall in diastolic blood pressure of >15% or a fall in creatinine of >20%) could be predicted by RFI in a group of 23 patients undergoing percutaneous angioplasty [34]. The RFI sensitivity to predict response to therapy was reasonable (91%), but specificity was low, suggesting a significant rate of unnecessary procedures. RFI <1.5 mL/min/cm^3 reached 100% sensitivity but had a 33% specificity that could be improved to 67% by combining RFI with clinical variables.

Autosomal Dominant Polycystic Kidney Disease

In 2003, King et al. used PC-MRI to measure RBF in 127 patients with early autosomal dominant polycystic kidney disease (ADPKD), showing that RBF had high accuracy and intra- and inter-observer reproducibility, strongly correlated with both renal volumes and GFR, and predicted GFR [18]. Another study by the same group demonstrated a negative correlation between RBF decrease over a 3-year follow-up, as well as total kidney volume (TKV) and total cyst volume slopes and a good correlation between baseline RBF and GFR slope in 131 patients with early ADPKD [17]. The latter suggests that RBF can predict structural and functional disease progression and may be considered as an outcome measure in ADPKD clinical trials. A small clinical trial used PC-MRI to investigate the short-term effects of Tolvaptan in patients with ADPKD on

RBF, alongside GFR and TKV; no RBF change was observed after 1 week of Tolvaptan treatment, but PC-MRI and PAH clearance flow measurements showed a good correlation [41]. More recently, RBF measurement by PC-MRI was further validated by comparison with continuous hippuran infusion. The study included a cohort of 91 ADPKD patients with a wide range of estimated GFR (eGFR) values. Although RBF was associated with ADPKD severity, technical problems in RBF quantification were predominantly reported in patients with lower eGFR (<70 mL/min). This suggests that RBF evaluation could be less feasible in patients with ADPKD at an advanced stage, likely due to the difficulty of identifying renal arteries and correctly setting the orthogonal planes for PC-MRI acquisition [42]. Kline et al. used PC-MRI as part of a comprehensive multi-parametric renal MRI protocol in a small cohort of young patients with early stage ADPKD and healthy controls [43]. The results showed no statistically significant difference in RBF between young ADPKD patients and the healthy controls. Nevertheless, the combination of PC-MRI with other quantitative renal MR techniques allowed a comprehensive characterization of the ADPKD kidney tissue and function.

Renal Transplantation

4D PC-VIPR MRI was recently used in association with non-contrast-enhanced MRA to depict renal artery branches and assess blood flow velocities in living transplant recipients, respectively. Blood flow velocities measured using 4D PC-VIPR and Doppler Ultrasonography demonstrated significant correlations, suggesting that 4D PC-VIPR in combination with MRA could be useful for evaluation of renal arteries in transplant recipients without the need for contrast media [44].

Common Issues and Artifacts

There are a number of common issues and possible artifacts to pay attention to during PC-MRI acquisition and processing in order to obtain accurate and reliable RBF measurements.

Noise

The SNR of the velocity map depends on the SNR of the magnitude image and the difference between the measured velocity and the encoded velocity (venc). The smaller the SNR of the magnitude image, the noisier the velocity map. The larger the difference between the actual velocity and the venc, the lower the SNR of the measurement. Since velocities much lower than venc cannot be measured reliably, venc should be kept as low as possible. RBF measurement precision can be increased by matching venc to the maximum velocity in the region of interest. Furthermore, noise is inversely proportional to the signal-to-noise ratio (SNR) of the magnitude image. Optimizing sequence parameters like slab thickness and voxel size, flip angle, echo time, and the receiver bandwidth results in optimal SNR [5]. A compromise should be reached between SNR, optimal image resolution to avoid partial voluming in the relatively small renal vessels, and short TE to minimize scan time [5].

Aliasing

Aliasing occurs when the phase difference exceeds $\pm\pi$. Since phase is essentially a polar angle, it is only uniquely defined within the range from $-\pi$ to π. If, due to choosing a venc that is too low, a spin gains a phase shift of more than π, say 1.5π, it is indiscernible from any spin gaining a phase of -0.5π (Fig. 15.8) and will be attributed an erroneous velocity of $-0.5v_{enc}$ [45].

Several approaches are available to choose the optimal venc. First, for optimizing an acquisition with low venc, it is necessary to acquire several PC-MRI scans until the peak velocity is free of aliasing. Acquiring images at multiple vencs within one breath-hold can help this iterative optimization; however, due to reduced spatial and temporal resolution, this approach can miss some aliasing. The latter issue can be solved by aggressive scan-time acceleration. It is also possible to correct flow-related aliased images using a post-processing technique called phase unwrapping [46–49]. In practice, some SNR is sacrificed to assure a venc sufficiently high to avoid aliasing. If aliasing still occurs and it cannot be corrected for, the PC-MRI acquisition should be repeated with a higher value of venc [45].

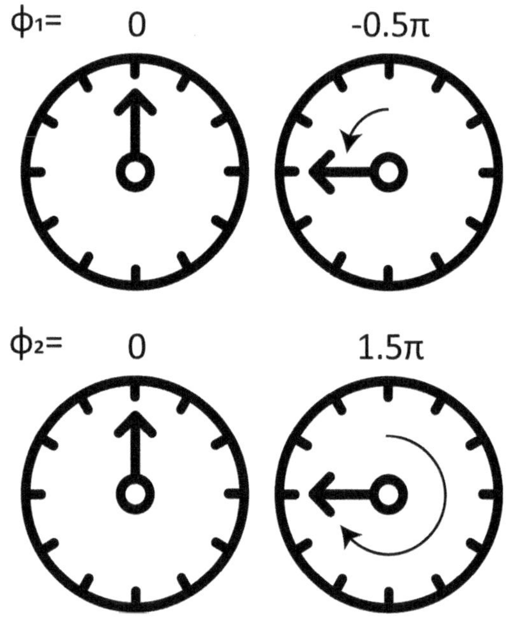

Fig. 15.8 Aliasing or phase wrapping. A phase shift of -0.5π radians cannot be discriminated from a phase of 1.5π (or any other phase that differs by a multiple of 2π). A phase shift of -0.5π radians corresponds to a velocity of $-0.5v_{enc}$, and a spin gaining a phase shift of 1.5π will also be attributed erroneously a velocity of $-0.5v_{enc}$, although it actually moved with a velocity of $1.5v_{enc}$

Deviation of Imaging Plane

In 2D PC-MRI, the imaging plane must be positioned perpendicular to the main direction of flow. Through-plane flow encoding must be used to assure that the flow is perpendicular to the image plane. In-plane flow encoding should not be used for quantification of flow due to increased partial volume effects and the inability of 2D PC-MRI to show the entire diameter of the vessel. Deviation of ±15° from the perpendicular imaging plane is acceptable for quantification of flow, while higher deviations may lead to significant underestimation of actual flow [5].

Inadequate Temporal Resolution

Inadequate temporal resolution (k-space line undersampling) may lead to missing the peak. Although possibly improving the temporal resolution of the measurement, interpolation (view sharing) will not be helpful to resolve the issue, since the true temporal resolution of the data collected will remain unchanged [5].

Inadequate Spatial Resolution

Significant partial volume effects, possibly generated by exceeding the vessel diameter by one-third and by acquiring MR data at low spatial resolution, cause underestimation of the flow and peak velocity [5].

Accelerated Flow and Spatial Misregistration

PC-MRI measurements are optimized for linear flow, while accelerated or turbulent flow may cause inaccurate flow measurement. This issue can be overcome by acquiring PC-MRI data with short TE. Possible spatial misregistration, for instance resulting from patient movement, can be avoided or minimized by electrocardiographic gating and breath-holding [5].

Phase Offset Errors

Every clinical MR imaging system unfortunately produces small phase offset errors, which are systematic phase errors of stationary as well as moving spins. The magnitude of phase offset errors largely depends on local magnetic field inhomogeneities or gradient imbalance. Phase offset errors are difficult to evaluate because they are usually not constant over the whole field of view. However, they could be detected using analysis softwares by performing a profile representation of the velocity images. They can be fixed by applying a thorough background subtraction, which compensates for phase offset errors as well as increased background noise or systematic motion of certain structures. To correct for phase offset errors, the user or the program itself defines an area representing either noise or the phase offset error, and the mean phase information of this area is subtracted from the vessel ROI. Since background compensation is a powerful tool, it should be used with caution, as it could introduce more phase errors than it compensates for. There is no simple way to evaluate the accuracy of background compensation performed in individual cases [5].

Magnetic Resonance Angiography of the Renal Arteries

MRA Physics and Acquisition Protocols

Contrast-Enhanced MRA

Contrast-enhanced techniques have long been dominant in depicting renal vasculature. The gain in signal obtained by contrast administration typically enables shorter scan times, higher spatial or temporal resolution, and larger anatomical coverage compared to non-contrast techniques [50].

Gadolinium-Based Contrast Agent-Enhanced MRA

Gadolinium-based contrast agents (GBCAs) are routinely used for renal MRA [50]. GBCAs consist of a gadolinium atom bound to a hydrophilic ligand. After intravenous administration, GBCAs distribute predominantly in the extracellular space, although some GBCAs exhibit more pronounced protein binding [51]. GBCAs used for renal imaging are excreted via renal filtration with dominant half-lives of <2 h in individuals with normal renal function [52]. The contrast-enhancing properties of GBCAs arise from its paramagnetism, resulting in shortening of T_1 relaxation time of the surroundings. Especially in T_1 weighted (short-TR) sequences, the diminished T_1 enhances regrowth of longitudinal magnetization within each repetition time, rendering more magnetization available for signal formation.

Typically, 3D spoiled gradient echo sequences are used for contrast-enhanced MRA, with low TE and TR to minimize scan time. Parallel imaging techniques (SENSE and GRAPPA) are used to limit acquisition time to one 10–20 s breath-hold. Thanks to the GBCA-induced T_1 shortening, relatively high flip angles can be used to enhance SNR. Spatial resolutions are typically below 1.5 mm. Timing is critical: in order to achieve optimal depiction of the renal arteries, image contrast (encoded in the center of k-space, see Fig. 15.9 [53]) should be acquired at peak contrast concentrations in the vessels of interest. If possible, a k-space sampling trajectory should be chosen that samples the center of k-space first (e.g., centric sampling [54]). To aid in timing of the main acquisition, a series of quick repeated test scans can be performed following injection of a small amount of contrast agent to determine the time-to-peak.

Ideally, contrast agent is injected at such a rate that the injection length equals the acquisition time of the scan. This avoids high peak contrast concentrations leading to T_2* decay and ensures a constant contrast influx during data acquisition. However, a too lengthy injection can result in venous enhancement. If breath-holding is challenging, for example in patients with pulmonary disease or in pediatric patients, motion-robustness can be increased by employing non-Cartesian schemes to sample k-space, such as radial or spiral imaging [44, 55]. A set of imaging parameters to get started is provided in Table 15.3, and an example image is shown in Fig. 15.10 [56].

If clinical interest is in blood flow rather than anatomical depiction of the vasculature, a shorter acquisition with lower spatial resolution or anatomical coverage can be repeated multiple times after contrast administration. The ultimate form of this "time-resolved" MRA is dynamic contrast-enhanced (DCE) imaging. Here, a quick (1–3 s) acquisition is repeated continuously to obtain a contrast enhancement curve, which is modeled to obtain quantitative information on blood flow and, specifically in renal imaging, glomerular filtration (see Chap. 19 "Gadolinium-based Dynamic Functional Imaging: MR Urography").

Ferumoxytol-Enhanced MRA

Ferumoxytol has been approved by the FDA since 2009 for iron supplementation in patients with chronic kidney disease, who often require intravenous suppletion of iron due to poor enteric absorption [57]. Originally however, it was developed as an intravenous MR contrast agent, thanks to its T_1 and T_2/T_2* shortening properties [58]. Unique to ferumoxytol is its long circulation time, with an intravascular half-life of 14–21 h. This effectively extends the time window available for image acquisition, allowing for high-resolution depiction of the arteriovenous

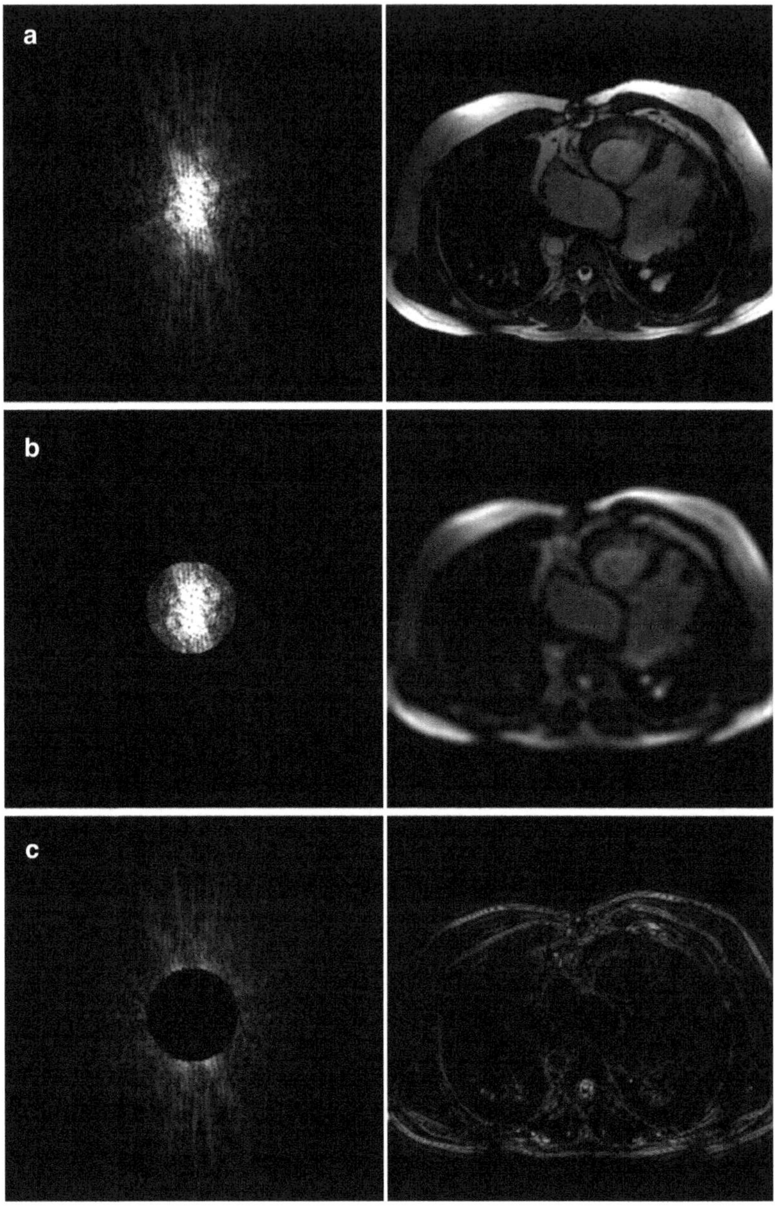

Fig. 15.9 K-space and associated MR image. MR data is acquired in k-space (**a**, left) and reconstructed using a Fourier transform (**a**, right). Low spatial frequencies are contained in the center of k-space (**b**, left). Note that reconstruction of the center of k-space only yields a blurred image (**b**, right). On the contrary, reconstruction of only the k-space periphery (high spatial frequencies) enhances image details and edges (**c**, right). (Reprinted from Moratal D et al. Biomed Imaging Interv J 2008 [53] under the terms of the Creative Commons Attribution License)

intravascular space. Thanks to its intravascular nature, there is a marked contrast between the lumen and vessel wall, which helps in discriminating them from each other (Fig. 15.11) [59]. Furthermore, the long steady-state allows for longer acquisitions with respiratory synchronization, omitting the need for breath-holding.

Ferumoxytol is metabolized mainly in the liver, spleen, and bone marrow after uptake by phagocytes. The carboxymethyldextran coating is cleaved and excreted by the kidneys as well as eliminated via the feces. The iron core enters the bodies' iron stores or is used for the production of hemoglobin.

Since it is excreted slowly, ferumoxytol associated signal changes can be present for several days following administration. Signal intensities in the liver, spleen, and bone marrow may be decreased for several months due to T_2 shortening [58]. Note that prior administration of

Table 15.3 Proposed scan parameters for gadolinium-based contrast agent (GBCA) imaging of the (native) renal arteries based on currently published literature

	GBCA-enhanced MRA
Field strength	1.5 T
2D/3D	3D
Base	T_1 weighted spoiled gradient echo
Respiratory compensation	Breath-hold
FOV	360–450 mm
Slice thickness	1–4 mm[a]
Slices	36–50
Voxel size	0.72–2.3 mm
Flip angle	25–40°
TR/TE	Shortest/shortest
Acquisition time	12–25 s
Timing after administration	Use test bolus for timing
Parallel imaging factor	2
Orientations	Coronal
k-space filling	Centric or Cartesian

FOV field of view, *GBCA* gadolinium-based contrast agent, *MRA* magnetic resonance angiography, *TE* echo time, *TR* repetition time

[a] The paper reporting a slice thickness of 3–4 mm used overcontiguous (overlapping) slices

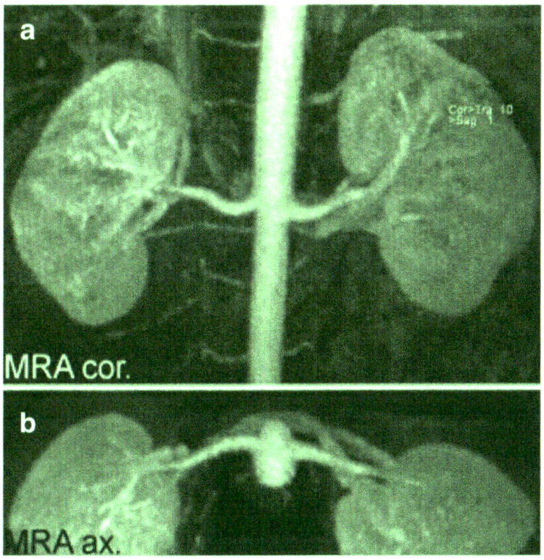

Fig. 15.10 Representative GBCA-enhanced MRA, in coronal (**a**) and axial (**b**) views, from an individual with an accessory right-sided renal artery. Reprinted from Slanina M et al. Contrast-enhanced MR angiography utilizing parallel acquisition techniques in renal artery stenosis detection. European Journal of Radiology 2010; 75:e46–e50 [56] with permission by Elsevier

ferumoxytol also obscures contrast enhancement from GBCAs for at least a few days up to 3 months [60].

Ferumoxytol first-pass imaging can be performed using similar sequences as used for GBCA-enhanced imaging. Its main strength lies in steady-state imaging, since the available intravascular time can be used to enhance image contrast and spatial resolution. When submillimeter voxels come into reach, appropriate respiratory compensation becomes even more crucial. To enhance motion-robustness, many authors use non-Cartesian sampling trajectories like spiral or radial imaging or centric sampling. Furthermore, currently advanced respiratory gating strategies are clinically available [61]. A set of imaging parameters to get started is provided in Table 15.4.

For vascular imaging, ferumoxytol dosages of 1 mg/kg up to 510 mg have been used for ferumoxytol-enhanced vascular imaging. In a study in CKD patients with eGFR <30 mL/min/1.73m^2, optimal SNR and contrast-to-noise ratio (CNR) in the aorta and inferior vena cava were found at a dose of 3 mL/kg, with higher dosages not resulting in a significant gain in SNR or CNR [62]. First pass images can be obtained after administration of part of this dosage as a bolus injection.

Safety Considerations Regarding the Use of Contrast Agents

As elaborated in Chap. 18 ("Gadolinium-based Contrast Agent Safety with Focus on Kidney MRI"), safety concerns exist with regard to GBCA administration, especially in patients with severe renal disease. In this population, GBCAs have been associated with the development of Nephrogenic Systemic Fibrosis (NSF), with the first reports dating from 2006 [63]. Since linear GBCAs were abandoned in favor of the more stable macrocyclic GBCAs (gadoteridol, gadoterate, and gadobutrol), NSF has largely been eliminated [64]. However, the pharmacokinetics of GBCAs in the human body are still not completely understood. Long-term deposition of GBCAs in multiple organs, especially brain, skin, and bone, has been reported in individuals with normal renal function, although clinical

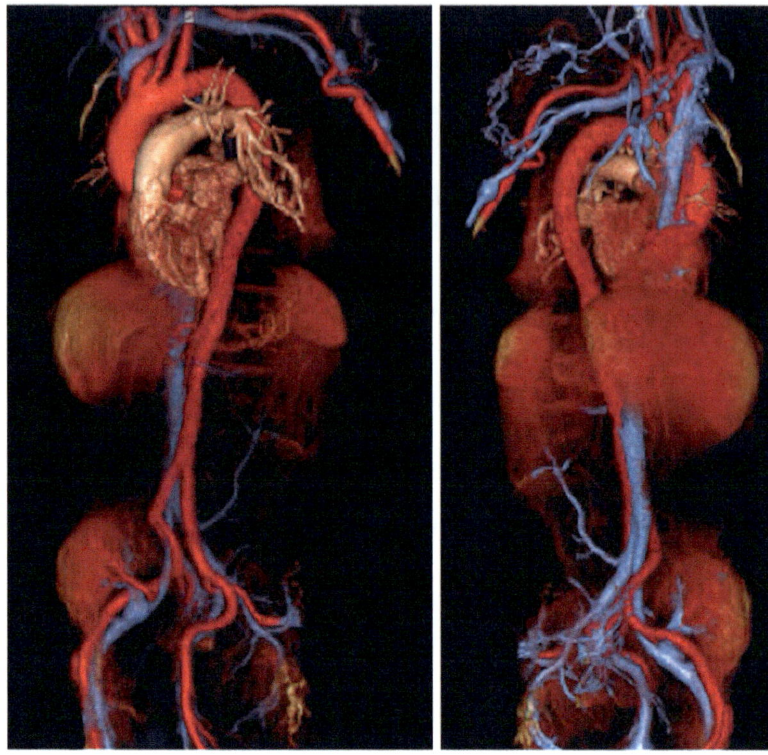

Fig. 15.11 Example of Ferumoxytol-enhanced MRA. Ferumoxytol enhanced steady-state MRA of an 87-year-old male patient with a renal transplant in situ after 3D volume rendering. (Reprinted from Finn JP et al. Clinical Radiology 2016; 71:796–806 [59] with permission by Elsevier)

Table 15.4 Proposed scan parameters for ferumoxytol imaging of a renal transplant kidney based on currently published literature

	First-pass	Steady-state
Field strength	1.5 T/3 T	1.5 T/3 T
2D/3D	3D	3D
Base	T_1 weighted spoiled gradient echo	T_1 weighted spoiled gradient echo
Respiratory compensation	Breathhold	Free breathing
FOV	340–400 mm	~250 mm
Slice thickness	~2.5 mm	0.5–1.5 mm
Slices	20–30	~30
Voxel size	1–2 mm	0.7–1.6 mm
Flip angle	5–30°	13–30
TR/TE	Shortest/shortest	2.4–6 ms/shortest
Acquisition time	15–20 s	4–12 min
Timing after administration	Use test bolus for timing	A few minutes up to hours after administration
Parallel imaging factor	2–3	
Orientations	Coronal	
k-space filling	Preferably non-Cartesian	

FOV field of view, *TE* echo time, *TR* repetition time

significance seems to be limited. Accumulation of GBCAs in a deep compartment and subsequent slow release has been hypothesized to explain these finding [65]. In the kidneys, gadobutrol is likely to be detectable a week after administration in healthy volunteers, supporting this theory [66]. However, these concerns should not lead to refraining from prescribing contrast-enhanced examinations in patients with a clinical indication. Even in those with a severely impaired kidney function, the small risk does not outweigh the possible harm of a missed or delayed diagnosis, as a recent consensus statement of the American College of Radiology and National Kidney Foundation emphasizes [51].

Unlike GBCAs, ferumoxytol is safe in patients with all stages of chronic kidney disease. However, intravenous suppletion of iron is generally associated with severe allergic reactions including anaphylaxis. For ferumoxytol, the latter is rare with an incidence of <0.2% [58], but in general, adverse events (mostly hypersensitivity reactions) occur 10 times more often than with GBCAs. As a precaution, ferumoxytol should be injected slowly: a single dose of 510 mg is administered in a 15-min time window, as advised by the FDA in March 2015. Note that older literature often describes ferumoxytol to be administered as a bolus injection, which is no longer the case. Furthermore, patients should be monitored for at least 30 min post administration, and trained personnel and appropriate medications should be available [58].

Common Issues and Artifacts

For an excellent overview of common pitfalls and artifacts in GBCA-enhanced MRA, including example images, we refer to the "Gadolinium-Enhanced MR Angiography" review, by Lee VS and colleagues [67]. Mistiming of the acquisition is a common issue and can be avoided by injecting a small test bolus prior to the actual acquisition to determine the time to peak enhancement. Timing the acquisition too early can result in a "Maki" artifact, with enhanced vessel walls and suppressed central regions. The artifact arises from acquisition of the center of k-space prior to contrast agent arrival. Contrarily, an overly delayed acquisition results in venous enhancement and background noise.

MR angiography has the tendency to overestimate artery stenosis. Arterial stenosis leads to turbulent flow, resulting in enhanced spin dephasing. Effectively, this leads to increased T_2 decay and signal loss. The effect can be exaggerated on maximum intensity projections, where the remaining vessel signal might get lost in the accumulated background signal.

Non-Contrast-Enhanced MRA

Non-contrast-enhanced MRA has several advantages over contrast-enhanced MRA but is not as routinely used in clinical practice as the latter. Most importantly, the risks associated with intravenous administration of contrast agents, either GBCAs or alternatives like ferumoxytol, are avoided. Contrast administration is furthermore associated with additional costs (the contrast agent itself, intravenous cannulas, and intravenous infusion parafernalia) and effort (installation of intravenous access and prior measurement of eGFR). Technically, non-contrast acquisitions can be repeated until diagnostic quality images are obtained; mistiming is not an issue. Furthermore, images in different image orientations, spatial settings, or patient positions can be obtained [68].

To obtain sufficient signal from the blood vessels for angiography, roughly four different contrast mechanisms can be employed. First, for arterial imaging, the inflow of fresh, previously unsaturated blood can be exploited to obtain a high intra-arterial signal. Those inflow-dependent techniques include time-of-flight (TOF) MRA and inflow-dependent inversion recovery (IFDIR). Second, non-contrast MRA can exploit the relatively long arterial T_1 and T_2, resulting in a high signal on balanced steady-state free precession (bSSFP) readouts. Third, arterial spin labeling as discussed in Chap. 16 ("Arterial Spin Labeling: Non-contrast Perfusion MRI of the Kidney") can also be used to increase intravascular signal. ASL, however, relies on the subtraction of a baseline and labeled image and is therefore prone to misalignment in organs moving with respiration, like the kidneys. Last, 4D phase contrast MRI (as described previously in this chapter) can be used for angiography. Although it requires longer acquisition time and advanced processing, it has the added advantage of providing quantitative information on blood flow.

As in contrast-enhanced MRA, non-contrast MRA might overestimate stenoses if turbulent flow causes accelerated T_2 dephasing. Furthermore, implants and stents can lead to artifacts, hampering diagnostic use. Typically, these artifacts are more severe on high field strengths.

In this section, we will focus on inflow-dependent techniques and bSSFP. Although ASL is commonly used to quantify renal perfusion, its application for renal angiography is scarce, probably due to its motion sensitivity. Phase contrast MRI is discussed extensively in a separate section of this chapter.

Time-of-Flight MRA

As one of the oldest non-contrast-enhanced MRA techniques, time-of-flight MRA relies on the inflow of fresh, unsaturated blood from outside the imaging volume. Due to the repetitive RF pulses applied inside the imaging volume, spins inside the imaging volume become magnetically

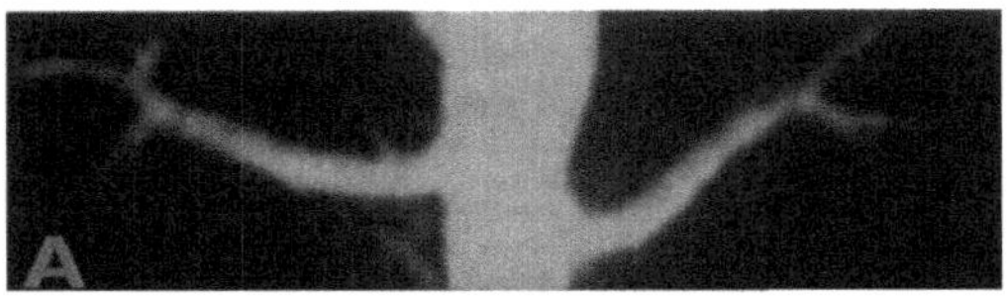

Fig. 15.12 Example of time-of-flight MRA of the renal arteries in a healthy volunteer. (Reprinted from King BF et al. Semin Ultrasound CT MR 1996;17(4):398–403 [69] with permission by Elsevier)

saturated. The longitudinal magnetization decreases with each RF pulse until it reaches a steady state. Arterial blood flowing through the aorta to the renal arteries however is not saturated yet and will therefore give a high signal and appear bright. However, the longer the blood travels through the imaging volume, the more RF-pulses it experiences and the more the magnetic saturation increases, ultimately ending up in a steady state. Therefore, the brightness of the vascular signal decreases further downstream and depends on flow velocity, which can be decreased distally of a severe stenosis—this is inherent to all inflow dependent techniques. TOF MRA therefore relies on relatively high flow velocities directed perpendicular to the imaging plane, and as a result is less suitable for depiction of the renal arteries (Fig. 15.12) [69]. It can be performed with a conventional spoiled gradient echo sequence, preferably with relatively high flip-angles and short repetition time to increase contrast between flowing blood and stationary tissue. Echo time is kept as short as possible to minimize T_2 decay. In 3D, due to saturation effects, slab thickness might be limited [70].

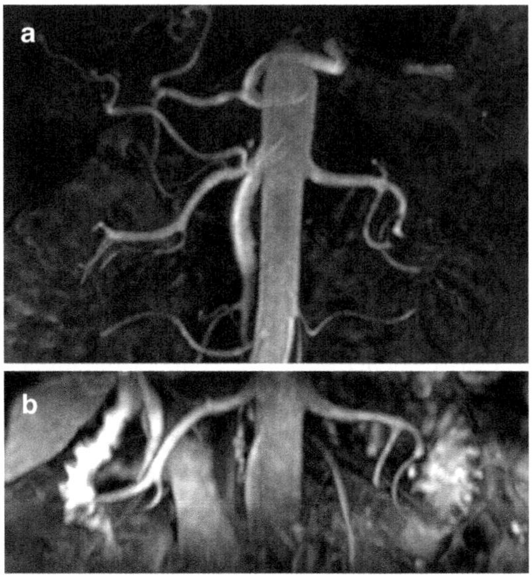

Fig. 15.13 GBCA-enhanced MRA of the renal arteries (**a**) versus bSSFP (**b**) in a hypertensive patient with normal renal arteris. (Reprinted from Gaudiano C et al. Eur Radiol 2014 [71] with permission by Springer Nature Customer Service Centre GmbH)

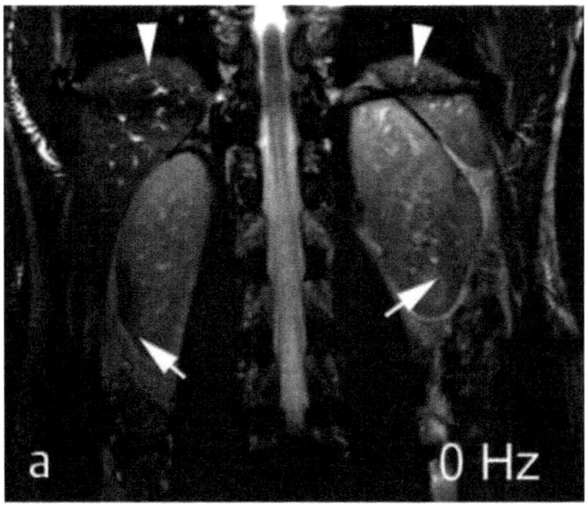

Fig. 15.14 Banding artifacts in SSFP imaging. (Excerpt from Boss A et al. Rofo 2005 [72], reprinted with permission by Georg Thieme Verlag KG)

bSSFP

Balanced steady-state free precession is an imaging sequence, which provides unique contrast depending on the ratio of T_2 to T_1. Compared to soft tissue, this ratio is relatively high in arterial blood, which facilitates its use for angiography (Fig. 15.13) [71]. Note however that this ratio is also relatively high in fat and other fluids like urine and cerebrospinal fluid. In the abdomen, bSSFP MRA is mostly performed at 1.5 T, due to the sensitivity of balanced sequences like bSSFP to field inhomogeneities. The proximity of the gastrointestinal tract can prove to be problematic in the abdomen especially at high field strengths, resulting in zebra-stripe and banding artifacts (Fig. 15.14) [72]. Furthermore, turbulent flow in stenosed arteries can lead to increased T_2 decay, resulting in signal loss and overestimation of severity [73]. High quality fat-suppression is

Table 15.5 Proposed scan parameters for balanced steady-state free precession (bSSFP) imaging of renal arteries

	bSSFP
Field strength	1.5 T
2D/3D	3D
Respiratory compensation	Breath-hold
FOV	250–340 mm
Slice thickness	1.5–2.4 mm
Slices	20–30
Voxel size	~1.5 mm
Flip angle	60–80°
TR/TE	3–4/1.5–2.2
Acquisition time	10–20 s
Parallel imaging factor	Not reported
Orientation	Variable
k-space filling	Centric
Fat suppression	Recommended

bSSFP balanced steady-state free precession, *FOV* field of view, *TE* echo time; *TR* repetition time

required for bSSFP MRA due to the inherently high fat signal.

Different vendors call bSSFP by different names: true fast imaging with steady-state precession (TrueFISP, Siemens), balanced fast field echo (bFFE, Philips), or fast imaging employing steady state acquisition (FIESTA, GE). For bSSFP, it is recommended to minimize TR and TE. A short TR minimizes sensitivity to banding artifacts [74], and with short TE, signal dephasing due to turbulent flow is minimized, avoiding overestimation of stenosis [73]. A set of typical imaging parameters in the literature is provided in Table 15.5. The use of parallel imaging is not always reported in the literature. Nevertheless, based on the authors' experience, parallel imaging is recommended to reduce acquisition time. In the abdomen, an acceleration factor of 2 should be achievable without deterioration of image quality. Fat suppression is recommended, as well as venous signal suppression by caudally placed saturation slabs.

IFDIR

For the renal arteries, inflow-dependent inversion recovery (IFDIR) is increasingly used. Here, image acquisition is preceded by a saturation pulse well around the imaging volume. After a waiting interval called the inversion time (TI) allowing for inflow of fresh blood, a 3D bSSFP readout is used for image formation for optimal depiction of the vasculature. Since it is an inflow-dependent technique, image quality depends on flow velocity, as discussed above. The bSSFP readout employs the inherent sensitivity of this sequence to arterial blood (Fig. 15.15) [75]. For an overview of commonly used acquisition parameters, see Table 15.6.

MRA Post-Processing and Data Analysis Methods

Maximum Intensity Projection

Maximum intensity projections (MIP) are used commonly in angiography since high intensity voxels, like contrast-filled vessels, are well displayed. In case of contrast-enhanced examinations, the non-enhanced images might be subtracted from the enhanced images. In the final image, for each voxel in the plane of choice, say coronal, only the voxel with the highest intensity in the orthogonal direction is shown (Fig. 15.16). The resulting image slightly resembles images obtained from conventional X-ray angiography. Although a MIP clearly displays the maximum diameter of the vessel of interest in each direction, all image depth is lost. For example, crossing vessels cannot be distinguished. To partly overcome this, MIPs can be created from different directions, resembling different points-of-view. In bSSFP imaging, high signal from other fluids can obscure the view of the renal arteries [73].

Due to partial voluming artifacts, marginal voxels containing both the lumen and vessel wall might not reach the MIP threshold, theoretically leading to overestimation of stenosis severity [76]. Furthermore, while large vessels with a high contrast-to-noise ratio are enhanced by the MIP algorithm, small vessels (or stenotic areas) are further obscured due to their inherently low contrast-to-noise ratio [77].

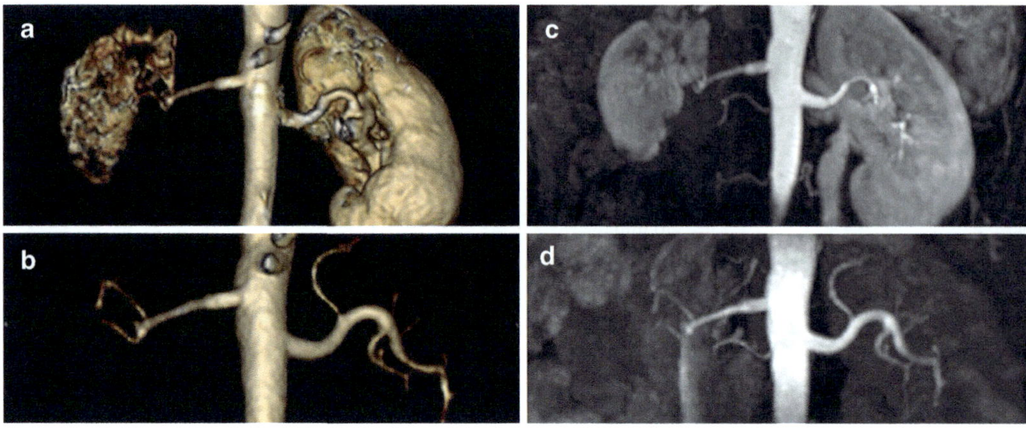

Fig. 15.15 GBCA-enhanced MRA volume rendering (**a**) and source image (**c**) versus IFDIR volume rendering (**b**) and source (**d**). The stenosis degree of the right renal artery was estimated to be 55% on contrast-enhanced MRA versus 45% on IFDIR. Note the superior depiction of intrarenal arteries on the IFDIR images. (Reprinted from Zhang W et al. J Comput Assist Tomogr. 2014 [75] with permission by Wolters Kluwer Health, Inc)

Table 15.6 Proposed scan parameters for inflow-dependent inversion recovery (IFDIR) imaging of renal arteries

	IFDIR
Field strength	Mostly 1.5
2D/3D	3D
Respiratory compensation	Navigator/triggering
FOV	320–400 mm
Slice thickness	1.1–2 mm
Slices	50–120
Voxel size	1–1.5 mm
Flip angle	70–120 (mostly 90)
TR/TE	4–5/1.5–2.5
TI	1200–1400
Acquisition time	2–5 min
Parallel imaging factor	2
Orientation	Axial, sometimes coronal
Fat suppression	Spectral
Venous suppression	Sometimes inversion/saturation

IFDIR inflow-dependent inversion recovery, *FOV* field of view, *TE* echo time, *TR* repetition time, *TI* inversion time

Multiplanar Reconstruction

On all clinical MR systems, multiplanar reconstruction (MPR) and maximum intensity projections are available. Multiplanar reconstruction allows for a dataset to be resampled in different directions, for example by adding a sagittal and axial view to a dataset acquired in the coronal plane [77]. The dataset should be acquired in 3D and with isotropic spatial resolution. For (isotropic) data acquired in 3D, MPR is lossless in both the phase- and the frequency-encoding direction. For other directions, note that resampling of data can slightly affect image quality.

Volume Rendering

Volume rendering is widely used in CT imaging to display renal CT angiography data. Based on a radiological property (for example X-ray attenuation), each voxel is assigned a brightness and opacity. Different algorithms exist to turn these brightness and opacity values into a volume model. Ultimately, the user is shown a 2D projection of this volume model of the image data. For CT data, the signal intensity as expressed in Hounsfield units is fairly constant over different examinations or patients for a given tissue. Therefore, look-up tables could be developed to pair each signal value to its corresponding brightness and opacity values. In MRI however, signal intensity is more or less arbitrary, rendering any look-up table useless. Therefore, these opacity and brightness values either have to be selected by an algorithm or based on some form of user input. Lastly, any opaque structure obscuring the view of the anatomy of interest must be removed, often manually [78]. For examples, see Figs. 15.11 and 15.15.

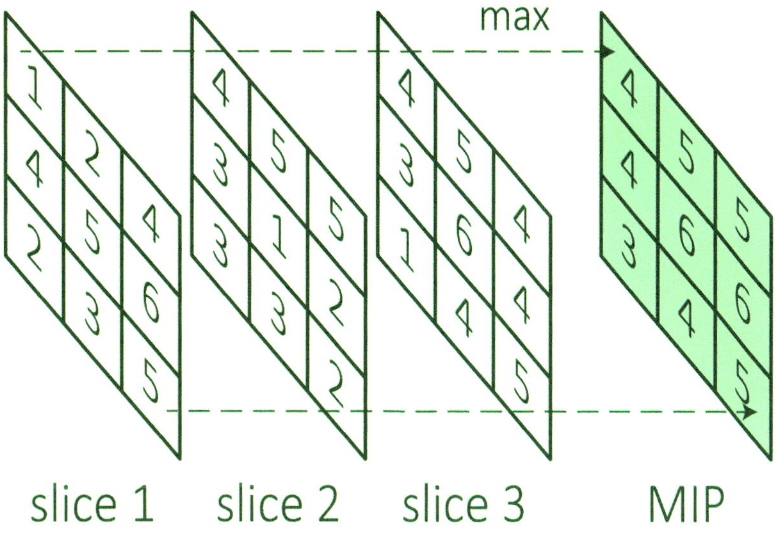

Fig. 15.16 Principle of maximum intensity projection (MIP). Imagine a simulated ray in one direction. The highest encountered signal value along the ray is displayed

Volume Rendering and MPR Compared to MIP

MIP and volume rendering have been compared in terms of their accuracy for diagnosing renal artery stenosis as compared to digital subtraction angiography (DSA), resulting in a slightly better performance for volume rendering compared to MIP, especially in terms of specificity [76, 77]. In both studies, observers were able to manually adjust volume rendering settings for each individual subject. In "Gadolinium-Enhanced 3D MR Angiography of Renal Artery Stenosis", by Baskaran and colleagues [77], MIP and volume rendering were compared to MPR as well, resulting in a comparable performance for MPR and volume rendering. MPR in this study was used in conjunction with MIP. Unsurprisingly, diagnostic performance of MPR aided by MIP was better than performance of MIP alone.

MIP and volume rendering have also been compared in the context of preoperative assessment of kidney donors, with a focus on the detection of accessory renal arteries. This study showed that assessment of source data, MIP, or volume renderings did not significantly differ in diagnostic accuracy compared to DSA [79].

To conclude, volume renderings and MPR seem not to be inferior to conventional MIP, and probably even provide additional information, improving diagnostic quality. As with all processing algorithms, it is advisable to use both MPR and volume renderings in conjunction with the original source data.

MRA Clinical Applications

Renovascular Hypertension

The kidneys are crucial in regulating the volume of the body's fluids and blood pressure. Based on the activity of the renin-angiotensin-aldosterone system (RAAS) and the sympathetic nervous system (SNS), salt and fluids are retained, increasing blood pressure. As described in 1934 by a pathologist named Goldblatt, stenosis of the renal artery leads to the affected kidney "sensing" a lower blood pressure. This triggers the kidneys to produce renin, increasing activity of the abovementioned RAAS and trigger the SNS via the efferent nerves leading from the kidney to the SNS ganglia. Consequently, fluid retention and vascular tone is increased and salt excretion diminished, leading to the so-called *renovascular hypertension* [80].

A stenosis in the renal artery in elderly or vascular impaired patients is often caused by atherosclerosis. In this case, treatment of the renal artery by stenting is not as beneficial for lowering of the blood pressure as one might expect considering the Goldblatt phenomenon described above.

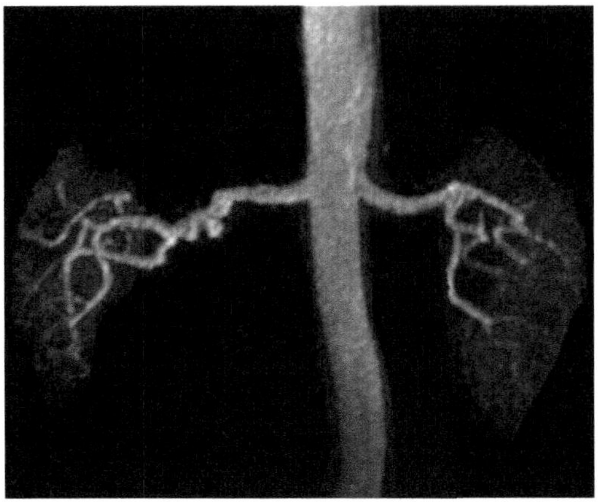

Fig. 15.17 Fibromuscular dysplasia of the mid and distal right renal artery. (Reprinted from Glockner JF et al. Abdom Imaging 2007 [82] with permission by Springer Nature Customer Service Centre GmbH)

The most likely explanation is that atherosclerosis is a systemic disease, probably affecting downstream vessels as well as the renal artery. Furthermore, the process of stenting itself might lead to formation of emboli and consequent microinfarctions of the treated kidney [81].

In most younger women up to 50 years of age, renal artery stenosis might be caused by fibromuscular dysplasia, a condition characterized by a typical *string-of-beads* appearance of the renal artery (Fig. 15.17) [82]. In those patients, renal artery stenting is indicated and beneficial [83]. Therefore, it is important to recognize fibromuscular dysplasia by angiography.

Currently, GBCA-enhanced MRA is mostly used in the assessment of patients suspected of renovascular disease. Several studies have compared the performance of GBCA-enhanced MRA to digital subtraction angiography, the reference standard for this diagnosis. Only considering recent (2005 or later) prospective studies including patients with a clinical suspicion of renovascular hypertension and aiming to perform both MRA and DSA in all patients, an average sensitivity of 85% and specificity of 91% can be calculated, weighting on the number of patients included in each study [56, 84, 85]. These studies considered a stenosis of >50–60% to be of hemodynamic significance. Note that this diagnostic accuracy is lower than what was reported in 2001 by Tan et al. [86], a meta-analysis of mostly small studies. The difference probably can be attributed to a combination of publication bias (studies with negative results are less likely to be published) and selection bias (the authors of the meta-analysis chose to include studies not only based on quality but also on size) [87].

Considering non-contrast-enhanced MRA, evidence of diagnostic quality compared to DSA is still limited. For bSSFP, a prospective study in 25 patients with suspected RAS found a sensitivity and specificity of 100% and 98%, respectively [73]. Only patients with a clinical indication for DSA based on a high suspicion of RAS were included. Another study performed a retrospective comparison of bSSFP to CE MRA and DSA, if available. Here, a sensitivity of 91.7% and a specificity of 100% were reported in 79 patients suspected of renal artery stenosis. A subset of patients with hemodynamically significant renal artery stenosis and an indication for renal artery stenting underwent DSA as well. In those 10 patients, bSSFP yielded a sensitivity of 88.2% and a specificity of 100%. However, four accessory arteries were missed due to the relatively small imaging volume [72]. A third and more recent study reported a sensitivity of 97% and 96% and a specificity of 90% and 91% for 1.5 T (49 patients) and 3.0 T (32 patients). However, data from large, prospective and blinded studies are required for definite conclusions.

Available evidence for IFDIR is also limited. Parienty et al. [88] were the first to report on the diagnostic accuracy of IFDIR in 23 patients suspected of RAS. Only patients with chronic kidney disease were included in this prospective study. Compared to DSA, a sensitivity and a specificity of 93% and 88%, respectively, were reported. Note however that patients were only included if a stenosis was detected on the IFDIR scan, which is a selection bias leading to an artificially high sensitivity. The other available study is retrospective, assessing 27 patients suspected of RAS and referred for DSA. A sensitivity of 100% and a specificity of 94% were reported [89]. Note however that also in this study prevalence of RAS was very high. IFDIR has been reported to be less reliable in fibromuscular dysplasia (Figs. 15.18 and 15.19) [90].

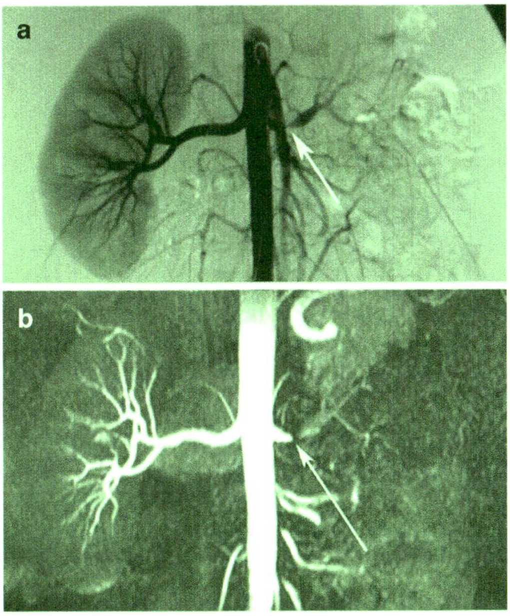

Fig. 15.18 DSA (**a**) and IFDIR (**b**) in the same patient showing subtotal occlusion of the left renal artery. Note that the artery seems completely occluded on the IFDIR image, despite some distal arteries are visible. Reprinted from Sebastià C et al. Accuracy of non-enhanced magnetic resonance angiography for the assessment of renal artery stenosis. European Journal of Radiology Open 2016; 3:200–206 [90] under the terms of Creative Commons CC-BY-NC-ND license

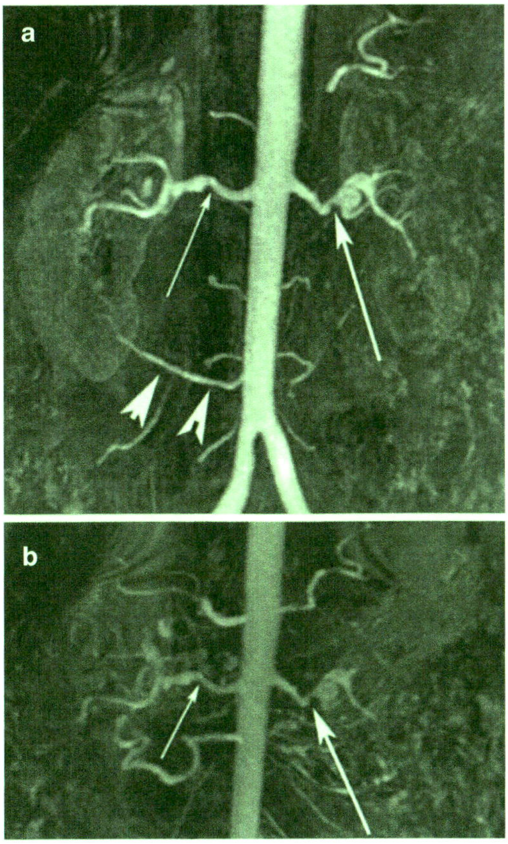

Fig. 15.19 CE-MRA (**a**) and IFDIR (**b**) in the same patient with a significant stenosis of the left renal artery in a subject with FMD. The notch in the right renal artery is considered significant at MRA and not significant by IFDIR. The accessory right renal artery on CE-MRA is not visualized on IFDIR. Reprinted from Sebastià C et al. Accuracy of non-enhanced magnetic resonance angiography for the assessment of renal artery stenosis. European Journal of Radiology Open 2016; 3:200–206 [91] under the terms of Creative Commons CC-BY-NC-ND license

Renal Transplantation

Regarding contrast-enhanced MRA of the renal artery, ferumoxytol has mostly been used to assess renal transplant vasculature (Fig. 15.20). For this application, agreement with DSA was shown to be excellent in a small study ($N = 33$, 1.5 T, ferumoxytol dose 3 mg/kg), although ferumoxytol-enhanced MRA had a slight tendency to overestimate stenosis severity [92]. This resulted in positive and negative predictive values of 94–97% and 100%, respectively, and a sensitivity and specificity of 100% and 75–88%, respectively [92].

GBCA-enhanced MRA has not been extensively used in kidney transplant recipients, probably due to the necessity of GBCA administration. Studies comparing its performance with DSA are equally scarce. Only one relatively recent (2011) study compared GBCA-enhanced MRA to DSA, yielding high specificity (94%) and moderate specificity (80%) in 30 patients with suspected transplant renal artery stenosis [91]. This confirms the results of older studies, showing that GBCA-enhanced MRA has the tendency to overestimate the degree of stenosis in this population [93, 94]. However, it justifies the use of GBCA-enhanced MRA as a screening instrument.

Regarding non-contrast-enhanced MRA, Lanzmann et al. performed bSSFP MRA in 20 kidney transplant recipients scheduled for DSA. bSSFP yielded excellent results with a sensitivity and specificity of 100% and 88%, respectively. One retrospective study compared IFDIR to DSA

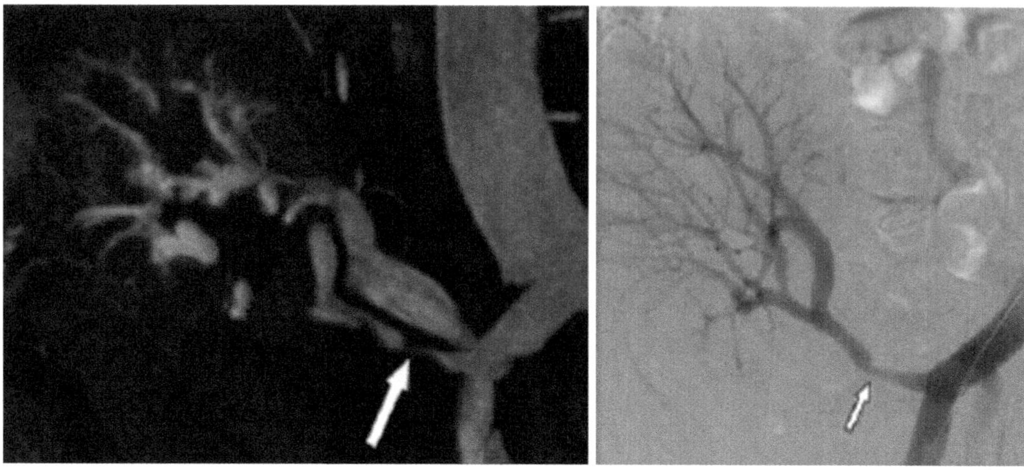

Fig. 15.20 Ferumoxytol-enhanced image of the vasculature of an allograft kidney, showing a significant stenosis. (Reprinted from Fananapazir G et al. J Magn Reson Imaging 2017 [92] with permission by John Wiley and Sons)

in renal transplants, but only patients with vascular complications on IFDIR (22 out of 330) were referred for DSA. On a per vessel base, a sensitivity of 100% and a specificity of 90% were reported [95]. Another study compared an IFDIR-based sequence to DSA and surgery in 15 patients, again selected by the non-enhanced MRA examination. A sensitivity of 100% was reported (specificity was not reported). The non-enhanced sequence was noted to slightly overestimate stenosis severity [96].

Conclusion

This chapter offered an overview of PC-MRI and MRA of the renal arteries, covering acquisition and post-processing details as well as clinical application. Despite PC-MRI not being routinely used in clinics yet, 2D PC-MRI is quite easy to implement and allows the measurement of RBF and derivative parameters, showing potential to support diagnosis and monitoring of early-stage renal diseases. 4D flow MRI technique, when possible acquired in combination with MRA, allows the investigation and visualization of blood flow dynamics in the vessel volume. More recent and more technically demanding than 2D PC-MRI, 4D flow MRI of the renal arteries is still in its infancy and requires proper clinical validation in renal disease. CE-MRA is routinely used for diagnosis of renal artery stenosis. Non-enhanced MRA and ferumoxytol-enhanced MRA are promising, although available evidence of clinical validity is still limited, suggesting the need for additional larger studies. Compared to DSA as a reference technique, MRI allows for a more comprehensive assessment of kidney structure and function. PC-MRI and MRA are likely to benefit from being combined with other promising renal MRI techniques (described in detail in the other chapters of this book) providing complementary information on renal microstructure and function and allowing complete assessment of the kidney, potentially improving renal disease diagnosis and monitoring.

Technical details provided in this and the other chapters of this book, along with recent standardization efforts (on PC-MRI [3] as well as on other kidney MRI techniques [97–100]) will hopefully promote more widespread adoption of renal PC-MRI, MRA, and multiparametric renal MRI and foster the initiation of multicenter studies using standardized MRI methods. Future multicenter studies are needed to define reliable and definitive reference ranges for PC-MRI of the renal arteries, to provide additional evidence of PC-MRI and novel MRA methods clinical validity, and to demonstrate their clinical potential as part of a multiparametric renal MRI protocol, ultimately allowing their transfer to clinical practice.

References

1. Villa G, Ringgaard S, Hermann I, Noble R, Brambilla P, Khatir DS, et al. Phase-contrast magnetic resonance imaging to assess renal perfusion: a systematic review and statement paper. MAGMA. 2020;33(1):3–21.
2. Davenport MS, Perazella MA, Yee J, Dillman JR, Fine D, McDonald RJ, et al. Use of intravenous iodinated contrast Media in Patients with kidney disease: consensus statements from the American College of Radiology and the National Kidney Foundation. Radiology. 2020;294(3):660–8.
3. de Boer A, Villa G, Bane O, Bock M, Cox EF, Dekkers IA, et al. Consensus-based technical recommendations for clinical translation of renal phase contrast MRI. J Magn Reson Imaging. 2020;55:323. https://doi.org/10.1002/jmri.27419.
4. Wymer DT, Patel KP, Burke WF, Bhatia VK. Phase-contrast MRI: physics, techniques, and clinical applications. Radiographics. 2020;40(1):122–40.
5. Lotz J, Meier C, Leppert A, Galanski M. Cardiovascular flow measurement with phase-contrast MR imaging: basic facts and implementation. Radiographics. 2002;22(3):651–71.
6. Bax L, Bakker CJG, Klein WM, Blanken N, Beutler JJ, Mali WPTRM. Renal blood flow measurements with use of phase-contrast magnetic resonance imaging: Normal values and reproducibility. J Vasc Interv Radiol. 2005;16(6):807–14.
7. Markl M, Frydrychowicz A, Kozerke S, Hope M, Wieben O. 4D flow MRI. J Magn Reson Imaging. 2012;36(5):1015–36.
8. Thunberg P, Karlsson M, Wigström L. Accuracy and reproducibility in phase contrast imaging using SENSE: phase contrast imaging using SENSE. Magn Reson Med. 2003;50(5):1061–8.
9. Alperin N, Lee SH. PUBS: Pulsatility-based segmentation of lumens conducting non-steady flow. Magn Reson Med. 2003;49(5):934–44.
10. Lalande A, Khau van Kien P, Salve N, Ben Salem D, Legrand L, Walker PM, et al. Automatic determination of aortic compliance with cine-magnetic resonance imaging: an application of fuzzy logic theory. Investig Radiol. 2002;37(12):685–91.
11. Kozerke S, Botnar R, Oyre S, Scheidegger MB, Pedersen EM, Boesiger P. Automatic vessel segmentation using active contours in cine phase contrast flow measurements. J Magn Reson Imaging. 1999;10(1):41–51.
12. Herment A, Kachenoura N, Lefort M, Bensalah M, Dogui A, Frouin F, et al. Automated segmentation of the aorta from phase contrast MR images: validation against expert tracing in healthy volunteers and in patients with a dilated aorta. J Magn Reson Imaging. 2010;31(4):881–8.
13. Oyre S, Ringgaard S, Kozerke S, Paaske WP, Scheidegger MB, Boesiger P, et al. Quantitation of circumferential subpixel vessel wall position and wall shear stress by multiple sectored three-dimensional paraboloid modeling of velocity encoded cine MR. Magn Reson Med. 1998;40(5):645–55.
14. Zöllner FG, Ankar Monssen J, Rørvik J, Lundervold A, Schad LR. Blood flow quantification from 2D phase contrast MRI in renal arteries using an unsupervised data driven approach. Z Für Med Phys. 2009;19(2):98–107.
15. Hackstein N, Schneider C, Eichner G, Rau WS. Effect of IV injection of radiographic contrast media on human renal blood flow. Am J Roentgenol. 2007;188(5):1367–72.
16. Khatir DS, Pedersen M, Jespersen B, Buus NH. Reproducibility of MRI renal artery blood flow and BOLD measurements in patients with chronic kidney disease and healthy controls: reproducibility of RABF and BOLD in CKD. J Magn Reson Imaging. 2014;40(5):1091–8.
17. Torres VE, King BF, Chapman AB, Brummer ME, Bae KT, Glockner JF, et al. Magnetic resonance measurements of renal blood flow and disease progression in autosomal dominant polycystic kidney disease. Clin J Am Soc Nephrol. 2006;2(1):112–20.
18. King BF, Torres VE, Brummer ME, Chapman AB, Bae KT, Glockner JF, et al. Magnetic resonance measurements of renal blood flow as a marker of disease severity in autosomal-dominant polycystic kidney disease. Kidney Int. 2003;64(6):2214–21.
19. van der Bel R, Verbree J, Gurney-Champion OJ, van Osch MJP, Stroes ESG, Nederveen AJ, et al. Sympathetic activation by lower body negative pressure decreases kidney perfusion without inducing hypoxia in healthy humans. Clin Auton Res. 2018;30(2):149–56. https://doi.org/10.1007/s10286-018-0570-7.
20. Maier SE, Scheidegger MB, Liu K, Schneider E, Bellinger A, Boesiger P. Renal artery velocity mapping with MR imaging. J Magn Reson Imaging. 1995;5(6):669–76.
21. van der Bel R, Coolen BF, Nederveen AJ, Potters WV, Verberne HJ, Vogt L, et al. Magnetic resonance imaging-derived renal oxygenation and perfusion during continuous, steady-state angiotensin-ii infusion in healthy humans. J Am Heart Assoc. 2016;5(3):e003185. https://doi.org/10.1161/JAHA.115.003185.
22. Markl M, Bammer R, Alley MT, Elkins CJ, Draney MT, Barnett A, et al. Generalized reconstruction of phase contrast MRI: analysis and correction of the effect of gradient field distortions. Magn Reson Med. 2003;50(4):791–801.
23. Bernstein MA, Zhou XJ, Polzin JA, King KF, Ganin A, Pelc NJ, et al. Concomitant gradient terms in phase contrast MR: analysis and correction. Magn Reson Med. 1998;39(2):300–8.
24. Walker PG. Semiautomated method for noise reduction and background phase error correction in MR phase velocity data. J Magn Reson Imaging. 1993;3(3):521–30.

25. Takayama T, Takehara Y, Sugiyama M, Sugiyama T, Ishii Y, Johnson KE, et al. Use of three-dimensional time-resolved phase-contrast magnetic resonance imaging with vastly undersampled isotropic projection reconstruction to assess renal blood flow in a renal cell carcinoma patient treated with sunitinib: a case report. BMC Res Notes. 2014;7(1):527.
26. Wentland AL, Grist TM, Wieben O. Repeatability and internal consistency of abdominal 2D and 4D phase contrast MR flow measurements. Acad Radiol. 2013;20(6):699–704.
27. Cortsen M, Petersen LJ, Ståhlberg F, Thomsen C, Søndergaard L, Petersen JR, et al. MR velocity mapping measurement of renal artery blood flow in patients with impaired kidney function. Acta Radiol. 1996;37(1):79–84.
28. Khatir DS, Pedersen M, Jespersen B, Buus NH. Evaluation of renal blood flow and oxygenation in CKD using magnetic resonance imaging. Am J Kidney Dis. 2015;66(3):402–11.
29. Cox EF, Buchanan CE, Bradley CR, Prestwich B, Mahmoud H, Taal M, et al. Multiparametric renal magnetic resonance imaging: validation, interventions, and alterations in chronic kidney disease. Front Physiol. 2017;8:696. https://doi.org/10.3389/fphys.2017.00696/full.
30. Michaely HJ, Schoenberg SO, Ittrich C, Dikow R, Bock M, Guenther M. Renal disease: value of functional magnetic resonance imaging with flow and perfusion measurements. Investig Radiol. 2004;39(11):698–705.
31. Khatir DS, Pedersen M, Ivarsen P, Christensen KL, Jespersen B, Buus NH. Effects of additional vasodilatory or nonvasodilatory treatment on renal function, vascular resistance and oxygenation in chronic kidney disease: a randomized clinical trial. J Hypertens. 2018;1:116.
32. Prowle JR, Molan MP, Hornsey E, Bellomo R. Measurement of renal blood flow by phase-contrast magnetic resonance imaging during septic acute kidney injury: a pilot investigation*. Crit Care Med. 2012;40(6):1768–76.
33. Lee VS, Rofsky NM, Ton AT, Johnson G, Krinsky GA, Weinreb JC. Angiotensin-converting enzyme inhibitor-enhanced phase-contrast MR imaging to measure renal artery velocity waveforms in patients with suspected Renovascular hypertension. Am J Roentgenol. 2000;174(2):499–508.
34. Binkert CA, Debatin JF, Schneider E, Hodler J, Ruehm SG, Schmidt M, et al. Can MR measurement of renal artery flow and renal volume predict the outcome of percutaneous transluminal renal angioplasty? Cardiovasc Intervent Radiol. 2001;24(4):233–9.
35. Binkert CA, Hoffman U, Leung DA, Matter H-G, Schmidt M, Debatin JF. Characterization of renal artery stenoses based on magnetic resonance renal flow and volume measurements. Kidney Int. 1999;56(5):1846–54.
36. Schoenberg SO, Knopp MV, Londy F, Krishnan S, Zuna I, Lang N, et al. Morphologic and functional magnetic resonance imaging of renal artery stenosis: a multireader Tricenter study. J Am Soc Nephrol. 2002;12:158.
37. Westenberg JJM, Wasser MNJM, van der Geest RJ, Pattynama PMT, de Roos A, Vanderschoot J, et al. Variations in blood flow waveforms in stenotic renal arteries by 2D phase-contrast cine MRI. J Magn Reson Imaging. 1998;8(3):590–7.
38. Schoenberg SO, Knopp MV, Bock M, Kallinowski F, Just A, Essig M, et al. Renal artery stenosis: grading of hemodynamic changes with cine phase-contrast MR blood flow measurements. Radiology. 1997;203(1):45–53.
39. Bock M, Schoenberg SO, Schad LR, Knopp MV, Essig M, van Kaick G. Interleaved gradient echo planar (IGEPI) and phase contrast CINE-PC flow measurements in the renal artery. J Magn Reson Imaging. 1998;8(4):889–95.
40. Schoenberg SO, Rieger JR, Michaely HJ, Rupprecht H, Samtleben W, Reiser MF. Functional magnetic resonance imaging in renal artery stenosis. Abdom Imaging. 2006;31(2):200–12.
41. Irazabal MV, Torres VE, Hogan MC, Glockner J, King BF, Ofstie TG, et al. Short-term effects of tolvaptan on renal function and volume in patients with autosomal dominant polycystic kidney disease. Kidney Int. 2011;80(3):295–301.
42. Spithoven EM, Meijer E, Borns C, Boertien WE, Gaillard CAJM, Kappert P, et al. Feasibility of measuring renal blood flow by phase-contrast magnetic resonance imaging in patients with autosomal dominant polycystic kidney disease. Eur Radiol. 2016;26(3):683–92.
43. Kline TL, Edwards ME, Garg I, Irazabal MV, Korfiatis P, Harris PC, et al. Quantitative MRI of kidneys in renal disease. Abdom Radiol. 2018;43(3):629–38.
44. Motoyama D, Ishii Y, Takehara Y, Sugiyama M, Yang W, Nasu H, et al. Four-dimensional phase-contrast vastly undersampled isotropic projection reconstruction (4D PC-VIPR) MR evaluation of the renal arteries in transplant recipients: preliminary results: 4D PC-VIPR in renal graft arteries. J Magn Reson Imaging. 2017;46(2):595–603.
45. Nayak KS, Nielsen J-F, Bernstein MA, Markl M, Gatehouse PD, Botnar RM, et al. Cardiovascular magnetic resonance phase contrast imaging. J Cardiovasc Magn Reson. 2015;17(1):71.
46. Xiang Q-S. Temporal phase unwrapping for cine velocity imaging. J Magn Reson Imaging. 1995;5(5):529–34.
47. Untenberger M, Hüllebrand M, Tautz L, Joseph AA, Voit D, Merboldt KD, et al. Spatiotemporal phase unwrapping for real-time phase-contrast flow MRI: phase unwrapping for real-time flow MRI. Magn Reson Med. 2015;74(4):964–70.
48. Carrillo H, Osses A, Uribe S, Bertoglio C. Optimal dual-VENC unwrapping in phase-

contrast MRI. IEEE Trans Med Imaging. 2019;38(5):1263–70.
49. Loecher M, Schrauben E, Johnson KM, Wieben O. Phase unwrapping in 4D MR flow with a 4D single-step laplacian algorithm: 4D Laplacian unwrapping for 4D flow MRI. J Magn Reson Imaging. 2016;43(4):833–42.
50. François CJ. Abdominal magnetic resonance angiography. Magn Reson Imaging Clin N Am. 2020;28(3):395–405.
51. Weinreb JC, Rodby RA, Yee J, Wang CL, Fine D, McDonald RJ, et al. Use of intravenous gadolinium-based contrast Media in Patients with kidney disease: consensus statements from the American College of Radiology and the National Kidney Foundation. Radiology. 2021;298(1):28–35.
52. McDonald RJ, Levine D, Weinreb J, Kanal E, Davenport MS, Ellis JH, et al. Gadolinium retention: a research roadmap from the 2018 NIH/ACR/RSNA workshop on gadolinium chelates. Radiology. 2018;289(2):517–34.
53. Moratal D, Valles-Luch A, Marti-Bonmati L, Brummer M. K-space tutorial: an MRI educational tool for a better understanding of k-space. Biomed Imaging Interv J. 2008;4(1):e15. http://www.biij.org/2008/1/e15/e15.pdf.
54. Wilman AH, Riederer SJ, King BF, Debbins JP, Rossman PJ, Ehman RL. Fluoroscopically triggered contrast-enhanced three-dimensional MR angiography with elliptical centric view order: application to the renal arteries. Radiology. 1997;205(1):137–46.
55. Timms L, Zhou T, Lyu Y, Qiao J, Mishra V, Lahoud RM, et al. Ferumoxytol-enhanced ultrashort TE MRA and quantitative morphometry of the human kidney vasculature. Abdom Radiol. 2021;46(7):3288–300.
56. Slanina M, Žižka J, Klzo L, Lojík M. Contrast-enhanced MR angiography utilizing parallel acquisition techniques in renal artery stenosis detection. Eur J Radiol. 2010;75(1):e46–50.
57. Warning: risk for serious hypersensitivity/anaphylaxis reactions. Revised 2018.
58. Toth GB, Varallyay CG, Horvath A, Bashir MR, Choyke PL, Daldrup-Link HE, et al. Current and potential imaging applications of ferumoxytol for magnetic resonance imaging. Kidney Int. 2017;92(1):47–66.
59. Finn JP, Nguyen K-L, Han F, Zhou Z, Salusky I, Ayad I, et al. Cardiovascular MRI with ferumoxytol. Clin Radiol. 2016 Aug;71(8):796–806.
60. McCullough BJ, Kolokythas O, Maki JH, Green DE. Ferumoxytol in clinical practice: implications for MRI. J Magn Reson Imaging. 2013;37(6):1476–9.
61. Courtier J, Rao AG, Anupindi SA. Advanced imaging techniques in pediatric body MRI. Pediatr Radiol. 2017;47(5):522–33.
62. Stoumpos S, Hennessy M, Vesey AT, Radjenovic A, Kasthuri R, Kingsmore DB, et al. Ferumoxytol magnetic resonance angiography: a dose-finding study in patients with chronic kidney disease. Eur Radiol. 2019;29(7):3543–52.
63. Grobner T. Gadolinium—a specific trigger for the development of nephrogenic fibrosing dermopathy and nephrogenic systemic fibrosis? Nephrol Dial Transplant. 2006;21(4):1104–8.
64. Attari H, Cao Y, Elmholdt TR, Zhao Y, Prince MR. A systematic review of 639 patients with biopsy-confirmed nephrogenic systemic fibrosis. Radiology. 2019;292(2):376–86.
65. Lancelot E. Revisiting the pharmacokinetic profiles of gadolinium-based contrast agents: differences in long-term biodistribution and excretion. Investig Radiol. 2016;51(11):691–700.
66. Boer A, Harteveld AA, Pieters TT, Blankestijn PJ, Bos C, Froeling M, et al. Decreased native renal T_1 up to one week after gadobutrol administration in healthy volunteers. J Magn Reson Imaging. 2020;52(2):622–31.
67. Lee VS, Martin DJ, Krinsky GA, Rofsky NM. Gadolinium-Enhanced MR Angiography: artifacts and pitfalls. AJR Am J Roentgenol. 2000;175:197–205.
68. Edelman RR, Koktzoglou I. Noncontrast MR angiography: an update: noncontrast MR angiography. J Magn Reson Imaging. 2019;49(2):355–73.
69. King BF. MR Angiography of the Renal Arteries. Semin Ultrasound CT MR. 1996;17(4):398–403. https://doi.org/10.1016/s0887-2171(96)90025-6.
70. Morita S, Masukawa A, Suzuki K, Hirata M, Kojima S, Ueno E. Unenhanced MR angiography: techniques and clinical applications in patients with chronic kidney disease. Radiographics. 2011;31(2):E13–33.
71. Gaudiano C, Busato F, Ferramosca E, Cecchelli C, Corcioni B, De Sanctis LB, et al. 3D FIESTA pulse sequence for assessing renal artery stenosis: is it a reliable application in unenhanced magnetic resonance angiography? Eur Radiol. 2014;24(12):3042–50.
72. Boss A, Martirosian P, Graf H, Claussen C, Schlemmer H-P, Schick F. High resolution MR perfusion imaging of the kidneys at 3 tesla without administration of contrast media. RöFo. 2005;177(12):1625–30.
73. Coenegrachts KL, Hoogeveen RM, Vaninbroukx JA, Bosmans HT, Bielen DJ, Maleux G, et al. High-spatial-resolution 3D balanced turbo field-Echo technique for MR angiography of the renal arteries: initial experience. Radiology. 2004;231(1):237–42.
74. Bultman EM, Klaers J, Johnson KM, François CJ, Schiebler ML, Reeder SB, et al. Non-contrast enhanced 3D SSFP MRA of the renal allograft vasculature: a comparison between radial linear combination and Cartesian inflow-weighted acquisitions. Magn Reson Imaging. 2014;32(2):190–5.
75. Zhang LJ, Peng J, Wen J, Schoepf UJ, Varga-Szemes A, Griffith LP, et al. Non-contrast-enhanced magnetic resonance angiography: a reliable clinical tool for evaluating transplant renal artery stenosis. Eur Radiol. 2018;28(10):4195–204.

76. Mallouhi A, Schocke M, Judmaier W, Wolf C, Dessl A, Czermak BV, et al. 3D MR angiography of renal arteries: comparison of volume rendering and maximum intensity projection algorithms. Radiology. 2002;223(2):509–16.
77. Baskaran V, Pereles FS, Nemcek AA, Carr JC, Miller FH, Ly J, et al. Gadolinium-enhanced 3D MR angiography of renal artery stenosis. Acad Radiol. 2002;9(1):50–9.
78. Smedby Ö, Öberg R, Åsberg B, Stenström H, Eriksson P. Standardized volume-rendering of contrast-enhanced renal magnetic resonance angiography. Acta Radiol. 2005;46(5):497–504.
79. Fink C, Hallscheidt P, Hosch W, Ott R, Wiesel M, Kauffmann G, et al. Preoperative evaluation of living renal donors: value of contrast-enhanced 3D magnetic resonance angiography and comparison of three rendering algorithms. Eur Radiol. 2003;13(4):794–801.
80. Goldblatt H, Lynch J, Hanzal RF. Summerville Studies on experimental hypertension. J Exp Med. 1934;59(3):347–79.
81. Morganti A, Bencini C, Del Vecchio C, Strata M. Treatment of atherosclerotic renal artery stenosis. J Am Soc Nephrol. 2002;13(suppl 3):S187–9.
82. Glockner JF, Vrtiska TJ. Renal MR and CT angiography: current concepts. Abdom Imaging. 2007;32(3):407–20.
83. Gornik HL, Persu A, Adlam D, Aparicio LS, Azizi M, Boulanger M, et al. First international consensus on the diagnosis and management of fibromuscular dysplasia. Vasc Med. 2019;24(2):164–89.
84. Rountas C, Vlychou M, Vassiou K, Liakopoulos V, Kapsalaki E, Koukoulis G, et al. Imaging modalities for renal artery stenosis in suspected Renovascular hypertension: prospective Intraindividual comparison of color Doppler US, CT angiography, GD-enhanced MR angiography, and digital Substraction angiography. Ren Fail. 2007;29(3):295–302.
85. Solař M, Žižka J, Krajina A, Michl A, Raupach J, Klzo L, et al. Comparison of duplex ultrasonography and magnetic resonance imaging in the detection of significant renal artery stenosis. Acta Med (Hradec Kralove). 2011;54(1):9–12.
86. Tan KT, van Beek EJR, Brown PWG, van Delden OM, Tijssen J, Ramsay LE. Magnetic resonance angiography for the diagnosis of renal artery stenosis: a meta-analysis. Clin Radiol. 2002;57(7):617–24.
87. Nicholson T. Magnetic resonance angiography for the diagnosis of renal artery stenosis. Clin Radiol. 2003;58(3):257.
88. Parienty I, Rostoker G, Jouniaux F, Piotin M, Admiraal-Behloul F, Miyazaki M. Renal artery stenosis evaluation in chronic kidney disease patients: nonenhanced time-spatial labeling inversion-pulse three-dimensional MR angiography with regulated breathing versus DSA. Radiology. 2011 May;259(2):592–601.
89. Liang K-W, Chen J-W, Huang H-H, Su C-H, Tyan Y-S, Tsao T-F. The performance of noncontrast magnetic resonance angiography in detecting renal artery stenosis as compared with contrast enhanced magnetic resonance angiography using conventional angiography as a reference. J Comput Assist Tomogr. 2017;41(4):619–27.
90. Sebastià C, Sotomayor AD, Paño B, Salvador R, Burrel M, Botey A, et al. Accuracy of unenhanced magnetic resonance angiography for the assessment of renal artery stenosis. Eur J Radiol Open. 2016;3:200–6.
91. Ismaeel MM, Abdel-Hamid A. Role of high resolution contrast-enhanced magnetic resonance angiography (HR CeMRA) in management of arterial complications of the renal transplant. Eur J Radiol. 2011;79(2):e122–7.
92. Fananapazir G, Bashir MR, Corwin MT, Lamba R, Vu CT, Troppmann C. Comparison of ferumoxytol-enhanced MRA with conventional angiography for assessment of severity of transplant renal artery stenosis: Ferumoxytol MRA of graft artery stenosis. J Magn Reson Imaging. 2017;45(3):779–85.
93. Chan YL, Leung CB, Yu SCH, Yeung DKW, Li PKT. Comparison of non-breath-hold high resolution gadolinium-enhanced MRA with digital subtraction angiography in the evaluation on allograft renal artery stenosis. Clin Radiol. 2001;56(2):127–32.
94. Huber A, Heuck A, Scheidler J, Holzknecht N, Baur A, Stangl M, et al. Contrast-enhanced MR angiography in patients after kidney transplantation. Eur Radiol. 2001;11(12):2488–95.
95. Zhang W, Lin J, Wang S, Lv P, Wang L, Liu H, et al. Unenhanced respiratory-gated magnetic resonance angiography (MRA) of renal artery in hypertensive patients using true fast imaging with steady-state precession technique compared with contrast-enhanced MRA. J Comput Assist Tomogr. 2014;38(5):700–4.
96. Tang H, Wang Z, Wang L, Hu X, Wang Q, Li Z, et al. Depiction of transplant renal vascular anatomy and complications: unenhanced MR angiography by using spatial labeling with multiple inversion pulses. Radiology. 2014;271(3):879–87.
97. Bane O, Mendichovszky IA, Milani B, Dekkers IA, Deux J-F, Eckerbom P, et al. Consensus-based technical recommendations for clinical translation of renal BOLD MRI. MAGMA. 2020;33(1):199–215.
98. Dekkers IA, de Boer A, Sharma K, Cox EF, Lamb HJ, Buckley DL, et al. Consensus-based technical recommendations for clinical translation of renal T1 and T2 mapping MRI. MAGMA. 2020;33(1):163–76.
99. Ljimani A, Caroli A, Laustsen C, Francis S, Mendichovszky IA, Bane O, et al. Consensus-based technical recommendations for clinical translation of renal diffusion-weighted MRI. MAGMA. 2020;33(1):177–95.
100. Nery F, Buchanan CE, Harteveld AA, Odudu A, Bane O, Cox EF, et al. Consensus-based technical recommendations for clinical translation of renal ASL MRI. MAGMA. 2020;33(1):141–61.

Quantitative Susceptibility Mapping of the Kidney

16

Eric Bechler, Alexey V. Dimov, Martin R. Prince, Yi Wang, and Alexandra Ljimani

Introduction

There has been an increasing research interest in functional renal MRI. Several previous studies have demonstrated great potential of MRI biomarkers for characterizing different pathological processes involved in the progression of chronic kidney disease (CKD). A histological hallmark of CKD is renal interstitial fibrosis, which is also a major cause of progressive renal function loss. The amount of interstitial fibrosis in renal tissue is an important indicator for determining the reversibility of kidney damage. Up to date, the only reliable clinical tool to evaluate the degree of tubulointerstitial fibrosis is the renal biopsy. However, since biopsies are invasive, impaired by sampling bias and not arbitrarily repeatable, a non-invasive imaging modality able to accurately assess the degree of renal interstitial fibrosis is highly desirable.

Quantitative susceptibility mapping (QSM) [1] is a novel MRI technique, which combines magnitude and phase of the gradient echo (GRE) to derive quantitative information about the magnetic properties of the underlying tissue. Conventionally, only the magnitude information has been used for diagnostic MR imaging, while the phase has been discarded. In QSM, signal phase is incorporated into rigorous biophysical modeling of the MRI signal [2]. QSM has been shown to be sensitive to changes in tissue microstructure and chemical composition and is, therefore, a promising, non-invasive approach for the assessment of renal interstitial fibrosis.

The phase of an MRI signal of a given voxel is influenced by the magnetic field inhomogeneity, which arises in part from the susceptibility of the surrounding tissue [3–5]. This magnetic susceptibility is an intrinsic electron-cloud property of matter that describes the extent to which a material is magnetized in an external field. The phase dispersion within a voxel also contributes to the T_2^* decay of the MRI signal magnitude. *Susceptibility-weighted imaging (SWI)* takes advantage of the intrinsic nonlocal properties of the phase to enhance the magnitude hypointensity (blooming artifact) of a T_2^*-weighted gradient echo sequence [6]. SWI has been widely applied in clinical diagnostics [7], for example, to detect cerebral microbleeds [8] and to visualize iron depositions in the human brain [9]. Although SWI can be used for qualitative assessment of tissue susceptibility, it cannot be used to determine a quantitative value for specific tissue structures [10].

E. Bechler · A. Ljimani (✉)
Department of Diagnostic and Interventional Radiology, Medical Faculty, Heinrich Heine University Düsseldorf, Düsseldorf, Germany
e-mail: Alexandra.ljimani@med.uni-duesseldorf.de

A. V. Dimov · M. R. Prince · Y. Wang
Department of Radiology, Weill Cornell Medicine, New York, NY, USA

S. D. Serai, K. Darge (eds.), *Advanced Clinical MRI of the Kidney*,
https://doi.org/10.1007/978-3-031-40169-5_16

It should be emphasized that the phase information in one voxel does not originate from the tissue in that voxel alone and is a combination of contributions from all surrounding magnetic susceptibility sources. Contribution of magnetic susceptibility depends on the displacement magnitude of the source to the voxel and the displacement orientation with respect to the applied magnetic field. Compared to tissue susceptibility contrasts, nearby tissue–air interfaces have much larger susceptibility contrasts and contribute to the large part of the phase measured on MRI.

QSM models the relationship between the measured MRI phase and the tissue susceptibility according to the dipole field. Unfortunately, the dipole kernel contains zeros and phase data contains noise, which make the phase to susceptibility inverse problem *ill-posed.* Additional information can be used to solve this inverse problem optimally through Bayesian inference. Accordingly, QSM requires several complex post-processing steps: phase unwrapping, background field removal, and finding an actual solution to the ill-posed inverse problem [11].

Clinical application of QSM has been overwhelmingly focused on the brain imaging [3, 4, 12, 13]. The main contributors to the magnetic susceptibility in the brain are iron, myelin, and calcium [11, 14–17]. Pathologic deposition of iron in the brain is often associated with various neurodegenerative diseases such as Parkinson's disease and multiple sclerosis (MS), and manifests as increase in measured susceptibility value [18, 19]. Myelin, on the other hand, is diamagnetic and thus leads to a decrease in the apparent tissue susceptibility. In the early stages of MS white matter lesions formation, demyelination-associated increase in magnetic susceptibility can be used as a biomarker for MS disease [4, 20].

Beyond the neuroimaging applications, QSM has been used to study liver iron content [21, 22] and fibrosis [23], prostate calcifications [24], cardiac oxygenation [25], knee cartilage [26], and carotid plaques [27]. Despite this progress, body QSM remains technically challenging. First, the presence of the interstitial and subcutaneous fat characterized by chemical shift complicates the estimation of the field map that is a critical step in the QSM algorithm [3, 22]. Second, respiratory movement of the upper abdominal organs blurs structural contrast, compromising the fidelity of the reconstructed susceptibility maps [22]. Third, the large susceptibility variations across the air–tissue interfaces and areas of low signal-to-noise ratio (SNR) cause severe streaking artifacts in QSM maps. Combined, these challenges make accuracy of the reconstructed susceptibility maps strongly dependent on reconstruction steps, such as unwrapping and background field removal [28].

QSM in the human kidney has not yet been adopted in clinical practice. However, existing body of research suggests that kidney inflammation and fibrosis lead to measurable decrease in susceptibility of kidney parenchyma in mice model [29]. Similar study in human subjects with severe kidney fibrosis [30] provided further support of diagnostic potential QSM in in vivo kidney imaging.

This chapter will take a closer look at the physics and concepts behind magnetic susceptibility and explain in detail how to calculate QSM from an MRI phase image. We will offer suggestions on best-suited sequences and post-processing algorithms, so that QSM can be successfully implemented for in vivo measurements in kidneys on clinical MRI scanners. The last part of this chapter will discuss selected clinical examples and possible applications of QSM in kidney pathologies.

MRI Physics and Acquisition Protocols

Magnetic Susceptibility

In electromagnetism, the magnetic susceptibility is a quantitative measure that describes the degree to which material is magnetized upon placement

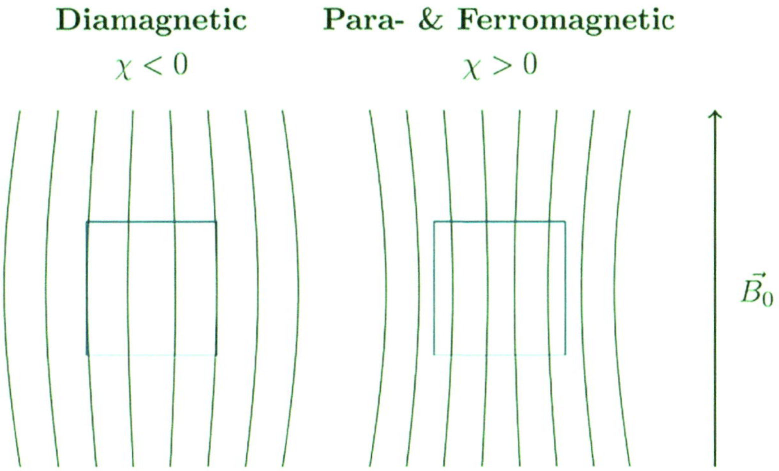

Fig. 16.1 Effect of a material (rectangle) with magnetic susceptibility χ on the magnetic field lines when exposed to an external magnetic field $\vec{B}$

in an external magnetic field. This dimensionless value is defined as the ratio between the material magnetization and the strength of the external field:

$$\chi = \frac{M}{H} \tag{16.1}$$

where M is the magnetization of the material and H is the magnetic field strength.

Based on the character of interaction between the matter and magnetic field, three major groups of materials could be defined (Fig. 16.1):

- Diamagnetics ($\chi < 0$) such as water, copper, and calcium oxalate repel magnetic field from themselves and develop an internal magnetization opposing the applied field (Fig. 16.1), leading to a decreased *magnetic flux density B* [31, 32].
- Paramagnetics ($\chi > 0$) such as manganese and deoxyhemoglobin attract magnetic field into the material and develop an internal magnetization in the direction of the applied field. Paramagnetic materials lead to an increased magnetic flux [31, 32].
- Ferromagnetics ($\chi \gg 1$) such as iron are similar to the paramagnetic substances in their interaction with magnetic field; however, the effect is much stronger. In general, ferromagnetic materials are not MR-safe and cannot be used in an MRI machine, since they would be pulled into the scanner bore like projectiles, creating safety issues [31, 32].

Most healthy human tissues are weakly diamagnetic, with the susceptibility comparable to that of water. However, in various pathologic conditions, this can be dramatically altered. Thus, deposition of excess iron within deep grey matter regions in Parkinson's disease, or in liver parenchyma in hemochromatosis, leads to strong increase of susceptibility of the affected tissues [19, 22]. Similarly, calcifications and protein deposits can result in strong shift towards diamagnetism [32, 33]. Accordingly, the susceptibility values measured on QSM should be interpreted with the underlying molecular processes in mind.

QSM Forward Problem

The magnetic field inhomogeneity ΔB_z induced by a magnetization distribution $M_z\left(\vec{r}'\right)$ in point $\vec{r}$ can be computed through a volume integral sans source location [3, 34, 35]:

$$\Delta B_z(\vec{r}) = \frac{\mu_0}{4\pi}\int_{V'}\left[\frac{3(z-z')^2}{|\vec{r}-\vec{r}'|^2} - 1\right]\frac{M_z(\vec{r}')}{|\vec{r}-\vec{r}'|^3}d^3r'. \quad (16.2)$$

where μ_0 is the vacuum permeability. Alternatively, this relationship can be reformulated as a convolution between the magnetization and the unit dipole field or *dipole kernel* $d(\vec{r})$:

$$\Delta B_z(\vec{r}) = \mu_0 M_z(\vec{r}) * d(\vec{r}), \quad (16.3)$$

with

$$d(\vec{r}) = \frac{1}{4\pi}\frac{3\cos^2(\Theta-1)}{r^3}. \quad (16.4)$$

where Θ is the angle between $\vec{r}$ and the z-axis. Using the Fourier convolution theorem and the assumption $\mu_0 M_z(\vec{r}) \approx B_0\chi(\vec{r})$ (true for $\chi \ll 1$), Eq. 16.3 can be re-written as multiplication in k-space:

$$\Delta B_z(\vec{r}) = B_0 \cdot FT^{-1}\left(X(\vec{k})\cdot D(\vec{k})\right). \quad (16.5)$$

Here FT^{-1} denotes the inverse Fourier transform, and $X(\vec{k})$ and $D(\vec{k})$ are the Fourier transforms of the susceptibility map and dipole kernel, respectively. $D(\vec{k})$ is explicitly defined as

$$D(\vec{k}) = \begin{cases} \frac{1}{3} - \frac{k_z^2}{k^2} & \text{for } k \neq 0 \\ 0 & \text{for } k = 0 \end{cases} \quad (16.6)$$

Due to the spatial extent of $d(\vec{r})$, field inhomogeneity $\Delta B_z(\vec{r})$ is *inherently nonlocal*, being a combination of two components caused by magnetic susceptibilities within (b_t, "tissue field") and outside (B_{bkg}, "background field") the region of interest [3, 5]:

$$\Delta B_z = b_t + B_{bkg} \quad (16.7)$$

The background fields can originate from a variety of sources, such as macroscopic currents in MRI shim coils, the inhomogeneity of the static main magnetic field, or simply the susceptibility change between air and tissue [36]. Usually, the contribution from the latter has the greatest impact on evolution of the signals phase.

Magnetic Field Mapping

Presence of the spatially varying field inhomogeneity ΔB_z (Eq. 16.3) causes the individual protons to sense a different magnetic field and thereby exhibit a spatially dependent precession frequency:

$$\Delta\omega(\vec{r}) = \gamma \cdot \Delta B_z(\vec{r}) \quad (16.8)$$

The induced magnetic field perturbation ΔB_z required for reconstruction of $\chi(\vec{r})$, therefore, can be estimated from $\Delta\omega$ measured from multi-echo GRE phase images:

$$\phi(\vec{r}, TE_j) = \gamma B_0 \cdot \Delta\omega(\vec{r}) \cdot TE_j \quad (16.9)$$

In the case of large SNR, $\Delta\omega(\vec{r})$ can be estimated through the linear regression of the signal phases at various TE. In a more general approach, $\Delta\omega(\vec{r})$ can be estimated iteratively using a gradient method, such as the Gauss–Newton or Levenberg–Marquardt.

Quantitative Susceptibility Mapping (QSM)

To calculate the underlying susceptibility, three major post-processing steps are typically used. First, the estimated field is unwrapped to remove 2π discontinuities. Second, the background field component is removed in order to estimate the tissue field dependent only on the underlying susceptibility. Third, the ill-posed inverse problem is solved to calculate the susceptibility map.

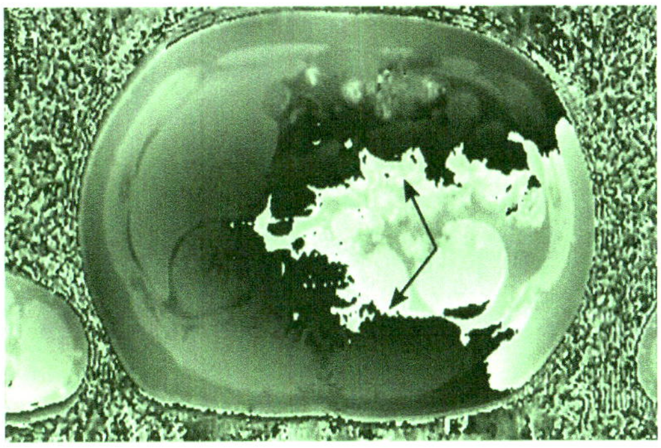

Fig. 16.2 Example of a phase image of the human abdomen with phase wraps (black arrows)

Phase Unwrapping

The field estimated from Eq. 16.9 might contain artificial jumps from voxel to voxel due to periodicity of the measured phase and its determination only up to a period such as $(-\pi, \pi]$ (Fig. 16.2). To map $\Delta\omega(\vec{r})$, these phase wraps have to be compensated through addition of integer multiples of 2π [37]:

$$\Delta\omega(\vec{r}) \cdot TE_j = \phi(\vec{r}, TE_j) + 2\pi \cdot k(\vec{r}, TE_j). \quad (16.10)$$

The voxel-dependent integer k is determined under assumption that the field map is spatially smooth. Multiple methods have been developed to impose this physical constraint via *path-following* and global minimization with *graph-cuts*. Unwrapping can also be rapidly achieved by the Fourier spectral solution of the Laplacian of the phase.

The path-following methods unwrap the phase along a specific path. First, several seed voxels within the ROI are heuristically selected. Then, adjacent voxel are iteratively added by minimizing the difference in phase with all previous voxels: if a difference of more than π is detected, the algorithm assumes that a phase wrap is present and adds or subtracts 2π to the candidate voxel. Path-following methods are prone to errors due to noise, and most algorithms use the so-called *quality map* to unwrap voxels along the paths with the highest signal-to-noise ratio (SNR) first [38].

The *graph-cuts* algorithms solve a global energy minimization problem, which assumes that adjacent voxels should not have a large difference in their phase values. The algorithm assigns a k-value for every voxel, repeating for multiple iterations to solve the equation above for the entire volume [39, 40].

Laplacian methods estimate the true phase from the measured wrapped phase by solving the Poisson equation [41]:

$$\nabla^2\phi_{true} = \cos(\phi_{wrapped}) \cdot \nabla^2 \sin(\phi_{wrapped}) - \sin(\phi_{wrapped}) \cdot \nabla^2 \cos(\phi_{wrapped}) \quad (16.11)$$

However, due to the properties of the Laplacian operator, solution of Eq. 16.11 determines estimate of ϕ_{true} only up to harmonic phase components, and application of boundary conditions is required to calculate the true underlying phase.

For a deeper understanding of the individual algorithms, we recommend the review by Robinson et al. [42].

Background Field Removal

After phase unwrapping, the resulting phase map is proportional to the magnetic field inhomogeneity $\Delta B_z(\vec{r})$. Since the background fields are often one to two orders of magnitude larger than tissue-related field variations within the ROI Ω, they are typically removed before the estimation of the susceptibility map [3].

By definition, the background fields are harmonic inside of Ω, i.e., $\nabla^2 B_{ext} = 0 \; in \; \Omega$. This property has been successfully utilized in a number of methods (e.g., *Sophisticated Harmonic Artifact Removal for Phase data (SHARP)* [43] and *Laplacian Boundary Value (LBV)* [44]) to separate the background and tissue field. A detailed explanation of background field removal for QSM and an overview of the different algorithms can be found in [36].

Solving the Ill-Posed Inverse Problem

In QSM, the inverse problem is solved by fitting measured field inhomogeneity to Eq. 16.5 in Fourier or to Eq. 16.4 in image domain to determine the susceptibility χ. This is an ill-posed problem because of the conic surface in k-space $k_x^2 + k_y^2 - 2k_z^2 = 0$ spanned by the *magic angle* ($\approx 54.7^{\circ}$) with respect to the main magnetic field where the dipole kernel is zero. Presence of this surface allows arbitrary k-space values in solutions $X(k)$ in the zero-cone neighborhood (Eq. 16.5).

Multiple approaches to overcome this problem have been developed to date. The closed-form *Truncated K-space Division (TKD)* substitutes values in $D(\vec{k})$ that fall below a certain threshold to avoid division by zero [45, 46]:

$$X(\vec{k}) = \frac{sign(D(\vec{k}))}{\max(\lambda, |D(\vec{k})|)} \cdot FT\left(\frac{\Delta B_z}{B_0}\right) \quad (16.12)$$

Alternatively, iterative optimization methods utilize physical priors to find the solution directly in image-space. For example, the *Morphology Enabled Dipole Inversion (MEDI)* algorithm exploits the structural consistency between the susceptibility map and the T_2^* w magnitude image of the same gradient echo. The algorithm penalizes erroneous unphysical solutions to Eq. 16.5 by putting additional minimization cost on the voxels that belong to edges in the susceptibility map but not to edges in the magnitude image [47].

Overall, there is a vast number of algorithms that try to tackle the ill-posed nature of the field-to-source inverse problem. The results of the latest challenge aimed to provide objective assessment of their performance can be found in [48].

Challenges in Body QSM

In comparison to the brain, everywhere else in the human body, there are additional challenges for QSM that must be addressed to successfully calculate the susceptibility. First, GRE phase includes additional contribution from electron cloud shielding ("chemical shift") of protons in fat molecules [22]. The chemical shift results in unphysical discontinuities at the boundaries between water- and fat-based tissues, and therefore, its influence must be removed before the susceptibility can be calculated. This can be achieved by the *Simultaneous Phase Unwrapping and Removal of chemical Shift (SPURS)* algorithm [3]. SPURS uses a combination of graph-cuts phase unwrapping and the *T_2^*-Iterative Decomposition of water and fat with Echo Asymmetry and Leas-squares estimation (T_2^*-IDEAL)* [49] to properly account for fat signals.

Second, breathing causes tissue motion during the MR imaging, creating artifacts in both the magnitude and the phase of the signal. These image artifacts have a negative effect on the computation of the magnetic field inhomogeneity resulting in low-fidelity susceptibility maps [22]. To prevent artifacts due to respiratory motion, breath-holding acquisition is typically used. However, this severely limits the acquisition time to below 30 s, allowing acquisition of ~30 thick (5 mm) slices. Alternatively, respiratory bellows gating or the navigator gating could be utilized [50–52]. Often, the latter works only with 2D sequences, which have proven to be insufficient for QSM [4, 10].

Third, the abdominal ROIs typically contain pockets of air and other strong susceptibility sources such as bones. Due to their closeness to the tissues of interest, their influence on magnetic field are hard to eliminate through background field removal techniques, which leads to artifacts in susceptibility maps [53]. Additionally, air leads to an increased amount of phase wraps that must be resolved. A recent analysis has shown that not every phase unwrapping algorithm is suitable for processing of the abdominal phase data. Methods based on graph-cuts tend to have better performance in body imaging, which make them highly applicable in kidney QSM [28].

MRI Sequence Parameters

The purpose of this section is to give the reader suitable sequence parameters for QSM in the abdomen, particularly the kidneys. These parameters are intended as a suggestion that could be further adapted to a specific research project. Here we will also describe some of the more important parameters for QSM in the kidneys and how they affect the measurement.

The first decision that must be made is whether the measurement should be performed in 2D or 3D. 2D acquisitions have the advantage of being less prone to patient movement. In addition, they provide the option to use a bellows or the navigator gating to account for respiratory movements of the kidneys. However, 2D measurements suffer from inter-slice inconsistencies, which result from large field variations [4]. Therefore, use of 3D sequences should be preferred. If the data is to be acquired with a 2D sequence, the inter-slice gap has to be set to zero to minimize the above-mentioned inconsistencies.

Separation of water and fat signals involves fitting of complex data with the minimum of five real-valued parameters [54]. Therefore, a minimum of three echoes is required for successful field mapping, although higher number of echoes is typically acquired (six echoes). For optimal phase SNR, the last acquired TE is typically limited by the characteristic T_2^* of the tissue of interest [2]. Thus, a recent study showed that susceptibility estimation in the abdomen reduces in inaccuracy when echo times larger than 15 ms are included [28]. Furthermore, for the abdominal imaging, the largest TE should be chosen relatively small (<15 ms) to achieve a short total scan time and facilitate a single breath-hold acquisition.

Voxel size has been reported as an important parameter for QSM accuracy [3, 55, 56]. It has been shown that a low in- and through-plane resolution leads to underestimated susceptibility values [56]. The reduced QSM accuracy at low resolutions is likely caused by dipole discretization errors. To maximize the resolution while keeping the acquisition time below 30 s, for abdominal QSM, 20–30 slices with thickness of 3–5 mm and in-plane resolution of $(1.5 - 2) \times (1.5 - 2)$ are typically acquired.

Lastly, the choice of readout bandwidth should be considered. Due to its chemical shift, the fat with ROI appears to be shifted; the magnitude of the shift is determined by the field strength, in-plane resolution, and readout bandwidth. Ideally, a fat water shift of below 1.5 voxels should be reached.

Table 16.1 MRI settings for successful measurement of QSM

Parameter	Value
FoV	$420 \times 315 \times 78$ mm^3
Resolution	$256 \times 192 \times 26$
Voxel size	$1.6 \times 1.6 \times 3$ mm^3
TE/ΔTE/TR	3.1/3.7/17 ms
Number of echoes	4
Readout bandwidth	1775 Hz
Parallel imaging factor (GRAPPA)	2

To summarize, the following kidney QSM protocol using an axial single breath-hold 3D multi-echo gradient echo sequence can be suggested: number of echoes = 4; $TE_1/\Delta TE/TR = 3.1/3.7/17$ ms; flip angle = 15°; acquisition matrix = 256 × 192 × 26; voxel size = 1.64 × 1.64 × 3 mm^3; bandwidth = 1775 Hz/pixel; slice and phase Fourier encoding = 6/8; parallel imaging acceleration factor = 2; acquisition time 33 s (Table 16.1). These parameters have been successfully applied for in vivo clinical studies [30].

Post-Processing Pipeline for QSM

The post-processing pipeline used in [30] can be utilized to calculate accurate susceptibility maps in the kidney (Fig. 16.3).

First, the measured data needs to be interpolated to artificially increase the resolution. This can be done by the so-called *zero-filling* or *zero-padding* in k-space. Earlier studies have shown that zero-padding prior to QSM calculation improves final image accuracy [57]. In the next step, the measured phase data needs to be unwrapped and the additional phase component due to the chemical shift of fat needs to be removed. In the abdomen, especially the kidneys, unwrapping algorithms based on the *graph-cuts* algorithm seem to be the most accurate solution [28]. The SPURS algorithm [3] is able to suc-

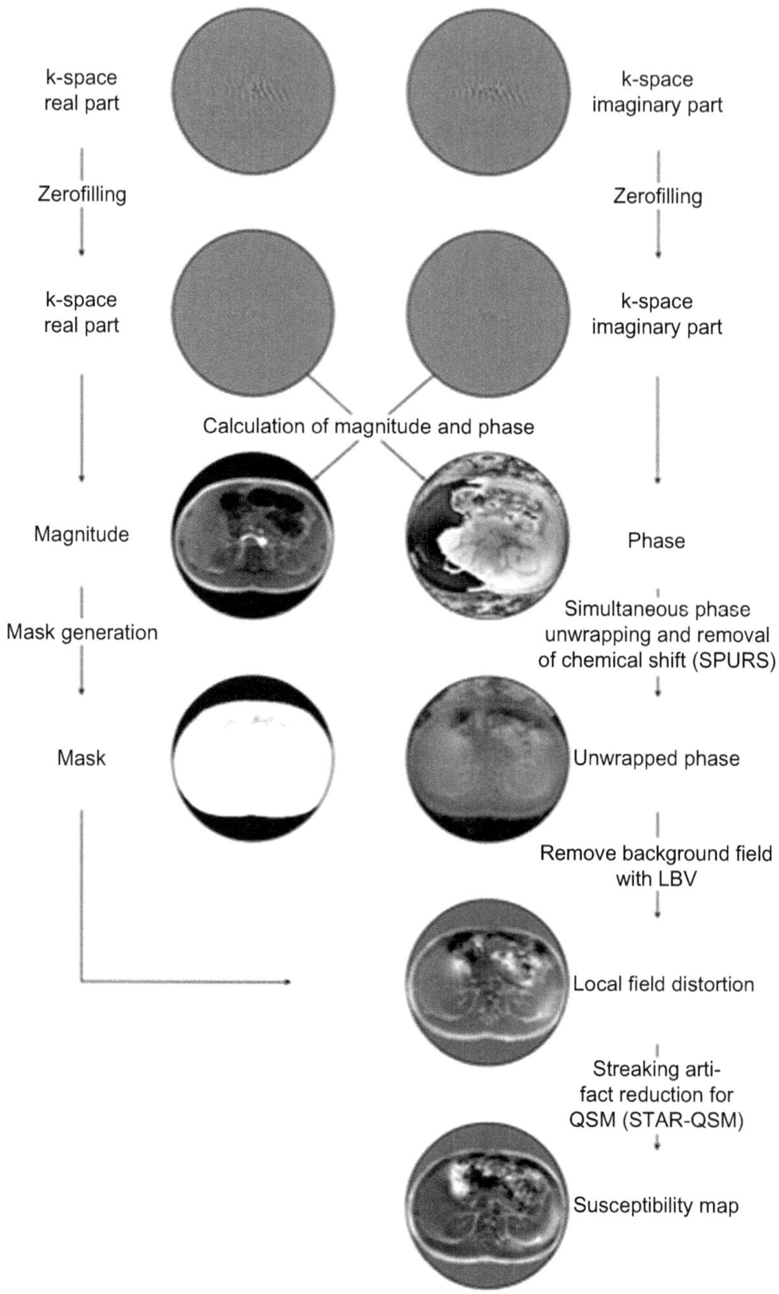

Fig. 16.3 Flowchart showing the post-processing steps for QSM quantification

cessfully unwrap kidney phase data and also remove the unwanted field distortions. It is a component of the MEDI toolbox [47] and can be run with default settings.

After unwrapping, the background field needs to be removed to calculate the local magnetic field distortion, which results from the underlying magnetic susceptibility. From the more commonly used algorithms, the *Laplacian Boundary Value (LBV)* showed the most promising results for regions with large susceptibility changes [28, 53]. It is also part of the MEDI-toolbox and is ready to be used with default parameters.

The last step is the actual susceptibility calculation by solving the ill-posed inverse problem. Among the available algorithms, the *streaking artifact reduction for QSM (STAR-QSM)* [58] algorithm is a good choice due to its ability to handle large variation in magnetic susceptibility characteristic to abdominal imaging. By employing a two-level reconstruction approach to handle strong and weak sources, STAR-QSM significantly reduced the streaking artifacts due to shart susceptibility interfaces while preserving the sharp boundaries and fine anatomical details in the final image. STAR-QSM is available in the STI-Suite, a Matlab toolbox [59].

Possible Clinical Application of Renal QSM

QSM is sensitive to changes in tissue microstructure and chemical composition. In the brain, QSM was shown to reflect tissue changes due to iron deposition or inflammation caused by MS [4, 20]. Inspired by these findings, QSM has been in a pilot study of systemic inflammatory diseases with renal involvement, e.g., systemic lupus erythematosus (SLE), and systemic diseases leading to protein deposits in the renal tissue, e.g., multiple myeloma, amyloidosis, or even the quantification of fibrosis degrees (Fig. 16.4) [30].

Another promising clinical application of QSM in kidney is autosomal dominant polycystic kidney disease (ADPKD) imaging. Presently, the commonly utilized biomarker for prediction of the renal function decline in ADPKD is height-adjusted total kidney volume (ht-TKV) [60–62]. Despite its utility, this measure only provides a surrogate marker, which does not take in account many other features of ADPKD and manifestations of kidney injury provided by abdominal MRI. Thus, recent findings suggest that the renal cyst hemorrhage is a significant predictor of rapid disease progression to End-Stage Renal Disease (ESRD) [63, 64]. Cystic hemorrhage can be detected as hyperintense on T_1-weighted images

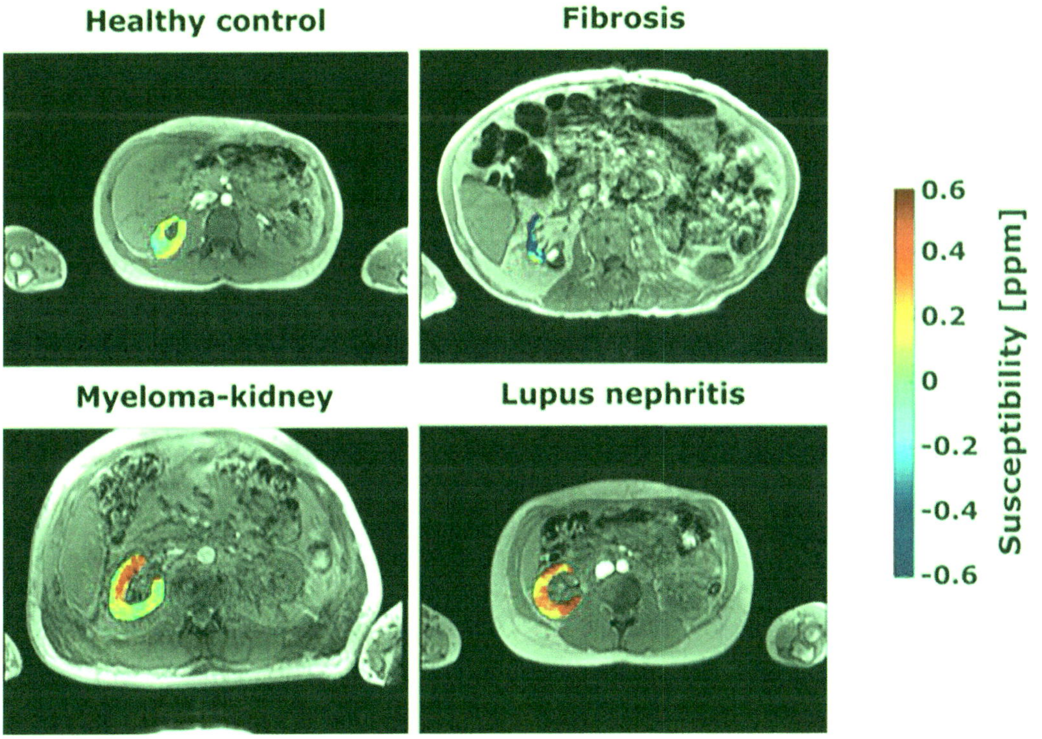

Fig. 16.4 Examples of QSM maps of a healthy volunteer, and subjects with high-degree renal fibrosis, kidney myeloma, and lupus nephritis. A noticeable difference in magnetic susceptibility can be seen between healthy and diseased renal parenchyma

acquired as a part of a multi-contrast abdominal MR examination, assuming erythrocytes have lysed releasing mobile iron [65]. However, the T_1-weighted signal intensity of hemorrhage is not hyperintense when erythrocytes have not lysed, or iron has been collected into large hemosiderin clusters. Thus, the T_1-weighted signal-intensity of hemorrhagic cysts is complicated and may lead to misdiagnosis. Due to its sensitivity to presence of paramagnetic iron particles, QSM is an attractive modality to enhance hemorrhagic cyst detection.

Kidney stones are common among the chronic kidney disease and ADPKD patients [66–70]. Patients with urinary stones should be followed up more closely for progression [69]. Non-contrast CT is a highly sensitive and specific technique for imaging kidney stones [71]. Once a partially obstructing ureteral stone has been identified on CT, following the gradually descent of the stone down the ureter is not practicable with CT due the cumulative radiation exposure of multiple scans [72]. QSM can exploit large differences in magnetic susceptibilities of blood products, mineral depositions, and normal kidney parenchyma to distinguish diagnostic features associated with the disease. QSM offers the potential to follow stones to see if they are progressing toward excretion or if the stone is stuck and an intervention will be required.

References

1. de Rochefort L, Liu T, Kressler B, et al. Quantitative susceptibility map reconstruction from MR phase data using Bayesian regularization: validation and application to brain imaging. Magn Reson Med. 2010;63(1):194–206.
2. Deistung A, Schafer A, Schweser F, Biedermann U, Turner R, Reichenbach JR. Toward in vivo histology: a comparison of quantitative susceptibility mapping (QSM) with magnitude-, phase-, and R2*-imaging at ultra-high magnetic field strength. NeuroImage. 2013;65:299–314.
3. Haacke EM, Liu S, Buch S, Zheng W, Wu D, Ye Y. Quantitative susceptibility mapping: current status and future directions. Magn Reson Imaging. 2015;33(1):1–25.
4. Schweser F, Deistung A, Reichenbach JR. Foundations of MRI phase imaging and processing for quantitative susceptibility mapping (QSM). Z Med Phys. 2016;26(1):6–34.
5. Liu C, Wei H, Gong NJ, Cronin M, Dibb R, Decker K. Quantitative susceptibility mapping: contrast mechanisms and clinical applications. Tomography. 2015;1(1):3–17.
6. Haacke EM, Xu Y, Cheng YC, Reichenbach JR. Susceptibility weighted imaging (SWI). Magn Reson Med. 2004;52(3):612–8.
7. Haacke EM, Reichenbach R Jr. Susceptibility weighted imaging in MRI: basic concepts and clinical applications, vol. xvi. Hoboken, NJ: Wiley-Blackwell; 2011. p. 743.
8. Ayaz M, Boikov AS, Haacke EM, Kido DK, Kirsch WM. Imaging cerebral microbleeds using susceptibility weighted imaging: one step toward detecting vascular dementia. J Magn Reson Imaging. 2010;31(1):142–8.
9. Liu Z, Shen HC, Lian TH, et al. Iron deposition in substantia nigra: abnormal iron metabolism, neuroinflammatory mechanism and clinical relevance. Sci Rep. 2017;7(1):14973.
10. Liu C, Li W, Tong KA, Yeom KW, Kuzminski S. Susceptibility-weighted imaging and quantitative susceptibility mapping in the brain. J Magn Reson Imaging. 2015;42(1):23–41.
11. Wang Y, Liu T. Quantitative susceptibility mapping (QSM): decoding MRI data for a tissue magnetic biomarker. Magn Reson Med. 2015;73(1):82–101.
12. Vinayagamani S, Sheelakumari R, Sabarish S, et al. Quantitative susceptibility mapping: technical considerations and clinical applications in neuroimaging. J Magn Reson Imaging. 2021;53(1):23–37.
13. Harada T, Kudo K, Fujima N, et al. Quantitative susceptibility mapping: basic methods and clinical applications. Radiographics. 2022;42(4):1161–76.
14. Duyn J. MR susceptibility imaging. J Magn Reson. 2013;229:198–207.
15. Reichenbach JR. The future of susceptibility contrast for assessment of anatomy and function. NeuroImage. 2012;62(2):1311–5.
16. Li X, Harrison DM, Liu H, et al. Magnetic susceptibility contrast variations in multiple sclerosis lesions. J Magn Reson Imaging. 2016;43(2):463–73.
17. Chen W, Zhu W, Kovanlikaya I, et al. Intracranial calcifications and hemorrhages: characterization with quantitative susceptibility mapping. Radiology. 2014;270(2):496–505.
18. Zivadinov R, Tavazzi E, Bergsland N, et al. Brain iron at quantitative MRI is associated with disability in multiple sclerosis. Radiology. 2018;289(2):487–96.
19. Li DTH, Hui ES, Chan Q, et al. Quantitative susceptibility mapping as an indicator of subcortical and limbic iron abnormality in Parkinson's disease with dementia. Neuroimage-Clin. 2018;20:365–73.
20. Deh K, Ponath GD, Molvi Z, et al. Magnetic susceptibility increases as diamagnetic molecules breakdown: myelin digestion during multiple sclerosis lesion formation contributes to increase on QSM. J Magn Reson Imaging. 2018;48(5):1281–7.
21. Sharma SD, Fischer R, Schoennagel BP, et al. MRI-based quantitative susceptibility mapping (QSM) and R2* mapping of liver iron overload: comparison

with SQUID-based biomagnetic liver susceptometry. Magn Reson Med. 2017;78(1):264–70.
22. Sharma SD, Hernando D, Horng DE, Reeder SB. Quantitative susceptibility mapping in the abdomen as an imaging biomarker of hepatic iron overload. Magn Reson Med. 2015;74(3):673–83.
23. Qu Z, Yang S, Xing F, et al. Magnetic resonance quantitative susceptibility mapping in the evaluation of hepatic fibrosis in chronic liver disease: a feasibility study. Quant Imaging Med Surg. 2021;11(4):1170–83.
24. Straub S, Laun FB, Emmerich J, et al. Potential of quantitative susceptibility mapping for detection of prostatic calcifications. J Magn Reson Imaging. 2017;45(3):889–98.
25. Wen Y, Weinsaft JW, Nguyen TD, et al. Free breathing three-dimensional cardiac quantitative susceptibility mapping for differential cardiac chamber blood oxygenation - initial validation in patients with cardiovascular disease inclusive of direct comparison to invasive catheterization. J Cardiovasc Magn Reson. 2019;21(1):70.
26. Dymerska B, Bohndorf K, Schennach P, Rauscher A, Trattnig S, Robinson SD. In vivo phase imaging of human epiphyseal cartilage at 7 T. Magn Reson Med. 2018;79(4):2149–55.
27. Nguyen TD, Wen Y, Du J, et al. Quantitative susceptibility mapping of carotid plaques using nonlinear total field inversion: initial experience in patients with significant carotid stenosis. Magn Reson Med. 2020;84(3):1501–9.
28. Bechler E, Stabinska J, Wittsack HJ. Analysis of different phase unwrapping methods to optimize quantitative susceptibility mapping in the abdomen. Magn Reson Med. 2019;82(6):2077–89.
29. Xie L, Sparks MA, Li W, et al. Quantitative susceptibility mapping of kidney inflammation and fibrosis in type 1 angiotensin receptor-deficient mice. NMR Biomed. 2013;26(12):1853–63.
30. Bechler E, Stabinska J, Thiel T, et al. Feasibility of quantitative susceptibility mapping (QSM) of the human kidney. MAGMA. 2021;34(3):389–97.
31. Bates LF. Modern magnetism, vol. ix. Cambridge Eng.: The University press; 1939. p. 331–9.
32. Schenck JF. The role of magnetic susceptibility in magnetic resonance imaging: MRI magnetic compatibility of the first and second kinds. Med Phys. 1996;23(6):815–50.
33. Luo J, He X, d'Avignon DA, Ackerman JJH, Yablonskiy DA. Protein-induced water H-1 MR frequency shifts: contributions from magnetic susceptibility and exchange effects. J Magn Reson. 2010;202(1):102–8.
34. Jackson JD. Classical electrodynamics, vol. xxi. New York: Wiley; 1999, 808 pp.
35. Marques JP, Bowtell R. Application of a Fourier-based method for rapid calculation of field inhomogeneity due to spatial variation of magnetic susceptibility. Concept Magn Reson B. 2005;25b(1):65–78.
36. Schweser F, Robinson SD, de Rochefort L, Li W, Bredies K. An illustrated comparison of processing methods for phase MRI and QSM: removal of background field contributions from sources outside the region of interest. NMR Biomed. 2017;30(4):e3604.
37. Ghiglia DC, Pritt MD. Two-dimensional phase unwrapping: theory, algorithms, and software, vol. xiv. New York: Wiley; 1998, 493 pp.
38. Witoszynskyj S, Rauscher A, Reichenbach JR, Barth M. Phase unwrapping of MR images using phi UN - a fast and robust region growing algorithm. Med Image Anal. 2009;13(2):257–68.
39. Bioucas-Dias JM, Valadao G. Phase unwrapping via graph cuts. IEEE T Image Process. 2007;16(3):698–709.
40. Dong JW, Chen F, Zhou D, Liu T, Yu ZF, Wang Y. Phase unwrapping with graph cuts optimization and dual decomposition acceleration for 3D high-resolution MRI data. Magn Reson Med. 2017;77(3):1353–8.
41. Schofield MA, Zhu YM. Fast phase unwrapping algorithm for interferometric applications. Opt Lett. 2003;28(14):1194–6.
42. Robinson SD, Bredies K, Khabipova D, Dymerska B, Marques JP, Schweser F. An illustrated comparison of processing methods for MR phase imaging and QSM: combining array coil signals and phase unwrapping. NMR Biomed. 2017;30(4):e3601.
43. Schweser F, Deistung A, Lehr BW, Reichenbach JR. Quantitative imaging of intrinsic magnetic tissue properties using MRI signal phase: an approach to in vivo brain iron metabolism? NeuroImage. 2011;54(4):2789–807.
44. Zhou D, Liu T, Spincemaille P, Wang Y. Background field removal by solving the Laplacian boundary value problem. NMR Biomed. 2014;27(3):312–9.
45. Shmueli K, de Zwart JA, van Gelderen P, Li TQ, Dodd SJ, Duyn JH. Magnetic susceptibility mapping of brain tissue in vivo using MRI phase data. Magn Reson Med. 2009;62(6):1510–22.
46. Wharton S, Schafer A, Bowtell R. Susceptibility mapping in the human brain using threshold-based k-space division. Magn Reson Med. 2010;63(5):1292–304.
47. Liu J, Liu T, de Rochefort L, et al. Morphology enabled dipole inversion for quantitative susceptibility mapping using structural consistency between the magnitude image and the susceptibility map. NeuroImage. 2012;59(3):2560–8.
48. Bilgic B, Langkammer C, Marques JP, et al. QSM reconstruction challenge 2.0: design and report of results. Magn Reson Med. 2021;86(3):1241–55.
49. Yu H, McKenzie CA, Shimakawa A, et al. Multiecho reconstruction for simultaneous water-fat decomposition and T2* estimation. J Magn Reson Imaging. 2007;26(4):1153–61.
50. Ehman RL, McNamara MT, Pallack M, Hricak H, Higgins CB. Magnetic resonance imaging with respiratory gating: techniques and advantages. AJR Am J Roentgenol. 1984;143(6):1175–82.
51. Klessen C, Asbach P, Kroencke TJ, et al. Magnetic resonance imaging of the upper abdomen using a free-breathing T2-weighted turbo spin echo sequence with navigator triggered prospective acquisition correction. J Magn Reson Imaging. 2005;21(5):576–82.
52. Vasanawala SS, Iwadate Y, Church DG, Herfkens RJ, Brau AC. Navigated abdominal T1-W MRI permits

free-breathing image acquisition with less motion artifact. Pediatr Radiol. 2010;40(3):340–4.
53. Fortier V, Levesque IR. Phase processing for quantitative susceptibility mapping of regions with large susceptibility and lack of signal. Magn Reson Med. 2018;79(6):3103–13.
54. Reeder SB, Pineda AR, Wen Z, et al. Iterative decomposition of water and fat with echo asymmetry and least-squares estimation (IDEAL): application with fast spin-echo imaging. Magn Reson Med. 2005;54(3):636–44.
55. Karsa A, Punwani S, Shmueli K. The effect of low resolution and coverage on the accuracy of susceptibility mapping. Magn Reson Med. 2019;81(3):1833–48.
56. Zhou D, Cho J, Zhang J, Spincemaille P, Wang Y. Susceptibility underestimation in a high-susceptibility phantom: dependence on imaging resolution, magnitude contrast, and other parameters. Magn Reson Med. 2017;78(3):1080–6.
57. Eskreis-Winkler S, Zhou D, Liu T, et al. On the influence of zero-padding on the nonlinear operations in quantitative susceptibility mapping. Magn Reson Imaging. 2017;35:154–9.
58. Wei H, Dibb R, Zhou Y, et al. Streaking artifact reduction for quantitative susceptibility mapping of sources with large dynamic range. NMR Biomed. 2015;28(10):1294–303.
59. Li W, Avram AV, Wu B, Xiao X, Liu CL. Integrated Laplacian-based phase unwrapping and background phase removal for quantitative susceptibility mapping. NMR Biomed. 2014;27(2):219–27.
60. Xue C, Zhou C, Mei C. Total kidney volume: the most valuable predictor of autosomal dominant polycystic kidney disease progression. Kidney Int. 2018;93(3):540–2.
61. Higashihara E, Yamamoto K, Kaname S, et al. Age- and height-adjusted total kidney volume growth rate in autosomal dominant polycystic kidney diseases. Clin Exp Nephrol. 2019;23(1):100–11.
62. Chapman AB, Bost JE, Torres VE, et al. Kidney volume and functional outcomes in autosomal dominant polycystic kidney disease. Clin J Am Soc Nephrol. 2012;7(3):479–86.
63. Cornec-Le Gall E, Audrezet MP, Rousseau A, et al. The PROPKD score: a new algorithm to predict renal survival in autosomal dominant polycystic kidney disease. J Am Soc Nephrol. 2016;27(3):942–51.
64. Riyahi S, Dev H, Blumenfeld JD, et al. Hemorrhagic cysts and other MR biomarkers for predicting renal dysfunction progression in autosomal dominant polycystic kidney disease. J Magn Reson Imaging. 2021;53(2):564–76.
65. Bradley WG Jr. MR appearance of hemorrhage in the brain. Radiology. 1993;189(1):15–26.
66. Kazancioglu R, Ecder T, Altintepe L, et al. Demographic and clinical characteristics of patients with autosomal dominant polycystic kidney disease: a multicenter experience. Nephron Clin Pract. 2011;117(3):c270–5.
67. Torres VE, Wilson DM, Hattery RR, Segura JW. Renal stone disease in autosomal dominant polycystic kidney disease. Am J Kidney Dis. 1993;22(4):513–9.
68. Nishiura JL, Neves RF, Eloi SR, Cintra SM, Ajzen SA, Heilberg IP. Evaluation of nephrolithiasis in autosomal dominant polycystic kidney disease patients. Clin J Am Soc Nephrol. 2009;4(4):838–44.
69. Ozkok A, Akpinar TS, Tufan F, et al. Clinical characteristics and predictors of progression of chronic kidney disease in autosomal dominant polycystic kidney disease: a single center experience. Clin Exp Nephrol. 2013;17(3):345–51.
70. Alexander RT, Hemmelgarn BR, Wiebe N, et al. Kidney stones and kidney function loss: a cohort study. BMJ. 2012;345:e5287.
71. Brisbane W, Bailey MR, Sorensen MD. An overview of kidney stone imaging techniques. Nat Rev Urol. 2016;13(11):654–62.
72. National Research Council (U.S.). Committee on health effects of exposure to low levels of ionizing radiations. Health effects of exposure to low levels of ionizing radiations: time for reassessment? vol. x. Washington, D.C.: National Academy Press; 1998, 76 pp.

MR Elastography for Evaluation of Kidney Fibrosis

17

Suraj D. Serai, Deep Gandhi, and Sudhakar K. Venkatesh

Part 1: Introduction and MRE Physics

Chronic kidney disease (CKD) is a collective term for kidney diseases that result in the progressive loss of renal function over time. Major causes of CKD include diabetic nephropathy, hypertensive nephrosclerosis, and glomerulonephritis. CKD leads to end stage renal disease, which requires dialysis or kidney transplant in most cases and could even lead to death if untreated or if treated after irreversible loss of renal function. CKD also leads to cardiovascular diseases, which are a major cause of deaths around the world. Renal fibrosis is an important pathway leading to the progression of CKD, marked by an abnormal increase in the interstitial extracellular matrix; as it progresses, renal tubules lose their function. Several studies have demonstrated the potential to curb and even reverse renal fibrosis if detected early before any significant permanent loss of renal function; therefore, diagnosis of renal fibrosis in the early stages is of paramount importance.

S. D. Serai (✉)
Children's Hospital of Philadelphia, University of Pennsylvania, Philadelphia, PA, USA
e-mail: serais@chop.edu

D. Gandhi · S. K. Venkatesh
Mayo Clinic, Rochester, MN, USA
e-mail: Gandhi.Deep@mayo.edu; Venkatesh.Sudhakar@mayo.edu

The current gold standard for assessing renal fibrosis is renal biopsy, which is generally done under ultrasound guidance [1]. Renal biopsy has several limitations such as sampling bias, and due to its invasive nature, pain risk of significant bleeding, risk of arteriovenous fistula, prolonged hospitalization, and secondary infections. Biopsy can also be technically challenging in obese individuals. Due to these factors, repeated biopsies for long-term monitoring and for evaluation in clinical trials for response assessment are typically not practical, and non-invasive tests are needed. While fibrosis can be directly visualized at histology, non-invasive techniques can provide surrogate biomarkers to indirectly assess fibrosis. Other non-invasive imaging techniques have the potential or have already been proven to diagnose renal fibrosis. Computed tomography (CT) has good overall diagnostic sensitivity for CKD, but it is limited for use in patients due to risk of higher radiation dose with repeated measurements. Although conventional ultrasound (US) imaging is a commonly used modality for diagnosing renal diseases, it is user-dependent, and has scanning limitations in obese patients. In recent years, US-based elastography methods such as transient elastography (TE), shear wave velocity imaging, acoustic radiation force impulse imaging (ARFI), and supersonic shear wave elastography (SWE) have been evaluated for diagnosing fibrosis in liver and kidneys [2]. However, US-based elastography methods pro-

S. D. Serai, K. Darge (eds.), *Advanced Clinical MRI of the Kidney*,
https://doi.org/10.1007/978-3-031-40169-5_17

vide only longitudinal one-dimensional stiffness, have lower penetration depth, and are highly dependent on body mass index, anisotropy of tissues, transducer force, and intra- and inter-observer variability. Also, US-based methods are typically insufficient for deeply seated abdominal organs such as kidneys due to the inability of ultrasound to penetrate deep inside the body.

Magnetic Resonance Imaging (MRI)-based methods are promising due to their non-invasive nature and lack of radiation as well as the ability to use them to perform repeated measurements for longitudinal monitoring without radiation risk to the patients. MRI-based methods also typically serve as a one-stop shop to answer the clinical questions that may pertain to the underlying pathology of the patient. The drawbacks of MRI in general are its access, especially in developing and underdeveloped countries, its cost, and relatively longer imaging time.

Magnetic Resonance Elastography

Magnetic Resonance Elastography (MRE) is a medical imaging technique that can non-invasively estimate the mechanical properties of soft tissue in vivo using a phase contrast sequence to image shear wave propagation within the tissues. MRE was developed in 1995 by Muthupillai and colleagues at Mayo Clinic as an imaging-based counterpart to physical palpation [3]. It is well known that mechanical properties of tissues change with pathological conditions. MRE has been shown to be effective for non-invasive assessment of tissue mechanical properties and used worldwide as a clinical tool to diagnose and stage liver fibrosis [4, 5]. Currently, MRE is also being investigated for clinical applications in brain, heart, lungs, pancreas, spleen, aorta, and intervertebral discs [6].

The principle of MRE is to induce harmonic vibrations of acoustic-range frequencies in the tissue of interest and image the propagation of these vibrations in the tissues to calculate quantitative values of mechanical parameters [7]. The desired output is to measure the stiffness value. The elastogram that is generated from the acquired images can differentiate if the tissue is hard or soft and can give diagnostic information about the presence of the disease. Since the mechanical properties of the renal tissues change with underlying pathologies, a non-invasive method such as MRE can be used to resolve the stiffness of renal tissues spatially. Thus, it could potentially be used for diagnosing renal fibrosis. MRE can be easily incorporated into standard clinical kidney MRI protocol [8]. Application of MRE for non-invasive evaluation of renal fibrosis has great potential for non-invasive assessment in patients with chronic kidney diseases. Development and applications of MRE in kidney are necessary primarily to validate the measurement against "gold-standard" invasive methods, to better understand physiology and pathophysiology, and to evaluate novel interventions for the management of CKD.

Modulus of Elasticity

Two parameters often used for describing tissue mechanical properties are shear modulus (μ) and Young's modulus (E). Poisson's ratio (ν), another widely used parameter, is the ratio of lateral strain to longitudinal strain. The shear modulus is known to be related to Young's modulus and one can be estimated from the other by knowing the Poisson's ratio. In general, soft tissues can be assumed to be incompressible and hence the Poisson's ratio can be assumed to be 0.5. The relationship between shear modulus and Young's modulus can be written as $E = 3\ \mu$, meaning that the calculation of E or μ provides the same information. This, however, applies to isotropic tissue. In anisotropic tissue such as renal tissue, ν has no bounds. It would therefore be incorrect to calculate E from μ in the kidney.

MRE is a dynamic elasticity imaging technique capable of calculating quantitative values of shear modulus of tissues. MRE generates shear waves in the organ of interest and then visualizes the shear waves by tracking tissue displacement using a modified phase contrast sequence. Then, it measures the speed of the propagating wave with specialized software called an inversion algorithm to produce stiffness maps.

The overall process of performing MRE can be divided into three main steps allowing for the measurement of the shear modulus:

1. Generation and transmission of mechanical waves into the tissues.
2. Imaging the propagation of shear waves using modified phase contrast sequence.
3. Generating a stiffness map that quantifies mechanical properties of the tissue.

Generation and Transmission of Mechanical Waves into Tissues

MRE uses low-frequency sound waves in the range of 40–150 Hz to induce shear waves in the tissue or organ of interest. In the commercial version of MRE on clinical MRI scanners supplied by Resoundant® Inc. (Rochester, MN, USA), the mechanical waves are generated by a subwoofer/speaker device ('active driver') placed outside the scanner room and are transmitted to a plastic disk ('passive driver') via a plastic tube passing through a wave guide (Fig. 17.1). The electrical signal for the active driver is created by a signal generator synchronized with the MRI pulse sequence triggered and is amplified by an audio amplifier before being fed into the mechanical driver.

The passive driver is secured by an elastic band over the abdominal organ of interest. In general, most patients can feel the vibrations generated by the disk but do not find them uncomfortable. After the mechanical excitation, a phase contrast-based pulse sequence known as the MRE sequence is used to encode the shear wave motion.

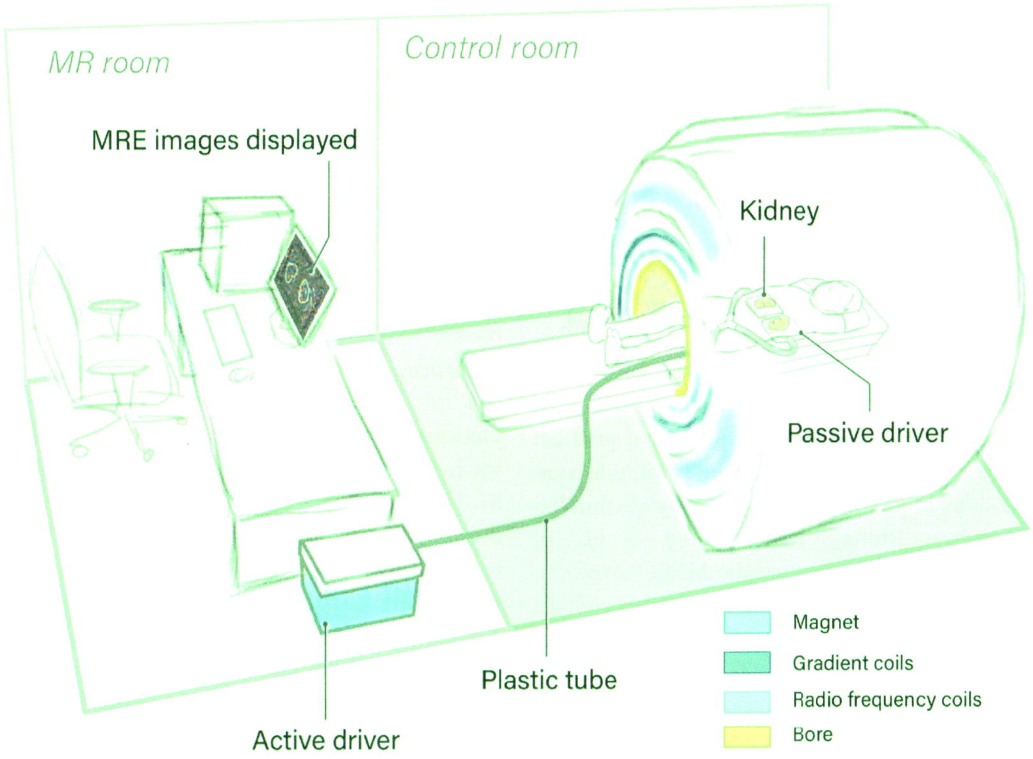

Fig. 17.1 Schematic of kidney MRE set up on a clinical MRI scanner (© [Suraj D. Serai, 2023. All Rights Reserved)

Imaging the Propagation of Mechanical Waves Using Modified Phase Contrast Sequence

To spatially map and measure the wave displacement patterns, a modified phase contrast MRE (PC-MRE) sequence is used to image the propagating waves in the tissues using a series of magnetic field gradients called motion-encoding gradients (MEG). These MEGs, synchronized with the mechanical excitations, are applied after radiofrequency (RF) excitation to image the propagating waves. MEG pairs oscillating at the same frequency as the external vibrations are imposed along a specific direction (usually in the Z-direction) and switched in polarity at an adjustable frequency. These MEG pairs are used to encode the motion of the tissues in the phase of an MR image. It is known that spins experience a change in phase in the presence of magnetic field gradients. Therefore, when these spins undergo continuous harmonic motion due to the application of shear waves in the presence of MEGs, a phase shift occurs in the obtained MR signal. MEGs can be applied in one or more directions to encode the motion in those specific directions. Trigger pulses synchronize an oscillator unit that drives a transducer, coupled with the surface of the target tissue to be imaged, to induce shear waves in the tissue at the same frequency as the MEGs. During MRE imaging, any cyclic motion of the spins in the presence of these MEGs causes a measurable phase shift, φ, in the received MR signal. The phase shift is also proportional to the period of the MEGs and the number of gradient pairs. High sensitivity to small amplitude synchronous motion can be achieved by accumulating phase shifts over multiple cycles of mechanical oscillation and the MEG waveform. The resulting MR image thus obtained is called a wave image and contains both the anatomical image and the propagating wave information (i.e., phase image). The phase image is typically derived by collecting two images with opposite MEG polarities and calculating a phase-difference image. Such wave images are obtained by tracking the external vibrations at different time points (or offsets) to visualize wave propagation. After post-processing, the information in the wave images are then converted into spatial stiffness maps known as elastograms using an inversion algorithm.

MRE acquisition sequences are based on either gradient recalled echo (GRE) (Fig. 17.2), or spin-echo echo planar imaging (SE-EPI) (Fig. 17.3) [9]. The MEG can be applied along a single spatial direction, i.e., the Z-direction, or along X, Y, and Z spatial directions to encode the propagating waves. The acquisition sequence, which applies MEG across a single spatial direction, is termed a 2D MRE acquisition sequence. The acquisition sequence, which applies MEG across all three spatial directions, is termed a 3D MRE acquisition sequence.

MRE is available as a hardware and software add-on to the existing or new MRI scanners from General Electric (GE Healthcare, Waukesha, WI, USA), Philips (Best, Netherlands), Siemens (Erlangen, Germany) and Cannon (Cannon Medical Systems, Tustin, CA, USA) at both 1.5 T and 3.0 T. Identical MRE hardware and inversion algorithms are commercially available on scanners manufactured by major MR vendors. Shear modulus is a mechanical property that is not dependent on MRI field strength, so kidney MRE can be performed on either a 1.5 T or 3 T clinical MR scanner. The shear stiffness measured on 1.5 T or 3.0 T magnets should be similar when all acquisition parameters (patient fasting status, breath holding, shear wave frequency, MRE sequence, and inversion algorithm) are the same. Multiple studies have demonstrated cross-platform and field strength compatibility of MRE for liver stiffness [10, 11]. As mentioned above, SE-EPI and GRE-based sequences are the two acquisition sequences that have been developed for MRE applications (Figs. 17.2 and 17.3). Historically, the technical failure rate has been slightly higher at 3.0 T with the 2D gradient recalled echo-MRE (2D GRE-MRE) sequence as the sequence is susceptible to T2* effects, resulting in poor signal-to-noise ratio (SNR) in tissues with short T2* relaxation times [12]. The use of SE-EPI-based MRE acquisition significantly improves the technical success at 3.0 T. The results from both GRE-MRE (Fig. 17.4) and

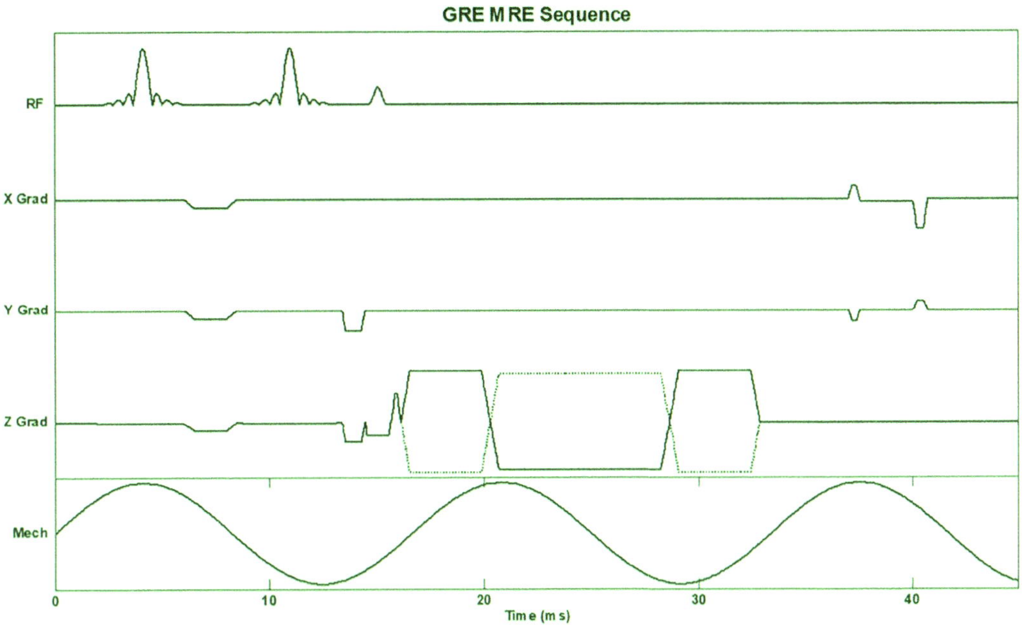

Fig. 17.2 Gradient-recalled echo acquisition sequence timing diagram. *RF* radiofrequency, *Grad* gradient, *ms* milliseconds, *Mech* mechanical excitation

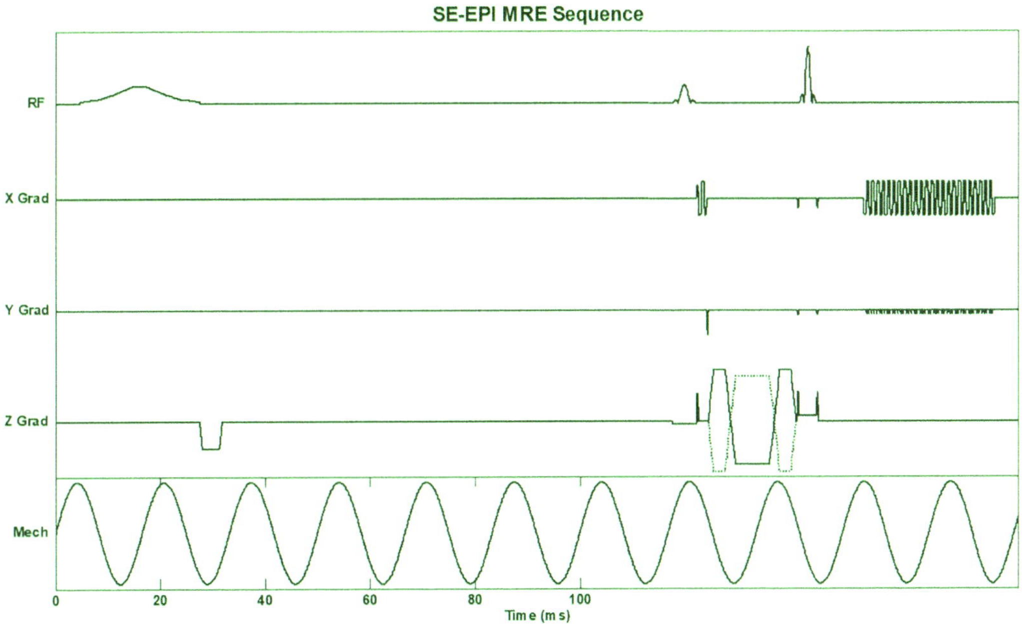

Fig. 17.3 Spin echo-echo planar imaging acquisition sequence timing diagram. *RF* radiofrequency, *Grad* gradient, *ms* milliseconds, *Mech* mechanical excitation

SE-EPI MRE (Fig. 17.5) are comparable [9, 13]. When selecting a scanner for the MRE application, kidney imaging at 1.5 T has an advantage due to less inhomogeneity and fewer distortion artifacts; however, both 1.5 T and 3.0 T will potentially yield precise, and reproducible

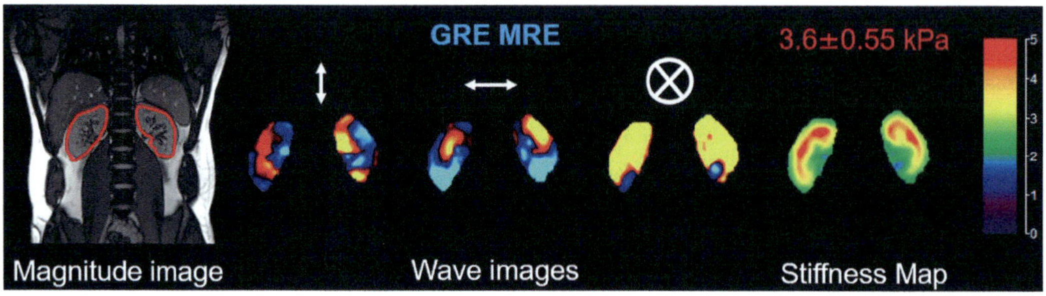

Fig. 17.4 Kidney MR elastography obtained on a volunteer using gradient-recalled echo acquisition method. Stiffness obtained was 3.6 ± 0.55 kPa

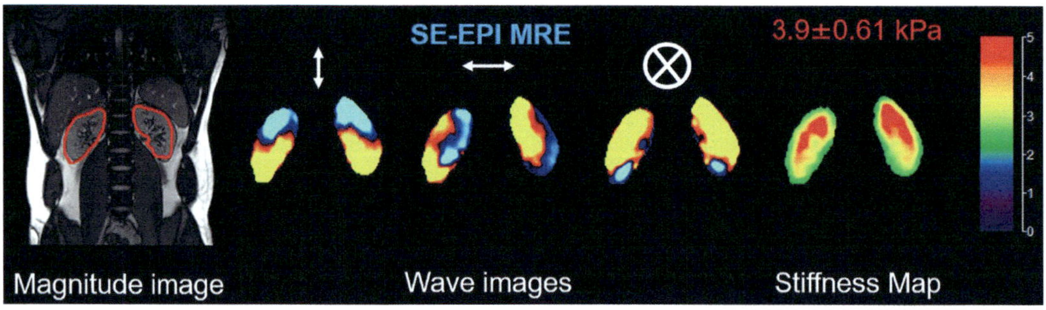

Fig. 17.5 Kidney MR elastography obtained on a volunteer using spin echo-echo planar imaging acquisition method. Stiffness obtained was 3.9 ± 0.61 kPa

results. SE-EPI MRE has several advantages over the current clinically used GRE-MRE sequence, such as faster scan times with multiple slices, fewer breath-holds, and high SNR [9, 13]. The GRE sequence requires separate breath-holds for each slice for a single-motion encoding direction, whereas SE-EPI-based sequences can acquire all the slices for a single-motion encoding direction in one breath-hold.

Generating a Stiffness Map That Quantifies Mechanical Properties of Tissue

In MRE, a measurable phase shift is induced by the motion-sensitizing gradient, which allows us to calculate the displacement at each voxel and directly image the acoustic waves. From the phase image that includes the phase shift or displacement data, it is possible to estimate tissue stiffness. As discussed, we already know by now, in the acquisition sequence, a measurable phase shift is induced by the motion-sensitizing gradient, which allows us to calculate the displacement at each voxel and directly image the acoustic waves. Now, from the principles of wave mechanics, we can estimate the shear modulus of a material by relating it to the shear wave speed. Wave length, λ, is defined as the wave speed (c) divided by frequency (f).

$$\lambda = \frac{c}{f}$$

Based on the principles of wave mechanics, the stiffness of an incompressible, isotropic, linear elastic material is directly related to wave speed, where the density in soft tissue (ρ) is assumed to be 1000 kg/m^3

$$\text{Shear modulus}, \mu = \rho c^2$$

Thus, if the shear wavelength can be estimated, the shear modulus can be calculated. In the simplest case, when a single shear wave is evident, this can be done manually. Alternatively, tissue stiffness can also be estimated by inverting the MRE displacement data. This can be accomplished using different algorithms such as local frequency estimation (LFE), the matched filter (MF), phase gradient (PG), and direct inversion (DI) [14]. The phase gradient method extracts the harmonic component of the shear wave at the driving frequency from experiments at multiple phase offsets of the shear wave, which yields the phase and amplitude of the propagating wave. If a single pure shear wave is present, the gradient of the phase can be used to calculate stiffness. This method, however, is very sensitive to noise and superposition of multiple waves (e.g., reflections). The LFE estimates the local spatial frequency of the shear wave propagation pattern and is relatively insensitive to noise; however, the LFE estimate is blurred at sharp boundaries and the correct estimate is reached only half a wavelength into a given region. The remaining methods are based on the equations of motion, which, under the assumptions above, reduce to the Helmholtz eq. [14]. These methods (and the LFE) are in principle capable of analyzing data from arbitrarily complex wave fields. DI algorithm inverts the Helmholtz equation by dividing a filtered estimate of the displacement by its spatial Laplacian at each point. The MF algorithm uses an adaptive filter based on a smoothed version of the data and its Laplacian to solve the Helmholtz equation. All the algorithms assume that the waves are propagating in a uniform, infinite, homogenous medium. Post-processing after the MRE data acquisition may be done on the scanner, or images may be taken offline for analysis. Magnitude and colored wave images are generated after a successful MRE acquisition (Fig. 17.6). The red to blue region (leading edge or red to the leading edge of next red) represents the wavelength of the propagating shear wave, and this wavelength becomes longer in the presence of a stiff region for a given excitation frequency. Technical failure of MRE is defined as the absence of visualized wave propagation on the wave images and/or no pixel value with a confidence index higher than 95% on the generated confidence maps. For image analysis, regions of interest (ROIs) should be drawn by a trained observer on the quantitative elastogram maps. ROIs for measurement of renal stiffness are drawn within the regions bound by the confidence maps in a manner to include as much of the kidney parenchyma as possible while staying approximately 2 mm within the outer kidney capsule and excluding the large vessels and renal

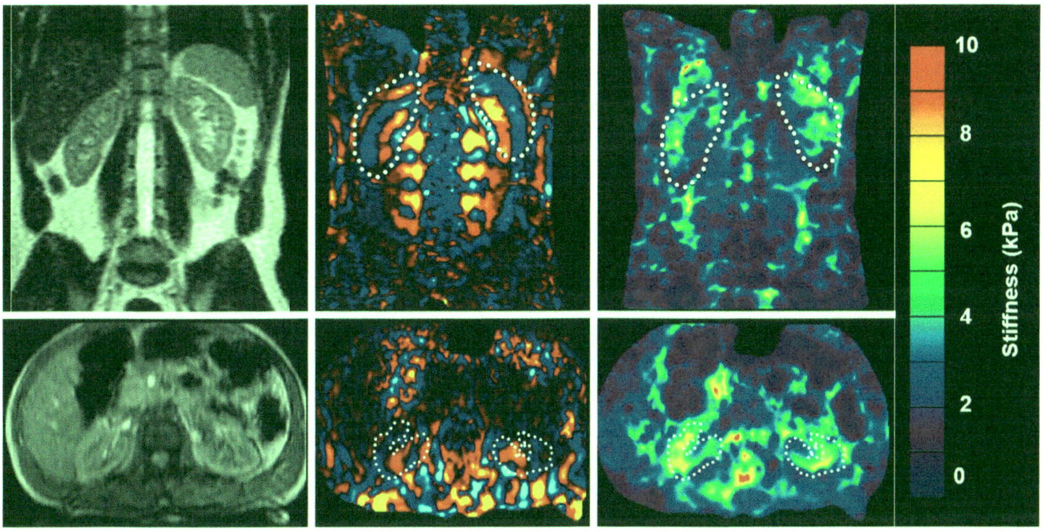

Fig. 17.6 MRE of kidneys performed in two normal healthy volunteers. MRE performed in coronal and axial planes. The dotted lines on the wave images and stiffness maps outline the kidneys. The stiffness of the normal kidneys ranged from 5 to 7.5 kPa

pelvis. The corresponding magnitude image and wave image are used as a guide. For each slice, the mean stiffness is calculated. The stiffness values are measured in kilopascals (kPa). Overall mean kidney stiffness is calculated as the average of stiffness values from each slice, weighted by the ROI area of each slice.

Part 2: Recommended Renal MRE Scanning Protocol

There is a great interest in assessment of tissue stiffness of the kidneys for evaluation of many disease processes affecting kidneys; however, the retroperitoneal location and small size of the native kidneys make it challenging to perform MRE of the kidneys. Because the kidneys lie on either side of the spine, which does not conduct shear waves well or impedes their propagation, modifications in driver technology is needed to deliver shear waves into both kidneys for good quality MRE. For kidney MRE, patients are set up in supine position head-first in the scanner (Fig. 17.7). As previously explained, the first step is to generate the shear wave inside the kidney. MRE relies on external vibrations generated by audio subwoofer magnets and transmitted to the kidney using a pneumatic pressure device, a plastic disk ("passive driver"), which is secured by an elastic band [15–17]. The pneumatic active-passive driver system (Resoundant Inc., Rochester, MN) is a similar set-up as that used for liver MRE. The plastic tube (polyvinyl chloride, 30 ft.) connecting the active driver and passive driver enters the room through the waveguide (a hole in the wall between the equipment room and the scanner). The connecting tube can be coiled and placed in a cabinet or on a shelf when not in use.

Initial training for performing MRE is usually provided by the MRI manufacturer application specialist. Although there are no standard training requirements to perform MRE, adequate training of MR technicians is essential for performing high-quality MRE scans. Similarly, radiologists reporting the MRE results would benefit from expert training to avoid interpretation errors. For the two kidneys, a 'Y-shaped' splitter is used to allow for two parallel passive drivers, one on each side of the spine (Fig. 17.7). Once positioned, the passive driver should be held firmly against the abdominal wall by a wide elastic band, placed around the torso. Check to ensure that the band is stretched sufficiently so that the driver is not loose during full expiration. Remember to check that the passive driver remains connected via a plastic tube to the active driver (vibration source), which is located outside the scan room. The passive driver disconnection with the active driver is a common reason for MRE failure.

Patient Preparation

Kidney MRE can be performed on sedated or non-sedated children. While in adults, it is recommended that MRE be performed after an over-

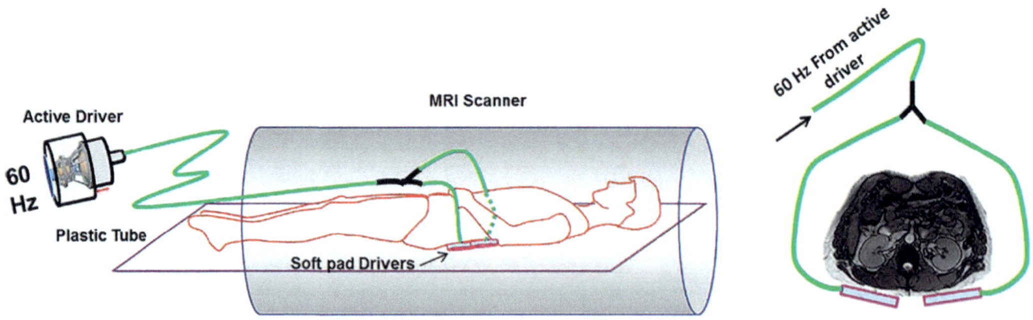

Fig. 17.7 Schematic of kidney MRE paddle positioning. The passive driver is positioned posteriorly to be relatively closer to the kidney from the dorsal side. A Y-shaped splitter is used to position two paddles in parallel under both kidneys (© [Suraj D. Serai, 2023. All Rights Reserved)

Table 17.1 Recommended kidney 2D MRE protocol parameters

Parameter	SE-EPI MRE
TR (ms)	1000
TE (ms)	30
Matrix size	100 × 100
Voxel size (mm)	1.5 × 1.5
Slice thickness (mm)	6
Bandwidth (Hz/px)	2380
No. of averages	1
No. of slices	4
No. of phases	4
MEG frequency (Hz)	60
MEG direction	Z axis (slice)
Echo spacing (ms)	0.5
EPI factor	100
Acceleration factor	2
Scan time (min:s)	0:11 (single breath-hold)

SE-EPI spin echo-echo planar imaging, *2D* two-dimensional, *TR* repetition time, *TE* echo time, *No.* number, *MEG* motion encoding gradients, *ms* milliseconds, *Hz* Hertz, *px* pixel, *mm* millimeter, *min* minutes, s seconds

Table 17.2 Recommended kidney 3D MRE protocol parameters

Parameter	SE-EPI MRE
TR (ms)	3200
TE (ms)	41
Matrix size	100 × 100
Voxel size (mm)	1.5 × 1.5
Slice thickness (mm)	3.5
Bandwidth (Hz/px)	2174
No. of averages	1
No. of slices	32
No. of phases	3
MEG frequency (Hz)	60
MEG direction	X, Y, Z axis
Echo spacing (ms)	0.5
EPI factor	100
Acceleration factor	2
Scan time (min:s)	1:09 (4 breath-holds)

night fast. In protocols for kidney MRE in children, we ask that they eat extremely lightly for at least 4 h before the MRE exam and that they stay normally hydrated before the MRE study.

MRE Protocol

Imaging protocol details for 2D MRE are listed in Tables 17.1 and 17.2. Coronal and sagittal localizer images are acquired to locate the anatomical position of the kidneys. We recommend acquiring kidney MRE in the coronal oblique plane, along the long axis of the kidney (Fig. 17.8). The advantage of this scan plane is that it provides a larger area of the kidney parenchyma, and better reproducibility. Acquired sections for MRE should be positioned at the level of the widest extent of the kidney. When possible, breath-holds must be performed at end-expiration to minimize motion artifacts. The scout or localizer image used for slice selection must also be performed at end-expiration. Additionally, the localizer image can typically be used to determine the location of the passive driver, visible as an indentation or flattening of the subcutaneous tissue. The driver should be repositioned before the MRE acquisition scan if not located over the kidney. Typically, four sections are obtained. Many of the pulse sequence parameters should be used as default and should not be adjusted, including the MEG vibration frequency, and MEG direction, the number of phase offsets, and the fractional encoding.

Abdominal organs such as the liver and kidney tissues are composed of viscoelastic material, and the stiffness calculated from the propagation of shear waves is dependent on the frequency of the applied motion. For clinical MRE, stiffness thresholds have been established and the frequency should not be changed, as an increase or decrease in frequency increases (decreases) measured shear wave speed. Similarly, the field of view should be kept consistent between repeat scans or for the course of a clinical trial. Currently, there is no consensus on the standard frequency for renal MRE, but several publications have used the standard 60 Hz as well as 90 Hz [15–17]. Higher frequency may have lower penetration. This is important to consider if patient groups that are being imaged are obese and the positioning paddle are relatively far away from the kidney. If comparisons are made, it is important that the stiffness values be compared against published series with the same frequency. For consistency, in our studies, we currently recommend to use the standard frequency of 60 Hz.

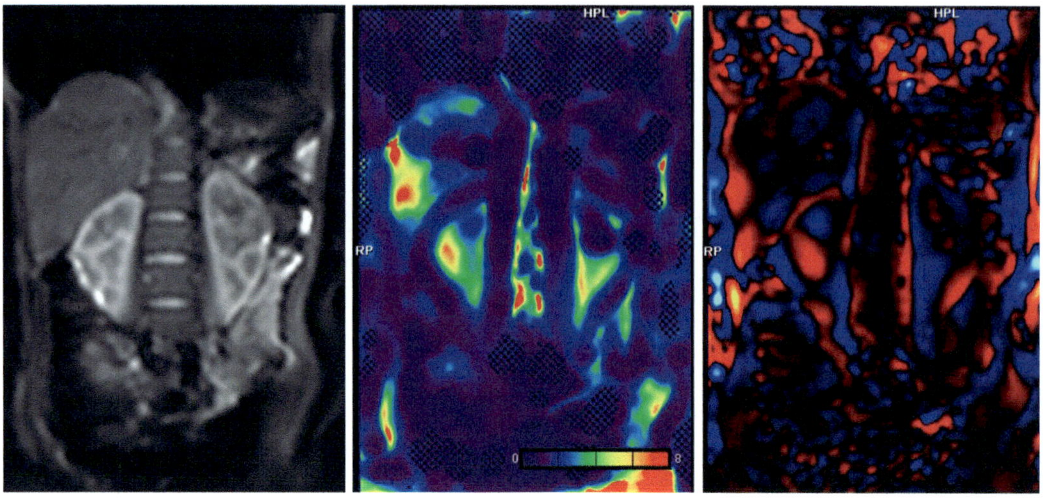

Fig. 17.8 Kidney MR elastography of an 8-year-old girl (healthy control). (**a**) Magnitude, (**b**) color stiffness map, and (**c**) wave image. A Y-shaped splitter is used to position two paddles in parallel under both kidneys. Mean stiffness = 3.6 kPa (© [Suraj D. Serai, 2023. All Rights Reserved)

The MRE protocol parameters that can be adjusted to improve image quality include the driver amplitude and the echo time (TE). The TE should be set to an in-phase value to improve signal, which may vary by pulse sequence and field strength. The driver amplitude determines the intensity of shear waves applied to the kidneys and can be increased or decreased depending on the body habitus of the patient and the passive driver used (rigid or flexible). If the amplitude setting is too low, shear wave penetration in the liver will be low and will result in a low-quality exam. Alternatively, if the amplitude setting is too high, the patient may experience some discomfort and the excessive motion in the liver can result in signal loss near the driver and a poor-quality exam. This is particularly important in small children.

MRE Quality Control

After completion of the exam, the performing MRI technologist (or the supervising MRI radiologist) should immediately review the images to ensure diagnostic quality and the MRE should be repeated if necessary. All the raw and post-processed images should be immediately reviewed to confirm the technical success of the acquisition. Following the acquisition, the magnitude and phase images are produced on the scanner and represent the raw data. The magnitude images provide anatomic information, and the phase images can be used to visually assess the presence of shear waves in the liver. Technologists should check the magnitude images for artifacts (ex: excessive respiratory motion) and the presence of a signal void in the subcutaneous tissue directly below the passive driver. Technologists should check the raw phase images for the presence of shear waves, the reconstructed wave images for adequate shear wave propagation, and the elastogram to confirm an adequate region of high confidence.

The phase images are the raw phase difference from the positive and negative motion encodings, displaying the tissue wave displacement. The reconstructed wave images are typically displayed in color and have been processed to remove phase wrapping (phase discontinuities). A critical step is to make sure that the shear waves are delivered and are propagating through the kidney. Planar wave propagation can be seen as parallel lines of shear wave motion (orange/blue lines in color image or light gray/dark gray in phase or grayscale wave image) and represents propagation of the waves in the imaging plane. If shear waves are present but the amplitude is low, denoted by visible waves in the phase/wave images but a small or absent region of high confidence in the elastogram, the exam should be repeated to obtain MRE with shear waves of adequate amplitude. Ensure a firm connection between the passive and active driver tubes. The belt securing the passive driver to the abdomen should be tightened at end-expiration. Additionally, if the subject is obese and/or has a large waist circumference, the amplitude can be increased. If no shear waves were visible, confirm the tube is connected, the active driver is on, and the amplitude settings are correct. The technician may consider standing next to the active driver during the scan to feel/listen for vibrations. If no vibrations are felt, contact the MR service engineer to help troubleshoot.

The most consistent output images are a grayscale elastogram (0–8 kPa) and a grayscale elastogram with confidence map overlay. The grayscale elastograms provide quantitative stiffness values and should be used for analysis. The confidence map is a tool used to assist in locating regions of reliable information for ROI placement. Additional post-processed images include grayscale and color wave images, a grayscale confidence map, and color elastograms with and without the confidence map overlay. Color elastograms are non-quantitative and should not be used to measure stiffness. They are useful for identifying hot spots, which should be avoided when making measurements. They also provide a qualitative overview of the kidney for a rapid visual assessment of whether the measured kidney stiffness will be normal or elevated. These post-processed images may require a manual step to generate on the scanner.

Stiffness Measurement

After assuring a high-quality exam, ROI can be drawn to measure stiffness. To reduce sampling error, the largest possible volume of tissue parenchyma should be included within the ROI. General guidelines for ROI drawing include avoiding the kidney edge, excluding the renal pelvicalyceal system and hilum, and within the parenchyma. When making manual stiffness measurements, this can be performed at the MR scanner or directly on PACS or a separate workstation for optimal workflow. The process for manual measurement varies slightly depending on the availability of images and features of the PACS/workstation such as availability of a copy/paste function.

We describe making manual measurements in three steps. For systems providing a confidence map and copy and paste function, the first step in making measurements is to draw an ROI on the elastogram with confidence map, while keeping the ROI within the valid or non-hashed-out region. Next, this ROI is copied to the magnitude image, where modifications can be made to ensure the ROI is within the liver and avoiding major vessels, kidney edge, and fissures. The ROI is then copied to the color wave image to ensure only high-quality waves are being sampled. Finally, the ROI is transferred to the grayscale elastogram to obtain the liver stiffness. With some vendors, the color stiffness map may be scaled so that stiffness measurement can be performed similar to that on a grayscale stiffness map. If no confidence map is obtained but a copy and paste function is available, the first step is drawing an ROI on the magnitude image. This ROI should then be copied to the color wave image, with modifications made to assure sampling of only high-quality waves. The final step is to copy the grayscale or color elastogram to obtain the stiffness measurement. On elastogram images, artifactual areas of elevated liver stiffness called hot spots are generally avoided. For systems that provide a confidence map but no copy and paste function, the first step in making measurements is to correlate the grayscale elastogram with confidence map image with the magnitude image. Ensure that appropriate areas in the kidney are excluded, such as the peripheral kidney and large blood vessels. Some systems provide a localizer function for this purpose. Next, the wave image should be reviewed to include only high-quality waves. Then, the color elastogram is reviewed to avoid hot spots created by wave distortion or the adjacent passive driver. After reviewing all four series, freehand ROI measurements are made on the grayscale elastogram image. This process is repeated for all four slices obtained. The weighted arithmetic mean is then calculated, which considers the kidney stiffness of each slice and the area sampled. The formula is as follows: weighted arithmetic mean = ($m1w1 + m2w2 + m3w3 + m4w4) \div (w1 + w2 + w3 + w4)$, where m equals the mean kidney stiffness for that particular slice and w equals the ROI size in pixels in mm^2 or cm^2.

The measurement technique described here includes both renal cortex and renal medulla. The stiffness thus measured is affected by pathological processes that occur in both medulla and cortex. With advances in the MRE technique, it may be possible to obtain stiffness measurements of renal cortex and medulla separately when a high resolution MRE is obtained. With such capability in the future, it may be possible to comprehensively evaluate glomerular diseases that affect the renal cortex predominantly and interstitial diseases that predominantly affect the renal medulla.

Part 3: Clinical Applications

In this section, we have described experimental procedures and step-by-step instructions to run MRE along with some illustrative applications. We also included information on how to perform data quality checks and analysis methods. In this section, we will review some of the clinical applications of kidney MRE.

Several studies have shown that MRE is a robust, reliable, repeatable, and reproducible technique for detection and staging of liver fibrosis [5, 10, 11]. The accuracy of MRE ranges from 0.85 to 0.99 for differentiating different stages of liver fibrosis. However, the performance of MRE for differentiating mild fibrosis (stage I) from normal liver or only inflammation is lower as inflammation also leads to increased stiffness. The performance of MRE is highest for diagnosis of cirrhosis (stage 4). Similarly, application of MRE for non-invasive evaluation of renal fibrosis has great potential for non-invasive assessment of fibrosis in patients with CKD. The two major kidney fibrotic pathologies where MRE may be clinically useful are CKD in native kidneys and interstitial fibrosis in allograft kidneys.

In CKD from various etiology, the final pathway is an increase in the extracellular matrix synthesis, with excessive fibrillary collagens, and characterizes the development of chronic lesions in the glomerular (glomerulosclerosis), interstitial (tubulointerstitial fibrosis) CKD and vascular compartments, leading progressively to end-stage renal failure. Mechanisms participating in these processes are increasingly being identified through research, and various therapeutic interventions have been shown to prevent or to favor regression of fibrosis in several experimental models. Therefore, development of new non-invasive MRE-based methods for identification and quantification of fibrosis is worthwhile.

Following the success of clinical use of MRE for liver fibrosis diagnosis and staging, several exploratory studies on kidney MRE have been performed in the last decade. Initial investigations using kidney MRE consisted of pilot studies focusing on feasibility and validation studies in preclinical populations as well as healthy volunteers. These studies successfully demonstrated that it is possible to generate and image shear waves in the kidneys. Soon, the focus quickly shifted to studies focusing on measurement of renal stiffness through two in vivo clinical applications: CKD in native kidneys and evaluation of interstitial fibrosis in kidney allografts. Renal allografts are much more easily accessible for shear wave propagation as they are usually placed in iliac fossa and less likely to move with respiration. Figure 17.9 shows representative images for 95% confidence intervals of MRE colored renal stiffness maps, with a color spectrum that codes for degree of stiffness (from 0 to 8 kPa), shown for a control participant and patients with Interstitial fibrosis and tubular atrophy in allografts. Anterior abdominal wall provides better contact with transplant kidney, and it is relatively easier to perform high frequency MRE on patients with renal allografts. Figure 17.10 shows kidney MRE of a 15-year-old male patient with dysplastic kidneys post renal transplant (Mean stiffness = 4.9 kPa): (a) sagittal anatomical image, (b) coronal anatomi-

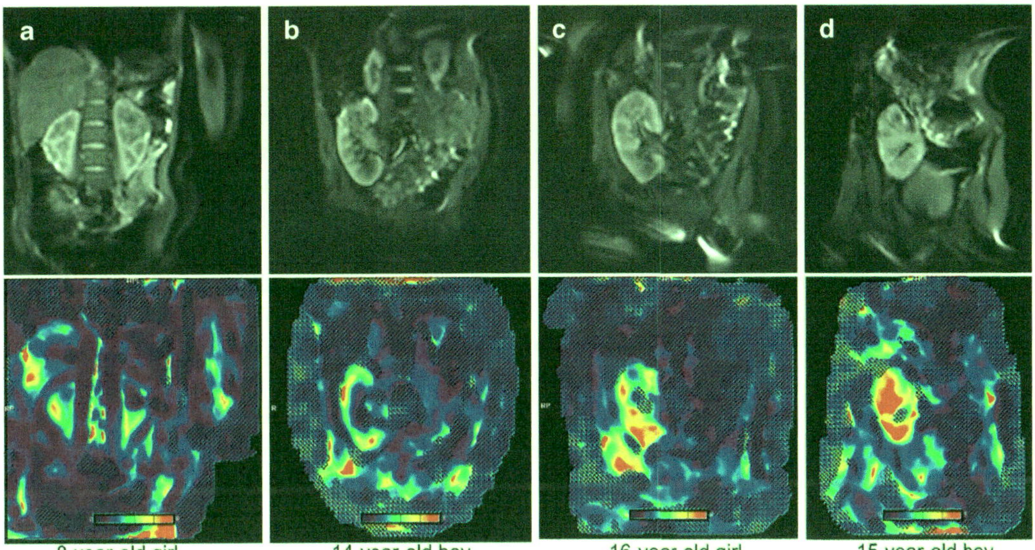

Fig. 17.9 MRE renal stiffness maps. Representative images for 95% confidence intervals of MRE colored renal stiffness maps, with a color spectrum that codes for degree of stiffness (from 0 to 8 kPa), shown for (**a**) an 8-year-old girl healthy control participant, (**b**) a 14-year-old boy with stable kidney allograft, (**c**) a 16-year-old girl with Grade 1 interstitial fibrosis and tubular atrophy allograft (IFTA), and (**d**) a 15-year-old boy with Grade 2 IFTA (© [Suraj D. Serai, 2023. All Rights Reserved)

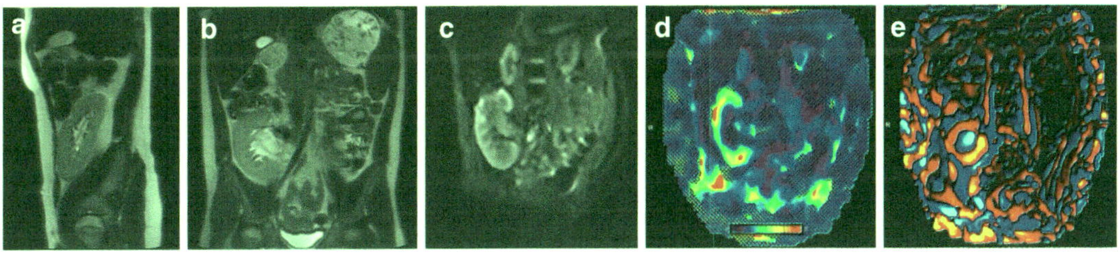

Fig. 17.10 Kidney MR elastography of a 15-year-old male patient with dysplastic kidneys post renal transplant. (**a**) Sagittal anatomical image, (**b**) coronal anatomical image, (**c**) magnitude, (**d**) color stiffness map, and (**e**) wave image. For patients with a single kidney, only one passive driver is sufficient for wave propagation. Mean stiffness = 4.9 kPa (© [Suraj D. Serai, 2023. All Rights Reserved)

cal image, (c) magnitude, (d) color stiffness map, and (e) wave image. For patients with a single kidney, only one passive driver is sufficient for wave propagation.

Although there are only a few published studies in the literature, these studies show promising results and set a path for using renal MRE for diagnosing as well as staging CKD in clinical settings. Here we will review studies investigating the use of renal MRE for two of the major clinical applications.

Evaluation of Fibrosis in Native Kidneys in CKD Patients

CKD results from a wide variety of causes including glomerular, tubulointerstitial, and vascular diseases. The tubulointerstitial compartment is almost always affected in renal disease from all causes. Chronic interstitial nephritis is characterized by interstitial fibrosis and tubular atrophy and accompanied by vascular changes of arterial and arteriolar sclerosis. Renal fibrosis is accompanied by loss of tubules, collapse of the interstitium around it, and reduced blood flow leading to overall loss of renal volume and renal blood flow. This complex change in composition of the tissue has effects on the tissue stiffness as described earlier. Although there is increased renal fibrosis as CKD progresses, the blood perfusion of the kidney reduces, and this greatly impacts the renal parenchymal stiffness measured.

Han et al. [8] conducted a pilot study using renal MRE in 25 clinically diagnosed CKD patients (five patients in each CKD stage) and five healthy volunteers, demonstrating that mean stiffness of the renal parenchyma increased in CKD patients compared to healthy controls. Moreover, the median stiffness of the renal parenchyma increased with an increase in CKD stage and finally, decreased for stage 5, although the range of stiffness values in stage 5 was very large. The diagnostic accuracy of renal MRE using mean area under the ROC was 0.82. Furthermore, Zhang et al. [2] also investigated renal MRE in 97 CKD patients and correlated the MRE-derived renal stiffness values with histology results. There was a negative correlation between renal stiffness and cortical extracellular matrix volume, indicating a decrease in renal stiffness as the CKD progressed. Stiffness measurements decreased with reduction in the renal function, whereas the cortical extracellular matrix volume increased with decrease in renal function.

A few other studies also investigated native kidneys in subjects with lupus nephritis (LN), diabetic nephropathy, and IgA nephropathy. Garcia et al. [3] used multifrequency MRE (tomoelastography) in 25 patients with LN. They observed a significant decrease in medullary stiffness of LN patients compared to healthy controls. In LN patients with normal renal function, the MRE-derived stiffness values decreased with increasing CKD stage in medulla and inner cortex compared to healthy controls. It was also observed that in LN patients with normal renal function, once the kidney is impaired, renal medulla is affected first, followed by inner cortex.

Finally, the diagnostic accuracy of CKD staging was increased when MRE results were paired with blood oxygen level-dependent (BOLD) MRI and diffusion weighted imaging (DWI) compared to just MRE, thereby highlighting the need for using multiparametric MRI for diagnosis of renal fibrosis [18]. Brown et al. investigated the use of renal MRE in 30 patients with CKD (all stages) due to diabetic nephropathy along with 13 healthy controls using 60 Hz and 90 Hz vibration frequency [19]. Significant decrease in cortical stiffness was observed in all stages of CKD compared to controls. For MRE with 60 Hz vibration frequency, there was no significant difference between stiffness values in healthy controls compared to stages 3, 4, and 5. However, in MRE with 90 Hz vibration frequency, they were able to distinguish CKD stage 3, 4, and 5 from healthy controls. In their recent work, the MRE team at Mayo Clinic recommend that a higher frequency (90 Hz) may be more suitable as kidneys are smaller in size and a 3D technique to evaluate shear wave propagation in a complex tissue structure in the kidney. MRE images are helpful to be obtained in the coronal plane that includes both kidneys for comparison. In general, tissue stiffness increases with collagen accumulation. Renal tissue stiffness is dependent on several components of the parenchyma. Approximately 25% of renal volume may be attributable to blood pressure, blood content, filtrate, and urine in the kidney. As kidneys are highly perfused organs, a possible fibrosis-induced increase in tissue stiffness might be masked by decreased renal perfusion pressure secondary to tubular and glomerular sclerosis and capillary rarefication. Changes in renal blood flow has been shown to affect renal stiffness, independent of the presence of fibrosis. It has been shown by MRE that atrophy of the renal parenchyma accompanied by reduced renal blood flow may reduce tissue stiffness in the absence of significant amount of fibrotic tissue (Fig. 17.11).

Finally, Lang et al. [5] investigated renal tomoelastography in 16 IgA nephropathy patients and 16 healthy controls. There was a significant

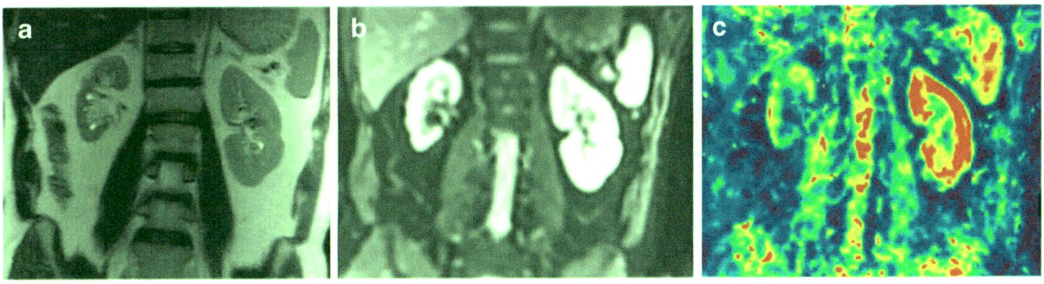

Fig. 17.11 3DMRE of the kidneys in a 36-year-old patient with primary hyperoxaluria type-1 with elevated plasma and urinary oxalates and eGFR >60 and serum creatinine of 0.8 mg/dL. Coronal T2 image (**a**) shows small and atrophic right kidney with compensatory hypertrophy of the left kidney. (**b**) Magnitude image and (**c**) stiffness maps obtained during the MRE show reduced tissue stiffness in the right kidney due to atrophy as compared to hypertrophied left kidney

decrease in the mean renal stiffness in IgA patients compared to healthy controls. MRE-derived stiffness values had higher diagnostic accuracy than DWI, with an area under ROC of 0.9.

These studies demonstrate that MRE can be used as a tool for diagnosing CKD with good accuracy as well as for successfully staging CKD levels. The important difference between increased stiffness in liver fibrosis patients compared to decreased stiffness in renal fibrosis in CKD patients can be attributed to the reduced renal blood flow and perfusion, leading to reduced renal turgor. Hence, as the CKD progresses to later stages, the increased tissue stiffness due to extracellular matrix deposition is offset by the reduced perfusion and blood flow to the kidneys, thereby reducing the renal turgor and leading to a decrease in overall parenchymal stiffness.

Interstitial Fibrosis in Renal Allografts

Renal allografts are at risk of chronic interstitial fibrosis and tubular atrophy (IFTA), which is thought to be mediated through immune and vascular processes leading to chronic allografts failure with most grafts having a lifespan of less than 10 years. Kirpalani et al. [6] used renal MRE to detect fibrosis in 16 allograft recipients who were more than 1-year post-transplant [20]. The whole kidney MRE stiffness correlated significantly with the biopsy-derived Banff fibrosis score, with the stiffer kidneys being more fibrotic. They also observed a negative correlation between MRE-derived renal stiffness values and eGFR, a measure of kidney function. Lee et al. imaged 11 patients with renal transplants using MRE. Three different vibration frequencies were used: 90 Hz, 120 Hz, and 150 Hz [21]. There were differences in renal stiffness values between kidneys with no fibrosis vs mild fibrosis vs moderate fibrosis, but these differences were not significant. The renal stiffness values also increased with increasing severity of fibrosis using all three frequencies between mild and moderately fibrotic kidneys. Finally, Garcia et al. used renal tomoelastography (40–70 Hz) in 22 renal transplant patients and 11 healthy controls [22]. It was observed that functioning transplants had higher stiffness values compared to non-functioning transplants and native kidneys. Renal stiffness was lowest in dysfunctional transplants with refined ROIs. The overall diagnostic accuracy of renal MRE in diagnosing renal allograft dysfunction, using area under the ROC curve, was 0.93. It is interesting to observe that in native kidneys, increased renal fibrosis in CKD show lower renal stiffness values, whereas in renal allografts, increased renal fibrosis show higher renal stiffness values.

However, these data have not been corrected for the renal perfusion pressure, which is usually maintained in the renal graft, and post transplantation changes in kidney microvasculature and perfusion may be responsible for differences in MRE-derived stiffness between native kidneys vs renal allografts. These differences, though interesting, have not yet been investigated in any of the studies. It must also be noted that all these studies were carried out using magnets of different field strength (1.5 T vs 3 T), vendors, pulse sequences, vibration frequencies, and in patients of different ages and under different hydration states.

The evaluation of the renal allografts with renal MRE is best assessed as changes in stiffness with a baseline stiffness available to compare. The change in stiffness (delta stiffness) is likely to have more clinical value than a single measurement for management. It is important to not perform baseline MRE of renal allografts in the immediate post-operative period or in the acute post transplantation period that could last 3–6 months. This period is often characterized by inflammation, possible allograft rejection, perigraft collections, and occasionally vascular complications, which can affect stiffness measurements. Renal MRE was still successfully able to differentiate between healthy and fibrotic kidneys as well as successfully stage the fibrosis in most cases. Therefore, renal MRE shows great promise in diagnosing fibrosis in renal allografts, even more with a standardized acquisition, post-processing, and analysis framework.

Multiparametric MRI including renal MRE with other MRI techniques such as BOLD MRI, arterial spin-labeling (ASL), DWI, susceptibility imaging, magnetization transfer (MT) imaging, and T1- and T2-weighted imaging can be used in a multi-parametric framework in a single MRI visit for non-invasive, accurate diagnosis and staging of renal fibrosis. The ASL and BOLD will provide the renal perfusion parametrics and therefore able to assess the influence of perfusion on stiffness. MT imaging may be useful in detecting increased amount of fibrosis in the kidneys. The multiparametric approach with quantitative information on different pathological processes will make it possible for correlation and clinical application.

Conclusions

Existing imaging technologies have been very successful in the non-invasive assessment of many focal diseases of the kidneys, but they have been somewhat less helpful for evaluating diffuse (medical) renal disease such as glomerulonephritis, and renal biopsy remains the diagnostic tool of choice in many situations. MRE is a powerful technology, which is capable of quantifying the mechanical properties of tissue. It is now feasible to quantitatively image the shear stiffness of both kidneys with a MRE employing, posteriorly located passive acoustic drivers. Wave images and the corresponding elastograms can be relatively easily acquired in axial, coronal, and sagittal planes. Preliminary results provide a basis and motivation for investigating the potential to use MRE as a diagnostic tool for characterizing renal parenchyma in diffuse diseases of the kidneys. MRE of the kidneys is promising for useful application in the evaluation of chronic renal disease and renal allografts. MRE has been shown to be capable of detecting alterations in the tissue mechanical properties of kidneys in vivo preclinical and clinical studies and helpful in early non-invasive detection and management of patients with chronic kidney disease (CKD). Continuing technology improvement and further studies are needed on clinical application of renal MRE.

Bibliography

1. Zhang J, Yu Y, Liu X, Tang X, Xu F, Zhang M, et al. Evaluation of renal fibrosis by mapping histology and magnetic resonance imaging. Kidney Dis (Basel). 2021;7(2):131–42.
2. Grossmann M, Tzschätzsch H, Lang ST, Guo J, Bruns A, Dürr M, et al. US time-harmonic Elastography for the early detection of glomerulonephritis. Radiology. 2019;292(3):676–84.
3. Muthupillai R, Lomas DJ, Rossman PJ, Greenleaf JF, Manduca A, Ehman RL. Magnetic resonance elastog-

raphy by direct visualization of propagating acoustic strain waves. Science. 1995;269(5232):1854–7.
4. Dillman JR, Trout AT, Costello EN, Serai SD, Bramlage KS, Kohli R, et al. Quantitative liver MRI-biopsy correlation in pediatric and young adult patients with nonalcoholic fatty liver disease: can one be used to predict the other? AJR Am J Roentgenol. 2018;210(1):166–74.
5. Serai SD, Obuchowski NA, Venkatesh SK, Sirlin CB, Miller FH, Ashton E, et al. Repeatability of MR Elastography of liver: a meta-analysis. Radiology. 2017;285(1):92–100.
6. Ehman RL. Magnetic resonance elastography: from invention to standard of care. Abdom Radiol (NY). 2022;47(9):3028–36.
7. Serai SD, Yin M. MR elastography of the abdomen: basic concepts. Methods Mol Biol. 2021;2216:301–23.
8. Han JH, Ahn J-H, Kim J-S. Magnetic resonance elastography for evaluation of renal parenchyma in chronic kidney disease: a pilot study. Radiol Med. 2020;125(12):1209–15.
9. Calle-Toro JS, Serai SD, Hartung EA, Goldberg DJ, Bolster BD, Darge K, et al. Magnetic resonance elastography SE-EPI vs GRE sequences at 3T in a pediatric population with liver disease. Abdom Radiol (NY). 2019;44(3):894–902.
10. Trout AT, Serai S, Mahley AD, Wang H, Zhang Y, Zhang B, et al. Liver stiffness measurements with MR Elastography: agreement and repeatability across imaging systems, field strengths, and pulse sequences. Radiology. 2016;281(3):793.
11. Trout AT, Anupindi SA, Gee MS, Khanna G, Xanthakos SA, Serai SD, et al. Normal liver stiffness measured with MR Elastography in children. Radiology. 2020;297:663.
12. Joshi M, Dillman JR, Towbin AJ, Serai SD, Trout AT. MR elastography: high rate of technical success in pediatric and young adult patients. Pediatr Radiol. 2017;47(7):838–43.
13. Serai SD, Dillman JR, Trout AT. Spin-echo echo-planar imaging MR Elastography versus gradient-echo MR Elastography for assessment of liver stiffness in children and young adults suspected of having liver disease. Radiology. 2017;282(3):761–70.
14. Ringleb SI, Chen Q, Lake DS, Manduca A, Ehman RL, An K-N. Quantitative shear wave magnetic resonance elastography: comparison to a dynamic shear material test. Magn Reson Med. 2005;53(5):1197–201.
15. Serai SD, Yin M. MR elastography of the abdomen: experimental protocols. Methods Mol Biol. 2021;2216:519–46.
16. Gandhi D, Kalra P, Raterman B, Mo X, Dong H, Kolipaka A. Magnetic resonance Elastography of kidneys: SE-EPI MRE reproducibility and its comparison to GRE MRE. NMR Biomed. 2019;32(11):e4141.
17. Dillman JR, Benoit SW, Gandhi DB, Trout AT, Tkach JA, VandenHeuvel K, et al. Multiparametric quantitative renal MRI in children and young adults: comparison between healthy individuals and patients with chronic kidney disease. Abdom Radiol (NY). 2022;47(5):1840–52.
18. Lang ST, Guo J, Bruns A, Dürr M, Braun J, Hamm B, et al. Multiparametric quantitative MRI for the detection of Iga nephropathy using tomoelastography, DWI, and BOLD imaging. Investig Radiol. 2019;54(10):669–74.
19. Brown RS, Sun MRM, Stillman IE, Russell TL, Rosas SE, Wei JL. The utility of magnetic resonance imaging for noninvasive evaluation of diabetic nephropathy. Nephrol Dial Transplant. 2020;35(6):970–8.
20. Kirpalani A, Hashim E, Leung G, Kim JK, Krizova A, Jothy S, et al. Magnetic resonance elastography to assess fibrosis in kidney allografts. Clin J Am Soc Nephrol. 2017;12(10):1671–9.
21. Lee CU, Glockner JF, Glaser KJ, Yin M, Chen J, Kawashima A, et al. MR elastography in renal transplant patients and correlation with renal allograft biopsy: a feasibility study. Acad Radiol. 2012;19(7):834–41.
22. Marticorena Garcia SR, Fischer T, Dürr M, Gültekin E, Braun J, Sack I, et al. Multifrequency magnetic resonance Elastography for the assessment of renal allograft function. Investig Radiol. 2016;51(9):591–5.

18 Microstructural Features and Functional Assessment of the Kidney Using Diffusion MRI

Suraj D. Serai, Sila Kurugol, Pim Pullens, Zhen Jane Wang, and Eric Sigmund

DWI in the Kidney: Background

Diffusion is a physical process that results from the thermally driven, random motion of water molecules. Diffusion-weighted imaging (DWI) provides an image contrast that is dependent on the molecular motion of water (diffusion), which is called Brownian motion. After Stejskal and Tanner [1] described a DW SE T2-weighted pulse sequence in NMR spectroscopy with two extra gradient pulses equal in magnitude and opposite in phase accumulation (Fig. 18.1), it took several decades for that sequence to become clinically feasible [2] due to limitations of MR equipment and imaging trajectories. In pure water, molecules undergo free, thermally agitated diffusion (with a three-dimensional Gaussian distribution). The width of the Gaussian distribution expands with the elapsed time, and the average square of this width per unit time gives the units of the apparent diffusion coefficient (ADC). In tissues, the term "apparent diffusion" is utilized since the movement of water molecules is modified by their interactions with cell membranes, macromolecules, and flow processes. Through measurement of this apparent diffusion, diffusion MRI provides insight into the microscopic details of tissue architecture and microcirculation.

DWI provides an image contrast using a "diffusion weighted" spin echo T2-weighted pulse sequence with two extra gradient pulses equal in magnitude and opposite in phase accumulation. This is done by modifying a standard T2-weighted imaging sequence by applying a symmetric pair of diffusion sensitizing gradients on either side of the 180° refocusing pulse. Moving water protons acquire a phase shift from the first diffusion-sensitizing gradient, which, as a consequence of motion, is not entirely rephased by the second gradient, resulting in attenuation of the measured signal intensity. Hence, the presence of water diffusion is observed as signal loss on diffusion-weighted MR images. However, it took several decades for that sequence to become clinically feasible [2] due to limitations of MR equipment, especially the gradient hard-

S. D. Serai (✉)
Children's Hospital of Philadelphia, University of Pennsylvania, Philadelphia, PA, USA
e-mail: serais@chop.edu

S. Kurugol
Harvard Medical School, Boston, MA, USA
e-mail: Sila.Kurugol@childrens.harvard.edu

P. Pullens
University of Antwerp, Antwerp University Hospital, Edegem, Belgium
e-mail: Pim.Pullens@uzgent.be

Z. J. Wang
University of California San Francisco, San Francisco, CA, USA
e-mail: Zhen.Wang@ucsf.edu

E. Sigmund
NYU Langone Health, New York, NY, USA
e-mail: Eric.Sigmund@nyulangone.org

S. D. Serai, K. Darge (eds.), *Advanced Clinical MRI of the Kidney*,
https://doi.org/10.1007/978-3-031-40169-5_18

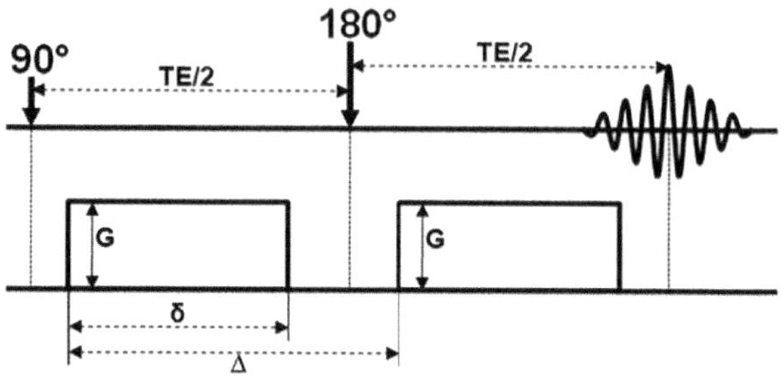

Fig. 18.1 Timing diagram of Stejskal–Tanner based diffusion acquisition sequence

ware. With recent advances in gradient hardware technology, high field scanners, RF coil design improvements, and image reconstruction innovations, DW MR imaging is reaching a potential for clinical use in the abdomen, particularly in the kidney. DW MR imaging is an attractive technique for multiple reasons: it can potentially add useful qualitative and quantitative information to conventional imaging sequences; it is rapid (performed within a breath-hold or can be performed free breathing with respiratory gating) and can be easily incorporated to existing clinical protocols.

Diffusion Measurements and ADC

In the most common and first approximation to the magnetization behavior with diffusion-weighting in tissue, the signal intensity (SI) of a diffusion-weighted image is best expressed as

$$\frac{S}{S_0} = \exp\left(-b \cdot ADC\right) \tag{1.1}$$

where S_0 is the signal intensity on a T2-weighted ($b = 0$) image, and b is the diffusion weighting factor, which is directly proportional to the square of the gyromagnetic ratio, the square of the magnitude of the gradient pulses, and three powers of gradient duration. The degree of diffusion weighting applied to an image is expressed by its *b*-value. The *b*-values are limited by the gradient hardware, but values of several hundreds to thousands are easily achievable on clinical MRI scanners (Fig. 18.2).

Diffusion is often not isotropic (same in all directions) in biological tissues since water diffuses more easily along the direction of globally aligned microstructural elements (such parallel tubules in renal medulla) rather than across them (diffusion anisotropy) [3, 4]. Because cellular structures are distributed anisotropically, the measurement of diffusion is also direction-dependent [4], emphasizing the need for measuring diffusion in several directions (Fig. 18.3). Thus, to obtain a rotationally invariant estimate of isotropic diffusion, diffusion-weighted images must be acquired in at least three orthogonal directions. The postprocessing of these images begins with the calculation of the natural logarithms of the images, which should be averaged to form a rotationally invariant (or "trace-weighted") resultant image. Using a linear least-squares regression on a pixel-by-pixel basis, the resultant image and the natural logarithm of the reference T2-weighted image are fitted to the *b*-values to calculate ADC, which is the negative slope of the fitted line.

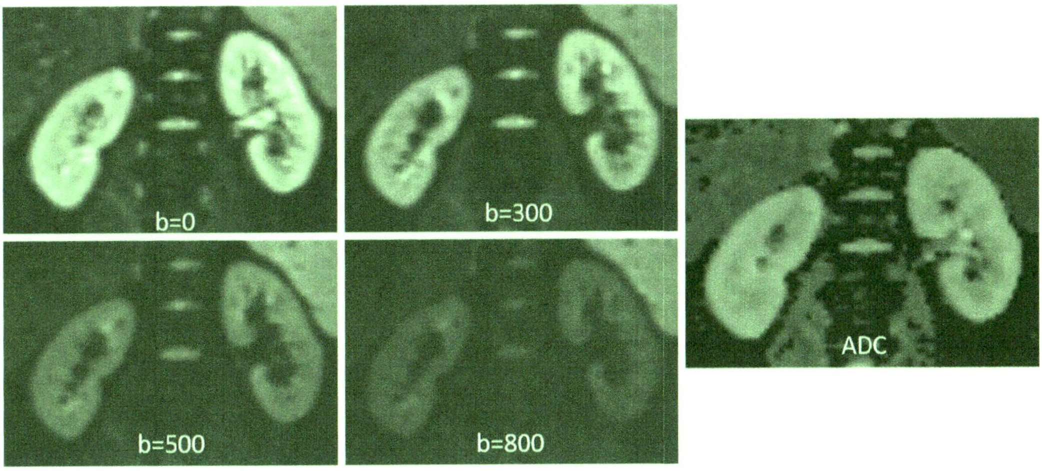

Fig. 18.2 Representative images of kidneys with increasing *b*-values and corresponding ADC map

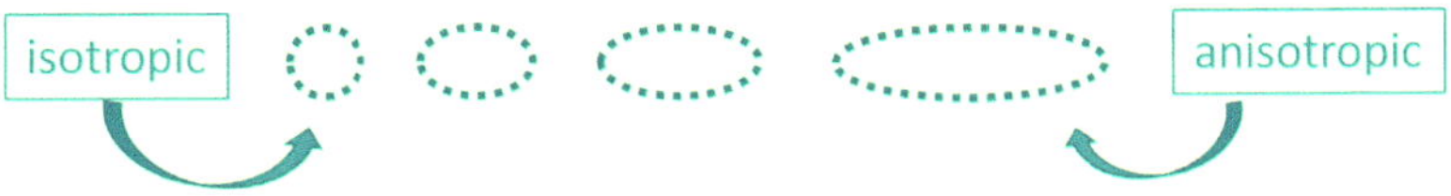

Fig. 18.3 Schematic representation of directionality. Rate of diffusion depends on the direction

IVIM (Microcirculation/Microstructure)

Given the prominent role that both perfusion and tubular flow play in the filtration process, one of the key extensions of the single compartment ADC representation for renal tissue is the inclusion of microcirculatory motion in addition to hindered Brownian motion. The most common approach to do so is the intravoxel incoherent motion (IVIM) model, one of the first signal descriptions in the history of DWI that has in the prior decade experienced a renaissance of use as technology has permitted its application to highly perfused organs [5–8]. The biophysical model of IVIM is a two-compartment description: molecular diffusion in tissues and microcirculatory motion in vessels/tubules. This approximation describes flow of blood through capillaries as a diffusion process (albeit a much faster one), due to the often-distributed orientations of flow within a capillary network. To separate the effects of diffusion and perfusion on the DW signal, a biexponential model is employed:

$$\frac{S}{S_0} = f\exp\left(-bD^*\right) + \left(1-f\right)\exp\left(-bD\right) \tag{18.2}$$

where f is the flowing blood fraction, D^* is the pseudo diffusion coefficient associated with blood microcirculation, and D the apparent diffusivity in the tissue space. In most cases, the pseudo diffusion coefficient associated with blood microcirculation is much larger (about ten times larger) than the water diffusion coefficient in tissues. The basic interpretation of the IVIM parameters are that (a) D reflects microstructure of the extravascular parenchymal space from restricted/hindered diffusion, (b) f represents flow volume, and (c) D^* reflects a combination of blood velocity and microcirculatory architecture.

The IVIM signature was observed in preclinical renal MRI as early as 1991 [9], and many subsequent studies explored its contrast in human kidney MRI. In particular, literature reviews [10–12] have indicated that much of the reported variability in renal ADC values can be traced to the use of variable *b*-values across studies. Since the single compartment ADC description does not capture the full IVIM signal behavior, measurements from different b-value combinations admit differing amounts of perfusion effects into the ADC parameter, which confounds study comparison. For this reason, among others, consensus statements have encouraged standardized b-value choices for studies that are to be pooled or compared to other trials.

As summarized in recent reviews [12, 13], IVIM metrics have been extensively reported in healthy and pathologic kidney tissue. Key findings include correlation of diffusion metrics (often D^* and f) with glomerular filtration rate (GFR), in some cases more strongly than that of ADC. Several disease processes (allograft dysfunction, acute pyelonephritis, polycystic disease, obstruction, renal artery stenosis, and chronic kidney disease) have been investigated with IVIM in smaller-scale studies, with trends of useful biomarkers from the IVIM model emerging. Conversely, diversity of acquisition/analysis parameters prevents large-scale conclusions given the current evidence, again supporting standardization efforts in the future.

DTI (Anisotropy)

Another microstructural feature beyond the ADC description is that of anisotropy. Due to the common orientation of microstructural barriers to transport in some tissue types such as renal medulla, the rate of apparent diffusion depends on direction, with largest diffusion occurring parallel to, and lowest diffusion perpendicular to, oriented structures such as renal tubules in medullary pyramids. The measurement and analysis framework that captures this behavior, as applied initially to the brain and later to many other organs (spine, muscle, breast, and kidney) is termed diffusion tensor imaging (DTI). DTI is based on the application of diffusion gradients in different directions in space, enabling the evaluation of the movement of water molecules in 3D and whether there is a dominant direction to diffusion restriction, which allows to determine fiber tracts according to the dominant direction of water movement in each voxel. DTI generalizes the ADC approach by incorporating images acquired with diffusion gradients in multiple directions to determine the directionality (i.e., anisotropy) of apparent diffusion. DTI metrics help provide rotationally invariant indices that describe the properties of the diffusion profile. DTI provides several quantitative parameters including fractional anisotropy (FA) and apparent diffusion coefficient (ADC) and also allows to generate primary eigenvector maps (Fig. 18.4). The amount of diffusion is characterized by ADC, and the anisotropy of diffusion is characterized by FA. FA is a normalized, dimensionless index that measures the properties of anisotropy of DTI. Mathematically, at least six noncollinear directions are required given the need to calculate six independent elements of the symmetric 3 × 3 diffusion tensor D_{ij} [14], an anisotropic but still Gaussian description of water motion. The tensor is then diagonalized to its principal frame

$$D_{ij} = \begin{pmatrix} \lambda_1 & 0 & 0 \\ 0 & \lambda_2 & 0 \\ 0 & 0 & \lambda_3 \end{pmatrix} \tag{18.3}$$

where its diagonal elements (eigenvalues) are the principal diffusivities, their average is the mean diffusivity (MD), and their corresponding eigenvectors (v_1, v_2, and v_3) define the principal diffusion directions [15]. The direction that corresponds to the largest eigenvalue (usually chosen to be λ_1) is called the axial or parallel direction, while the other two directions are called the radial or perpendicular directions. The axial diffusivity is given by

$$D_{\parallel} \equiv \lambda_1, \tag{18.4}$$

and the radial diffusivity is given by

$$D_{\perp} \equiv \frac{1}{2}(\lambda_2 + \lambda_3) \tag{18.5}$$

Anisotropy indices are different combinations of the directional diffusion coefficients, such as the normalized variance called fractional anisotropy (FA),

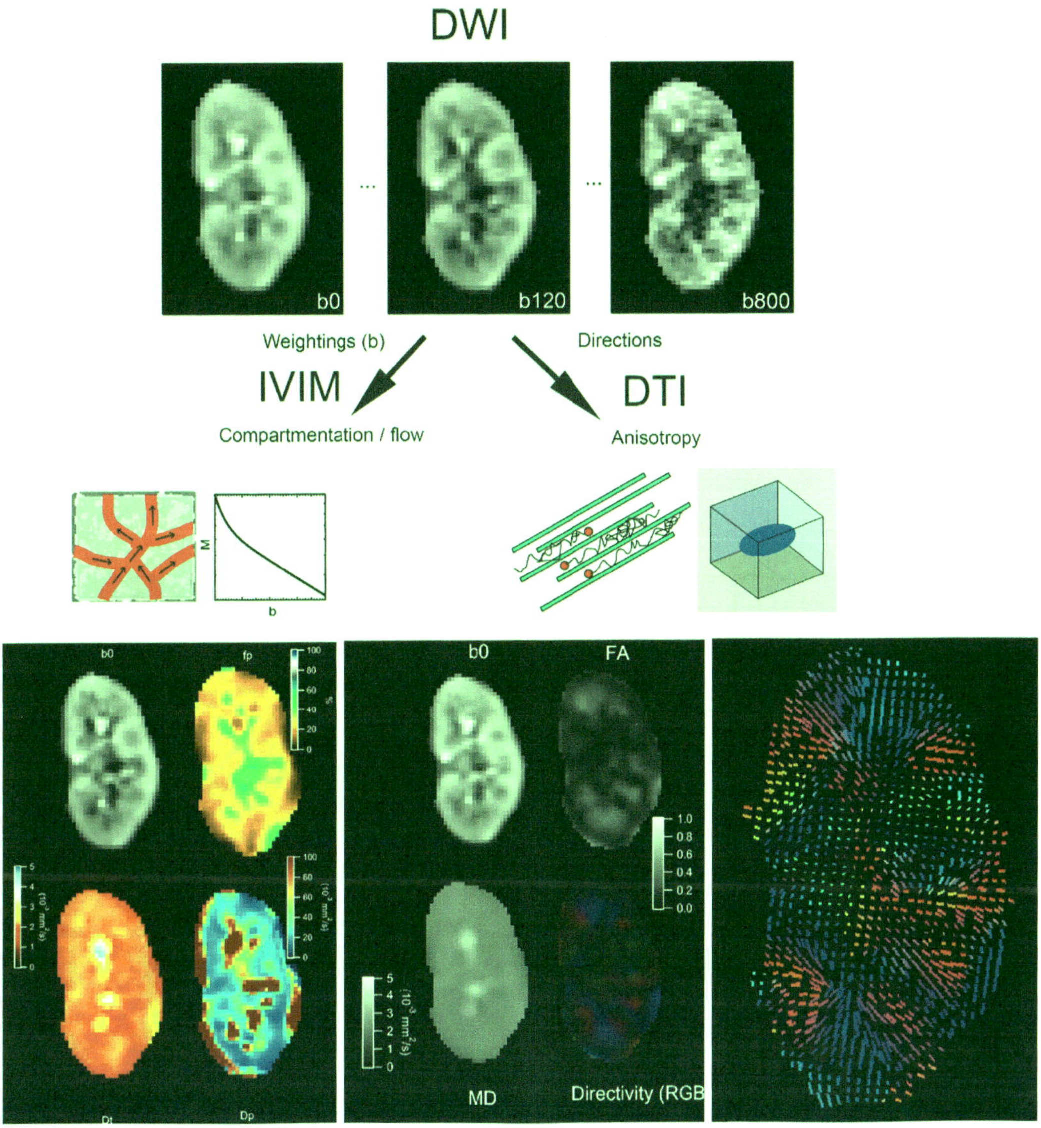

Fig. 18.4 Example intravoxel incoherent motion (IVIM) and diffusion tensor imaging (DTI) maps from a healthy volunteer left kidney. Left: biexponential IVIM fitting of multiple b-value data provides maps of perfusion fraction (f_p), tissue diffusion (D_t), and pseudo diffusity (D_p). Right: DTI tensor fitting of multidirectional data provides maps of mean diffusivity (MD), fractional anisotropy (FA), directivity, and principal diffusion orientation (v1)

$$\mathrm{FA} = \sqrt{\frac{3}{2}\frac{\sum_{i=1}^{3}(\lambda_i - \mathrm{MD})^2}{\sum_{i=1}^{3}\lambda_i^2}} \tag{18.6}$$

The FA varies from 0 to 1 and quantifies the degree to which a tissue is anisotropic. FA reflects how dominant one particular water movement direction in a voxel is and is measured from 0 to 1; while ADC measures the directionally averaged diffusivity. Low FA values imply similar diffusion along all directions, while higher FA implies that there is a marked directional dependence such that diffusion occurs preferentially along one dominant direction.

In other organs such as the brain or skeletal muscle, optimization studies have been conducted to determine b-value and number of directions choices to minimize noise-induced bias or uncertainty [16, 17]; a minimum of 20 or 30 directions are typically recommended, but it is advised to apply diffusion-weighted images in many directions as allowed by scan time limitation [17, 18].

The "radial" pattern of tubule/duct orientation in the renal medulla is well known in diffusion tensor imaging [19–23] following an initial demonstration by Ries et al. [24]. In addition to depiction of this pattern in discrete images, another application of DTI is tractography, which generates continuous streamlines as virtual representation of the anisotropic structures influencing apparent diffusion. While only a few examples have been published [20, 22], they clearly illustrate the radial path from medullary pyramids through renal pelvis and ureter.

A wide range of studies have probed DTI methods in both healthy and diseased kidney [25, 26]. Quantitatively, common findings are that glomerular filtration rate (GFR) correlates significantly with both mean diffusion MD and fractional anisotropy FA, consistent with their partial sensitivity to the vascular/tubular flow that affects filtration. Pathologic tissue often shows decreases in MD and FA, and often a decrease in corticomedullary differentiation in these parameters (Figs. 18.5 and 18.6).

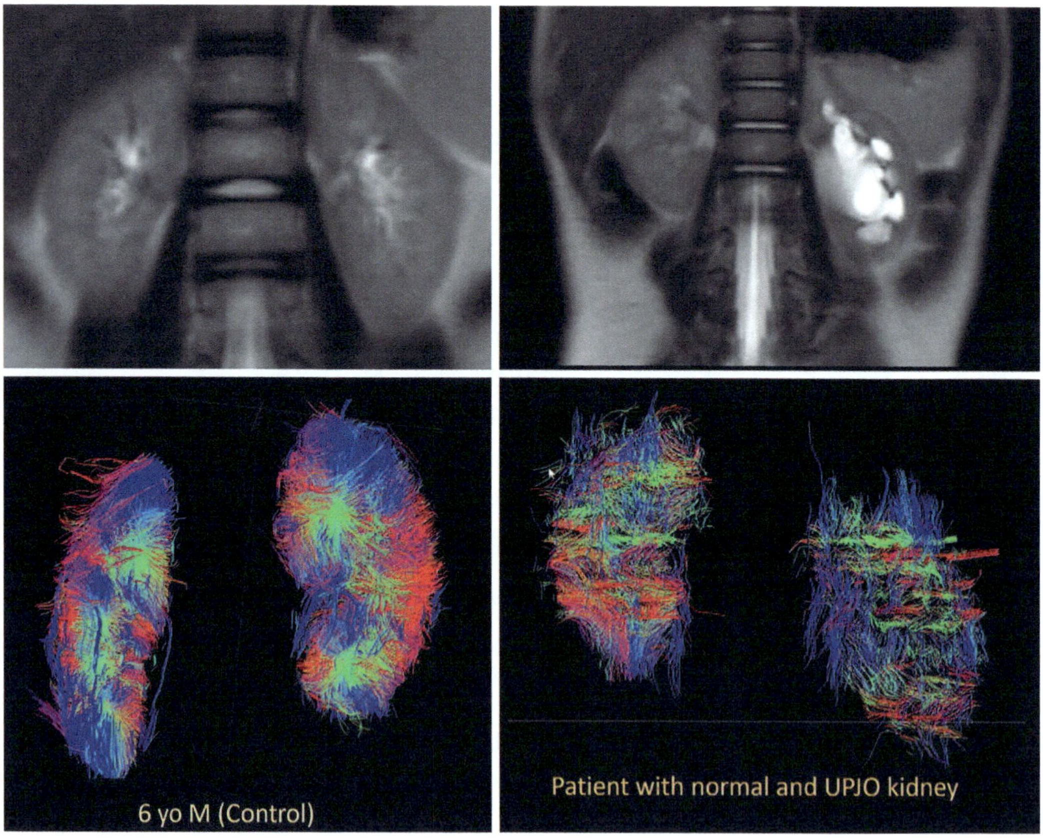

Fig. 18.5 DTI-based tractography shows microstructural disarrangement in kidneys with ureteropelvic junction obstruction [25]

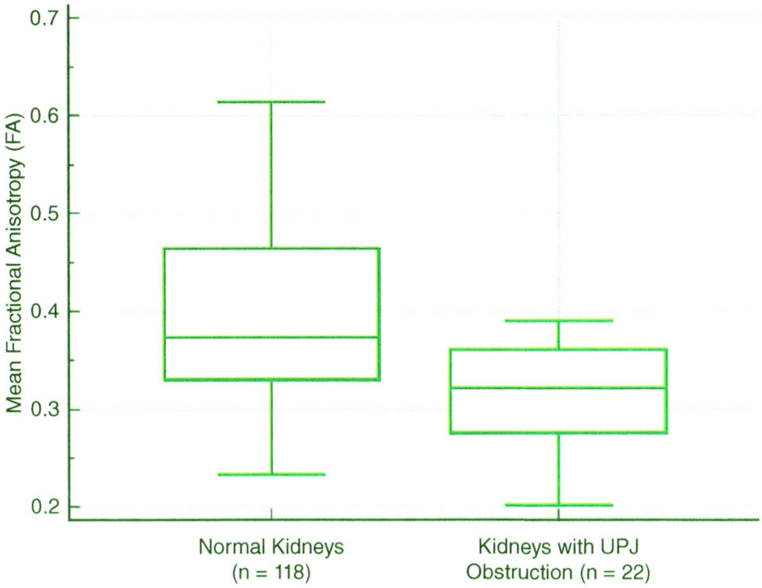

Fig. 18.6 Box and whisker plot of mean FA in normal kidneys vs patients with ureteropelvic junction (UPJ) obstruction. Horizontal lines within boxes represent medians, and vertical lines and whiskers represent the lowest and highest observations within 1.5 interquartile ranges of lower and upper quartiles, respectively. Mean FA values were significantly lower (0.31 ± 0.07; $n = 22$) in kidneys with UPJ obstruction than normal kidneys (0.40 ± 0.08; $n = 118$) [25]

Advanced/Hybrid Models

While signatures of microcirculation and anisotropy are now unmistakable in renal DWI, their interpretation, biologic validation, and modification by disease remain topics of research. In particular, multiple circulatory networks coexist in renal cortex and medulla (glomeruli, vasa recta, proximal/distal tubules, loops of Henle, and collecting ducts) and disentangling their individual contributions to the DWI signal is nontrivial. A variety of advanced approaches have been pursued to do so, either combining existing methods (IVIM and DTI) or varying acquisition parameters (echo time, diffusion time, cardiac phase, and gradient waveform).

Flow Anisotropy

Intuitively, microscopic flow contributes to medullary anisotropy just as microstructure does, as indirectly suggested by DTI studies showing elevated anisotropy when lower *b*-values were employed [23]. Directly, several studies have now shown that the flow term shows a similar orientation pattern. One experimental demonstration employed multiple *b*-value, multiple direction data to illustrate this collinear anisotropy of structural, and pseudo diffusion in a combined IVIM/DTI scheme [27], showing a pseudo diffusion anisotropy comparable to that of microstructure. This approach also yielded diagnostic potential in the assessment of renal function in pre-surgical renal mass patients [28]. One of the measures most sensitive to asymmetric laterality in kidney diffusion—reflecting the compensatory redistribution of flow in response to a neoplasm—was axial medullary pseudo diffusion. Another approach employed an intravoxel oriented flow (IVOF) model incorporating an apparent flow fraction tensor to capture the microcirculation and microstructural anisotropy in medullary tissue [29]. Another study employed a separate tensorial description for all three IVIM parameters (D, f, D^*) and showed high fractional anisotropy for all three in the medullary compartment [30]. These studies have confirmed that the best representation of water transport in kidney should incorporate directionality in both flow and structural degrees of freedom.

Encoding Variations

As with other organs, diffusion contrast varies with various MRI encoding or acquisition parameters, in a way that may be exploited to improve the biophysical interpretation of the approach. Not surprisingly, given the strong role of perfusion in renal DWI, the cardiac phase has been shown to be a powerful modulator of renal DWI metrics in cardiac-gated imaging studies. These have included ADC [31, 32], IVIM [33, 34], and DTI [35] studies that show pseudo diffusion, perfusion fraction, and anisotropy all maximizing in systolic phase compared to diastolic phase.

Diffusion time, or the duration allotted for water spins to explore the microenvironment, is another variable that affects diffusion contrast. Microstructural barriers reduce water diffusion below the thermodynamic free diffusion value, such that apparent diffusion tends to decrease with increasing diffusion time. If the timescale associated with dominant hindrance scales l ($t \sim l^2/2D$) approximates accessible diffusion times, this provides a means of contrast modulation and potential biophysical modeling. Conversely, microcirculatory flow that gives rise to pseudo diffusion effects can also induce a diffusion time dependence as spins advance through the network. This trend is typically opposite to the microstructural one as pseudo diffusion increases in a short-time ballistic limit and finally saturates in a long-time pseudo diffusive limit. While very little systematic variation of diffusion time has been performed for renal DWI, recent work [36] employing both spin echo and stimulated echo DTI measurements suggests that in the diffusion time range of 20–125 ms, microcirculation effects predominate and apparent diffusion and anisotropy increase with diffusion time. This observation, which could be further explored with quantitative modeling or increased sampling, is another example of the key importance of microcirculation in renal tissue water transport.

Finally, as discussed above, the known physiology of renal tissue clearly indicates that the conventional IVIM representation of one microcirculatory and one parenchymal compartment is only a first-order approximation to the reality. Multiple sources of microcirculation, both vascular (arteries, veins, capillaries, glomeruli, and vasa recta) and tubular (proximal/distal convoluted tubule, loops of Henle, and collecting ducts), contribute to pseudo diffusion, and separating their influences might dramatically improve specificity. One approach to doing so is via rate of pseudo diffusion, and several studies have shown that three compartments [37] or more generally a spectrum of diffusion coefficients [38, 39] are more descriptive of renal tissue than the conventional IVIM model. In these studies, the fastest component is typically assigned to vascular volume, while the intermediate rate compartment is interpreted as tubular flow.

Another effect on DWI contrast is through gradient waveform, which can be chosen to modulate the degree of sensitivity to steady flow (i.e., flow encoding or compensation). Specifically, constant velocity motion induces a phase shift proportional to the first moment of the gradient waveform (M_1), and in the presence of heterogeneous flow, these phase shifts interfere and induce IVIM contrast. Gradient waveforms, by varying or nulling M_1 (flow compensated, $M_1 = 0$), can correspondingly vary this attenuation, which can aid IVIM signal analysis and biophysical modeling. Flow compensated IVIM measurements have been shown in phantom [40–42], brain [43–45], liver [46–48], placenta [49], and heart [50] studies; in one study of the liver, a continuous range of gradient moments M_1 was implemented for more complete contrast variation and tissue modeling [46]. In the case of renal tissue, only pilot studies have been performed [47, 51] that modulate M_1, and their analysis regarding multiple flow compartments is still in development. However, this variable may prove promising in disentangling renal flow compartments.

Both evidence generation and modeling in the space of advanced kidney DWI continue to evolve, as does their interpretation. However, it seems likely the conventional IVIM description will eventually give way to a more nuanced treatment for maximum biological specificity.

Advanced Readouts (SMS, RS-EPI, rFOV, Non-Cartesian)

The most common readout for kidney DWI is single shot echo-planar imaging (ss-EPI), in which all required lines of k-space are acquired in a single echo train, typically in a Cartesian pattern. The EPI technique is used to achieve very fast image acquisition in order to minimize the effects of subject motion and to retain high SNR [52, 53]. As EPI is a 2D imaging technique, volumes are acquired slice-by-slice with repetition times (TR) being set sufficiently long to both minimize T1 contrast and accommodate the whole volume of interest. Due to the length of the echo train in comparison with the transverse relaxation time T2*, however, ss-DWI suffers blurring, distortion, and ghosting, which limit spatial resolution and reduce image quality. Image post-processing can ameliorate these issues to some extent, such as EPI image dewarping via reversed phase encoding acquisition as has been shown in several kidney DWI studies [54–56]. Beyond correcting EPI, however, a variety of alternatives has therefore been deployed throughout the body, some of which have been applied to kidney imaging. Some are based on single-shot turbo spin echo (TSE) acquisitions, to avoid the gradient echo-based sensitivities of EPI [57, 58]. Multiband approaches such as simultaneous multi-slice (SMS) acquisition have been used to accelerate the slice dimension [59–65], as in other organs [66–68]. Reduced field of view (rFOV) DWI captures a smaller subvolume to limit EPI echo train length and associated artifacts, providing high resolution DWI in the kidney [58, 69–71].

Multi-shot DWI EPI techniques offer higher spatial resolution but are susceptible to motion-induced phase errors since each individual shot may have suffered different slight coherent motions from pulsation, respiration, etc. Without correction, this results in ghosting artifacts, pixel misregistration, and low image resolution with poor diffusion contrast in the reconstructed images [72], resulting in inaccurate measurements. Readout-segmented EPI (rs-EPI) alters the conventional EPI trajectory by acquiring all phase encodes but restricting the readout acquisition in each shot as a means of limiting susceptibility artifacts [73, 74]. Each of these methods, either as modifications or alternatives of standard EPI-DWI, broadens the available toolbox of kidney DWI and provides hope for higher spatial resolution, which is often crucial for proper quantification when corticomedullary differentiation deteriorates with reduced renal function. However, the variability in execution, parameter choice, and interpretation limits their broad utility now such that concerted efforts for broad translation of one alternative or another would be a valuable next step.

Diffusion Data Acquisition Methods

Acquisition method standardization is an important milestone in the validation of DWI-based parameters as imaging biomarkers for renal disease. The international collaboration on renal imaging (PARENCHIMA) has proposed technical recommendations on three variants of renal DWI, mono-exponential DWI, IVIM, and DTI, as well as associated MRI biomarkers (ADC, D, D^*, f, FA, and MD) to aid ongoing international efforts on methodological harmonization. In their recommendations, reported DWI biomarkers from 194 prior renal DWI studies were extracted and Pearson correlations between diffusion biomarkers and protocol parameters were computed. Based on the literature review, surveys were designed for the consensus building. Survey data were collected via Delphi consensus process on renal DWI preparation, acquisition, analysis, and reporting (Table 18.1). Consensus was defined as ≥75% agreement. Summary of the literature and

Table 18.1 Imaging protocol recommendations for image acquisition of renal diffusion dataset

Protocol option	Recommendation		
Patient preparation	Normal hydration status		
Field strength	1.5 T or 3 T		
Sequence	Single shot EPI		
Orientation	Oblique coronal		
Matrix size	>128		
In-plane resolution	2–3 mm		
Slice thickness	>4 mm		
Coverage	Full kidney		
Parallel imaging factor	2		
Fat suppression	SPAIR		
TR (s)	4		
TE (msec)	Minimum (<100)		
No. of averages	3		
Breathing mode	Respiratory gated		
Cardiac gating	Not required		
Diffusion gradients	Monopolar		
	ADC	IVIM	DTI
No. of *b*-values	4 or 5	>6	2 or more
Suggested *b*-values	0, 100, 200, 400, 800	0, 30, 70, 100, 200, 400, 800	0, 400, 800
No. of directions	3	3	12 or more
Distortion correction	Yes		
Image registration	Yes		
Diffusion units	10^{-3} mm²/s		

survey data as well as recommendations for the preparation, acquisition, processing, and reporting of renal DWI were then provided in a published manuscript [12]. Diffusion tensor properties among field strength 1.5 T and 3 T were also highlighted (Fig. 18.7).

The following sections contain guides for carrying out each of these protocols on clinical scanners; these guides are stated in general terms as precise implementations may vary amid different vendor solutions.

DW-EPI for ADC

Sequence: Select a spin echo-based sequence with echo-planar imaging (EPI) readout with a diffusion preparation module. While single refocused monopolar is suggested for consensus, twice-refocused spin echo (TRSE) with bipolar gradients is acceptable.

b-values: The diffusion weighting factors b and gradient sensitizing directions are then adjusted.

Choose your *b*-values to the following values: 0, 100, 200, 400, 800 s/mm^2 over three orthogonal directions; this is often labeled as Trace-weighted or three-scan trace encoding.

Repetition time (TR): choose at least 4 s for sufficient signal-to-noise per time (SNR/t) efficiency. TR will be limited by the length of the excitation pulse, length of echo train, and the number of slices you acquire.

Echo time (TE): use the shortest TE allowable given all *b*-values selected.

Acquisition bandwidth (BW): This should be chosen as a balance between short inter-echo spacing and therefore minimum echo time on the one hand, and sufficient signal-to-noise ratio on the other. If the bandwidth is too slow, long readout duration will lead to T2-weighted signal loss; if it is too high, then high frequency noise can overwhelm the primary signal. For clinical renal MRI, a typical compromise is ~2 kHz/pixel.

Fat saturation: Choose a method of fat saturation, using chemical shift contrast, T1 contrast, or both. The recommended approach is spectral adiabatic inversion recovery (SPAIR) to combine both chemical shift and T1 contrast for fat suppression.

Respiratory gating: This is essential to reduce motion artifacts, motion blurring, and unwanted intensities variations among the images acquired with different *b*-values. If this is not available, consider retrospective motion correction with dedicated software (see section below).

Geometry: Choose as phase-encoding direction the L-R direction and adapt the geometry so

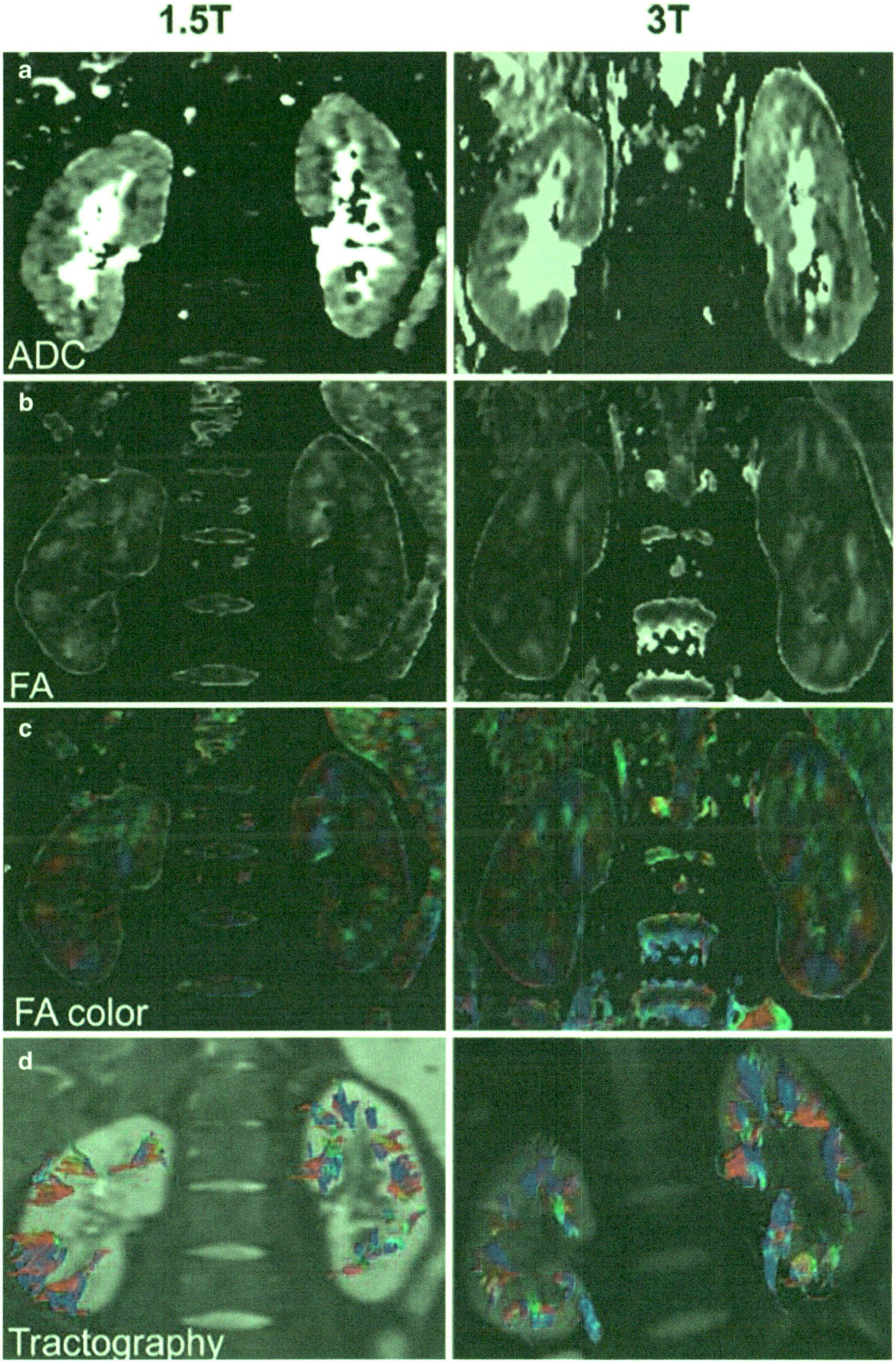

Fig. 18.7 Diffusion properties at 1.5 T and 3 T do not show significant differences. (**a**) ADC maps: ADC of the cortex is significantly higher than ADC of the medulla both at 1.5 T and 3 T. (**b**) FA maps: FA of the medulla is significantly higher than of the cortex both at 1.5 T and 3 T. In FA maps, the renal pelvis appears smaller, because cortex and pelvis both exhibit an almost isotropic diffusion, so that discrimination between both compartments is hampered. (**c**) The color-coded FA maps allows identification of the diffusion direction (red: left-right; blue: head-foot; green: anterior-posterior). (**d**) Tractography reveals a typically radial diffusion direction in the medulla reflecting the radial organization of anatomic structures like vessels and tubules [75]

that the FOV in this direction includes the entire region. Use frequency encoding in head-feet (rostral-caudal) direction to avoid severe aliasing.

Averages: Increase the number of averages to improve signal-to-noise ratio by a factor of $\sqrt{\text{averages}}$, especially important for higher *b*-values (use three averages as a recommendation).

DW-EPI for IVIM

Load the DW-EPI sequence with the same parameters as DWI-EPI for ADC (TE, TR, matrix size, averages, and bandwidth). Increase the number of *b*-values to at least 6 (e.g., 0, 30, 70, 100, 200, 400,800 s/mm^2) to probe fast diffusion from microcirculation.

DW-EPI for DTI

For DTI acquisitions, employ the same imaging parameters as suggested for ADC imaging above, use several *b*-values (suggested 0, 400, 800 s/mm^2), and select multiple gradient directions for each *b*-value. At least six noncollinear directions are required for DTI analysis, with more typically acquired for improved tensor estimation (recommended at least 12 for kidney DTI).

Motion Management

Kidney DW-MRI is sensitive to physiological motion (respiratory, peristaltic, and pulsatile). For instance, when using multi-shot acquisitions where different portions of k-space are obtained following separate signal excitations, severe artifacts may appear, due to the presence of inconsistent motion-related phase offsets across shots [76]. Therefore, kidney DW-MRI acquisition is typically performed with rapid single shot echo planar imaging sequences. With this type of acquisition, each image is acquired very fast, minimizing the effect of motion within a slice. However, rapid pulsatile motion may still lead to artifacts and signal void in the image [77]. Also, during the acquisition of the entire set of DW-MR images, respiratory motion causes displacement of the kidneys and misalignment of slices acquired at the same position across different repetitions and diffusion encodings. This misalignment reduces the accuracy and robustness of quantitative parameter maps obtained from DW-MR images. Also, image quality degrades due to blurring because of motion, when averaging multiple repetitions of misaligned images to increase signal-to-noise ratio.

To minimize the effects of motion, DW-MR images are commonly either acquired during a breath-hold period, at the expense of the signal-to-noise ratio and spatial coverage, which may not even be feasible for some patients, or using respiratory triggering methods at the expense of increased scan time and remaining effect of motion in triggered acquisitions [78]. Respiratory triggering can be performed either using a respiratory belt type sensor wrapped around the abdomen or with an image navigator located at the diaphragm [79]. The triggering technique does not always perform well if the respiratory rhythm is irregular as in the case of anxious awake children who are breathing rapidly or irregularly. Residual motion artifacts may remain in respiratory triggered scans, and triggered scans have low efficiency as no data is acquired in most parts of the breathing cycle.

Another alternative approach used to compensate for respiratory motion is to either retrospectively perform triggering by accepting data from a certain phase of the breathing cycle and discarding the rest or sort each repetition into discrete motion states over the breathing cycle [80] based on the trajectory of periodic respiratory motion from the navigator signal. However, inaccuracies of the navigator signal can hinder correct sorting of the data into motion states. Also, volumes for certain motion states can have missing slices due to lower sampling rate per motion state. Irregular respiratory rhythm or rapid breathing can exacerbate these problems.

Another approach is non-rigid image registration of individual images for alignment. A simple approach is using non-rigid registration of a single image slice in 2D to the corresponding slice in the reference volume. A normalized mutual information metric may be used to register images acquired with different diffusion encodings and therefore have different contrast. However, single slice registration methods cannot correct for the motion between slices.

A more accurate approach is using a rigid 3D slice-to-volume image registration separately for each kidney. This approach uses the image features of 2D slices, each acquired in about 200 ms [81]. This rapid acquisition of each slice allows effective estimation of physiological motion via a slice-to-volume image registration algorithm [55], which was first developed for the brain [82]. A 3D motion-free reference volume is registered to each 2D slice including the region of interest for each kidney using a rigid transform (Fig. 18.8). The approach is most effective in coronal acquisitions where the motion is happening mostly in plane, and a motion-free reference volume is selected among one of the acquired $b = 0$ volumes. However, slice to volume registration is an ill-posed problem. Therefore, the rigid motion parameters can be tracked and regularized based on the information content of the sequentially acquired DW-MRI slices, using a robust state estimation with Kalman filtering instead of predicting the motion parameters for each slice independently [81]. The estimated motion parameters are then applied to correct the position of each slice in 3D. As a result of applying the estimated transformation to each 2D slice for motion correction, a scattered 3D point cloud is obtained for each 3D volume. It is possible to resample these scattered points to a regular 3D grid to reconstruct a motion-corrected 3D volume. Alternatively, a quantitative model such as IVIM or DTI can be fitted using a 3D neighborhood of points around each grid point using a kernel function for weighting each point based on their distance to the grid center and using least squares fitting to estimate the model parameters. The rigid 3D SVR will correct for the rigid

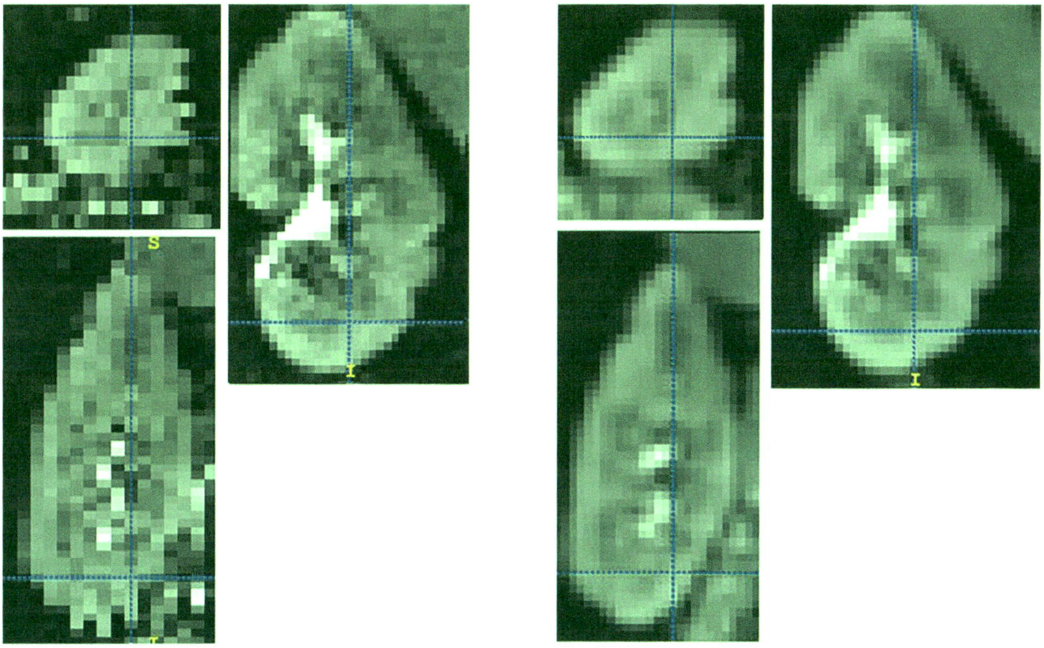

Fig. 18.8 Left panel shows an original $b = 0$ image acquired in coronal plane. The axial and sagittal views show that the slices in the original image are misaligned due to motion. Right panel shows the resultant motion-corrected $b = 0$ image. The rigid motion parameters are estimated with 3D slice to volume registration and regularized based on the information content of the sequentially acquired DW-MRI slices using Kalman filtering. The resultant 3D rigid transforms are then applied to each slice and the data is reformatted to a grid. On the right panel, both axial and sagittal views show that the slices are aligned after motion correction

motion for each kidney. However, remaining non-rigid motion such as pulsatile motion may need to be corrected by a non-rigid transformation.

Motion compensation using 3D non-rigid image registration can also be used to bring the volumes acquired at different repetitions and diffusion encodings into the same physical coordinate space before fitting a signal decay model [83, 84]. However, each *b*-value image has different contrast; as a result, independent registration of different *b*-value images to a reference image (usually $b = 0$ image) can be challenging, especially for high *b*-value images where the signal is significantly attenuated and the signal-to-noise ratio is low. In [85], quantitative MR images are registered without using any predefined model by utilizing a PCA-based groupwise image registration technique. However, the PCA-based representation is only applicable to data from a simplified single exponential decay rather than data with an underlying complex signal decay composed of a bi-modal distribution of fast and slow diffusion components. Alternatively, signal decay model (such as IVIM) driven registration methods that perform simultaneous image registration and model estimation were proposed to account for this problem [86]. These approaches jointly solve for the image registration and quantitative parameter estimation problems. The images are registered to the corresponding volume reconstructed from the signal decay model at each *b*-value, which eliminates the problem of contrast differences between the moving image and the reference image during registration. Note that non-rigid registration can be challenging for acquisitions with axial slice orientation with a slice thickness of around 5–6 mm as these acquisitions have low resolution in the main direction of respiratory motion. On the other hand, acquisitions with coronal slice orientation are affected by susceptibility artifacts leading to image distortion and moreover, distortion fields change with motion; therefore, motion and distortion correction needs to be addressed simultaneously to correct such acquisitions [55].

Common techniques for distortion correction for DW-MRI assumes that there is no motion throughout the acquisition of DW-MR images with different diffusion encodings, and therefore, the distortion field is static. The distortion field is then estimated once from a single pair of images acquired with opposite phase encoding directions and, hence, have opposite distortion effects [56, 87]. This assumption does not hold for kidney DW-MRI acquired during free-breathing due to presence of motion. Distortion field changes across images acquired at different positions of the organs. A distortion field then needs to be computed for each slice. A dual echo EPI acquisition can be used where two EPI readouts of the same slice can be acquired with opposite phase encoding directions at two echo times and used to estimate a distortion field and a distortion-corrected image for each slice [88]. This technique has been applied to DW-MRI of kidneys [55], where two EPI readouts of the same slice with left to right (L- > R) and right to left (R- > L) directions were acquired and used to estimate a distortion field for each slice. Figures 18.9 and 18.10 show how this technique was corrected for distortion in kidneys for each coronal slice. After distortion correction, the 3D slice to volume registration and motion tracking was applied to correct for the effect of motion retrospectively for all slices. Fig. 18.11 shows the effect of motion compensation and the estimated rigid motion parameters for all slices. Figure 18.12 shows IVIM and DTI parameters estimated on the original data without processing and after distortion and motion compensation (top rows) for a representative subject.

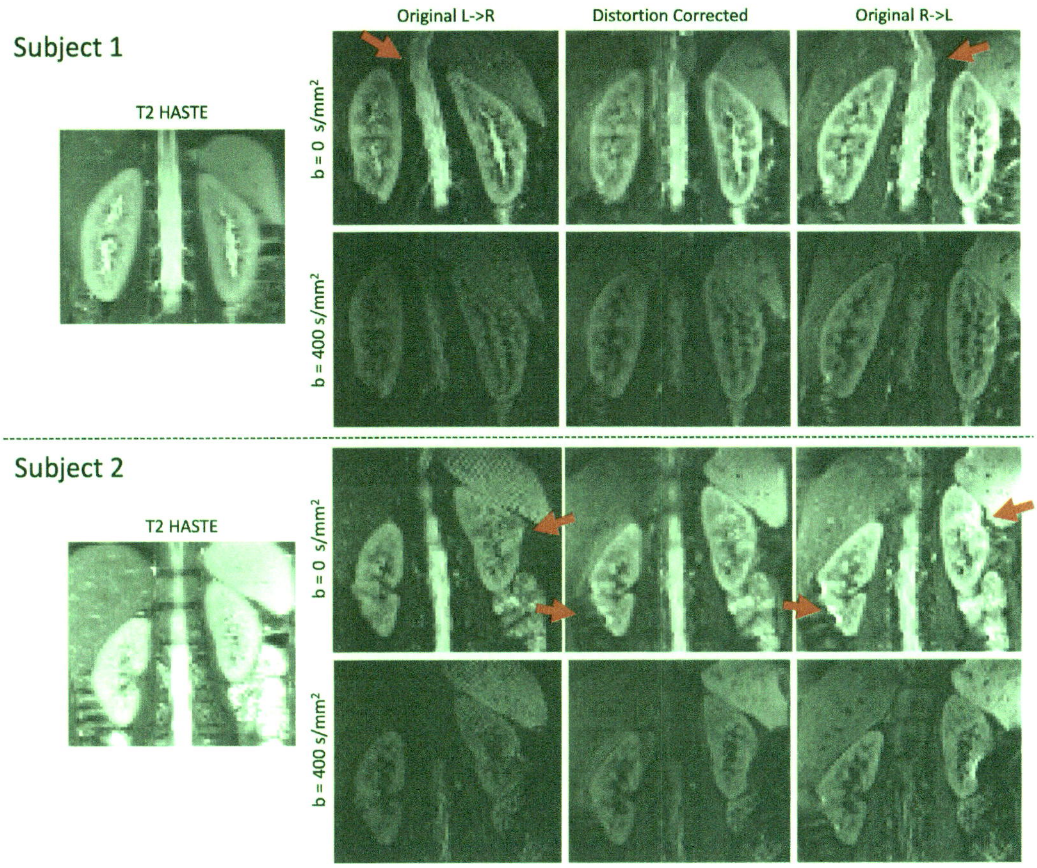

Fig. 18.9 The comparison of the reference T_2-HASTE image of two subjects and DW-MR images (for two *b*-values) before and after distortion correction for two representative subjects. The T_2-HASTE reference (left column), original L- > R image (middle left), original R- > L image (right), and distortion-corrected image (middle right) are shown. Red arrows indicate areas where distortion is present. The original images present large distortion, particularly in the upper part of the kidneys and near the bowel, indicated with red arrows. After distortion correction, the distortion is reduced in most of the kidney, although there are some remaining errors in the right kidney of subject 2 near the bowel, also indicated by the red arrows

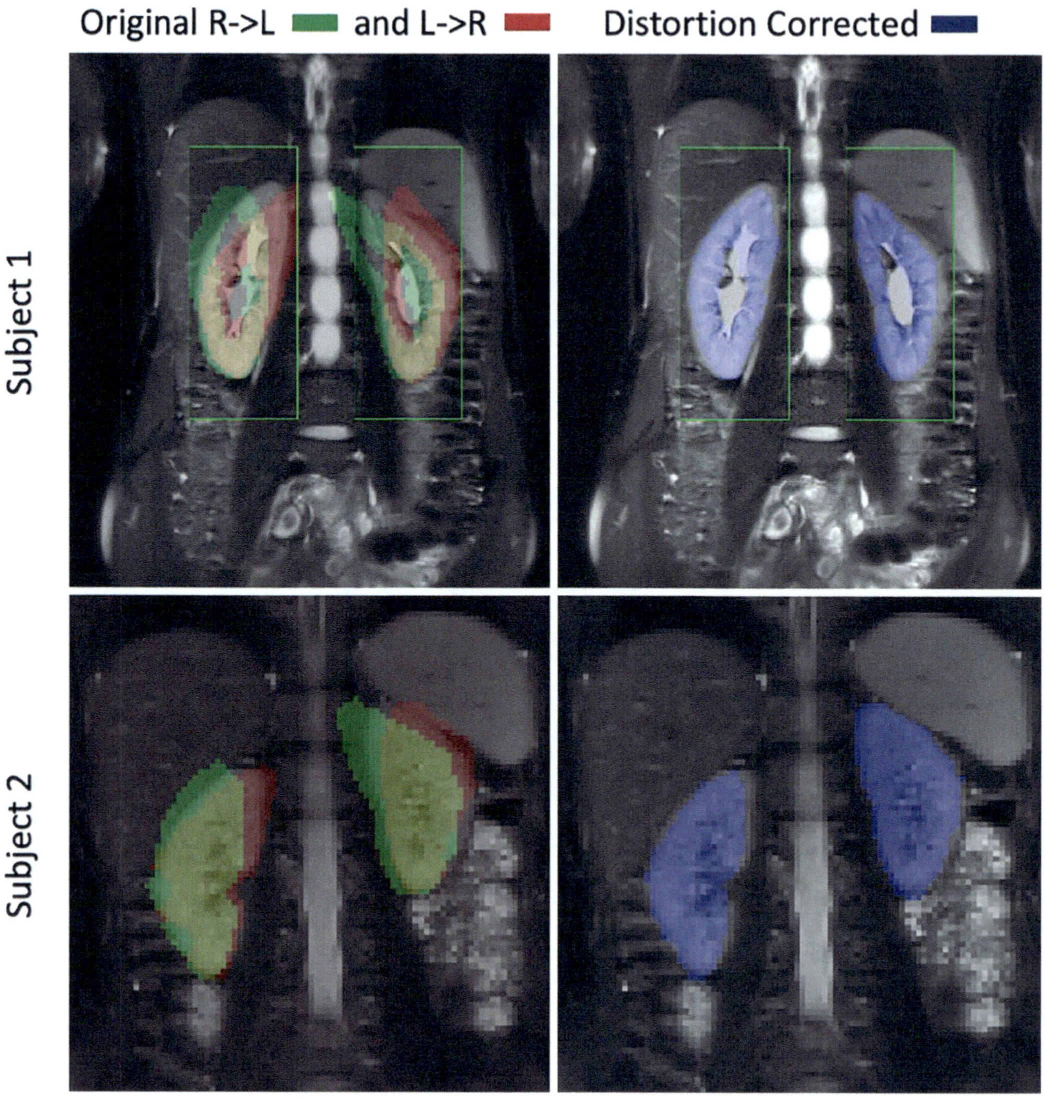

Fig. 18.10 Reference T_2-HASTE image and the segmented kidney masks from the DW images are shown for the L- > R and R- > L images without correction on the left and for the distortion-corrected image on the right. Each row corresponds to one representative subject. The kidneys are severely distorted in the original DW images. After distortion correction, the kidneys are in good alignment with the reference image

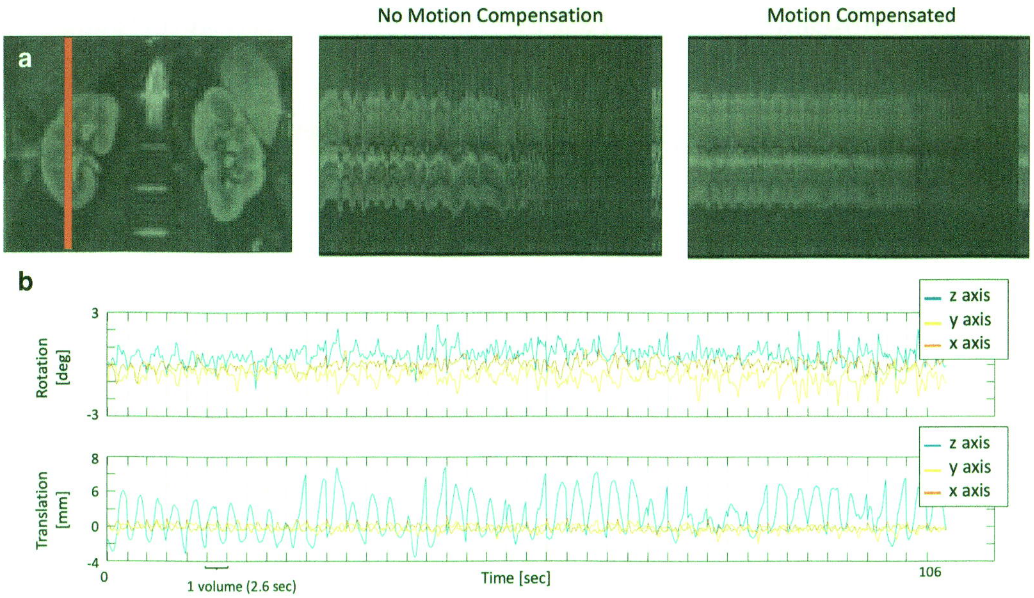

Fig. 18.11 Temporal evolution of a line of voxels from one kidney over different DW acquisitions and the registration parameters of the consecutively acquired slices during the first 1.8 min for a representative subject. The leftmost column in (**a**) shows the images of the cropped kidneys with a red line indicating the selected line of voxels plotted on the right. The middle panel shows the line plot for the volume with distortion correction, but no motion compensation and right panel shows the line plot for the distortion and motion-corrected volume. Panel (**b**) shows the rotation and translation parameters (top and bottom). The time to acquire each volume (2.6 s) is indicated with vertical lines. Without motion compensation, the line plot shows large oscillations due to breathing. On the other hand, motion compensation corrects these oscillations and aligns the DW-MR volumes in the acquired sequence

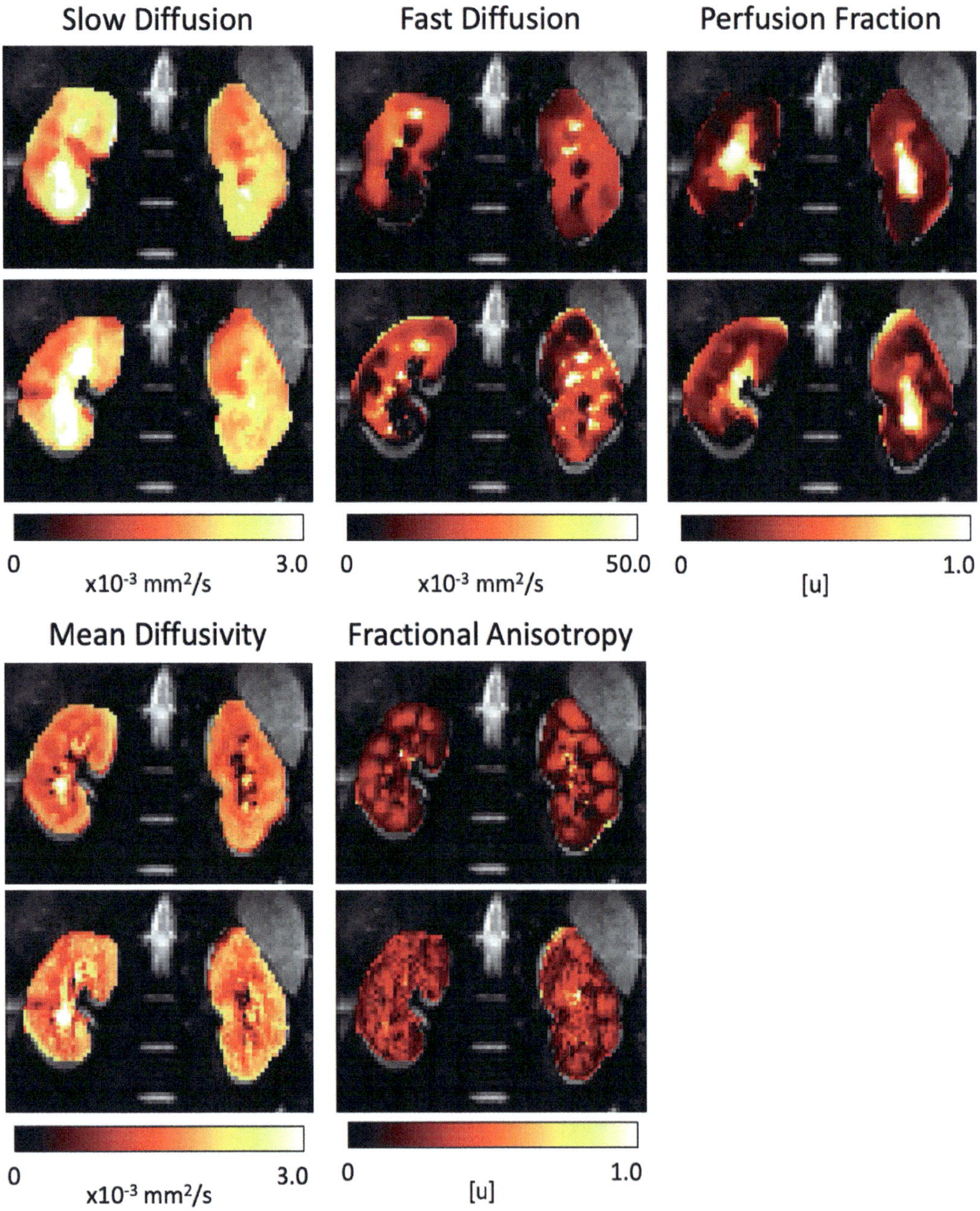

Fig. 18.12 IVIM and DTI parameters estimated on the original data without processing (no correction—bottom rows) and after distortion and motion compensation (top rows) for a representative subject. The columns correspond to the slow diffusion (D), fast diffusion (D^*), perfusion fraction (f) of the IVIM model and the mean diffusivity (MD), and fractional anisotropy (FA) parameters of the DTI model. The parameter maps obtained after distortion and motion compensation processing have fewer outliers and discontinuities. Moreover, the medulla and cortex can be better identified in the perfusion fraction (f) and fractional anisotropy (FA) maps of corrected images

Clinical Applications of Renal DWI

Chronic Kidney Disease

Chronic kidney disease (CKD) is a global health problem, affecting more than 10% of the world's population and more than half of adults over 70 years of age [89]. Present treatment strategies focus on slowing the progression of CKD, which requires accurate monitoring of renal function in patients with CKD. Current clinical methods of estimating renal function, such as creatine and estimated glomerular filtration rate (eGFR), have limitations as these indicators cannot reliably assess early injury and they do not reflect morphological changes in the kidneys.

There are numerous studies investigating the role of DWI in patients with CKD. A meta-analysis of DWI for staging CKD, as defined by eGFR, showed that patients with stage 1–2 CKD had lower renal ADC values than healthy subjects, and those with stage 3 CKD had higher ADC than the ones with stages 4–5 CKD [90]. There was, however, no differences in ADC values between stage 3 and stages 1–2 CKD [90]. The studies included in the analysis were heterogeneous with respect to *b* values, scanning parameters and methods for defining region of interests (ROIs), and reliable threshold levels could not be derived from the analysis. Nonetheless, this meta-analysis provides evidence for DWI in the assessment of renal function in CKD. In addition to ADC measurement, other more advanced DWI techniques have also been investigated for assessing renal function. For example, preliminary study of DTI in renal disease patients showed that fractional anisotropy (FA) was significantly lower in CKD patients than healthy controls, regardless of whether eGFR was reduced (Fig. 18.13) [91]. This may be related to the early changes in tissue microstructure and suggests the potential of DTI for early diagnosis of CKD.

A hallmark of CKD is the presence of interstitial fibrosis, which is critical for early diagnosis and treatment adaptation, and prognosis. Several clinical studies have demonstrated a good correlation between renal ADC values and histopathological fibrosis scores [73, 92–94], supporting the usefulness of DWI as a noninvasive tool for assessing renal fibrosis and monitoring CKD. Additionally, measuring the differences

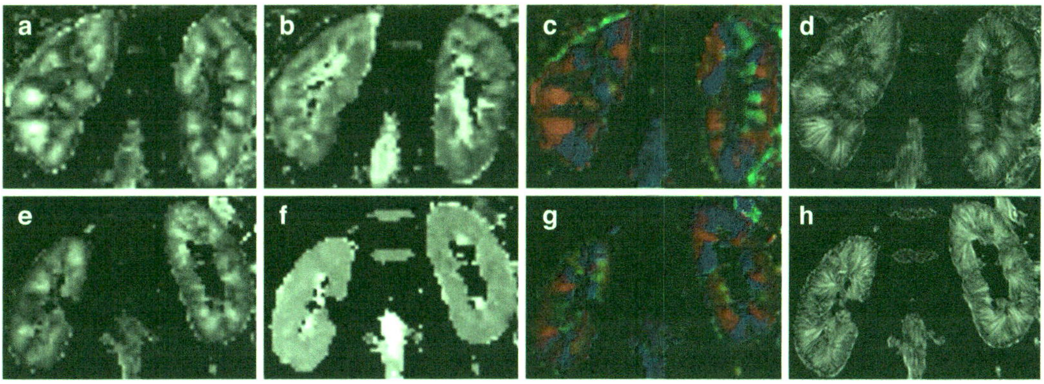

Fig. 18.13 Diffusion properties in healthy kidneys of the control group (**a**–**d**) and impaired kidneys of the study group (**e**–**h**). The coronal FA maps (**a** and **e**); A shows a higher cortico-medullary differentiation than E. The ADC maps show similar signal intensity in the cortex and medulla (**b** and **f**). The color-coded FA maps allow the identification of the direction of diffusion (red: left-right; blue: head-foot; green: anterior-posterior) (**c** and **g**). The FA maps illustrate by texture (**d** and **h**). Figure taken with permission

between cortical and medullary ADC, termed delta-ADC, has been shown to decrease inter-individual variability and to better correlate with fibrosis in CKD [73]. In human kidneys, perfusion-induced water mobility has been reported to be much larger than the true water diffusivity [21]. Thus, IVIM imaging, which separates the true water diffusion from pseudo diffusion induced by vascular perfusion and tubular flow, has also been utilized to interrogate renal fibrosis. For example, in a study of 85 CKD patients who underwent renal biopsy, all of the IVIM parameters had a significant negative correlation with the histopathological fibrosis score [95].

The experience and promising results of DWI in kidney disease from prior studies have led to a number of ongoing multicenter clinical studies of DWI in CKD. The AFiRM (Application of Functional Renal MRI to Improve Assessment of Chronic Kidney Disease) will recruit 450 participants to investigate if multi-parametric renal MRI including DWI can characterize patients with and without CKD progression (NCT04238299). As new therapies are being developed to treat CKD, DWI is also being utilized for therapy response monitoring. The TOP-CKD (Trial of Pirfenidone to Prevent Progression in Chronic Kidney Disease) study is an ongoing clinical trial (NCT04258397) where DWI is used as a biomarker for monitoring renal fibrosis in 200 participants with CKD treated with Pirfenidone, an anti-fibrotic drug.

DWI has shown an overall outstanding potential in CKD, from early diagnosis of disease before renal functional decline to evaluation of the degree of tissue fibrosis and monitoring microstructure changes after treatment. To enable wider clinical adoption, standardizations of DWI acquisition and processing protocols, as well as large multi-center studies are necessary.

Kidney Transplant

Kidney transplantation is the most effective way to treat end stage renal disease. However, chronic allograft injury remains one of the biggest challenges in kidney transplantation, resulting in 20–30% of the allografts failing by 10 years [96]. While several etiologies lead to chronic allograft injury, similar to native kidney diseases, the final common pathway is interstitial fibrosis and tubular atrophy. Currently, biopsy remains the standard for assessing kidney allograft pathology, either via surveillance or indication biopsies. Improved monitoring and timely diagnosis of allograft injury are needed to improve long-term allograft survival.

Several studies have demonstrated the potential of DWI to detect allograft fibrosis. In a study including 118 patients with kidney allograft who had undergone allograft biopsy, delta ADC was highly correlated with interstitial fibrosis and eGFR [97]. In a separate study of 27 patients, ADC was shown to differentiate functioning kidney allografts from fibrotic ones [98]. In addition, cortical ADC had good performance at predicting an eGFR decline of ≥4 mL/min/1.73 m^2 per year at 18 months [98]. In another study of 103 patients with renal allograft and who underwent indication biopsies, ADC was negatively correlated with interstitial fibrosis and was able to differentiate patients with versus without 50% fibrosis with an area under the curve of 0.88 [99]. Another recent study also investigated IVIM imaging in kidney transplant and found that IVIM-derived parameters allowed the stratification of patients into categories in which kidney allograft biopsy results are or are not likely to change clinical management [98]. Thus, DWI may have a role in guiding clinical management of patients with kidney transplant by selecting those most likely to benefit from allograft biopsies.

Kidney Cancer

The incidence of renal tumors has risen significantly in the last 20 years, largely due to the increased utilization of imaging with incidental discovery of many localized tumors [100]. One unmet clinical need is to noninvasively and reliably distinguish benign tumors from renal cell carcinomas (RCCs) pre-operatively. Another unmet need is to noninvasively distinguish low grade indolent RCCs, which are amenable to active surveillance from high grade aggressive RCCs that require timely surgery or other definitive treatment.

DWI has been evaluated extensively in renal tumor characterization. In a meta-analysis including nine publications with 11 datasets encompassing 988 ADC measurements, DWI showed a relatively good diagnostic accuracy in differentiating malignant (RCCs and transitional cell carcinomas) from benign renal lesions (oncocytomas, angiomyolipomas, and cysts), with pooled weighted sensitivity and specificity of 88% and 72%, respectively [101]. Interestingly, the performance of ADC did not differ significantly in subgroup analysis including versus excluding renal cysts (Bosniak I-IIF cysts), despite the fact that cysts are known to demonstrate high ADC values. Also notably, a subgroup analysis found that studies, which excluded renal angiomyolipomas, had an obvious improvement in specificity from 63% to 84%, likely related to the observation that angiomyolipomas have restricted diffusion due to muscle and fat components [102]. IVIM has also been utilized for subtyping renal tumors. Perfusion fraction (f) and tissue diffusivity (D) derived from IVIM have been shown to differentiate among clear cell, papillary, chromophobe, and cystic RCCs, as well as benign entities like oncocytoma and angiomyolipoma [102–104]. A recent study also compared the performance of ADC and IVIM derived parameters in differentiating between malignant and benign renal tumors, and found tissue diffusivity (D) derived from IVIM is the best parameter for differentiating clear cell RCCs from benign renal tumors, and perfusion fraction (f) is the best parameter for differentiating non-clear cell RCCs from benign renal tumors(Figs. 18.14 and 18.15) [105].

Clear cell RCCs are the most common subtype of RCCs, and noninvasive differentiation between low and high grade clear cell RCCs can help guide the selection of patients who may benefit from active surveillance versus surgery. A meta-analysis including eight DWI studies with 397 clear cell RCCs showed moderate diagnostic performance of ADC for differentiating low from high grade tumors, with pooled sensitivity and specificity of 0.78 and 0.86, respectively [105]. Substantial heterogeneity was observed among the studies included in the analysis, mainly attributed to the threshold effects with regard to the ADC cutoff value used to determine high grade tumors [105].

Similar to the case of diffuse renal disease, DWI has shown substantial promise for noninvasive characterization of localized renal tumors, which in turn will help guide clinical management to match treatment to those most likely to benefit. Standardized protocols are necessary to better establish its performance and assess impact on patient outcomes.

DTI of the kidney in children: comparison between normal kidneys and those with ureteropelvic junction (UPJ) obstruction.

In a study by Serai et Al., 118 normal kidneys from 102 patients were compared to 22 kidneys from 16 patients with UPJ obstruction [25]. Mean FA values were significantly lower (0.31 ± 0.07; $n = 22$) in kidneys with UPJ obstruction than normal kidneys (0.40 ± 0.08; $n = 118$). The study suggests that DTI derived metrics are potential biomarkers to differentiate kidneys with UPJ obstruction and assess renal parenchymal damage.

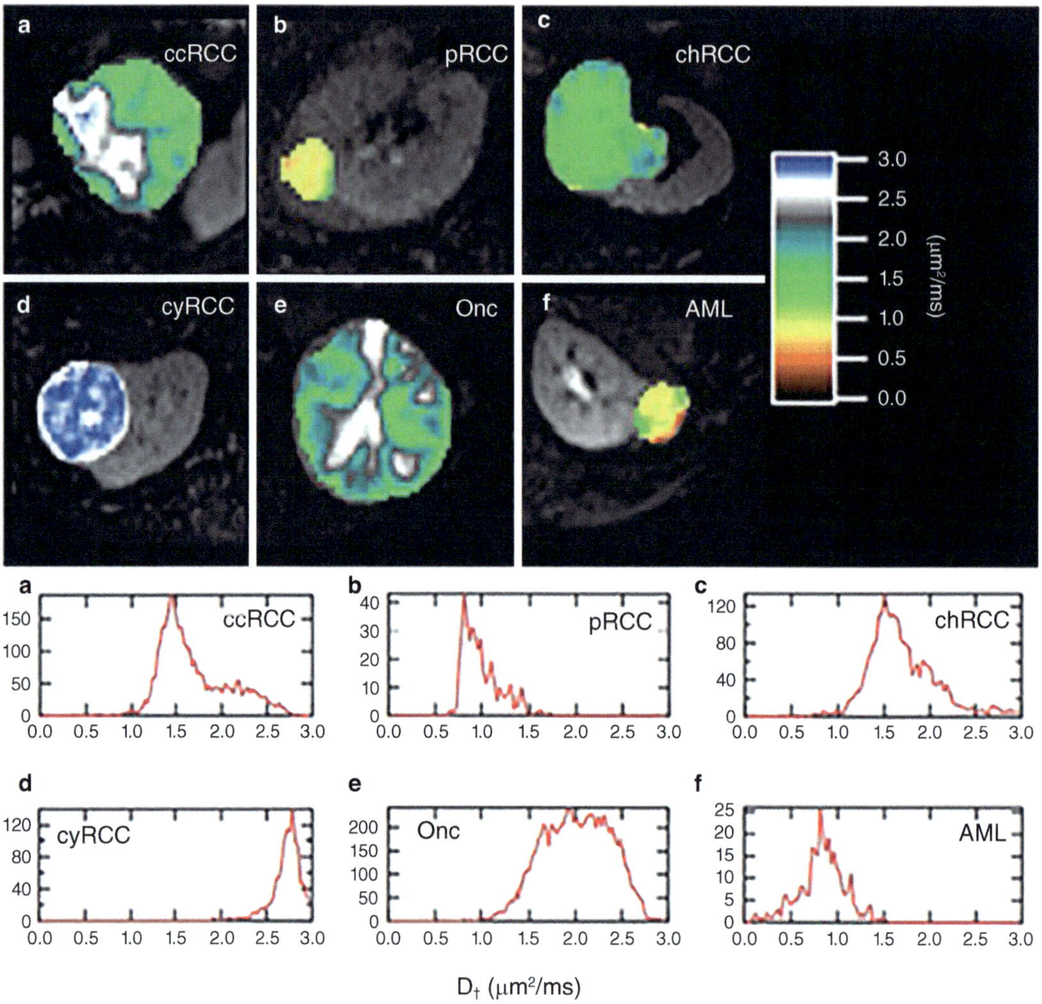

Fig. 18.14 D_t maps and corresponding voxel-wise histograms of six representative renal lesions. (**a**) ccRCC, (**b**) pRCC, (**c**) chRCC, (**d**) cyRCC, (**e**) Onc, and (**f**) AML. Although ccRCC, chRCC, and Onc have similar mean D_t values, their distribution around the means are different, reflecting varying skewness (Reproduced with permission)

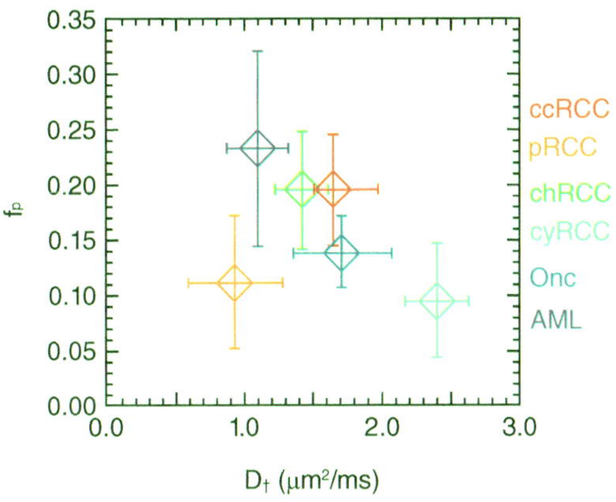

Fig. 18.15 Mean f_p values plotted against mean D_t values among six renal tumor subtypes. Data points represent mean values and error bars represent standard deviation (Reproduced with permission)

Summary

This chapter has summarized the current state of renal DWI and its most common variants, as well as highlighted the next generation of innovations in the pipeline. Recent consensus efforts by the community have also begun to migrate the growing but heterogeneous evidence base for renal DWI to the next level of translation, so that techniques and clinical data may soon be acquired sufficient to include renal DWI confidently in clinical trials of renal dysfunction (chronic kidney disease, etc.). The educational basis provided herein should help promote literacy of renal DWI within the renal community (physicists, radiologists, physiologists, and nephrologists) to further facilitate this migration.

References

1. Stejskal EO, Tanner JE. Spin diffusion measurements: spin echoes in the presence of a time-dependent field gradient. J Chem Phys. 1965;42(1):288–92.
2. Le Bihan D, Breton E, Lallemand D, Grenier P, Cabanis E, Laval-Jeantet M. MR imaging of intravoxel incoherent motions: application to diffusion and perfusion in neurologic disorders. Radiology. 1986;161(2):401–7.
3. Harada K, Fujita N, Sakurai K, Akai Y, Fujii K, Kozuka T. Diffusion imaging of the human brain: a new pulse sequence application for a 1.5-T standard MR system. AJNR Am J Neuroradiol. 1991;12(6):1143–8.
4. Sakuma H, Nomura Y, Takeda K, Tagami T, Nakagawa T, Tamagawa Y, et al. Adult and neonatal human brain: diffusional anisotropy and myelination with diffusion-weighted MR imaging. Radiology. 1991;180(1):229–33.
5. Bihan DL, lima M, Federau C, Sigmund EE. Intravoxel incoherent motion (IVIM) MRI: principles and applications. 1st ed. Jenny Stanford Publishing; 2018.
6. Englund EK, Reiter DA, Shahidi B, Sigmund EE. Intravoxel incoherent motion magnetic resonance imaging in skeletal muscle: review and future directions. J Magn Reson Imaging. 2022;55(4):988–1012.
7. Federau C. Intravoxel incoherent motion MRI as a means to measure in vivo perfusion: a review of the evidence. NMR Biomed. 2017;30(11):e3780.
8. Li YT, Cercueil J-P, Yuan J, Chen W, Loffroy R, Wáng YXJ. Liver intravoxel incoherent motion (IVIM) magnetic resonance imaging: a comprehensive review of published data on normal values and applications for fibrosis and tumor evaluation. Quant Imaging Med Surg. 2017;7(1):59–78.
9. Müller MF, Prasad PV, Edelman RR. Can the IVIM model be used for renal perfusion imaging? Eur J Radiol. 1998;26(3):297–303.
10. Thoeny HC, De Keyzer F. Diffusion-weighted MR imaging of native and transplanted kidneys. Radiology. 2011;259(1):25–38.
11. Zhang JL, Sigmund EE, Chandarana H, Rusinek H, Chen Q, Vivier P-H, et al. Variability of renal apparent diffusion coefficients: limitations of the monoexponential model for diffusion quantification. Radiology. 2010;254(3):783–92.
12. Ljimani A, Caroli A, Laustsen C, Francis S, Mendichovszky IA, Bane O, et al. Consensus-based technical recommendations for clinical translation of renal diffusion-weighted MRI. MAGMA. 2020;33(1):177–95.
13. Caroli A, Schneider M, Friedli I, Ljimani A, De Seigneux S, Boor P, et al. Diffusion-weighted magnetic resonance imaging to assess diffuse renal pathology: a systematic review and statement paper. Nephrol Dial Transplant. 2018;33(suppl_2):ii29–40.
14. Le Bihan D, Mangin JF, Poupon C, Clark CA, Pappata S, Molko N, et al. Diffusion tensor imaging: concepts and applications. J Magn Reson Imaging. 2001;13(4):534–46.
15. Basser PJ, Pierpaoli C. Microstructural and physiological features of tissues elucidated by quantitative-diffusion-tensor MRI. J Magn Reson B. 1996;111(3):209–19.
16. Froeling M, Nederveen AJ, Nicolay K, Strijkers GJ. DTI of human skeletal muscle: the effects of diffusion encoding parameters, signal-to-noise ratio

and T2 on tensor indices and fiber tracts. NMR Biomed. 2013;26(11):1339–52.
17. Jones DK. The effect of gradient sampling schemes on measures derived from diffusion tensor MRI: a Monte Carlo study. Magn Reson Med. 2004;51(4):807–15.
18. Jones DK, Horsfield MA, Simmons A. Optimal strategies for measuring diffusion in anisotropic systems by magnetic resonance imaging. Magn Reson Med. 1999;42(3):515–25.
19. Lanzman RS, Ljimani A, Pentang G, Zgoura P, Zenginli H, Kröpil P, et al. Kidney transplant: functional assessment with diffusion-tensor MR imaging at 3T. Radiology. 2013;266(1):218–25.
20. Gaudiano C, Clementi V, Busato F, Corcioni B, Orrei MG, Ferramosca E, et al. Diffusion tensor imaging and tractography of the kidneys: assessment of chronic parenchymal diseases. Eur Radiol. 2013;23(6):1678–85.
21. Sigmund EE, Vivier P-H, Sui D, Lamparello NA, Tantillo K, Mikheev A, et al. Intravoxel incoherent motion and diffusion-tensor imaging in renal tissue under hydration and furosemide flow challenges. Radiology. 2012;263(3):758–69.
22. Hueper K, Gutberlet M, Rodt T, Gwinner W, Lehner F, Wacker F, et al. Diffusion tensor imaging and tractography for assessment of renal allograft dysfunction-initial results. Eur Radiol. 2011;21(11):2427–33.
23. Notohamiprodjo M, Glaser C, Herrmann KA, Dietrich O, Attenberger UI, Reiser MF, et al. Diffusion tensor imaging of the kidney with parallel imaging: initial clinical experience. Investig Radiol. 2008;43(10):677–85.
24. Ries M, Jones RA, Basseau F, Moonen CT, Grenier N. Diffusion tensor MRI of the human kidney. J Magn Reson Imaging. 2001;14(1):42–9.
25. Otero HJ, Calle-Toro JS, Maya CL, Darge K, Serai SD. DTI of the kidney in children: comparison between normal kidneys and those with ureteropelvic junction (UPJ) obstruction. MAGMA. 2020;33(1):63–71.
26. Serai SD, Otero HJ, Calle-Toro JS, Berman JI, Darge K, Hartung EA. Diffusion tensor imaging of the kidney in healthy controls and in children and young adults with autosomal recessive polycystic kidney disease. Abdom Radiol (NY). 2019;44(5):1867–72.
27. Notohamiprodjo M, Chandarana H, Mikheev A, Rusinek H, Grinstead J, Feiweier T, et al. Combined intravoxel incoherent motion and diffusion tensor imaging of renal diffusion and flow anisotropy. Magn Reson Med. 2015;73(4):1526–32.
28. Liu AL, Mikheev A, Rusinek H, Huang WC, Wysock JS, Babb JS, et al. Renal flow and microstructure anisotropy (REFMAP) MRI in normal and peritumoral renal tissue. J Magn Reson Imaging. 2018;48(1):188–97.
29. Hilbert F, Bock M, Neubauer H, Veldhoen S, Wech T, Bley TA, et al. An intravoxel oriented flow model for diffusion-weighted imaging of the kidney. NMR Biomed. 2016;29(10):1403–13.
30. Phi van V, Reiner CS, Klarhoefer M, Ciritsis A, Eberhardt C, Wurnig MC, et al. Diffusion tensor imaging of the abdominal organs: influence of oriented intravoxel flow compartments. NMR Biomed. 2019;32(11):e4159.
31. Lanzman RS, Ljimani A, Müller-Lutz A, Weller J, Stabinska J, Antoch G, et al. Assessment of time-resolved renal diffusion parameters over the entire cardiac cycle. Magn Reson Imaging. 2019;55:1–6.
32. Ito K, Hayashida M, Kanki A, Yamamoto A, Tamada T, Yoshida K, et al. Alterations in apparent diffusion coefficient values of the kidney during the cardiac cycle: evaluation with ECG-triggered diffusion-weighted MR imaging. Magn Reson Imaging. 2018;52:1–8.
33. Wittsack H-J, Lanzman RS, Quentin M, Kuhlemann J, Klasen J, Pentang G, et al. Temporally resolved electrocardiogram-triggered diffusion-weighted imaging of the human kidney: correlation between intravoxel incoherent motion parameters and renal blood flow at different time points of the cardiac cycle. Investig Radiol. 2012;47(4):226–30.
34. Milani B, Ledoux J-B, Rotzinger DC, Kanemitsu M, Vallée J-P, Burnier M, et al. Image acquisition for intravoxel incoherent motion imaging of kidneys should be triggered at the instant of maximum blood velocity: evidence obtained with simulations and in vivo experiments. Magn Reson Med. 2019;81(1):583–93.
35. Heusch P, Wittsack H-J, Kröpil P, Blondin D, Quentin M, Klasen J, et al. Impact of blood flow on diffusion coefficients of the human kidney: a time-resolved ECG-triggered diffusion-tensor imaging (DTI) study at 3T. J Magn Reson Imaging. 2013;37(1):233–6.
36. Stabinska J, Ljimani A, Frenken M, Feiweier T, Lanzman RS, Wittsack H-J. Comparison of PGSE and STEAM DTI acquisitions with varying diffusion times for probing anisotropic structures in human kidneys. Magn Reson Med. 2020;84(3):1518–25.
37. van Baalen S, Leemans A, Dik P, Lilien MR, Ten Haken B, Froeling M. Intravoxel incoherent motion modeling in the kidneys: comparison of mono-, bi-, and triexponential fit. J Magn Reson Imaging. 2017;46(1):228–39.
38. Periquito JS, Gladytz T, Millward JM, Delgado PR, Cantow K, Grosenick D, et al. Continuous diffusion spectrum computation for diffusion-weighted magnetic resonance imaging of the kidney tubule system. Quant Imaging Med Surg. 2021;11(7):3098–119.
39. Stabinska J, Ljimani A, Zöllner HJ, Wilken E, Benkert T, Limberg J, et al. Spectral diffusion analysis of kidney intravoxel incoherent motion MRI in healthy volunteers and patients with renal pathologies. Magn Reson Med. 2021;85(6):3085–95.
40. Cho GY, Kim S, Jensen JH, Storey P, Sodickson DK, Sigmund EE. A versatile flow phantom for intravoxel incoherent motion MRI. Magn Reson Med. 2012;67(6):1710–20.

41. Maki JH, MacFall JR, Johnson GA. The use of gradient flow compensation to separate diffusion and microcirculatory flow in MRI. Magn Reson Med. 1991;17(1):95–107.
42. Schneider MJ, Gaass T, Ricke J, Dinkel J, Dietrich O. Assessment of intravoxel incoherent motion MRI with an artificial capillary network: analysis of biexponential and phase-distribution models. Magn Reson Med. 2019;82(4):1373–84.
43. Ahlgren A, Knutsson L, Wirestam R, Nilsson M, Ståhlberg F, Topgaard D, et al. Quantification of microcirculatory parameters by joint analysis of flow-compensated and non-flow-compensated intravoxel incoherent motion (IVIM) data. NMR Biomed. 2016;29(5):640–9.
44. Wu D, Zhang J. The effect of microcirculatory flow on oscillating gradient diffusion MRI and diffusion encoding with dual-frequency orthogonal gradients (DEFOG). Magn Reson Med. 2017;77(4):1583–92.
45. Wu D, Zhang J. Evidence of the diffusion time dependence of intravoxel incoherent motion in the brain. Magn Reson Med. 2019;82(6):2225–35.
46. Moulin K, Aliotta E, Ennis DB. Effect of flow-encoding strength on intravoxel incoherent motion in the liver. Magn Reson Med. 2019;81(3):1521–33.
47. Wetscherek A, Stieltjes B, Laun FB. Flow-compensated intravoxel incoherent motion diffusion imaging. Magn Reson Med. 2015;74(2):410–9.
48. Kuai Z-X, Liu W-Y, Zhang Y-L, Zhu Y-M. Generalization of intravoxel incoherent motion model by introducing the notion of continuous pseudodiffusion variable. Magn Reson Med. 2016;76(5):1594–603.
49. Jiang L, Sun T, Liao Y, Sun Y, Qian Z, Zhang Y, et al. Probing the ballistic microcirculation in placenta using flow-compensated and non-compensated intravoxel incoherent motion imaging. Magn Reson Med. 2021;85(1):404–12.
50. Spinner GR, Stoeck CT, Mathez L, von Deuster C, Federau C, Kozerke S. On probing intravoxel incoherent motion in the heart-spin-echo versus stimulated-echo DWI. Magn Reson Med. 2019;82(3):1150–63.
51. Sigmund EE, Mikheev A, Brinkmann IM, Gilani N, Babb JS, Basukala D, et al. Cardiac phase and flow compensation effects on renal flow and microstructure anisotropy MRI in healthy human kidney. J Magn Reson Imaging. 2022;58(1):221–2.
52. Partridge SC, Nissan N, Rahbar H, Kitsch AE, Sigmund EE. Diffusion-weighted breast MRI: clinical applications and emerging techniques. J Magn Reson Imaging. 2017;45(2):337–55.
53. Mansfield P. Real-time echo-planar imaging by NMR. Br Med Bull. 1984;40(2):187–90.
54. Borrelli P, Cavaliere C, Basso L, Soricelli A, Salvatore M, Aiello M. Diffusion tensor imaging of the kidney: design and evaluation of a reliable processing pipeline. Sci Rep. 2019;9(1):12789.
55. Coll-Font J, Afacan O, Hoge S, Garg H, Shashi K, Marami B, et al. Retrospective distortion and motion correction for free-breathing DW-MRI of the kidneys using dual-Echo EPI and slice-to-volume registration. J Magn Reson Imaging. 2021;53(5):1432–43.
56. Lim RP, Lim JC, Teruel JR, Botterill E, Seah J-M, Farquharson S, et al. Geometric distortion correction of renal diffusion tensor imaging using the reversed gradient method. J Comput Assist Tomogr. 2021;45(2):218–23.
57. Hilbert F, Wech T, Neubauer H, Veldhoen S, Bley TA, Köstler H. Comparison of turbo spin Echo and Echo planar imaging for intravoxel incoherent motion and diffusion tensor imaging of the kidney at 3Tesla. Z Med Phys. 2017;27(3):193–201.
58. Jin N, Deng J, Zhang L, Zhang Z, Lu G, Omary RA, et al. Targeted single-shot methods for diffusion-weighted imaging in the kidneys. J Magn Reson Imaging. 2011;33(6):1517–25.
59. Kenkel D, Barth BK, Piccirelli M, Filli L, Finkenstädt T, Reiner CS, et al. Simultaneous multislice diffusion-weighted imaging of the kidney: a systematic analysis of image quality. Investig Radiol. 2017;52(3):163–9.
60. Phi Van VD, Becker AS, Ciritsis A, Reiner CS, Boss A. Intravoxel incoherent motion analysis of abdominal organs: application of simultaneous multislice acquisition. Investig Radiol. 2018;53(3):179–85.
61. Taron J, Weiß J, Martirosian P, Seith F, Stemmer A, Bamberg F, et al. Clinical robustness of accelerated and optimized abdominal diffusion-weighted imaging. Investig Radiol. 2017;52(10):590–5.
62. Tavakoli A, Krammer J. Attenberger UiI, Budjan J, Stemmer a, nickel D, et al. simultaneous multislice diffusion-weighted imaging of the kidneys at 3 T. Investig Radiol. 2020;55(4):233–8.
63. Xu H, Zhang N, Yang D-W, Ren A, Ren H, Zhang Q, et al. Scan time reduction in Intravoxel incoherent motion diffusion-weighted imaging and diffusion kurtosis imaging of the abdominal organs: using a simultaneous multislice technique with different acceleration factors. J Comput Assist Tomogr. 2021;45(4):507–15.
64. Zhang G, Sun H, Qian T, An J, Shi B, Zhou H, et al. Diffusion-weighted imaging of the kidney: comparison between simultaneous multi-slice and integrated slice-by-slice shimming echo planar sequence. Clin Radiol. 2019;74(4):325.e1–8.
65. Tabari A, Machado-Rivas F, Kirsch JE, Nimkin K, Gee MS. Performance of simultaneous multi-slice accelerated diffusion-weighted imaging for assessing focal renal lesions in pediatric patients with tuberous sclerosis complex. Pediatr Radiol. 2021;51(1):77–85.
66. Blaimer M, Choli M, Jakob PM, Griswold MA, Breuer FA. Multiband phase-constrained parallel MRI. Magn Reson Med. 2013;69(4):974–80.
67. Duan F, Zhao T, He Y, Shu N. Test-retest reliability of diffusion measures in cerebral white matter: a multiband diffusion MRI study. J Magn Reson Imaging. 2015;42(4):1106–16.

68. Schmitter S, Adriany G, Waks M, Moeller S, Aristova M, Vali A, et al. Bilateral multiband 4D flow MRI of the carotid arteries at 7T. Magn Reson Med. 2020;84(4):1947–60.
69. Chan RW, Von Deuster C, Stoeck CT, Harmer J, Punwani S, Ramachandran N, et al. High-resolution diffusion tensor imaging of the human kidneys using a free-breathing, multi-slice, targeted field of view approach. NMR Biomed. 2014;27(11):1300–12.
70. Schneider JT, Kalayciyan R, Haas M, Herrmann SR, Ruhm W, Hennig J, et al. Inner-volume imaging in vivo using three-dimensional parallel spatially selective excitation. Magn Reson Med. 2013;69(5):1367–78.
71. Xie Y, Li Y, Wen J, Li X, Zhang Z, Li J, et al. Functional evaluation of transplanted kidneys with reduced field-of-view diffusion-weighted imaging at 3T. Korean J Radiol. 2018;19(2):201–8.
72. Wu W, Miller KL. Image formation in diffusion MRI: a review of recent technical developments. J Magn Reson Imaging. 2017;46(3):646–62.
73. Friedli I, Crowe LA, de Perrot T, Berchtold L, Martin P-Y, de Seigneux S, et al. Comparison of readout-segmented and conventional single-shot for echo-planar diffusion-weighted imaging in the assessment of kidney interstitial fibrosis. J Magn Reson Imaging. 2017;46(6):1631–40.
74. Wu C-J, Wang Q, Zhang J, Wang X-N, Liu X-S, Zhang Y-D, et al. Readout-segmented echo-planar imaging in diffusion-weighted imaging of the kidney: comparison with single-shot echo-planar imaging in image quality. Abdom Radiol (NY). 2016;41(1):100–8.
75. Notohamiprodjo M, Dietrich O, Horger W, Horng A, Helck AD, Herrmann KA, et al. Diffusion tensor imaging (DTI) of the kidney at 3 tesla-feasibility, protocol evaluation and comparison to 1.5 tesla. Investig Radiol. 2010;45(5):245–54.
76. Hernando D, Zhang Y, Pirasteh A. Quantitative diffusion MRI of the abdomen and pelvis. Med Phys. 2022;49(4):2774–93.
77. Binser T, Thoeny HC, Eisenberger U, Stemmer A, Boesch C, Vermathen P. Comparison of physiological triggering schemes for diffusion-weighted magnetic resonance imaging in kidneys. J Magn Reson Imaging. 2010;31(5):1144–50.
78. Kataoka M, Kido A, Yamamoto A, Nakamoto Y, Koyama T, Isoda H, et al. Diffusion tensor imaging of kidneys with respiratory triggering: optimization of parameters to demonstrate anisotropic structures on fraction anisotropy maps. J Magn Reson Imaging. 2009;29(3):736–44.
79. Li Q, Wu X, Qiu L, Zhang P, Zhang M, Yan F. Diffusion-weighted MRI in the assessment of split renal function: comparison of navigator-triggered prospective acquisition correction and breath-hold acquisition. AJR Am J Roentgenol. 2013;200(1):113–9.
80. Liu Y, Zhong X, Czito BG, Palta M, Bashir MR, Dale BM, et al. Four-dimensional diffusion-weighted MR imaging (4D-DWI): a feasibility study. Med Phys. 2017 Feb;44(2):397–406.
81. Kurugol S, Marami B, Afacan O, Warfield SK, Gholipour A. Motion-robust spatially constrained parameter estimation in renal diffusion-weighted MRI by 3D motion tracking and correction of sequential slices. Mol Imaging Reconstr Anal Mov Body Organs Stroke Imaging Treat. 2017;10555:75–85.
82. Marami B, Scherrer B, Afacan O, Erem B, Warfield SK, Gholipour A. Motion-robust diffusion-weighted brain MRI reconstruction through slice-level registration-based motion tracking. IEEE Trans Med Imaging. 2016;35(10):2258–69.
83. Guyader J-M, Bernardin L, Douglas NHM, Poot DHJ, Niessen WJ, Klein S. Influence of image registration on apparent diffusion coefficient images computed from free-breathing diffusion MR images of the abdomen. J Magn Reson Imaging. 2015;42(2):315–30.
84. Mazaheri Y, Do RKG, Shukla-Dave A, Deasy JO, Lu Y, Akin O. Motion correction of multi-b-value diffusion-weighted imaging in the liver. Acad Radiol. 2012;19(12):1573–80.
85. Huizinga W, Poot DHJ, Guyader JM, Klaassen R, Coolen BF, van Kranenburg M, et al. PCA-based groupwise image registration for quantitative MRI. Med Image Anal. 2016;29:65–78.
86. Kurugol S, Freiman M, Afacan O, Domachevsky L, Perez-Rossello JM, Callahan MJ, et al. Motion-robust parameter estimation in abdominal diffusion-weighted MRI by simultaneous image registration and model estimation. Med Image Anal. 2017;39:124–32.
87. Andersson JLR, Skare S, Ashburner J. How to correct susceptibility distortions in spin-echo echo-planar images: application to diffusion tensor imaging. NeuroImage. 2003;20(2):870–88.
88. Afacan O, Hoge WS, Wallace TE, Gholipour A, Kurugol S, Warfield SK. Simultaneous motion and distortion correction using dual-Echo diffusion-weighted MRI. J Neuroimaging. 2020;30(3):276–85.
89. Levey AS, Coresh J. Chronic kidney disease. Lancet. 2012;379(9811):165–80.
90. Liu H, Zhou Z, Li X, Li C, Wang R, Zhang Y, et al. Diffusion-weighted imaging for staging chronic kidney disease: a meta-analysis. Br J Radiol. 2018;91(1091):20170952.
91. Liu Z, Xu Y, Zhang J, Zhen J, Wang R, Cai S, et al. Chronic kidney disease: pathological and functional assessment with diffusion tensor imaging at 3T MR. Eur Radiol. 2015;25(3):652–60.
92. Inoue T, Kozawa E, Okada H, Inukai K, Watanabe S, Kikuta T, et al. Noninvasive evaluation of kidney hypoxia and fibrosis using magnetic resonance imaging. J Am Soc Nephrol. 2011;22(8):1429–34.

93. Zhao J, Wang ZJ, Liu M, Zhu J, Zhang X, Zhang T, et al. Assessment of renal fibrosis in chronic kidney disease using diffusion-weighted MRI. Clin Radiol. 2014;69(11):1117–22.
94. Xu X, Palmer SL, Lin X, Li W, Chen K, Yan F, et al. Diffusion-weighted imaging and pathology of chronic kidney disease: initial study. Abdom Radiol (NY). 2018;43(7):1749–55.
95. Mao W, Zhou J, Zeng M, Ding Y, Qu L, Chen C, et al. Intravoxel incoherent motion diffusion-weighted imaging for the assessment of renal fibrosis of chronic kidney disease: a preliminary study. Magn Reson Imaging. 2018;47:118–24.
96. Stegall MD, Gaston RS, Cosio FG, Matas A. Through a glass darkly: seeking clarity in preventing late kidney transplant failure. J Am Soc Nephrol. 2015;26(1):20–9.
97. Berchtold L, Friedli I, Crowe LA, Martinez C, Moll S, Hadaya K, et al. Validation of the corticomedullary difference in magnetic resonance imaging-derived apparent diffusion coefficient for kidney fibrosis detection: a cross-sectional study. Nephrol Dial Transplant. 2019;35:937.
98. Bane O, Hectors SJ, Gordic S, Kennedy P, Wagner M, Weiss A, et al. Multiparametric magnetic resonance imaging shows promising results to assess renal transplant dysfunction with fibrosis. Kidney Int. 2020;97(2):414–20.
99. Wang W, Yu Y, Wen J, Zhang M, Chen J, Cheng D, et al. Combination of functional magnetic resonance imaging and histopathologic analysis to evaluate interstitial fibrosis in kidney allografts. Clin J Am Soc Nephrol. 2019;14(9):1372–80.
100. Hollingsworth JM, Miller DC, Daignault S, Hollenbeck BK. Rising incidence of small renal masses: a need to reassess treatment effect. J Natl Cancer Inst. 2006;98(18):1331–4.
101. Zhang H, Gan Q, Wu Y, Liu R, Liu X, Huang Z, et al. Diagnostic performance of diffusion-weighted magnetic resonance imaging in differentiating human renal lesions (benignity or malignancy): a meta-analysis. Abdom Radiol (NY). 2016;41(10):1997–2010.
102. Tanaka H, Yoshida S, Fujii Y, Ishii C, Tanaka H, Koga F, et al. Diffusion-weighted magnetic resonance imaging in the differentiation of angiomyolipoma with minimal fat from clear cell renal cell carcinoma. Int J Urol. 2011;18(10):727–30.
103. Chandarana H, Kang SK, Wong S, Rusinek H, Zhang JL, Arizono S, et al. Diffusion-weighted intravoxel incoherent motion imaging of renal tumors with histopathologic correlation. Investig Radiol. 2012;47(12):688–96.
104. Gaing B, Sigmund EE, Huang WC, Babb JS, Parikh NS, Stoffel D, et al. Subtype differentiation of renal tumors using voxel-based histogram analysis of intravoxel incoherent motion parameters. Investig Radiol. 2015;50(3):144–52.
105. Woo S, Suh CH, Kim SY, Cho JY, Kim SH. Diagnostic performance of DWI for differentiating high- from low-grade clear cell renal cell carcinoma: a systematic review and meta-analysis. AJR Am J Roentgenol. 2017;12:W1–8.

Arterial Spin Labeled MRI for Quantitative Non-Contrast Perfusion Measurement of the Kidneys

19

Ananth J. Madhuranthakam and Maria A. Fernandez-Seara

Abbreviations

AKI	Acute kidney injury
ASL	Arterial spin labeling
BGS	Background suppression
bSSFP	Balanced steady state free precession
CASL	Continuous arterial spin labeling
CKD	Chronic kidney disease
DCE	Dynamic contrast-enhanced
DSC	Dynamic susceptibility contrast
FAIR	Flow alternating inversion recovery
FOCI	Frequency offset corrected inversion
FSE	Fast spin echo
GraSE	Gradient and spin echo
GRE	Gradient echo
MRI	Magnetic resonance imaging
NSF	Nephrogenic systemic fibrosis
PASL	Pulsed arterial spin labeling
pCASL	Pseudo continuous arterial spin labeling
PET	Positron emission tomography
PLD	Post-label delay
RCC	Renal cell carcinoma
SE-EPI	Spin-echo echo-planar imaging
SNR	Signal to noise ratio
SPECT	Single photon emission computed tomography
SShTSE	Single-shot turbo spin echo
TSE	Turbo spin echo

A. J. Madhuranthakam (✉)
Department of Radiology, UT Southwestern Medical Center, Dallas, TX, USA
e-mail: Ananth.Madhuranthakam@UTSouthwestern.edu

M. A. Fernandez-Seara
Radiology Department, Clínica Universidad de Navarra, University of Navarra, Pamplona, Spain
e-mail: mfseara@unav.es

Introduction

Perfusion is the delivery of oxygen and nutrients to the tissue and helps with the removal of carbon-dioxide and waste products. Perfusion is well regulated in a normal physiological state, but alterations to perfusion can lead to pathology. Decreased or lack of perfusion can be observed in conditions such as stroke [1] or myocardial infarction [2], while elevated perfusion can be observed in the tumors due to angiogenesis [3]. In kidneys, decreased perfusion can be observed in acute kidney injury (AKI) or chronic kidney disease (CKD) [4], and increased perfusion can be observed in renal cell carcinoma (RCC) [5]. Measuring perfusion can be beneficial for longitudinal monitoring and for the assessment of therapy response.

Noninvasive perfusion measurement can be performed with different imaging modalities including: (1) positron emission tomography (PET) using ^{15}O-labeled water [6]; (2) single photon emission computed tomography (SPECT) using ^{99m}Tc [7]; (3) computed tomography using

S. D. Serai, K. Darge (eds.), *Advanced Clinical MRI of the Kidney*,
https://doi.org/10.1007/978-3-031-40169-5_19

iodinated contrast agent [8]; and (4) magnetic resonance imaging (MRI) either using gadolinium contrast agent [9] or non-contrast perfusion using arterial spin labeled (ASL) MRI [10]. Among all these methods, ASL-MRI is the one imaging modality that can be performed without the administration of exogenous contrast agent. Furthermore, ASL-MRI provides the assessment of perfusion in quantitative physiological units of milliliters per 100 grams of tissue per minute (mL/100 g/min), and can facilitate intrasubject and inter-subject comparisons.

ASL-MRI was originally developed for the measurement of brain perfusion [11, 12]. Since its introduction in the early 1990s, there have been several technical innovations to improve the robustness and reliability of ASL-MRI. Over the past two decades, the advancements in preparation and data acquisition have enabled ASL-MRI to become one of the mainstream methods for the measurement of brain perfusion [13]. Some of these developments have been translated and further refined to enable kidney perfusion measurement. The ability to measure perfusion without the administration of exogenous contrast agent is very appealing for kidney imaging since many kidney diseases result in compromised renal function and could be contraindicated for exogenous contrast agent.

This chapter is divided into three main components. In part 1 of this chapter, the principles of ASL-MRI and acquisition protocols are reviewed. In part 2, the post-processing and data analysis methods are reviewed. Finally, in part 3, some of the clinical applications of ASL-MRI to measure kidney perfusion are presented.

Part 1: MRI Physics and Acquisition Protocols

ASL-MRI uses highly permeable water as a tracer by magnetically labeling the water protons in the arterial blood and measuring their accumulation in the tissue of interest. Various versions of ASL-MRI have been validated in animals using microspheres, and in humans using the gold standard PET with ^{15}O-labeled water in the brain [14]. Compared to dynamic contrast-enhanced (DCE) or dynamic susceptibility contrast (DSC) perfusion measurements, ASL has several advantages. Specifically, ASL does not require the administration of an exogenous contrast agent, thus alleviating the concerns of gadolinium accumulation in the brain [15] or nephrogenic systemic fibrosis (NSF) in patients with impaired renal function [16]. Unlike DCE/DSC, the contribution of vascular permeability to ASL measured perfusion is negligible [17], enabling absolute perfusion quantification in physiological units of mL/100 g/min.

ASL-MRI consists of three distinct steps to achieve absolute quantification of tissue perfusion [18] (Fig. 19.1). First is the acquisition of two images: a labeled image and a control image. In the labeled image, only the inflowing blood is selectively inverted while the static tissue is maintained at its full magnetization. In the control image, the inflowing blood and the static tissue are maintained at their full magnetization. The second step is to generate the perfusion-weighted image by subtracting the labeled image from the control image. Since the inflowing blood is inverted in the labeled image, the signal intensity of the blood is lower in the labeled image than in the control image, while the signal intensity of the static tissue remains the same between the two images. The third step is the generation of the perfusion quantification from the perfusion-weighted image, using the corresponding proton-density (M0) image with the same acquisition parameters to account for tissue characteristics. This generates a quantitative perfusion map in physiological units of mL/100 g/min.

The ASL-MRI pulse sequence generally consists of three different steps (Fig. 19.2): labeling, post-label delay (PLD), and data acquisition. First, the inflowing blood is selectively inverted upstream of the imaging region of interest in the labeling period. Second, this labeled blood is allowed to accumulate in the imaging region during the PLD. Third, images are subsequently acquired that capture the labeled blood and the static tissue in the imaging region. This entire

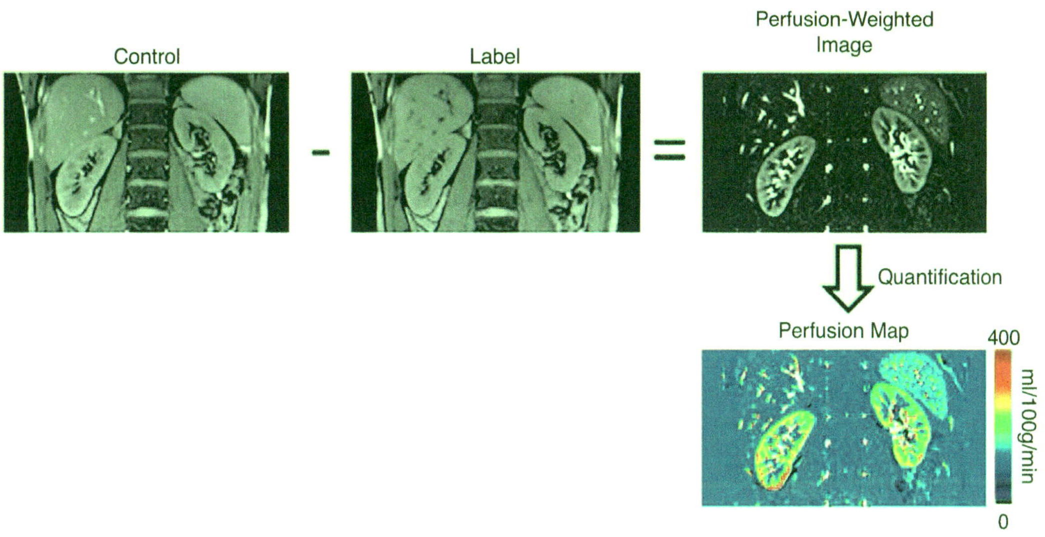

Fig. 19.1 Schematic of the steps involved in acquiring kidney ASL perfusion images. The acquisition includes a control image, where the magnetization is maintained at its equilibrium, and a labeled image, where the inflowing blood is selectively inverted. The subtraction of the labeled image from the control image generates the perfusion-weighted image. Using a separately acquired proton-density image and the perfusion quantification model, absolute perfusion maps in physiological units of mL/100 g/min can be generated (Reproduced with permission from Wolters Kluwer Health Inc. from ref. [18])

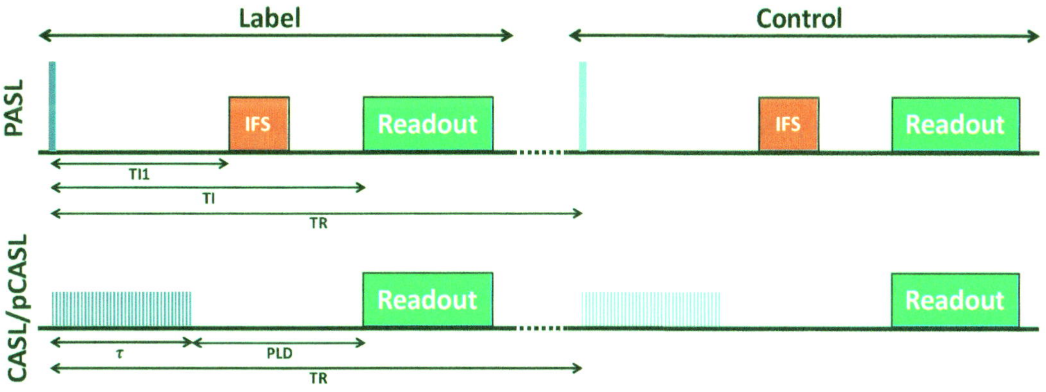

Fig. 19.2 Schematic of ASL pulse sequence timing diagram for PASL (top) and CASL/pCASL (bottom), depicting both label (left) and control (right) conditions. Labeling pulses are shown in blue and the green blocks represent the readout. The red block represents the inflow saturation (IFS) to define the bolus temporal width for PASL. TR is the repetition time. PASL variables include inversion time (TI) and bolus duration (TI1) and CASL/pCASL variables include label duration (τ) and post-label delay (PLD)

process is repeated for the control image, without inverting the inflowing blood. During the PLD, the inverted blood in the labeled image starts recovering towards its full magnetization and hence its signal will be lower than the signal of the control image, depending upon the labeling duration and PLD.

Labeling Schemes

There are broadly two different labeling schemes that have been predominantly used for kidney imaging: pulsed arterial spin labeling (PASL), which is based on a single inversion pulse applied for a short duration to label the blood, and continuous arterial spin labeling (CASL), which uses one or more pulses for a longer duration to label the blood.

Pulsed Arterial Spin Labeling

The most commonly used and well-established PASL method for kidney imaging is based on flow alternating inversion recovery (FAIR) [19]. This approach uses a selective inversion pulse applied across the imaging slice for the control image, and a non-selective inversion pulse for the labeled image (Fig. 19.3). With this approach, the imaging slice is inverted in both the control and the labeled image and maintains the same intensity between the two images. However, the inflowing blood from outside of the selective inversion slab is only inverted in the labeled image due to non-selective inversion. Hence, the difference between the control and the labeled image provides the perfusion-weighted image. The inversion is often accomplished using adiabatic hyperbolic secant (HS) pulses, which are robust to B1 inhomogeneities, or frequency offset corrected inversion (FOCI) pulses, which are more robust to both B1 and B0 inhomogeneities [20].

Pseudo Continuous Arterial Spin Labeling (pCASL)

Continuous labeling is achieved using a constant radiofrequency (RF) pulse along with a selective gradient for longer durations to invert the inflowing blood upstream of the imaging region of interest. The original ASL was demonstrated using CASL in the brain [12], immediately followed by its application in the kidneys [10]. Since CASL enables inverting the inflowing blood for longer durations, it has better signal to noise ratio (SNR) compared to PASL [21]. However, it is challenging to apply the continuous RF pulses for prolonged durations on commercially available whole-body MR scanners since these scanners are designed for the execution of pulsed RF waveforms. This challenge has been overcome by the introduction of pCASL, which replaces the continuous RF waveform by a train of pulsed RF waveforms [22]. The train of RF pulses that are typically applied axially across the descending aorta for the labeled image, in combination with the gradients, selectively invert the inflowing blood (Fig. 19.4). The RF pulses are phase-cycled for the control image such that the inflowing blood is not inverted, but the magnetization transfer (MT) effects due to the RF pulses in the imaging slice are maintained between the control and the labeled image (Fig. 19.5). The application of pulsed RF waves with pCASL enables labeling for prolonged durations on the order of seconds on commercial whole-body MR scanners.

Acquisition Methods

Various methods have been used to acquire the ASL kidney images, independent of the labeling strategies. These include spin-echo echo-planar imaging (SE-EPI), fast or turbo spin echo (FSE/

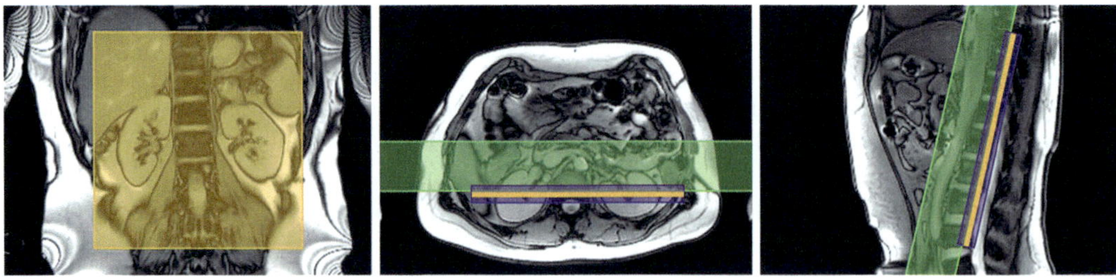

Fig. 19.3 Labeling scheme with FAIR shown on anatomical images in the coronal (left), axial (middle), and sagittal (right) orientations. The imaging slice in the coronal orientation is shown in orange, while the FAIR selective inversion slab is shown in purple. The green box over the abdominal aorta represents the inflow saturation slab used for QUIPSS II or Q2TIPS (Reproduced from the open access article, ref. [30], under the creative commons license (http://creativecommons.org/licenses/by/4.0/))

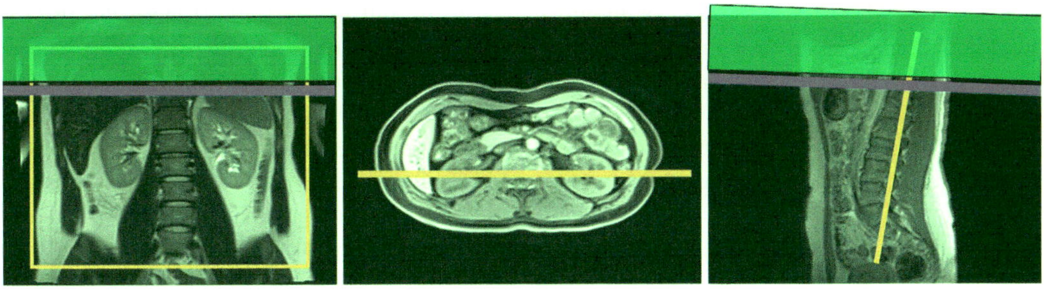

Fig. 19.4 Labeling scheme with pCASL shown on anatomical images in the coronal (left), axial (middle), and sagittal (right) orientations. The imaging slice in the coronal orientation is shown in orange, while the pCASL selective inversion slab is shown in purple. The green box shows the inflow saturation slab (Reproduced from the open access article, ref. [30], with some modifications under the creative commons license (http://creativecommons.org/licenses/by/4.0/))

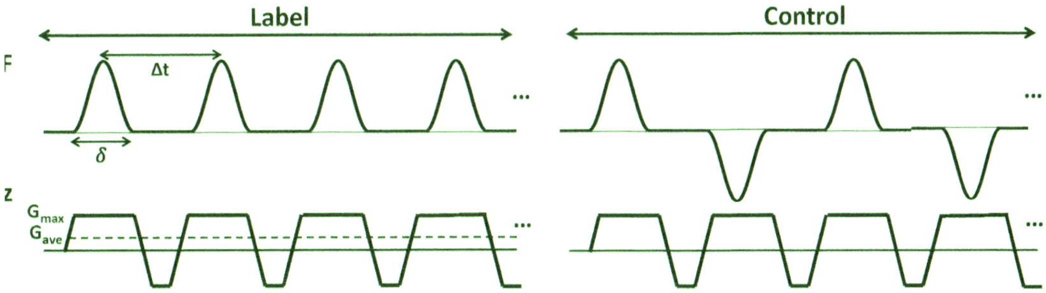

Fig. 19.5 Schematic of the pCASL pulse sequence showing the successive radiofrequency (RF) pulses on the top along with the slice selection gradient (Gz) on the bottom for the label (left) and control (right) schemes. δ—RF pulse duration, Δt—RF pulse spacing, G_{max}—amplitude of the slice selection gradient, and G_{ave}—net average gradient

TSE), gradient echo (GRE), balanced steady state free precession (bSSFP), and the combined gradient and spin echo (GraSE) imaging. Kidney ASL images have been predominantly acquired as a single-slice 2D image; however, multi-slice 2D images as well as 3D images have also been successfully demonstrated.

2D Acquisitions

The primary methods for the majority of 2D acquisitions have been using either SE-EPI [23] or single-shot TSE (SShTSE) [24], which due to their fast acquisition can be often performed in less than a second. In addition, the use of a single excitation pulse to acquire the entire slice is particularly important due to its compatibility with background suppression (BGS), described in more detail below. Furthermore, SE-EPI and SShTSE acquisitions allow an increased number of signal averages (NSAs) to be acquired in relatively shorter scan times. This is significant since ASL images are low in SNR and require multiple NSAs to achieve good image quality. While both SE-EPI and SShTSE acquisitions have been successfully demonstrated, each approach has advantages and disadvantages. For example, SE-EPI images are more prone to B0 inhomogeneities and suffer from geometric distortions, which can significantly affect the image quality. Hence, 2D SE-EPI images are often acquired with parallel imaging or partial Fourier to shorten the readout durations, which improves the image quality. SShTSE images are more robust to B0 inhomogeneities due to the multiple refocusing pulses, but these images often suffer from increased image blurring due to longer readout durations. Although parallel imaging methods such as SENSE, GRAPPA, or Compressed Sense

(CS) can be used to shorten the readout durations for SShTSE, they are not recommended for ASL images since parallel imaging further reduces the SNR. Nevertheless, SE-EPI and SShTSE acquisition methods can also be extended to multiple 2D slices [25], albeit at slightly longer scan times and particularly so with SShTSE since each slice needs to be acquired with multiple NSAs. Kidney 2D ASL images have also been demonstrated using bSSFP [26], although to a lesser extent.

3D Acquisitions

There are several advantages of acquiring kidney ASL images using a 3D acquisition compared to 2D acquisition. (1) 3D acquisitions allow volumetric coverage that can be used to image the entire kidneys. (2) The increased number of slices with 3D acquisition can be used instead of the higher number of signal averages with 2D acquisition, which allows volumetric coverage with similar SNR in the same acquisition time. (3) The volumetric excitation makes the 3D acquisition readily amenable to the BGS pulses, enabling uniform BGS throughout the volume.

These advantages are the driving force for the research community to adopt 3D acquisitions for volumetric kidney ASL. However, there are several challenges in achieving good image quality with 3D acquisition. To date, the majority of 3D acquisitions for kidney ASL use either 3D rapid acquisition with relaxation enhancement (RARE) [27, 28], also known as FSE/TSE, or 3D GraSE [29]. This is currently an active area of research focused on improving the robustness of volumetric kidney ASL images. Further developments and optimizations are needed before the routine use of 3D acquisitions for volumetric kidney ASL images can be realized [30].

Post-Label Delay (PLD)

The ASL pulse sequence consists of a PLD in pCASL or inversion time (TI) in FAIR to allow the labeled blood from the upstream to accumulate in the tissue of interest (Fig. 19.2). During this PLD, the inverted blood also partially recovers to its full magnetization. Thus, the PLD is chosen such that it is long enough for the labeled blood to flow into the tissue of interest but also short enough such that the blood is not completely recovered to its full magnetization. For kidney imaging, the PLD often ranges from 1.2 to 2.0 s depending upon the labeling strategy (i.e., FAIR vs. pCASL) and the magnetic field strength. This is because the longitudinal relaxation time of the blood ($T1_{blood}$) is longer at 3 T (1.65 s) compared to 1.5 T (1.48 s) [31], and hence longer PLDs are often used at 3 T. During this PLD, two important functionalities need to be incorporated for successful quantitative kidney ASL images: background suppression and inflow saturation.

Background Suppression (BGS)

ASL is a subtraction technique, and hence, it is imperative to maintain the signal intensities between the control and labeled images as close as possible, except for the differences in the labeled blood. Additionally, the contribution of labeled blood in a given voxel amounts to only 2–5% of the background signal. Hence, any additional difference between the control and labeled images leads to substantial artifacts on the subtracted perfusion-weighted images. This problem is accentuated in the kidney ASL images due to respiratory motion combined with the increased propensity of B0 inhomogeneities in the body. A major solution to address this challenge uses BGS, which can be accomplished using pairs of inversion pulses. It is well-known that a single inversion pulse can be used to null the signal from a given tissue based on its T1 relaxation time. For example, short tau inversion recovery (STIR) uses shorter inversion times (e.g., 150–200 ms) to null the fat signal, while fluid attenuated inversion recovery (FLAIR) uses longer inversion times (e.g., 2200 ms) to null the signal from the cerebrospinal fluid (CSF). Similarly, the application of 4–5 inversion pulses with optimal inversion times can achieve signal suppression from tissues across a wide range of T1 relaxation times [32]. Based on this principle, the signal intensities of the static tissue between the control and the labeled images can be sufficiently suppressed using pairs of inversion pulses. Typically, 4 BGS pulses with either HS or FOCI are applied during the PLD to achieve optimal suppression (Fig. 19.6). While this substantially reduces the signal intensities of the static tissues across a wide range of T1s, it also necessitates the use of complex subtraction between the control and the labeled images to produce the blood signal difference. The complex subtraction is not always readily feasible when SE-EPI or GraSE readouts are used due to the additional phase corrections required during reconstruction. In such instances, either 2 BGS pulses or 4 BGS pulses, with suboptimal inversion times, are used such that the background signal is considerably reduced. At the same time, the control and the labeled blood signals are maintained on the positive magnetization, allowing magnitude subtraction. The application of BGS pulses substantially improves the image quality and is highly recommended for kidney ASL images (Fig. 19.7) [24, 33].

Inflow Saturation

In addition to the labeled blood that flows into the tissue of interest, fresh blood continues to flow after the labeling has ended. Since the transit time of this fresh blood is relatively short, it often ends up in the major vessels and does not lead to perfusion signal during the data acquisition. In an ideal scenario, this fresh blood signal should be identical between the control and labeled images, and hence subtracted in the final perfusion-weighted image. However, due to variations in the cardiac cycle and the transit delays, this fresh blood signal is not always subtracted and leads to signal in the major vessels in the perfusion-weighted images. Hence, inflow saturation pulses are applied upstream to the imaging region of interest during PLD to suppress this fresh blood signal. These inflow saturation pulses can be interleaved with the BGS pulses.

In addition to suppressing the fresh blood signal, the inflow saturation pulses also serve the purpose of defining the bolus width with pulsed

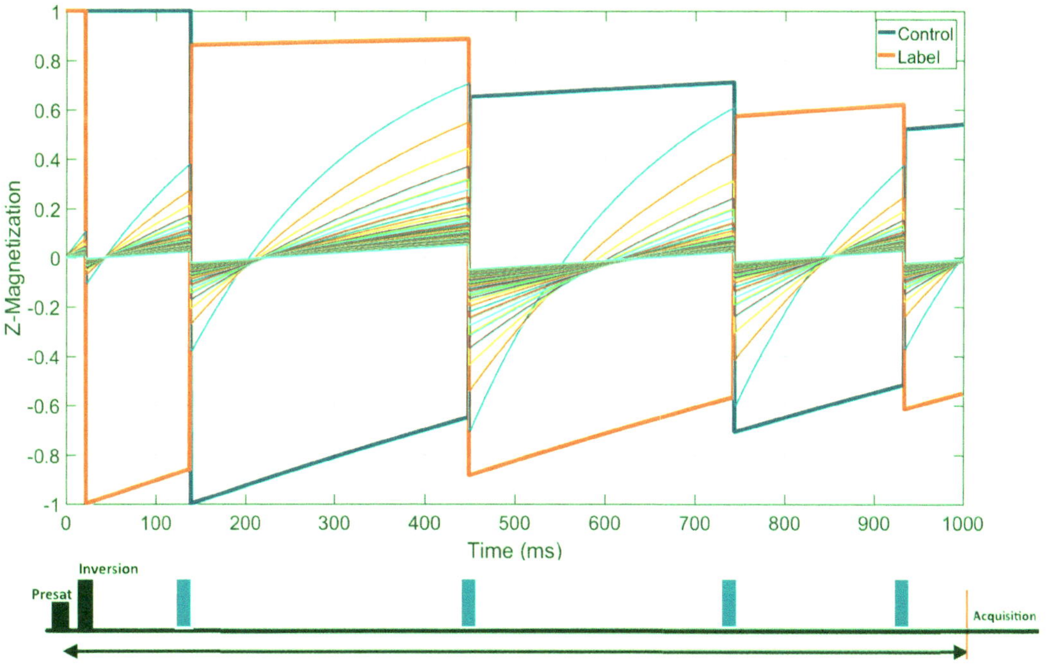

Fig. 19.6 Demonstration of background suppression using four non-selective inversion pulses (blue) applied during the post-label delay. The solid red line represents the blood signal in the labeled image, while the solid blue line represents the blood signal in the control image. The static tissues within the imaging slice with a broad range of T1 (e.g., 200–4200 ms) experience different relaxations and will be close to zero at the time of acquisition, while the blood signal maintains the difference between the control and labeled images

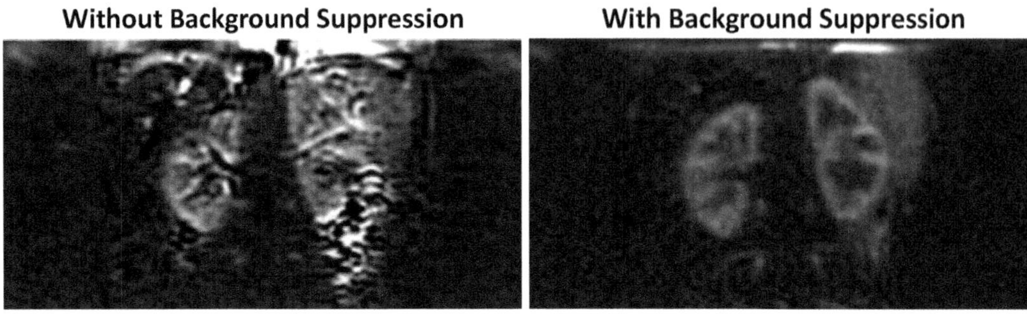

Fig. 19.7 Significance of background suppression (BGS) to minimize artifacts in kidney ASL images. The additional signal differences between control and labeled images due to systemic errors including respiratory motion and B0 inhomogeneities contribute to artifacts (left), which are substantially reduced with BGS (right) (Reproduced from ref. [24] with permission from John Wiley & Sons with some modifications)

labeling such as FAIR. Unlike pCASL, which selectively labels the blood and defines the bolus at the end of the labeling duration, the labeled bolus is not defined with FAIR due to the non-selective inversion pulse. Thus, the inflow saturation pulses applied during the PLD using schemes such as QUIPPS II saturation or Q2-TIPS [34] define the cut-off time, and the blood that has flown before this cut-off time is considered the labeled bolus. This is particularly important to perform quantitative perfusion measurements [35].

ASL Acquisition Protocol

This section describes the practical considerations and the parameters required to successfully acquire kidney ASL images. This includes patient preparation, hardware considerations, parameters for both FAIR and pCASL labeling schemes, readout parameters for commonly used acquisition methods, and other sequence considerations.

Patient Preparation

It is well-recognized that the hydration status of the subjects affects kidney perfusion. Several studies have shown that the kidney ASL perfusion varies significantly when subjects were challenged with water loading as well as protein loading, adenosine, and furosemide [36, 37]. Measuring hydration status, however, is challenging, and there are no universally accepted reference standards. Hence, it is desirable to scan subjects in their normal hydration status when appropriate.

Hardware Considerations

The commonly used MR scanners at both 1.5 T and 3 T can be used for kidney ASL imaging. Imaging at 3 T is advantageous for ASL, since it provides higher SNR combined with longer T1 relaxation times of the labeled blood and the kidney tissue. However, susceptibility-induced B0 inhomogeneities are more pronounced at 3 T and this may lead to image distortions and signal loss. In addition, the greater specific absorption rate (SAR) at 3 T may pose limits on slice coverage or longer acquisition times. Nevertheless, successful kidney ASL images using both FAIR and pCASL have been shown at both 1.5 T and 3 T field strengths [24, 27]. For signal transmission, the integrated body coil can be used and the abdominal phased-array coil, combined with the spine coil that may often be embedded in the patient table, can be used for signal reception.

FAIR Labeling Parameters

The RF pulses used for selective inversion should have sharp inversion profile edges, and adiabatic FOCI pulses can achieve this with increased robustness to both B0 and B1 inhomogeneities. The selective inversion slab needs to be centered on the imaging slice and should be carefully positioned to exclude the feeding arteries (i.e., descending aorta for kidney ASL). This ensures that the inflowing blood is inverted only in the labeled image and not in the control image, and maximizes the signal difference between the control and labeled images to yield high perfusion signal (Fig. 19.3). The thickness of the selective inversion slab typically should be 10–20 mm larger than the imaging slab thickness. This avoids a mismatch between the locations of the selective inversion slab and the imaging slab, which could occur due to motion between the labeling and the signal readout. However, when prescribing this additional thickness, extra precaution needs to be taken such that the selective inversion slab does not include the descending aorta. An inversion time (TI) of 1.8–2.0 s provides sufficient time for the labeled blood to reach the kidneys at 3 T; a slightly lower TI of 1.5–1.8 s can be used at 1.5 T due to the shorter T1 of blood at 1.5 T. The temporal width of the labeled bolus can be defined using QUIPSS II or Q2TIPS saturation pulses applied approximately 1.0–1.2 s after the inversion pulse. This defines the bolus duration (or TI1) and allows sufficient labeled blood to enter the kidneys before the tail of the bolus is saturated.

pCASL Labeling Parameters

There are two different versions of pCASL that have been reported in the literature: balanced pCASL and unbalanced pCASL. Both versions have been successfully used to acquire kidney ASL images. However, unbalanced pCASL has demonstrated greater robustness to B0 inhomogeneities [38] and is particularly recommended for kidney ASL due to the proximity of the labeling plane to the lungs [39] (Fig. 19.4). Although the following parameters are not typically available to the end-user, the recommended pCASL labeling parameters include (Fig. 19.5): RF pulse duration (δ) = 0.5 ms; RF pulse gap (Δt) = 1.0–1.5 ms; average gradient (G_{ave}) = 0.4–0.6 mT/m; ratio of maximum to average gradients (G_{max}/G_{ave}) = 7; and the average RF pulse amplitude = 1.6 μT over time. These values maximize the labeling efficiency in the descending aorta even in the presence of pulsatile blood flow. The pCASL labeling plane should be positioned approximately perpendicular to the descending aorta, above the highest kidney to prevent direct saturation, while also avoiding the heart. If constrained by the subject's size and anatomy, it is often recommended to place the labeling plane below the lungs to minimize B0 inhomogeneities. A labeling duration of 1.5–1.8 s and a PLD of 1.2–1.5 s allow all labeled blood to arrive at the renal parenchyma before image acquisition in most subjects. In some patient cohorts, where the transit time could be abnormally long (e.g., in renal artery stenosis), a longer PLD can be used, albeit at the expense of reduced SNR due to T1 decay.

Readout Parameters

While both 2D and 3D acquisitions can be used for kidney ASL images, the majority of research and clinical applications to date have been primarily based on single-slice 2D acquisitions. The readout parameters for the commonly used single-slice 2D acquisitions based on SE-EPI and single-shot turbo spin echo (SShTSE) are included here. Images can be generally acquired in coronal oblique slices, along the major axis of the kidneys. This is particularly necessary for FAIR to avoid labeling of the inflowing blood in the descending aorta. This orientation also has the advantage of containing the most kidney movement due to the respiratory cycle within the imaging plane, such that registration algorithms can be used during post-processing. Typical readout parameters for both SE-EPI and SShTSE include: FOV = 240–300 mm along the foot-head (F/H) and 300–360 mm along the right-left (R/L); slice thickness = 4–8 mm; in-plane resolution = 2–4 mm; TE = shortest possible using partial Fourier; acceleration factors = not more than 2 to minimize SNR loss; TR (including labeling and readout) = 5–6 s; number of signal averages (NSAs) = 16–20 pairs of label and control; and total scan time = 3–4 min. Fat suppression is recommended for SE-EPI and can also be beneficial for SShTSE readouts. Readers are referred to refs. [27, 40] for 3D RARE and to ref. [29] for 3D GraSE readout parameters.

Other Sequence Considerations

To minimize systemic errors caused by imperfect inversion profiles and residual magnetization between repetitions, pre-saturation of the imaging slab is recommended at the beginning of the sequence before labeling for both FAIR and pCASL. This also helps to reduce the background signal in combination with BGS pulses, which can be achieved by the use of two or four carefully timed non-selective inversion pulses. The timings of these BGS pulses depend upon the labeling duration and the PLD [41, 42]. The inflow saturation pulses (typically three to four) are applied above the kidneys after TI1 with FAIR and during the last 1.0 s of the PLD with pCASL. Since the acquisition occurs over several minutes, respiratory triggering or guided breathing is recommended for data acquisition and breath-hold is not recommended. If using respiratory triggering, care must be taken such that the data are acquired during the end-expiration, which can occur after 2–3 s from the initial trigger. The alternative strategy includes guided-breathing, where the subjects are instructed to breathe during the labeling and PLD (2–3 s) and to hold their breath at end-expiration during the data acquisition (<1 s) [24]. Finally, a proton-density weighted (M0) image should be acquired using exactly the same readout parameters but without any labeling, BGS, or inflow saturation pulses to facilitate perfusion quantification.

Part 2: Post-Processing and Data Analysis Methods

Data Processing

After the data are acquired, perfusion-weighted images are generated by subtracting the control and labeled images. Prior to this step, some retrospective processing methods can be employed to improve image quality. The standard operation includes voxel-wise signal averaging of the multiple control-label measurements with both FAIR and pCASL. This addresses the inherently low SNR of ASL images and also provides a degree of motion robustness when the images are acquired using respiratory-triggering or guided-breathing approaches. Additional steps can be taken to reduce the effects of motion. These include removing or providing low weights for outlier measurements that are often mis-aligned with the majority of the images due to kidney motion, retrospective sorting of kidney ASL images using data from external sensors such as respiratory bellows, and using motion correction techniques based on image registration or the combination of both [43]. These post-processing steps help to reduce image artifacts, reduce partial volume effects between cortex and medulla, and improve the SNR of the perfusion-weighted signal and the repeatability of perfusion measurements. When using rigid/affine transformations for motion correction, each kidney should be processed separately since they move independently [44]. Finally, these methods should be used to not only align ASL control and labeled images but also the corresponding M0 images required for perfusion quantification.

Perfusion Quantification

The next step in processing ASL images is to convert the perfusion-weighted images into quantitative perfusion values in physiological units of mL/100 g/min. Accurate quantification enables comparison of perfusion values across scans, subjects, MR scanners, and even with non-MRI blood flow measurements. Furthermore, quantification also removes sensitivity to technical and physiologic factors that are not directly related to perfusion. The perfusion quantification can be performed with a single compartment model that neglects MRI signal relaxation differences between blood and tissue and uses only the corresponding M0 image. This approach provides tissue perfusion, also commonly referred to as renal blood flow (RBF), at each image voxel using the following equations [30]:

$$\mathrm{RBF}_{\mathrm{FAIR}} = \frac{\Delta M}{M_0} \cdot \frac{6000 \cdot \lambda}{2 \cdot \alpha \cdot \mathrm{TI1}} \cdot \exp\left(\mathrm{TI} / \mathrm{T1}_{\mathrm{blood}}\right) \tag{19.1}$$

$$\mathrm{RBF}_{\mathrm{pCASL}} = \frac{\Delta M}{M_0} \cdot \frac{6000 \cdot \lambda}{2 \cdot \alpha \cdot \mathrm{T1}_{\mathrm{blood}}} \cdot \frac{\exp\left(\frac{\mathrm{PLD}}{\mathrm{T1}_{\mathrm{blood}}}\right)}{(1 - \exp\left(-\frac{\tau}{\mathrm{T1}_{\mathrm{blood}}}\right))} \tag{19.2}$$

The FAIR-specific variables include inversion time (TI) and bolus duration defined by the first inflow saturation pulse (TI1), while the pCASL-specific variables include label duration (τ) and PLD. Other variables that are common to both methods include blood-tissue partition coefficient (λ) = 0.9 mL/g; labeling efficiency (α) = 0.95 for FAIR without BGS, 0.85 for pCASL without BGS, and α should be multiplied by an additional factor of 0.93 for each BGS inversion pulse; ΔM is the measured perfusion difference signal between label and control and M0 is the measured proton-density signal using same readout parameters without any preparation pulses. For the single-compartment model, the longitudinal relaxation time of blood ($\mathrm{T1}_{\mathrm{blood}}$) of 1.65 s at 3 T and 1.48 s at 1.5 T is assumed for all tissues, removing the necessity of accurately measuring the T1 of the tissues. The units of mL/g/s are typically converted to the customary physiological literature units of mL/100 g/min by multiplying with a factor of 6000. These variables can be used for a single-slice 2D and 3D acquisitions. For 2D multi-slice imaging, the values of TI (for FAIR) and PLD (for pCASL) should be adjusted for each slice due to the time delay between slice acquisitions.

Data Analysis

From the quantitative RBF maps, renal perfusion values can be calculated on a voxel basis. However, it is generally recommended to use region of interest (ROI) analysis to estimate the average perfusion values in the renal cortex and medulla. The measurement of perfusion in the renal cortex is more reliable due to its high blood flow combined with minimal artifacts, since the renal cortex is located far from the collecting system and major arteries. The ROIs should be drawn manually on an anatomic image such as an M0 image or a spatially co-registered higher resolution image. (Semi-) automated methods can be used to segment the cortex and medulla; however, there are no known robust methods available at this time. Recent studies have explored the use of machine learning algorithms for automated segmentation of the cortex and medulla, but these require further validation [45]. The ROIs should be adjusted to avoid hyperintense signals on the perfusion images since they are more likely to represent the vessels.

Several studies have shown that a lower cortical thickness is associated with reduced renal function as measured by estimated glomerular filtration rate (eGFR) [46]. The reduction in cortical thickness can be severe enough in some advanced diseases that it approaches the typical dimensions of the ASL image voxel size. This significantly reduces the number of pure renal cortex voxels and may underestimate the perfusion in the renal cortex due to partial volume mixing of the lower perfusion signal in the renal medulla. In such instances where cortical thinning is evident, the interpretation of perfusion values in the renal cortex should be performed with caution.

The medullary perfusion can also be measured from the RBF maps; however, this measure is less reliable because of its lower perfusion (and hence lower signal) and its proximity to the renal cortex, which makes it susceptible to partial volume contamination [47]. Furthermore, the kinetics of labeled water are also uncertain since the arterial water is divided between filtrate and smaller arterioles. This labeled water may also exchange with the surrounding tissue before penetrating deep into the medulla. In spite of these limitations, a carefully selected ROI that includes the medulla combined with optimized acquisitions using increased NSAs can potentially provide an estimate of the medullary perfusion, when it is of research or clinical interest.

For data analysis and reporting of renal perfusion values, it is recommended to use the mean and standard deviation of cortical RBF values at the subject level and at the group level. In the presence of skewed RBF distributions, the inclusion of median values will also be helpful. Furthermore, the analysis should be performed separately for the right and left kidneys.

Part 3: Clinical Applications

In the kidneys, there is a complex interaction between renal perfusion, renal oxygen delivery, renal oxygen consumption, and glomerular filtration [48]. The kidneys are unique since the majority of the oxygen consumption (>80%) is used to power tubular sodium reabsorption. Hence, the oxygen consumption in the kidneys and thus the RBF varies with the glomerular filtration rate (GFR). All of the blood that flows to the kidneys passes through the glomeruli in the renal cortex of both kidneys. This accounts for approximately 25% of the cardiac output at rest, which is about 1200 mL/min or 400 mL/100 g/min in a 70 kg adult with a 300 g kidney. The renal medullary circulation arises from the subpopulation of glomeruli at the corticomedullary junction and involves only about 10% of the RBF. Thus, the renal circulation comprises two independent cortical and medullary circulations. It is becoming increasingly evident that the renal tissue ischemia and the associated hypoxia are critical factors in the initiation and progression of both AKI and CKD, irrespective of the underlying etiology [49]. Hence, the measurement of RBF using ASL-MRI allows a noninvasive means to understand the physiological regulation of renal perfusion and the role of its dysregulation in kidney disease and injury. Furthermore, the ASL-MRI has the advantage of measuring the RBF at the individual kidney level as well as at the regional level without the need for exogenous contrast injection.

Renal ASL has been applied in a variety of kidney diseases including CKD, AKI, diabetes, hypertension, lupus nephritis, and renovascular disease [50]. All of the studies have consistently shown that the RBF in the renal cortex is reduced in CKD compared to healthy volunteers [51] (Fig. 19.8). Furthermore, the RBF decreases with increasing stages of CKD and correlates to eGFR. Renal ASL is also well-suited for the assessment of renal transplants, since 28% of the transplants from deceased donors and 15% from living donors undergo chronic rejection within

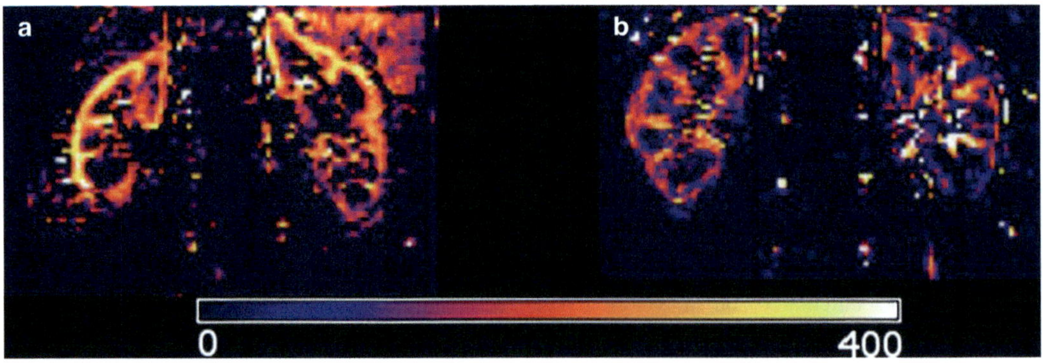

Fig. 19.8 ASL-MRI measured renal blood flow (RBF) maps show decreased perfusion in a diabetic patient (**b**) compared to a healthy volunteer (**a**). The colorbar represents RBF values in mL/100 g/min (Reproduced from ref. [51] with permission from John Wiley & Sons)

5 years after transplantation. Percutaneous biopsy is often used to monitor renal transplants; however, it is invasive and provides information from only a small sample that may not be representative of the entire transplant function. Renal ASL along with other functional MRI parameters including blood oxygenation level-dependent (BOLD), diffusion-weighted imaging (DWI), and MR elastography (MRE) can provide regional assessment of the entire renal transplant. Studies have shown that RBF measured by ASL-MRI in the renal cortex differs between patients with early and delayed graft function and correlates with allograft function [52] (Fig. 19.9). ASL-MRI has also been used to determine filtration fraction that could potentially be employed as a biomarker of renal functional reserve in potential living kidney donors [53].

ASL-MRI can also be used to estimate perfusion in renal masses. In patients with CKD, this could potentially obviate the need for exogenous contrast injection. When measured by ASL-MRI, perfusion has been shown to correlate with micro-vessel density in clear cell RCC [54], validating the use of ASL-MRI to measure perfusion in renal tumors (Fig. 19.10). ASL-MRI has also been demonstrated to differentiate tumor types in primary RCC [5] and to assess therapy response in metastatic RCC [55]. Many RCC patients may also have compromised kidney function and are contraindicated for gadolinium-based contrast agents, and hence, ASL would be an ideal choice for non-contrast perfusion measurement. The increasing role of anti-angiogenic therapies in patients with advanced malignancies has highlighted the need to develop prognostic and predictive imaging biomarkers based on the mechanistic effects of these drugs (i.e., changes in tumor vascularity). Studies have illustrated the potential to assess tumor response based on ASL-measured tumor perfusion: generally, the response to anti-angiogenic drugs is associated with a decrease in tumor vascularity. Furthermore, high pre-treatment tumor vascularity measured at baseline may be predictive of response to these therapies.

Renal ASL-MRI has great potential in clinical applications; however, the repeatability and reproducibility of the technique should be carefully evaluated to increase confidence in its objective measurements [56]. ASL perfusion phantoms with highly reproducible measurements over long periods [57] and across multiple sites [58], and standardization of the acquisition and data processing methods could potentially enable the translation of ASL as an imaging biomarker into clinical settings. As a first step towards standardization, a group of 23 interna-

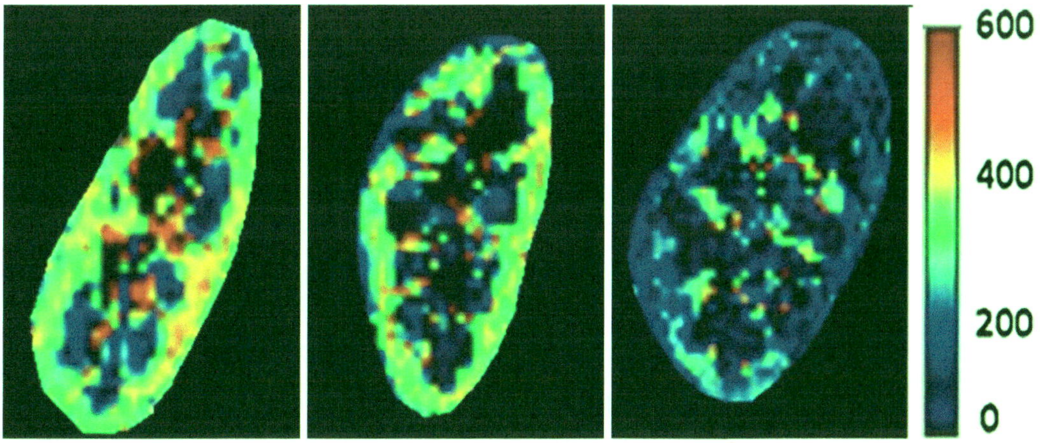

Fig. 19.9 ASL-MRI measured renal blood flow (RBF) maps in a healthy volunteer (left) compared to renal transplant patients with stable allograft function (middle) and impaired allograft function (right). Perfusion values appear to be low in the allograft with impaired function. The colorbar represents RBF values in mL/100 g/min (Reproduced from ref. [52] with permission from Elsevier with some minor modifications)

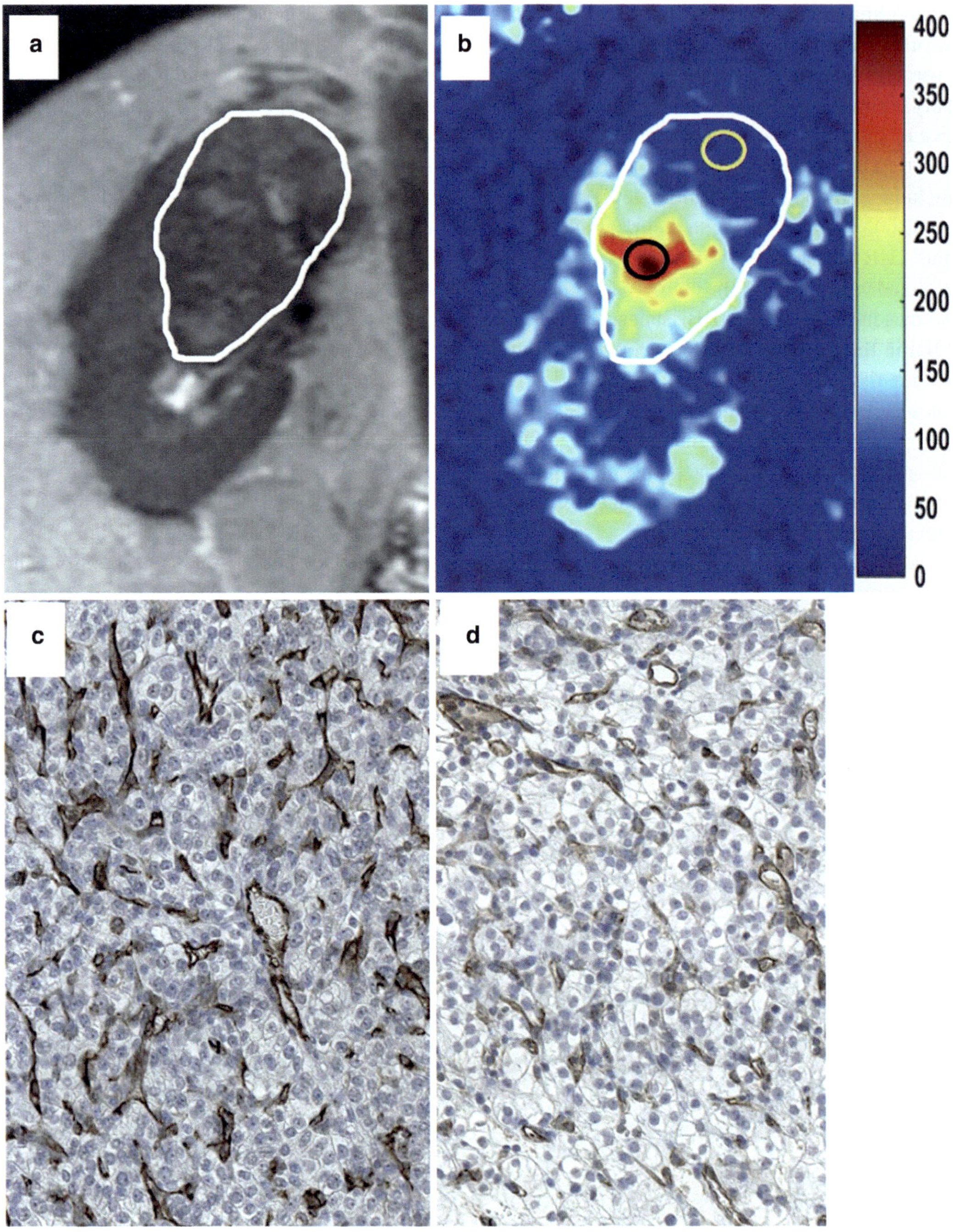

Fig. 19.10 ASL-MRI shows high perfusion in clear cell renal cell carcinoma. Coronal T2-weighted image (**a**) shows a relatively homogeneous mass (white circle) isointense to the renal parenchyma, while ASL measured perfusion map (**b**) shows heterogeneous vascularity in the mass. Black and yellow circles on (**b**) denote regions of interest in high and low perfusion areas and the corresponding photographs of CD31 immunochemistry slides show high (**c**) and low (**d**) microvessel density. The colorbar represents perfusion values in mL/100 g/min (Reproduced from ref. [54] with permission from Elsevier with some minor modifications)

tional clinical and non-clinical experts in the field have developed guidelines for data acquisition, processing, and analysis [30], which were summarized in parts 1 and 2 of this chapter. These guidelines will pave the way for the use of ASL in clinical trials and ultimately clinical practice.

Conclusion

In conclusion, ASL-MRI has gone through several technical innovations and has become almost a mainstream method to measure renal perfusion. The advantages of ASL-MRI include the capability to measure renal perfusion in physiological units of mL/100 g/min without the need for exogenous contrast agent. This enables repeated measurements and longitudinal assessment that can be readily incorporated into clinical settings.

References

1. Ma H, Campbell BCV, Parsons MW, Churilov L, Levi CR, Hsu C, et al. Thrombolysis guided by perfusion imaging up to 9 hours after onset of stroke. N Engl J Med. 2019;380(19):1795–803.
2. Greenwood JP, Maredia N, Younger JF, Brown JM, Nixon J, Everett CC, et al. Cardiovascular magnetic resonance and single-photon emission computed tomography for diagnosis of coronary heart disease (CE-MARC): a prospective trial. Lancet. 2012;379(9814):453–60.
3. Folkman J. Tumor angiogenesis: therapeutic implications. N Engl J Med. 1971;285(21):1182–6.
4. Breidthardt T, Cox EF, Squire I, Odudu A, Omar NF, Eldehni MT, et al. The pathophysiology of the chronic cardiorenal syndrome: a magnetic resonance imaging study. Eur Radiol. 2015;25(6):1684–91.
5. Lanzman RS, Robson PM, Sun MR, Patel AD, Mentore K, Wagner AA, et al. Arterial spin-labeling MR imaging of renal masses: correlation with histopathologic findings. Radiology. 2012;265(3):799–808.
6. Wong CY, Thie J, Gaskill M, Ponto R, Hill J, Tian HY, et al. A statistical investigation of normal regional intra-subject heterogeneity of brain metabolism and perfusion by F-18 FDG and O-15 H2O PET imaging. BMC Nucl Med. 2006;6:4.
7. Berman DS, Kiat H, Maddahi J. The new 99mTc myocardial perfusion imaging agents: 99mTc-sestamibi and 99mTc-teboroxime. Circulation. 1991;84(3 Suppl):I7–21.
8. Kambadakone AR, Sahani DV. Body perfusion CT: technique, clinical applications, and advances. Radiol Clin N Am. 2009;47(1):161–78.
9. Sourbron SP, Michaely HJ, Reiser MF, Schoenberg SO. MRI-measurement of perfusion and glomerular filtration in the human kidney with a separable compartment model. Investig Radiol. 2008;43(1):40–8.
10. Roberts DA, Detre JA, Bolinger L, Insko EK, Lenkinski RE, Pentecost MJ, et al. Renal perfusion in humans: MR imaging with spin tagging of arterial water. Radiology. 1995;196(1):281–6.
11. Detre JA, Leigh JS, Williams DS, Koretsky AP. Perfusion imaging. Magn Reson Med. 1992;23(1):37–45.
12. Williams DS, Detre JA, Leigh JS, Koretsky AP. Magnetic resonance imaging of perfusion using spin inversion of arterial water. Proc Natl Acad Sci U S A. 1992;89(1):212–6.
13. Alsop DC, Detre JA, Golay X, Günther M, Hendrikse J, Hernandez-Garcia L, et al. Recommended implementation of arterial spin-labeled perfusion MRI for clinical applications: a consensus of the ISMRM perfusion study group and the European consortium for ASL in dementia. Magn Reson Med. 2015;73(1):102–16.
14. Ye FQ, Berman KF, Ellmore T, Esposito G, van Horn JD, Yang Y, et al. H(2)(15)O PET validation of steady-state arterial spin tagging cerebral blood flow measurements in humans. Magn Reson Med. 2000;44(3):450–6.
15. McDonald RJ, McDonald JS, Kallmes DF, Jentoft ME, Murray DL, Thielen KR, et al. Intracranial gadolinium deposition after contrast-enhanced MR imaging. Radiology. 2015;150025:772.
16. Saleh L, Juneman E, Movahed MR. The use of gadolinium in patients with contrast allergy or renal failure requiring coronary angiography, coronary intervention, or vascular procedure. Catheter Cardiovasc Interv. 2011;78(5):747–54.
17. Wolf RL, Wang J, Wang S, Melhem ER, O'Rourke DM, Judy KD, et al. Grading of CNS neoplasms using continuous arterial spin labeled perfusion MR imaging at 3 tesla. J Magn Reson imaging: JMRI. 2005;22(4):475–82.
18. Madhuranthakam AJ, Yuan Q, Pedrosa I. Quantitative methods in abdominal MRI: perfusion imaging. Top Magn Reson Imaging. 2017;26(6):251–8.
19. Kim SG, Tsekos NV. Perfusion imaging by a flow-sensitive alternating inversion recovery (FAIR) technique: application to functional brain imaging. Magn Reson Med. 1997;37(3):425–35.
20. Wang X, Greer JS, Dimitrov IE, Pezeshk P, Chhabra A, Madhuranthakam AJ. Frequency offset corrected inversion pulse for B0 and B1 insensitive fat suppression at 3T: application to MR Neurography of brachial plexus. J Magn Reson Imaging. 2018;48(4):1104–11.
21. Wang J, Zhang Y, Wolf RL, Roc AC, Alsop DC, Detre JA. Amplitude-modulated continuous arterial spin-labeling 3.0-T perfusion MR imaging

with a single coil: feasibility study. Radiology. 2005;235(1):218–28.
22. Dai W, Garcia D, de Bazelaire C, Alsop DC. Continuous flow-driven inversion for arterial spin labeling using pulsed radio frequency and gradient fields. Magn Reson Med. 2008;60(6):1488–97.
23. Gardener AG, Francis ST. Multislice perfusion of the kidneys using parallel imaging: image acquisition and analysis strategies. Magn Reson Med. 2010;63(6):1627–36.
24. Robson PM, Madhuranthakam AJ, Dai W, Pedrosa I, Rofsky NM, Alsop DC. Strategies for reducing respiratory motion artifacts in renal perfusion imaging with arterial spin labeling. Magn Reson Med. 2009;61(6):1374–87.
25. Buchanan CE, Cox EF, Francis ST. Evaluation of 2D imaging schemes for pulsed arterial spin labeling of the human kidney cortex. Diagnostics (Basel). 2018;8(3)
26. Martirosian P, Klose U, Mader I, Schick F. FAIR true-FISP perfusion imaging of the kidneys. Magn Reson Med. 2004;51(2):353–61.
27. Greer JS, Wang X, Wang Y, Pinho MC, Maldjian JA, Pedrosa I, et al. Robust pCASL perfusion imaging using a 3D Cartesian acquisition with spiral profile reordering (CASPR). Magn Reson Med. 2019;82(5):1713–24.
28. Robson PM, Madhuranthakam AJ, Smith MP, Sun MR, Dai W, Rofsky NM, et al. Volumetric arterial spin-labeled perfusion imaging of the kidneys with a three-dimensional fast spin Echo Acquisition. Acad Radiol. 2016;23(2):144–54.
29. Nery F, De Vita E, Clark CA, Gordon I, Thomas DL. Robust kidney perfusion mapping in pediatric chronic kidney disease using single-shot 3D-GRASE ASL with optimized retrospective motion correction. Magn Reson Med. 2019;81(5):2972–84.
30. Nery F, Buchanan CE, Harteveld AA, Odudu A, Bane O, Cox EF, et al. Consensus-based technical recommendations for clinical translation of renal ASL MRI. MAGMA. 2020;33(1):141–61.
31. Zhang X, Petersen ET, Ghariq E, De Vis JB, Webb AG, Teeuwisse WM, et al. In vivo blood T(1) measurements at 1.5 T, 3 T, and 7 T. Magn Reson Med. 2013;70(4):1082–6.
32. Dixon WT, Sardashti M, Castillo M, Stomp GP. Multiple inversion recovery reduces static tissue signal in angiograms. Magn Reson Med. 1991;18(2):257–68.
33. Taso M, Guidon A, Alsop DC. Influence of background suppression and retrospective realignment on free-breathing renal perfusion measurement using pseudo-continuous ASL. Magn Reson Med. 2019;81(4):2439–49.
34. Luh WM, Wong EC, Bandettini PA, Hyde JS. QUIPSS II with thin-slice TI1 periodic saturation: a method for improving accuracy of quantitative perfusion imaging using pulsed arterial spin labeling. Magn Reson Med. 1999;41(6):1246–54.
35. Song R, Loeffler RB, Hillenbrand CM. Improved renal perfusion measurement with a dual navigator-gated Q2TIPS fair technique. Magn Reson Med. 2010;64(5):1352–9.
36. Shirvani S, Tokarczuk P, Statton B, Quinlan M, Berry A, Tomlinson J, et al. Motion-corrected multiparametric renal arterial spin labelling at 3 T: reproducibility and effect of vasodilator challenge. Eur Radiol. 2019;29(1):232–40.
37. Wang J, Zhang Y, Yang X, Wang X, Zhang J, Fang J, et al. Hemodynamic effects of furosemide on renal perfusion as evaluated by ASL-MRI. Acad Radiol. 2012;19(10):1194–200.
38. Zhao L, Vidorreta M, Soman S, Detre JA, Alsop DC. Improving the robustness of pseudo-continuous arterial spin labeling to off-resonance and pulsatile flow velocity. Magn Reson Med. 2017;78(4):1342–51.
39. Zhou L, Wang Y, Madhuranthakam AJ, editors. Improving the robustness of pseudo-continuous arterial spin labeling for renal perfusion imaging. Proceedings of the 29th Annual Meeting of ISMRM; 2021; Virtual.
40. Taso M, Zhao L, Guidon A, Litwiller DV, Alsop DC. Volumetric abdominal perfusion measurement using a pseudo-randomly sampled 3D fast-spin-echo (FSE) arterial spin labeling (ASL) sequence and compressed sensing reconstruction. Magn Reson Med. 2019;82(2):680–92.
41. Garcia DM, Duhamel G, Alsop DC. Efficiency of inversion pulses for background suppressed arterial spin labeling. Magn Reson Med. 2005;54(2):366–72.
42. Maleki N, Dai W, Alsop DC. Optimization of background suppression for arterial spin labeling perfusion imaging. MAGMA. 2012;25(2):127–33.
43. Cox EF, Buchanan CE, Bradley CR, Prestwich B, Mahmoud H, Taal M, et al. Multiparametric renal magnetic resonance imaging: validation, interventions, and alterations in chronic kidney disease. Front Physiol. 2017;8:696.
44. Song R, Tipirneni A, Johnson P, Loeffler RB, Hillenbrand CM. Evaluation of respiratory liver and kidney movements for MRI navigator gating. J Magn Reson Imaging. 2011;33(1):143–8.
45. Philbrick KA, Weston AD, Akkus Z, Kline TL, Korfiatis P, Sakinis T, et al. RIL-contour: a medical imaging dataset annotation tool for and with deep learning. J Digit Imaging. 2019;32(4):571–81.
46. Noda Y, Ito K, Kanki A, Tamada T, Yamamoto A, Kazuya Y, et al. Measurement of renal cortical thickness using noncontrast-enhanced steady-state free precession MRI with spatially selective inversion recovery pulse: association with renal function. J Magn Reson Imaging. 2015;41(6):1615–21.
47. Wu W-C, Su M-Y, Chang C-C, Tseng W-YI, Liu K-L. Renal perfusion 3-T MR imaging: a comparative study of arterial spin labeling and dynamic contrast-enhanced techniques. Radiology. 2011;261(3):845–53.

48. Evans RG, Ince C, Joles JA, Smith DW, May CN, O'Connor PM, et al. Haemodynamic influences on kidney oxygenation: clinical implications of integrative physiology. Clin Exp Pharmacol Physiol. 2013;40(2):106–22.
49. Ow CPC, Ngo JP, Ullah MM, Hilliard LM, Evans RG. Renal hypoxia in kidney disease: cause or consequence? Acta Physiol (Oxf). 2018;222(4):e12999.
50. Odudu A, Nery F, Harteveld AA, Evans RG, Pendse D, Buchanan CE, et al. Arterial spin labelling MRI to measure renal perfusion: a systematic review and statement paper. Nephrol Dial Transplant. 2018;33(suppl_2):ii15–21.
51. Mora-Gutierrez JM, Garcia-Fernandez N, Slon Roblero MF, Paramo JA, Escalada FJ, Wang DJ, et al. Arterial spin labeling MRI is able to detect early hemodynamic changes in diabetic nephropathy. J Magn Reson Imaging. 2017;46(6):1810–7.
52. Ren T, Wen CL, Chen LH, Xie SS, Cheng Y, Fu YX, et al. Evaluation of renal allografts function early after transplantation using intravoxel incoherent motion and arterial spin labeling MRI. Magn Reson Imaging. 2016;34(7):908–14.
53. Cutajar M, Hilton R, Olsburgh J, Marks SD, Thomas DL, Banks T, et al. Renal blood flow using arterial spin labelling MRI and calculated filtration fraction in healthy adult kidney donors pre-nephrectomy and post-nephrectomy. Eur Radiol. 2015;25(8):2390–6.
54. Zhang Y, Kapur P, Yuan Q, Xi Y, Carvo I, Signoretti S, et al. Tumor vascularity in renal masses: correlation of arterial spin-labeled and dynamic contrast-enhanced magnetic resonance imaging assessments. Clin Genitourin Cancer. 2016;14(1):e25–36.
55. Tsai LL, Bhatt RS, Strob MF, Jegede OA, Sun MRM, Alsop DC, et al. Arterial spin labeled perfusion MRI for the evaluation of response to tyrosine kinase inhibition therapy in metastatic renal cell carcinoma. Radiology. 2021;298(2):332–40.
56. Zhou L, Wang Y, Pinho MC, Pan E, Xi Y, Maldjian JA, et al. Intrasession reliability of arterial spin-labeled MRI-measured noncontrast perfusion in glioblastoma at 3 T. Tomography. 2020;6(2):139–47.
57. Wang Y, Zhou L, Udayakumar D, Madhuranthakam AJ, editors. Reproducibility and repeatability of quantitative pCASL measurements in a 3D-printed perfusion phantom. Proceedings of the 29th Annual Meeting of ISMRM; 2021; Virtual.
58. Oliver-Taylor A, Hampshire T, Mutsaerts HJMM, Clement P, Warnert E, Harteveld AA, et al., Editors. A multi-site round-robin assessment of ASL using a perfusion phantom. Proceedings of the 27th annual meeting of ISMRM; 2019; Montreal, Canada.

Gadolinium-Based Functional MR Urography: From Image Acquisition to Interpretation

20

Erika A. Rincon-Escobar, Dmitry Khrichenko,
and Hansel J. Otero

Abbreviations

CTT	Calyceal transit time
DRF	Differential renal function
eGFR	Estimated glomerular filtration rate
fMRU	Functional magnetic resonance urography
MTT	Mean transit time
RTT	Renal transit time

Introduction

There are many clinical indications for qualitative and quantitative renal imaging function tests; a common one is to differentiate between urinary tract functional obstruction and dilatation, which at times might persist even after decompressive surgery. Furthermore, renal function can be assessed in adults and children to identify and stage renal disease and, during surgical planning and at follow-up, to assess treatment response [1, 2].

E. A. Rincon-Escobar · D. Khrichenko
Department of Radiology, Children's Hospital of Philadelphia, Philadelphia, PA, USA

H. J. Otero (✉)
Department of Radiology, Children's Hospital of Philadelphia, Philadelphia, PA, USA

Perelman School of Medicine at the University of Pennsylvania, Philadelphia, PA, USA
e-mail: Oteroh@chop.edu

Gadolinium-based functional MR urography (fMRU) offers significant advantages in functional evaluations, providing high spatial, contrast, and temporal resolution and allowing to characterize anatomic anomalies not thoroughly evaluated with conventional anatomic imaging (i.e., ultrasound and/or computed tomography). fMRU uses renal parenchymal signal changes in dynamic T1-weighted images related to uptake and excretion after intravenous administration of a gadolinium-based contrast agent to estimate renal function and contrast clearance times. This technique has been proved to give equivalent information to nuclear medicine renal scans and intravenous urograms without the use of ionizing radiation and with increased anatomic detail. fMRU is increasingly being used to evaluate the urinary tract with both anatomic and functional information [2–4]. However, fMRU has several limitations, including longer acquisition time than other imaging modalities, higher costs, and high susceptibility to motion artifacts, often requiring sedation or anesthesia in patients unable to cooperate. Also, the functional analysis of the MRU scan requires the interpreting clinician to be familiar with postprocessing assumptions and software [1, 5–7]. MRU might be ideal to assess the urinary tract in many cases but may be limited in cases with altered renal function and severe urinary tract obstruction [8]. In this chapter, we describe patient preparation, imaging acquisition, and postprocessing including com-

S. D. Serai, K. Darge (eds.), *Advanced Clinical MRI of the Kidney*,
https://doi.org/10.1007/978-3-031-40169-5_20

mon quantitative parameters to assist further dissemination and adoption of this technology.

Patient Preparation

Patients undergoing MRU require special preparation, including proper hydration and administration of a loop diuretic (furosemide). Hydration can be done orally or intravenously. However, it is usually administered intravenously [9]. Furosemide is intravenously administered at the start of the examination, approximately 15 min before contrast injection (1 mg/kg, a maximum of 20 mg). Both are used to (1) reduce the concentration of gadolinium-contrast in the collecting system. It is well known that the relationship between signal intensity and gadolinium concentration is relatively linear at low concentrations. At higher concentrations, in addition to T1 shortening, which increases the T1 signal intensity, it also shortens T2/T2* that results in loss of signal. The competing effects result in loss of signal at high contrast concentrations [10–13]; (2) evaluate the excretory function during diuresis; and (3) ensure rapid filling of the urinary tract, hence reducing study time.

A bladder catheter is usually placed to allow free drainage of the bladder during the study and avoid overdistension. An overdistended bladder increased the pressure on the collecting system, which could artifactually delay quantitative drainage parameters. Increased pressure can further alter quantitative analysis in the presence of vesicoureteral reflux. Additionally, a bladder catheter improves patient comfort and helps decrease motion. It also eliminates the possible urgency of voiding and consequent interruption of the study [5, 14].

For postcontrast imaging and functional analysis, a number of gadolinium-based contrast agents that are approved for routine clinical use can be utilized. However, more recently, due to safety concerns related to the reported deposition of gadolinium in the brain, and higher risk of nephrogenic systemic fibrosis (NSF), macrocyclic agents have been preferred [8, 15, 16]. At the authors' institution, an ionic agent is routinely used, as it theoretically results in improved uptake and faster excretion in the kidney (Gadoterate Meglumine, Dotarem®; Guerbet LLC, Villepinte, France). Gadolinium-contrast agents are administered at a standard dose of 0.1 mmol/kg (0.2 mL/kg) with a maximum dose of 20 mL. To ensure the linear relationship between signal intensity and gadolinium concentration, avoiding T2*-related signal loss mentioned above, in addition to hydration and diuretics, the contrast agent is administered through a power injector at speed between 0.1 mL/s and 0.25 mL/s [5, 9, 11–14]. Standard gadolinium-contrast agents guidelines in terms of safety, contraindications, and risk/benefit analysis are followed [16].

Sedation is generally required in children older than 6 months but younger than 7 years of age, depending on the MR institutional practices. Newborn and young infants can be imaged with a "feed and wrap" approach to avoid anesthesia use [8].

Image Acquisition

The acquisition protocol varies between groups, and there is no established consensus protocol; a generally suggested protocol is shown in Table 20.1. In general, it starts with 2D localizer images and sagittal T2 images to determine the positioning of the kidneys and bladder and to plan an oblique coronal plane angled parallel to the long axis of the kidneys. The field of view goes from the diaphragm and through the pelvis to include the urethra [9, 14].

Table 20.1 fMRU image acquisition protocol

	Localizers	SS-T2-w (SSFSE/HASTE/SSTSE)	T1-w 3D GRE dynamic Gd (LAVA/VIBE/THRIVE)
Plane	3 planes	Sagittal	Coronal
Fat saturation	No	Yes	Yes
Respiratory compensation	No	No	No
Number of slices	3 + 3 + 3	~60	20–32
Field of view	450 mm	160–380 mm	200–400 mm
Slice thickness	10 mm	3 mm	2 mm
Matrix	256 × 256	256 × 256	256 × 256
TR	15	1100	3.6
TE	5	100	1.2
Flip angle	40	177	15
Receiver bandwidth	180 mHz	476 mHz	650 mHz
Turbo factor		150	
Parallel acquisition tech	No	No	GRAPPA [2]

GRE gradient recalled-echo, *TE* echo time, *TR* repetition time, *w* weighted

MRU imaging is performed using a 3D, coronal oblique, dynamic, gradient-echo sequence orientated along the axis of the kidneys, and the acquisition volume includes kidneys and abdominal aorta, and bladder (Fig. 20.1). In general, any gradient echo sequence that has a linear relationship between contrast concentration and signal intensity, and a "fast enough" acquisition time with sufficient resolution can be utilized. Examples of major MRI manufacturers include VIBE for Siemens, LAVA for GE, and THRIVE for Philips. The sequence is optimized with parameters to obtain a short acquisition time (i.e., <10 s per phase). The dynamic T1 sequences is then repeated at increasing intervals to assess contrast; usually, six volumes/minute during the first 5 min from the time contrast is injected until 10–15 min after the injection. Doing that allows a formal functional analysis and grants evaluation of renal perfusion with parenchymal enhancement and time of contrast material excretion into the renal collecting system [2, 8]. Motion reduction is most relevant for the first 3 min after contrast injection because the functional analysis is based primarily on the postcontrast images acquired during this period, which show the initial enhancing of the parenchyma and passage of contrast into the calyces. Preliminary results for fMRU using a Golden-angle RAdial Sparse Parallel (XD GRASP) sequence were reported recently. This type of sequence is more robust against motion, and its continuous acquisition allows for detailed functional analysis. Other similarly faster and motion-robust T1-weighted sequences are becoming available and can likely be adopted for fMRU [17, 18].

Clinically, additional delayed postcontrast imaging with higher resolution might be advantageous for anatomical detail. Delayed postcontrast images can also be used to generate 2D reformations that allow for optimal visualization of anatomic structures of interest [8]. However, additional images are not used for functional analysis.

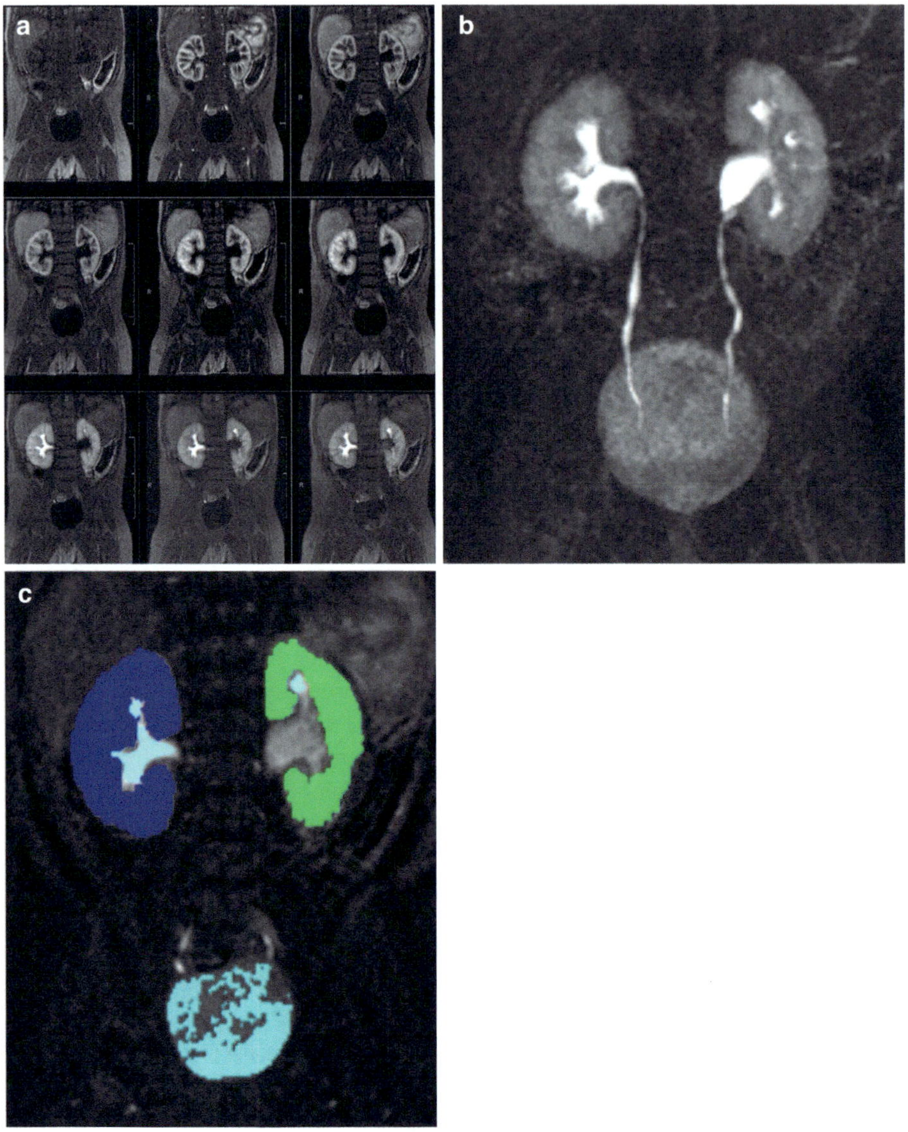

d	Right Kidney	Left Kidney
CTT [min, sec]	1m 59s	2m 29s
RTT [min, sec]	2m 9s	2m 49s
TTP [min, sec]	2m 19s	2m 39s
Volume [mL]	38.21	29.60
vDRF [%]	56.35	43.65
pDRF [%]	49.27	50.73
vpDRF [%]	55.63	44.37
Patlak [(mL/min)/mL]	0.50910	0.52420

Fig. 20.1 (**a**) Dynamic coronal oblique T1-w GRE images of the kidneys and bladder before and after gadolinium-based contrast administration showing the contrast transit from the cortex to the medulla and asymmetrically faster excretion of contrast into the left collecting system. (**b**) Volumetric maximum intensity projection from sources images shown in (**a**) demonstrated bilateral patent collecting systems with normal caliber of the ureters. (**c**) Coronal oblique image with color overlay showing the results from semiautomated segmentation of the included renal (blue = right and green = left) parenchyma, collecting systems and bladder used for functional analysis. (**d**) Postprocessing quantitative analysis results (explain in the section below) from the same study

Postprocessing

fMRU uses postcontrast images to estimate differential renal function and several quantitative parameters. The basis of this functional analysis is to generate enhancement curves related to the passage of contrast material through the kidneys and collecting systems to give information similar to renal scintigraphy [8]. To achieve this, regions of interest are drawn in the aorta and renal parenchyma, and the average signal intensity over time is calculated. Each curve represents the relative enhancement of the segmented tissue over time from the baseline.

Segmentation of the kidneys is required to assess renal function with MRU because it provides the renal volume to estimate filtration, and it is also useful as a mask that determines the pixels that contribute to the average time course for the kidney (Fig. 20.1c) [19]. It is possible to do a manual segmentation; however, this technique is very time-consuming. The easiest way to perform the segmentation is to select the dynamic sequences the moment the renal cortex and medulla are isointense, but before the contrast medium is seen in the collecting system. Different time points are selected for each kidney in the nonsymmetric excretion of contrast agents [20].

The aorta must also be segmented because some data on its signal intensity are required. For this, the point with the maximum enhancement of the aorta is selected, and from this, the segmentation is performed. Although the segmentation of the aorta is relatively robust because it has significant signal changes compared with the surrounding tissue, the measured signal can be distorted by pulsatility and/or turbulence [20].

The first step is to generate enhancement curves that represents the relative enhancement of the segmented tissue over time from the baseline (i.e., precontrast) signal intensity.

Signal Intensity–Transit Time Curves

Deriving the mean signal from the segmented volumes and converting the signal values to concentrations allows the generation of renal parenchymal signal intensity-time versus time curves, similar to nuclear medicine renal scans. It is generally included an aortic curve as well as curves representing the passage of the contrast agent through each kidney. These curves give information about renal function by measuring perfusion, uptake, and excretion of contrast medium [1, 8]. Each data point is the relative aorta and parenchymal enhancement vs. time, where enhancement is *Enhancement [time] = (signal_intensity [time]—baseline)/baseline* and baseline is the average signal intensity before contrast injection (Fig. 20.2a). As such, an enhancement value of 2.0 means that the signal intensity at that instance is 2 × precontrast signal intensity.

The aortic curve is characterized by an initial peak corresponding to the injection of the contrast medium and a rapid decrease in its concentration secondary to the filtration from the vascular compartment and renal excretion [1].

The curve of the kidneys begins with a rapid upward slope after the peak of the aortic curve. Subsequently, there is a more gradual increase, and finally, after the concentration peak, the contrast concentration begins to fall, and the curve of the kidneys becomes parallel to that of the aorta.

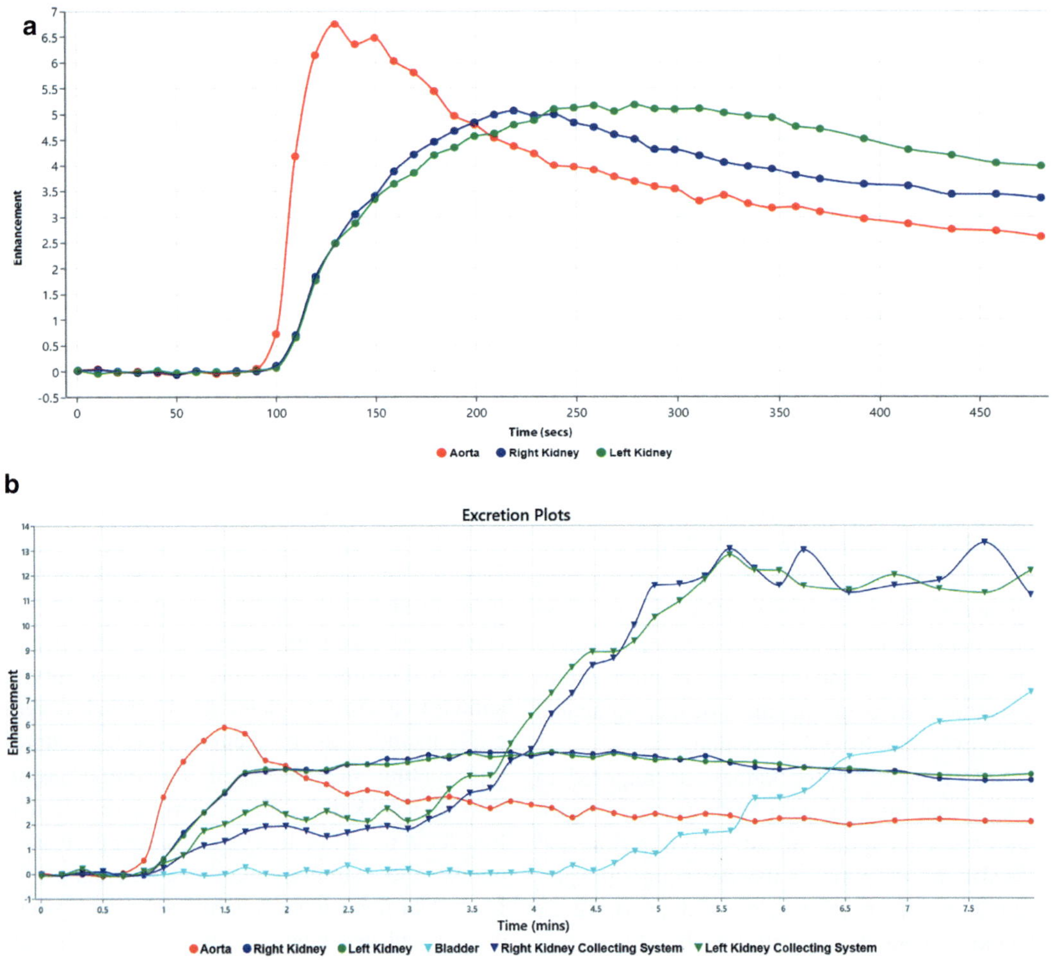

Fig. 20.2 (**a**) Normal average enhancement vs. time curve: Each data point is the relative aorta and parenchymal enhancement vs. time, where enhancement is *Enhancement [time] = (signal_intensity [time]—baseline)/baseline* (aorta: red; right kidney: blue; and left kidney: green). The aorta shows a characteristic fast enhancement and early peak (dependent on the injection of contrast) followed by a rapid decrease in its contrast concentration (due to filtration away from the vascular compartment from renal excretion), while the kidneys show rapid upward slope following the aortic enhancement peak and a more gradual increase. Overtime, the contrast concentration begins to fall, and the curve of the kidneys becomes parallel to that of the aorta. (**b**) Excretion plot: These curves show time versus signal intensity of the segmented collecting systems and urinary bladder

This curve represents the initial renal perfusion. Subsequently, it reflects the contrast in the nephrons, secondary to glomerular filtration. After the concentration peak, the contrast leaves the nephrons in the collecting system, and it reaches the steady state with the aorta [1]. These curves are generally symmetrical between both kidneys, and when an asymmetry is found, a possible pathology should be investigated [5, 19].

Similar to the enhancement curves, described above, excretion curves can be derived. These curves are the time versus signal intensity of the segmented collecting systems and urinary bladder (Fig. 20.2b).

Temporal Parameters (Fig. 20.1d)

Time to Peak

The first temporal parameter and the easiest to derive is the time to peak, which just identifies the lapse in seconds to maximum intensity of the enhancing parenchyma and can serve as a rough estimate of renal function when asymmetrically delay in the affected kidney.

Calyceal Transit Time

The calyceal transit time is defined as the time required for the contrast medium to pass from the renal cortex to the proximal ureter, at the level of the lower pole of the kidney. This parameter allows differentiating between an obstructed kidney and a normal kidney when evaluated together with the morphological images [5].

In normal kidneys, this time is symmetrical, and if asymmetry is found, a renal lesion should be investigated. When the CTT is found to be decreased, this may be secondary to renal damage leading to a tubular concentration defect, a long-standing partial obstruction, an intermittent obstruction, or after surgical repair of an obstruction. Occasionally, rapid CTT occurs in cases of glomerular hyperfiltration. When the CTT is increased, an acute obstruction should be suspected; however, CTT can also be delayed in patients with hypotension, renal artery stenosis, and dehydration [1, 5, 21].

Renal Transit Time (RTT)

Renal transit time (RTT) is the time needed in seconds for the contrast to reach the proximal ureter (below the level of the lower pole of the kidney). RTT is prolonged in obstructed kidneys. However, it can also be prolonger in capacious unobstructed kidneys and can be influenced by patient position and the morphology of the ureteropelvic junction. In kidneys without excretion, the RTT cannot be calculated.

The RTT is delayed in cases of obstruction; however, it can also be a false positive in cases with severe dilatation and stasis that causes slow drainage of the contrast medium in the absence of obstruction or in cases with a nondependent anteriorly positioned ureteropelvic junction. When this occurs, the gadolinium accumulates in the dependent portions of the collecting system and causes delayed RTT. In such cases, prone imaging generally facilitates the drainage of the contrast medium [1, 8]. Jones et al. found good agreement between MR urography and renal scintigraphy and concluded that an RTT greater than 490 s suggests obstruction [22]. Viteri et al. found that decreasing the RTT cutoff to 360 s results in a 5% increased sensitivity [23].

Functional Parameters

Differential Renal Function (DRF)

One of the essential quantitative parameters is the DRF, which expresses the results of functional measurements for each kidney as a percentage of total function. DRF can be calculated by two different methods; the first one is the easiest and is based on the volumetric segmentation of the enhancing renal parenchyma (*volumetric differential renal function—vDRF*) compared to adjacent structures such as the collecting system and vessels. The functional parenchymal volume is reported in mL (*renal volume*). Then, the relative contribution that each kidney contributes to the total enhancing renal parenchyma volume is reported as *vDRF*. The main disadvantage of this method is that it interprets all areas of enhancing renal parenchyma as having the same function and therefore may have difficulty reflecting differences in renal function between enhancing regions of the same kidney or between both kidneys [8].

The second way to calculate the DRF is the Patlak-Rutland method, which is currently the reference technique used for functional analysis (*Patlak differential renal function—pDRF*). The Patlak method uses a mathematical formula that transforms the signal from the renal parenchyma and aorta to generate a specific graph for each kidney based on the estimated glomerular filtration rate; these graphs allow for estimation of differential renal function. The way Patlak method works by assuming that the change in renal parenchymal signal intensity in the postcontrast sequences has a proportional and linear relationship with gadolinium concentration. Based on the differential renal function calculated by the Patlak method, parametric maps can be obtained that allow the evaluation of renal function [2, 8, 24].

A combination of both vDRF and pDRF can also be calculated as vpDRF. It represents the relative total function of right versus left (NOT per unit tissue). This number is also the most comparable to the functional numbers in nuclear medicine renal scans (MAG3). While for severely dilated kidneys, the DRF estimated by fMRU is lower than the results from nuclear medicine renal scan (MAG3), making simultaneous comparisons, inaccurate [2]; these two tests are similar and clinically equivalent with high specificity to detect obstruction [23].

Patlak Plots

The Patlak plot technique describes a two-compartment model with one-way flow from the vasculature (compartment 1) to the parenchyma (compartment 2). As such, changes in signal intensity that approximate the amount of contrast that abandons the vascular space and enters the parenchyma can be used to estimate "clearance" [25, 26] (Fig. 20.3a). As mentioned above, the underpinning assumption is that signal changes are proportional to the concentration of gadolinium in a particular voxel and that this relationship is linear. It is also assumed that the contrast is evenly distributed in the blood pool and that the concentration of contrast (as well as the hematocrit) is always the same in the aorta and renal arteries. Under these assumptions, the amount of contrast in any given voxel is the sum of the vascular contrast plus the contrast in the nephron (thus neglecting the interstitium). Moreover, because it is assumed that the aorta and renal vasculature have equals amounts of contrast at all times (and that the contrast determines the signal intensity), the amount of contrast filtered into the nephron can be calculated as a proportion to the integral of the gadolinium concentration curve of the aorta in the first 60–180 s after injection. If all assumptions were in fact true, the resulting Patlak plot results in a straight line. Additionally, two values can be extracted from the Patlak plot. The slope, which equals the Patlak number and can be presented in a pixel-by-pixel basis, as a "Patlak map" (Fig. 20.3b) and the intercept, which equals the blood volume reaching the kidneys, a pixel-by-pixel representation of the renal tissue with equivalent signal intensity to that of the aorta (an estimate of cortical function/perfusion relative to the aorta) presented as "blood volume maps" (Fig. 20.3c).

The calculated Patlak number, reported in [(mL/min)/mL], can be theoretically converted to GFR, and hence, reporting GFR per kidney (or moiety/pole) is possible by adjusting by contrast concentration, hematocrit, and body surface area. However, this method shows marked variability, and it is prompt to error given the limitations in temporal and spatial resolution of the fMRU images with conflicting reports on its accuracy in the literature [27].

Patlak Maps

These are renal parametric maps based on Patlak differential renal function that allows for regional assessment of renal function (including upper versus lower moieties in the context of a duplex kidney). The map is the first Patlak parameter (slope) on a pixel-by-pixel basis calculated relative to the aorta and an estimation of glomerular filtration rate (GFR). Such information can assist in presurgical planning, for example, when deciding whether to perform upper pole nephrectomy or ureteric reimplantation in the context of a duplex kidney with an obstructed upper moiety.

Fig. 20.3 (**a**) Patlak plots: These plots represent the fit of the two-compartment model (vasculature and parenchyma). The assumption is that the signal/contrast relationship is linear and that the aorta and renal vasculature have equals amounts of contrast at all times, and hence, the amount of contrast filtered into the nephron can be calculated as a proportion to the integral of the contrast concentration curve of the aorta. (**b**) Patlak map: it is the graphic representation in a pixel-by-pixel basis of the Patlak number (estimated glomerular filtration rate) derived from the slope of the Patlak curve. (**c**, **d**) Blood volume maps: It is a map of the second Patlak parameter (intercept) on a pixel-by-pixel basis calculated relative to the aorta

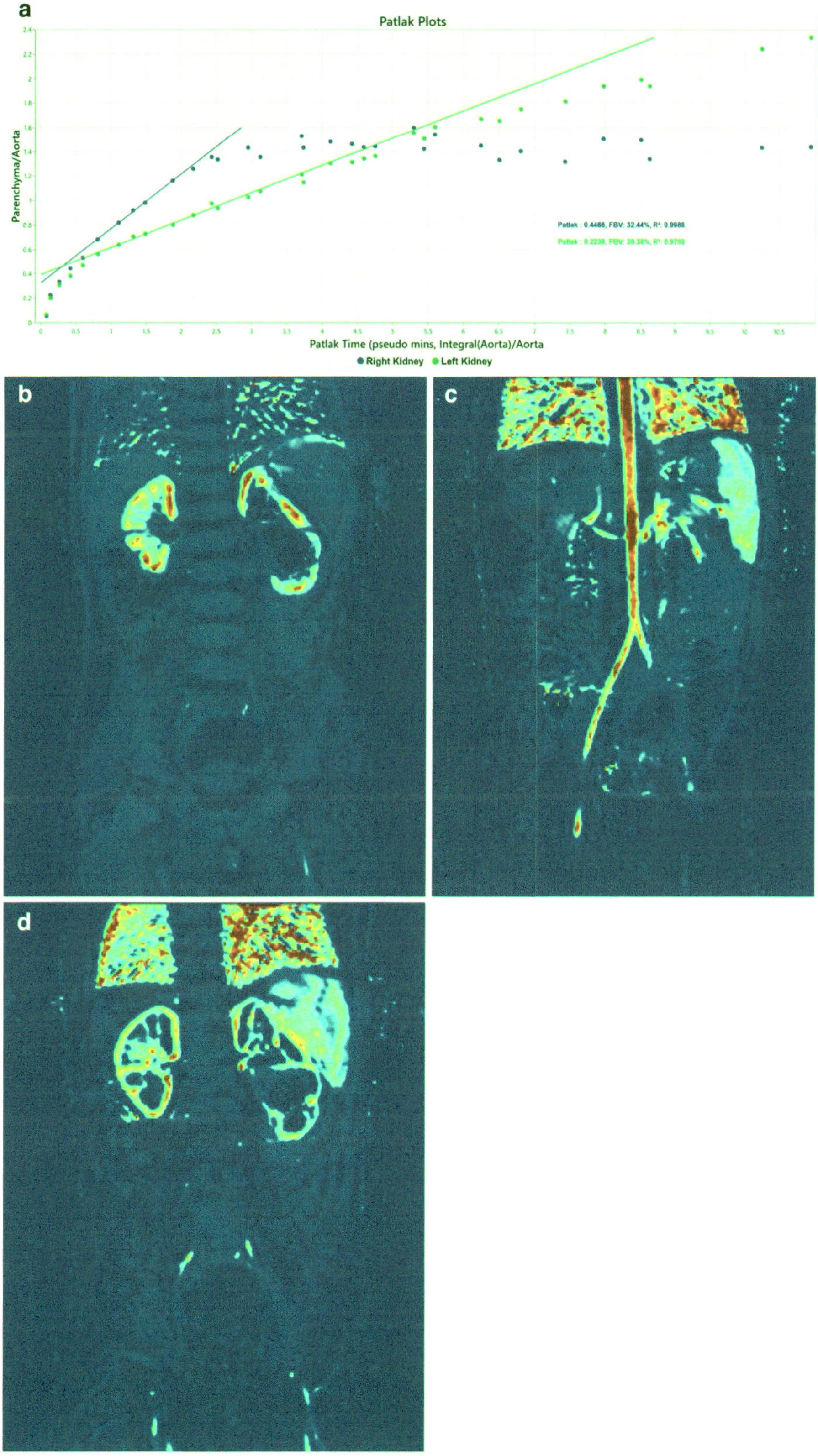
a
Patlak Plots
Parenchyma/Aorta
Patlak : 0.4466, FBV: 32.44%, R²: 0.9988
Patlak Time (pseudo mins, Integral(Aorta)/Aorta)
Right Kidney
Left Kidney
b
c
d

Blood Volume Maps

These are renal parametric maps based on enhancement and allow for regional assessment of blood flow (i.e., regions of equivalent signal intensity/gadolinium concentration between the aorta and the kidney). It is a map of the second Patlak parameter (intercept) on a pixel-by-pixel basis calculated relative to the aorta and a visual tool to differentiate vessels and renal cortex from the medulla under the aforementioned assumptions.

Normal Curves

To generate these curves, several steps were taken. First, the time of injection (timeinjection) was calculated by finding the x-intercept of the line containing the first and second postcontrast enhancement point. A temporally interpolated and shifted enhancement (TISE) curve is calculated by linearly interpolating to a 1-s temporal resolution, truncating at 6 min postcontrast, and shifting the x-axis by timenormalized = timeoriginal—timeinjection, so the first data point is at time of injection (Fig. 20.4a).

Then, the TISE curves are used to generate a normalized temporally interpolated and shifted enhancement (NTISE) curves (Fig. 20.4b). NTISE curves are calculated by scaling the TISE curve by its area under the curve (AUC), which is calculated using the midpoint method, and multiplying by the total time in seconds (360 s) to produce an average NTISE value of 1.0 throughout the duration.

A version of these curves, generated from normal studies and including a shaded area of two standard deviations above and below are then superimposed on the individual curves allowing for visual identification of kidneys functioning above or below the expected "normal" values (Fig. 20.4c). It is also a visual guide of relative function in patients with single or functionally single kidneys.

Three quantitative parameters are reported, scale, average σ, and quality. Scale gives an estimate of the amount of contrast absorbed and is defined as

$$\text{Scale} = 100\% \frac{\text{AUC}_{\text{TISE}}}{\text{AUC}_{\text{MEAN TISE}}} \tag{20.1}$$

Where $\mathbf{AUC_{TISE}}$ is the area under the curve of the TISE curve and $\mathbf{AUC_{MEAN\ TISE}}$ is the area under the curve of the mean TISE curve for the proper age group. Mean σ is the average deviation of the NTISE curve from the normal MEAN NTISE curve and is defined as

$$\text{Mean}\,\sigma = \frac{1}{N}\sum_{t=1}^{N}\left|\frac{\text{NTISE}_t - \text{MEAN NTISE}_t}{\sigma_t}\right| \tag{20.2}$$

Where N is the number of NTISE points, **NTISE**t is the NTISE value at time = t, **MEAN NTISE**t is the MEAN NTISE value at time = t, and $\boldsymbol{\sigma}$t is the standard deviation of the MEAN NTISE at time = t. Quality is a measure of uptake and excretion (higher if uptake is faster and excretion is faster than normal; lower or negative if uptake is slower and excretion is slower than normal) and is defined as

$$\text{Quality} = \frac{1}{N}\left(\sum_{t=1}^{t_{\text{peak}}}\frac{\text{NTISE}_t - \text{MEAN NTISE}_t}{\sigma_t} + \sum_{t=t_{\text{peak}}}^{N}\frac{\text{MEAN NTISE}_t - \text{NTISE}_t}{\sigma_t}\right) \tag{20.3}$$

Where $\boldsymbol{t_{\text{peak}}}$ is the peak time of the normal mean NTISE curve.

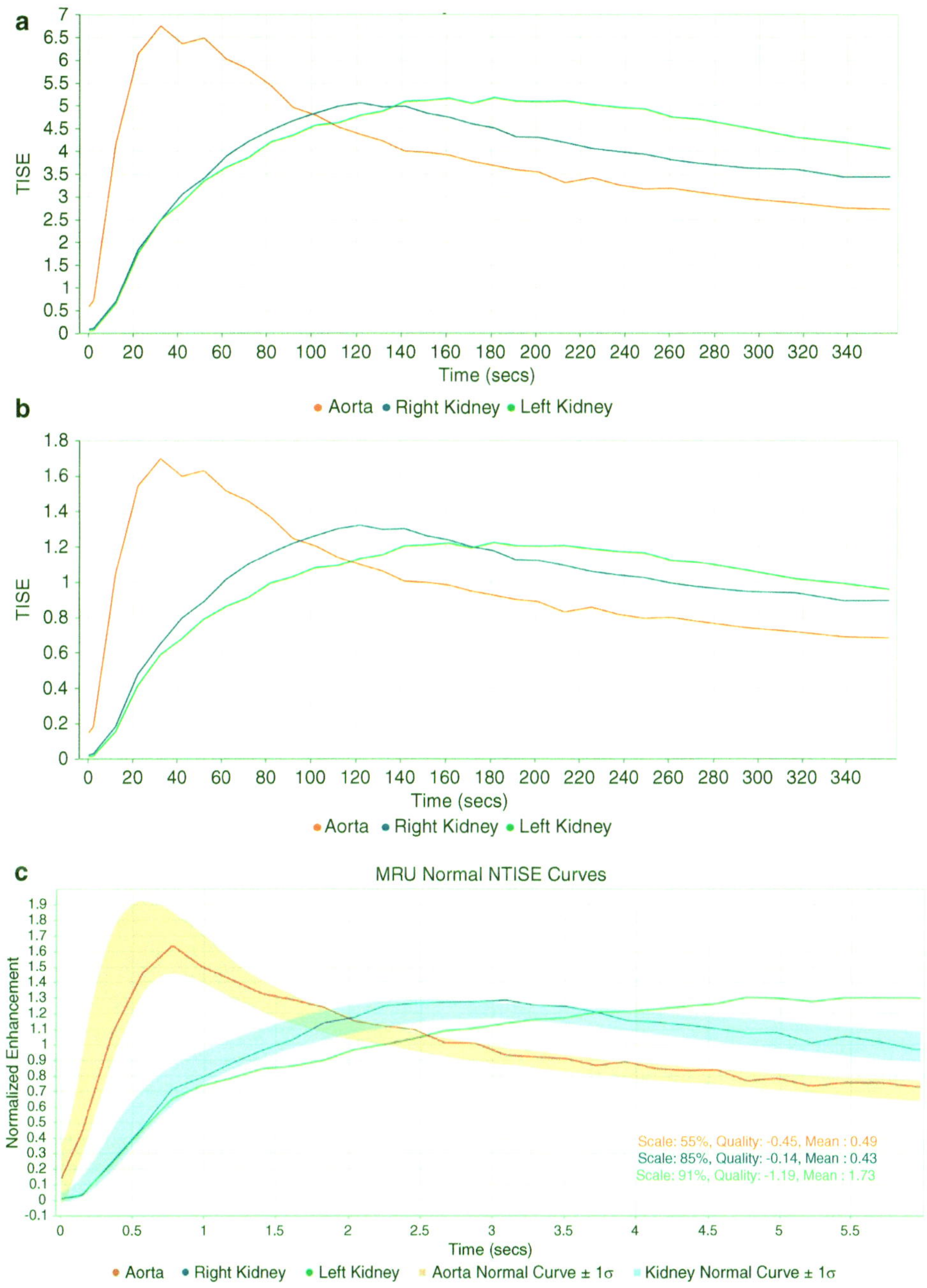

Fig. 20.4 (**a**) Temporally interpolated and shifted enhancement (TISE) curve: a normalize curve calculated by linearly interpolating to a 1-s temporal resolution, truncating at 6 min postcontrast, and shifting the x-axis so the first data point is the time of injection. (**b**) Normalized temporally interpolated and shifted enhancement (NTISE): These curves were calculated by scaling the TISE curve by its area under the curve (AUC) using the midpoint method. (**c**) NTISE curves are incorporated to every study adding a shaded area of two standard deviations above and below normal values and then superimposed on the individual curves of the study. In this case showing the curves from an MRU in a patient with left ureteropelvic junction obstruction. The abnormal left kidney shows delayed enhancement (shifted rightward) without the characteristic early peak and with no decrease over time as the contrast continues to accumulate instead of been excreted

Clinical Applications and Interpretation

The pathophysiology of specific renal diseases is beyond the scope of this chapter; however, it is essential to keep in mind that a systematic approach should be performed to get the most out of fMRU by integrating morphologic and functional findings. In the morphological evaluation, both kidneys' presence and location must be assessed. Also, renal ectopia, dysplastic kidneys, and anatomic alterations such as renal fusion (e.g., horseshoe kidney or crossed-fused renal ectopia) must be identified. The renal parenchyma should be evaluated to rule out the presence of acute inflammatory processes such as pyelonephritis or focal thinning that may be the result of chronic pathological processes such as scarring from reflux [8, 20]. fMRU has been shown to help identify severely dysplastic kidneys that are still functional and are not identified on ultrasound or nuclear medicine renal scans [8, 28].

As such, to correctly interpret the functional analysis, it is essential to start with a visual or qualitative evaluation of the kidneys. This visual analysis is performed with dynamic sequences and evaluates contrast excretion and symmetry in both kidneys. If any abnormality is found, it is necessary to confirm whether these pathological findings are unilateral or bilateral. In general, the quantitative analysis is easier [1]. In the case of dysplastic kidneys or with uropathy, a heterogeneous enhancement will be found in the postcontrast dynamic sequences reflecting chronic damage in the microvasculature, glomeruli, and tubules; however, these findings can also be secondary to acute changes in the GFR [1].

When used for the evaluation of urinary tract dilation, one of the most frequent indications in children, fMRU is able to appropriately differentiate ureteropelvic obstruction, vesicoureteral junction obstruction, and vesicoureteral reflux nephropathy from functional or transient dilation [29]. fMRU can also identify crossing vessels or other causes of extrinsic mass effect, resulting in obstruction at or near the ureteropelvic junction [30]. The UPJ obstruction is a partial or intermittent blockage of the flow of urine that causes the upper tracts to overfill and exceed their physiological capacity [31]. fMRU is the best method for the evaluation of function in duplex kidneys because it can assess each fraction separately and can also define the cortex between the upper and lower pole as well as differentiate between duplex kidneys and its mimics, such as cysts, diverticula, and segmental dysplastic multicystic kidneys [1].

In summary, fMRU is a robust relatively simple MR technology based on universally available sequences. However, attention to patient preparation, imaging parameters, and postprocessing are needed to satisfy the underpinning assumptions that allow for the calculation of quantitative parameters including differential renal function, contrast clearance, and estimation of GFR.

Commercial sequences labels are listed for Siemens Healthcare, GE Healthcare, and Philips Healthcare MRI systems, respectively. SSFSE: single-shot fast spin echo; HASTE: half-Fourier acquisition single-shot turbo spin-echo; SSTSE: single-shot turbo spin-echo; LAVA: liver acquisition with volume acceleration; VIBE: volumetric interpolated breath-hold examination; THRIVE: T1-weighted high-resolution isotropic volume examination.

References

1. Grattan-Smith JD, Chow J, Kurugol S, Jones RA. Quantitative renal magnetic resonance imaging: magnetic resonance urography. Pediatr Radiol. 2022;52(2):228–48.
2. Claudon M, Durand E, Grenier N, Prigent A, Balvay D, Chaumet-Riffaud P, et al. Chronic urinary obstruction: evaluation of dynamic contrastenhanced MR urography for measurement of split renal function. Radiology. 2014;273(3):801–12.
3. Damasio MB, Bodria M, Dolores M, Durand E, Sertorio F, Wong MCY, et al. Comparative study between functional MR urography and renal scintigraphy to evaluate drainage curves and Split renal function in children with congenital anomalies of kidney and urinary tract (CAKUT). Front Pediatr. 2020;7:7(January).
4. Karaveli M, Katsanidis D, Psarrakos K, Sioundas A, Dimitriadis A, Haritanti A, et al. MR urography: anatomical and quantitative information on congenital malformations in children. Niger Med J. 2013;54(2):136.

5. Khrichenko D, Darge K. Functional analysis in MR urography - made simple. Pediatr Radiol. 2010;40(2):182–99.
6. Bo S, Sedaghat F, Devi Pavuluri K, Rowe SP, Cohen A, Kates M, et al. Dynamic contrast enhanced-mr cest urography: an emerging tool in the diagnosis and management of upper urinary tract obstruction. Tomography. 2021;7(1):80–94.
7. Abreu-Gomez J, Udare A, Shanbhogue KP, Schieda N. Update on MR urography (MRU): technique and clinical applications. Abdom Radiol. 2019;44(12):3800–10.
8. Dickerson EC, Dillman JR, Smith EA, Dipietro MA, Lebowitz RL, Darge K. Pediatric MR urography: indications, techniques, and approach to review. Radiographics. 2015;35(4):1208–30.
9. Riccabona M. Pediatric urogenital radiology. Third edit. Springer International Publishing; 2018. p. 34.
10. Jones RA, Easley K, Little SB, Scherz H, Kirsch AJ, Grattan-Smith JD. Dynamic contrast-enhanced MR urography in the evaluation of pediatric hydronephrosis: part I, functional assessment. Am J Roentgenol. 2005;185(6):1598–607.
11. Lee MJ, Kim MJ, Yoon CS, Song SY, Park K, Kim WS. The T2-shortening effect of gadolinium and the optimal conditions for maximizing the CNR for evaluating the biliary system: a phantom study. Korean J Radiol. 2011;12(3):358;/pmc/articles/PMC3088853/.
12. Elster AD, Sobol WT, Hinson WH. Pseudolayering of Gd-DTPA in the urinary bladder. Radiology. 1990;174(2):379–81; https://pubmed.ncbi.nlm.nih.gov/2296649/.
13. May DA, Pennington DJ. Effect of gadolinium concentration on renal signal intensity: an in vitro study with a saline bag model. Radiology. 2000;216(1):232–6;https://pubmed.ncbi.nlm.nih.gov/10887253/.
14. Delgado J, Bedoya MA, Adeb M, Carson RH, Johnson AM, Khrichenko D, et al. Optimizing functional MR urography: prime time for a 30-minutes-or-less fMRU. Pediatr Radiol. 2015;45(9):1333–43.
15. Altun E, Martin DR, Wertman R, Lugo-Somolinos A, Fuller ER, Semelka RC. Nephrogenic systemic fibrosis: change in incidence following a switch in gadolinium agents and adoption of a gadolinium policy - report from two U.S. universities. Radiology. 2009;253(3):689–96.
16. ACR manual on contrast media 2022: ACR Committee on drugs and contrast media. 2022.
17. Runge VM, Richter JK, Heverhagen JT. Motion in magnetic resonance: new paradigms for improved clinical diagnosis. Invest Radiol. 2019;54(7):383–95;https://pubmed.ncbi.nlm.nih.gov/30946182/.
18. Feng L. Golden-angle Radial MRI: basics, advances, and applications. J Magn Reson Imaging. 2022;56(1):45–62;https://pubmed.ncbi.nlm.nih.gov/35396897/.
19. Jones RA, Grattan-Smith JD, Little S. MR urography in children. Milan: Springer; 2014. p. 295–310.
20. Jones RA, Schmotzer B, Little SB, Grattan-Smith JD. MRU post-processing. Pediatr Radiol. 2008;38(1 SUPPL):18–27.
21. Little SB, Jones RA, Grattan-Smith JD. Evaluation of UPJ obstruction before and after pyeloplasty using MR urography. Pediatr Radiol. 2008;38(1 SUPPL):106–24.
22. Jones RA, Perez-Brayfield MR, Kirsch AJ, Grattan-Smith JD. Renal transit time with MR urography in children. Radiology. 2004;233(1):41–50.
23. Viteri B, Calle-Toro JS, Ballester L, Darge K, Furth S, Khrichenko D, et al. Potential benefits of functional magnetic resonance urography (fMRU) over MAG3 renal scan in children with obstructive uropathy. J Pediatr Urol. 2021;17(5):659.e1–7.
24. Patlak CS, Blasberg RG. Graphical evaluation of blood-to-brain transfer constants from multiple-time uptake data. J Cereb Blood Flow Metab. 1985;5(4):584–90.
25. Hackstein N, Heckrodt J, Rau WS. Measurement of single-kidney glomerular filtration rate using a contrast-enhanced dynamic gradient-Echo sequence and the Rutland-Patlak plot technique. J Magn Reson Imaging. 2003;18(6):714–25.
26. Hackstein N, Kooijman H, Tomaselli S, Rau WS. Glomerular filtration rate measured using the Patlak plot technique and contrast-enhanced dynamic MRI with different amounts of gadolinium-DTPA. J Magn Reson Imaging. 2005;22(3):406–14; https://pubmed.ncbi.nlm.nih.gov/16106358/.
27. Mendichovszky I, Pedersen M, Frøkiær J, Dissing T, Grenier N, Anderson P, et al. How accurate is dynamic contrast-enhanced MRI in the assessment of renal glomerular filtration rate? A critical appraisal. J Magn Reson Imaging. 2008;27(4):925–31.
28. McMann LP, Kirsch AJ, Scherz HC, Smith EA, Jones RA, Shehata BM, et al. Magnetic resonance urography in the evaluation of prenatally diagnosed Hydronephrosis and renal dysgenesis. J Urol. 2006;176(4 SUPPL):1786–92.
29. Grattan-Smith JD, Jones RA. Magnetic resonance urography in children. Magn Reson Imaging Clin N Am. 2008;16(3):515–31.
30. Park JM, Bloom DA. The pathophysiology of UPJ obstruction: current concepts. Urol Clin North Am. 1998;25(2):161–9.
31. Farrugia MK, Whitaker RH. The search for the definition, etiology, and effective diagnosis of upper urinary tract obstruction: the Whitaker test then and now. J Pediatr Urol. 2019;15(1):18–26.

21 Tools and Techniques to Map Glomerular Distribution and Nephron Function Using MRI

Edwin J. Baldelomar and Kevin M. Bennett

Introduction

Nephron Number and Cationic Ferritin–Enhanced MRI

The kidneys maintain filtration, blood pressure, and electrolyte homeostasis. These functions are performed by the combined action of individual nephrons. The number of nephrons in a kidney is fixed at birth, and human nephron number varies by an order of magnitude individuals [1–5]. Nephrons are damaged or lost due to injury, aging, or disease. A reduced or low nephron number at birth likely predicts susceptibility to kidney disease and functional decline [5–7]. The potential clinical value of biomarkers at the scale of individual nephrons is highlighted by recent reports estimating nephron number and single nephron glomerular filtration rate (GFR) in large population studies using biopsies [8, 9]. In these studies, nephron loss and an altered estimated single nephron GFR were associated with factors leading to chronic kidney disease. However, the methods used in these population studies cannot be directly applied to measure nephron function or count nephrons in individuals [10]. Directly and non-destructively detecting human nephron number and nephron loss in individuals would facilitate earlier diagnostics of kidney disease and aid potential new therapies.

MRI is a sophisticated tool that has allowed the first examinations of the entire, intact kidney at the level of the individual nephron, in vivo [11–13]. A number of targeted and non-targeted contrast agents have been developed for contrast enhancement of various morphology and lesions using MRI in the body [14]. Cationic ferritin–enhanced MRI was proposed in 2008 as the first tool to three-dimensionally map glomeruli and glomerular size throughout the intact kidney [11]. Since then, CFE-MRI has been applied in pre-clinical models in mice [15, 16], rats [17], rabbits [18], and in human kidneys [19, 20]. CFE-MRI has also been applied in vivo in rats [13] and mice [12], providing a new tool to monitor nephron number longitudinally.

CFE-MRI relies on a modified form of the MRI-detectable protein ferritin (Fig. 21.1). Ferritin is an iron storage protein endogenous in all mammals and most other living organisms. Iron is typically stored within the ferritin core as a super-paramagnetic iron oxide nano-crystal. Iron-oxide nano-crystals within ferritin distort the local magnetic field during MRI. Aggregation of many ferritin molecules at a local site and within an image voxel will induce negative (dark) contrast in T2- or T2*-weighted MR images. Cationic ferritin (CF) is formed by conjugating a cationic

E. J. Baldelomar (✉) · K. M. Bennett
Washington University School of Medicine in St. Louis, St. Louis, MO, USA

Biomedical MR Center—Mallinckrodt Institute of Radiology, Washington University School of Medicine in St. Louis, St. Louis, MO, USA
e-mail: e.baldelomar@wustl.edu; kmbennett@wustl.edu

S. D. Serai, K. Darge (eds.), *Advanced Clinical MRI of the Kidney*,
https://doi.org/10.1007/978-3-031-40169-5_21

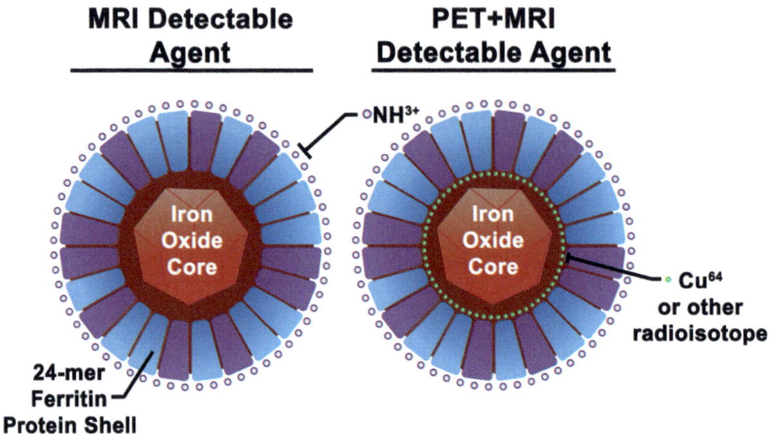

Fig. 21.1 Ferritin is an iron storage protein endogenous in all mammals and most other living organisms. Mammalian ferritin contains two sub-units, heavy and light chain ferritin, that forms a 24-mer spherical shell. Iron is typically stored inside as super-paramagnetic iron oxide crystal. Cationic ferritin (CF) is formed by conjugating amines to the surface of the protein shell. Intravenously injected CF transiently binds to the anionic proteoglycans on the glomerular basement membrane. After accumulation with an MR detectable dose, kidney glomeruli are visible against tissue background in vivo and ex vivo. CF can be further modified with the addition of a radioisotope (previously Copper-64, Cu^{64}) for use with positron emission tomography

crosslinker to its outer surface [21]. CF binds transiently to the glomerular basement membrane after intravenous injection (Fig. 21.2a–f). CF appears to be non-toxic in healthy rodents in MRI-detectable doses, and labeled glomeruli are typically clear of CF after several days [22, 23].

CFE-MRI has been used alone and in combination with other pulse sequences to map other structural and functional features of the kidney. Other features have been mapped in relation to individual nephrons and regions of nephron loss for multi-parametric studies [19, 24]. These features include vascular morphology [24], gross cortical and medullary anatomy [19, 20], glomerular distribution [20], and filtration at the scale of the individual nephron [25].

Applications in Pre-clinical Models of Human Disease

Kidney Phenotyping with CFE-MRI

Kidney Preparation and Ex Vivo Imaging

High-resolution ex vivo CFE-MRI has been used to map and count functioning nephrons throughout the kidney [15–17, 20]. The image of the CF-labeled kidney can also be used to measure whole kidney volume, cortical volume, and the distribution of glomerular volumes (Fig. 21.2g).

CF is typically administered in up to three intravenous injections, at 90-min intervals. It is possible to administer only one injection, but the total dose must be sufficient for detection with the MRI system, and the concentration of CF in the bolus must be low enough to avoid arterial clogging in microcapillaries when administered intravenously. These factors should be considered each time a new experimental protocol is developed. A total CF dose of 5.75-mg/100-g bodyweight has been the most common dose used in pre-clinical studies in rodents (1.92-mg/100-g bodyweight for each injection). Most previous published studies were imaged at 7 T. We have also delivered CF by intraocular injection, which reduces sensitivity to bolus concentration and may reduce acute toxicity [15]. Ninety minutes after final CF injection, animals are transcardially perfused [26] with 0.15 M NaCl followed by 10% formalin. Kidneys are resected and stored in 10% formalin. For ex vivo imaging, a good perfusion is important because remnant blood will appear as negative contrast, similar to CF, and could confound detection of glomeruli. Before imaging, kidneys are washed

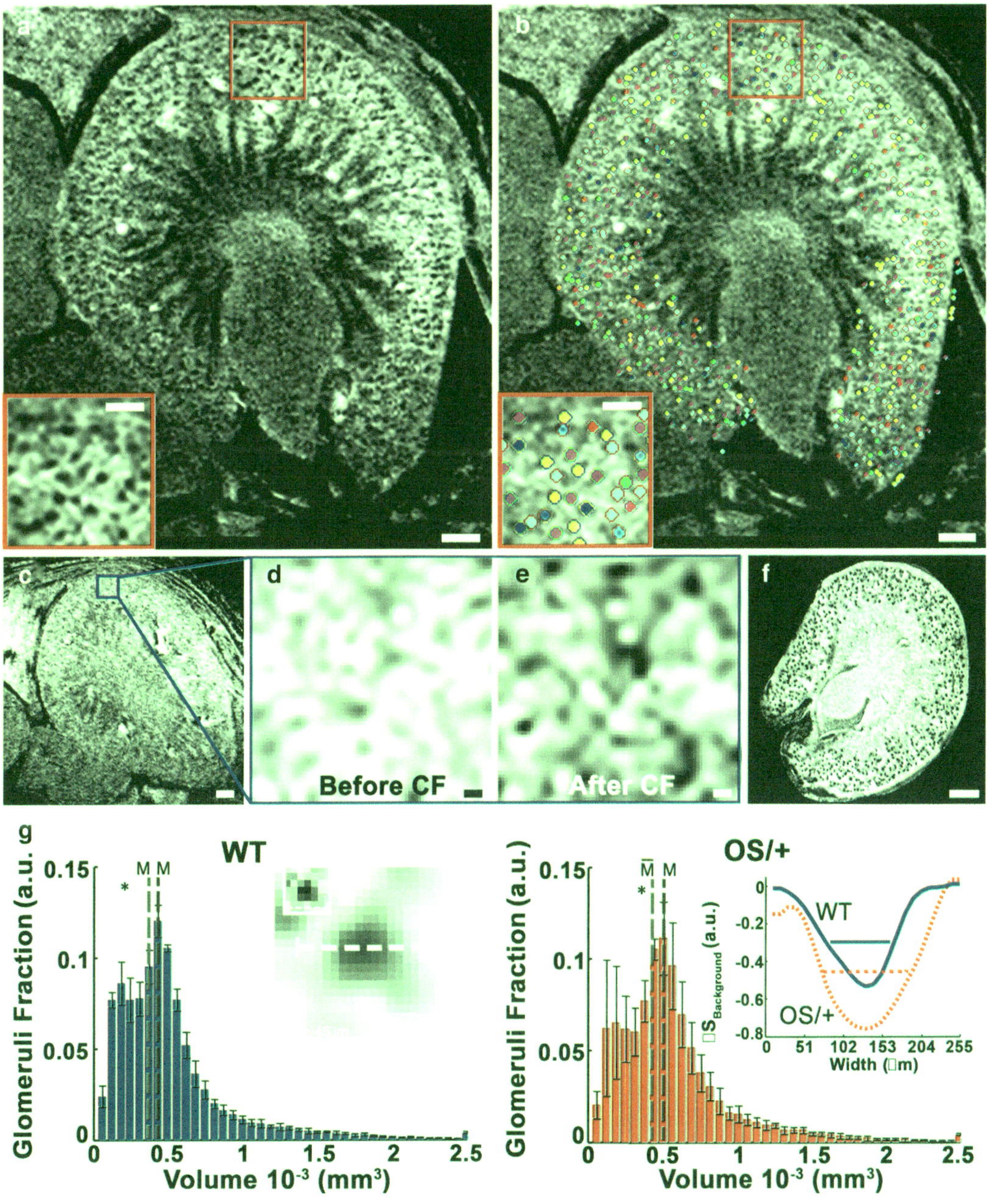

Fig. 21.2 (**a–e**) In vivo 3D CFE-MRI and custom software detect and map rat kidney glomeruli. A rat kidney after injection of CF revealed dark punctate labeling in the kidney cortex, consistent with CF labeling on the glomerular basement membrane. (**f**) CF labeling and glomerular morphology can be also be validated by high-resolution ex vivo CFE-MRI. (**g**) Distributions of glomerular volume detected with CFE-MRI in normal mice (WT) and in a mouse model of congenital renal hypoplasia leading to a reduced nephron mass (OS/+). CFE-MRI detected gross glomerular hypertrophy in OS/+ mice. Adapted from Baldelomar et al. [13, 15]

for 24 h in phosphate-buffered saline and then imaged in phosphate-buffered saline.

Custom imaging holders were fabricated using software (e.g. AutoCAD) and 3D printers to image multiple kidneys together. We have imaged as many as 16 mouse kidneys in a single 3D data set. We recommend using a quadrature volume coil for uniform signal across the sample and good signal-to-noise ratio. We recommend B_0 shimming and a line width of approximately

50–100 Hz. Published studies used a three dimensional gradient recalled echo (GRE) pulse sequence and typical imaging parameters at 7T are: echo time (TE)/repetition time (TR) = 20/80, flip angle = 30°, and bandwidth = 75 Hz/pixel. We typically use image resolutions less than the average diameter of the glomeruli. Mouse kidneys are typically imaged with a near isotropic resolution around 40 um [15, 16]. Rat kidneys are typically imaged with a near isotropic resolution around 50 μm [13, 17].

In Vivo CFE-MRI

CF-labeled glomeruli have been detected and mapped in vivo and longitudinally [12, 13].

Hardware and Experimental Preparations

In vivo imaging of the rodent kidney requires a well-designed radiofrequency (RF) coil. Published studies have used a custom transmit-receive (TxRx) coil for CFE-MRI. It may be possible to perform CFE-MRI using transmit-only (Tx) RF coil combined with a receive-only (Rx) coil for excitation. However, testing and validation should be performed before a full study. The expected kidney size and coil loading influence the design of the tuning and matching circuit [27]. Previously, multi-ring coils were developed for in vivo studies of rats (number of loops, $N_{\text{loops}} = 4$) and mice ($N_{\text{loops}} = 3$) [27]. Coil diameter was designed to account for rodent kidney volume. We have typically used a coil diameter that is ~1.5 times the longest dimension of kidney.

In vivo imaging is strongly affected by motion artifacts due to respiration and pulse. To minimize this, we used respiratory gating and built a custom animal bed. The animal was laid on the bed such that the kidney lies inside the inner diameter of the RF coil rings. The coil was tuned and matched to each animal during each imaging session.

B1 field mapping [28, 29] is required to ensure that the kidney is completely imaged and that the spatial variation of flip angle is minimal (<10%) across the kidney.

In Vivo Imaging

For in vivo imaging, a total CF dose of 5.75-mg/100-g bodyweight as been used in rats, and a total dose of 7.68-mg/100-g bodyweight has been used in mice, administered in multiple injections as described in Section "Kidney Preparation & Ex vivo Imaging". To date, published in vivo studies have all been performed using a field strength of 7 T, using a three-dimensional gradient recalled echo (GRE) pulse sequence with flow compensation in the read direction. Rat studies were performed using echo time (TE)/repetition time (TR) = 14/70; flip angle (FA) = 25°; resolution = 70.2 × 70.2 × 140 μm^3; and partial Fourier = 6/8. The number of averages (N_{averages}) is adjusted based on SNR in individual 3D images and capability to detect glomeruli above noise fluctuation ($N_{\text{averages}} = 2$ was used, on average, in published studies). Mouse studies were carried out with the following parameters: TE/TR = 14/70; FA = 30°; resolution = 54.7 × 109.4 × 50 μm^3; and partial Fourier = 6/8; N_{averages} was adjusted based on SNR in individual 3D images and capability to detect glomeruli above noise. $N_{\text{averages}} = 3$ was used in published studies.

Respiratory gating was used during imaging to minimize motion. The pneumatic pillow was placed near the kidney. To minimize motion further, we also developed a custom imaging bed with an insert for the RF coil to be fixed with the bed so the animal lies on the bed and RF coil. The animal was positioned such that the kidney rests within the inner diameter of the rings of custom RF coil. A few adjustments to animal position are typically required to optimize the placement of the kidney with respect to the RF coil.

Imaging Kidney Function in Isolated Perfused Kidneys with MRI

The isolated perfused kidney is an important model to investigate local kidney physiology without systemic effects [30, 31]. The kidney from an animal model was isolated with renal vasculature and ureter intact and blood or a blood substitute perfusate is perfused through the kidney to maintain healthy function for a limited time (~1 h). MRI offers the potential to study perfusion and filtration, providing measurements throughout the whole isolated kidney. Targeted and non-targeted contrast agents have been used to visualize contrast agent kinetics within the isolated perfused kidney [25]. We detail the use of dynamic MRI and using two contrast agents within the isolated perfused rat kidney: cationic ferritin (CF) as a targeted agent to investigate the dynamic uptake of targeted macromolecules onto the glomerular basement membrane; and gadolinium diethylenetriamine penta-acetic acid (Gd-DTPA) as non-targeted, freely filtrating, agent to investigate kidney physiology at the scale of the individual nephron.

Preparing the Kidney

We adapted the technique to isolate and resect the rat kidney from Czogalla, et al. [32]. Ligatures were placed around vasculature and a MR compatible catheter was secured within the renal artery by both a tied ligature and glue to the hub of the catheter and renal artery. We used a preservative solution (Lifor) comparable to clinical preservative solutions [33] to preserve the kidney in transport on ice between resection and MR imaging.

Hardware Considerations

A custom MR frame was fabricated to hold the kidney during imaging, secure the RF coil over the kidney, and allow for excess perfusate to be collected and removed. A custom TxRx RF coil was designed similarly as described in the previous Section "Hardware and Experimental Preparations". Coil diameter and number of loops was adjusted to ensure coverage over the kidney (typically N_{loop} =4). One should be careful in placing the coil over the kidney to not let the coil occlude the perfusion line into the kidney.

Perfusion medium containing rodent red blood cells [32, 34] is the most ideal to mimic in vivo conditions and optimize oxygenation to the kidney. However, cell-free perfusion medium has been used in numerous published studies and was chosen for previous published studies [25, 31, 35, 36]. We used a physiological medium containing Krebs-Ringer solution with Fraction V BSA (5.5 g/100 mL), select amino acids [35, 36], and 95/5% O_2/CO_2 by bubbling to mimic physiological conditions. We used perfusion setup that did not re-circulate perfusate. CF was infused with the perfusion medium at a rate of 0.2 mg/min (0.033 mg/mL). Gd-DTPA bolus of 12.5 μmol was administered in 2 mL of perfusate.

Harvard Apparatus offers a Universal Perfusion System that entails a complete setup and offer options for MR compatible transducers. Other custom setups can be used as long as the following are controlled for: pressure (and thus controlling flow), temperature, bubble trap, injection of contrast agents, and are MR compatible.

Imaging

Imaging of both agents used a 3D gradient recalled echo (GRE) protocol with the following parameters: field of view = 20.000 × 13.125 × 14 .080 mm^3, matrix size = 192 × 126 × 64, and resolution = 104.2 × 184.9 × 220.0 μm^3. To image CF dynamics, we used T2*-weighted GRE with the following parameters: TE/TR = 12.6/45, FA = 45°, and acquisition time of = 2.83 min. To image Gd-DTPA kinetics, we used T1-weighted GRE with TE/TR = 3.23/22 ms, FA = 45°, and acquisition time of = 1.38 min. A reduced FOV either with 3D or 2D GRE could be used to achieve higher temporal resolutions.

Following is a description of the imaging experiment we carried out as an example: *Part I, Binding kinetics of macromolecules targeted to the glomerular basement membrane*—Acquire three T2*-weighted image volumes before infusion of CF to establish baseline signal. Begin infusion of CF (0.2 mg/min) for 10 min with continuous imaging occurring. Acquire two image volumes after ceasing CF infusion. *Part II, Free filtration through individual nephrons*—Acquire three T1-weighted image volumes to establish baseline signal. Injection bolus of Gd-DTPA into the perfusion line and acquire continuous image volumes for at least 20 min after injection. The kidney was removed from the perfusion line and manually perfused with fixative.

Post-processing, Analysis, and Validation

CFE-MRI is often used to measure glomerular number (N_{glom}), the distribution of individual glomerular volume (IGV), and the median or mean glomerular volume (V_{glom}). MATLAB (The MathWorks) was used for the majority of published studies [12, 13, 15]. Other software such as Amira (Fisher Scientific) were used for visualization and 3D rendering of data.

There are many approaches to segment CF-labeled glomeruli in MR images. A local adaptive threshold has been used in recent animal studies, imaged at high resolution with respect to glomerulus size in that model. Threshold parameters were optimized in a representative region of interest (ROI) from the image data set. Threshold parameters have also been adjusted between data sets using comparative metrics between data sets, such as the mean value of kidney tissue background or contrast-to-noise ratio (CNR) of labeled glomeruli with respect to tissue background. However, this approach was not robust to image or tissue artifacts. More robust and semi-automated approaches have been developed [19, 20, 37–39]. A semi-automated software package is available online to segment mouse kidney glomeruli [40].

A few methods have been used to determine Individual glomerular volumes: (1) the product of the number of voxels in the segmented glomerulus and the voxel dimensions; (2) model the signal intensity of each CF-labeled glomerulus artifact to a 2D (using just two orthogonal dimensions of the artifact) or 3D Gaussian (using all three orthogonal dimensions of the artifact) and determine the artifact diameter based on the model parameters; and (3) measure line profiles in orthogonal directions from the CF-labeled glomerulus artifact and determine the glomerulus diameter from the width of the profile at half height. Glomerular volume in (2) and (3) is then determined using a spherical model of the glomerulus. Average glomerular volume was previously validated by direct measurement of glomeruli, typically performed by optical imaging and either serial sections or random sampling [15, 41–46] from a representative kidney. Optical clearing and imaging are another potential option to validate MR measurements [47]. Tissue shrinkage should be considered as factor influencing tissue volume in each of these methods for validation [42, 43, 48, 49].

Similar methods as described above were used to analyze dynamic MR signal magnitude and measure kidney function at the scale of individual nephrons. The software AFNI (NIH), originally developed for functional MRI studies in the brain, combined with MATLAB were used to process and analyze 4D (3D + time) MRI data. Time courses in individual voxels were fitted to exponential models to extract information such as glomerulus perfusion and uptake rate of CF. Single nephron filtration fraction and filtration rate were measured through modeling and direct measurement of the time course kinetics. Filtration fraction was determined using area under the curve analysis in a setup where perfusate was not re-circulated and contrast enhancement of Gd-DTPA was visible in nephrons at the time of bolus and again later when the filtered fraction of Gd-DTPA re-appeared in the distal tubule after filtration and passage through the nephron. Grenier et al. have reviewed methods to measure in vivo glomerular filtration rate in the individual kidney using gadolinium contrast agents injected intravenously [50]. These methods could be useful in an isolated perfused kidney apparatus where contrast agents are re-circulated.

Applications in the Human Kidney

Assessment of Human Allografts with CFE-MRI

CFE-MRI has been applied to human kidneys rejected for transplantation to measure the number of functional nephrons and the distribution of glomerular volumes [20]. CFE-MRI was recently used to show the high variability of using biopsies to estimate nephron number [10]. Biopsy-based studies are useful in large population studies, but the factor of high variability significantly impacts measurements in individuals [51]. Human kidneys rejected for transplantation and donated for research were obtained through national and local procurement organizations. Investigators can screen potential kidneys based on donor demographics, disease, and medical history.

Preparing the Kidney

All work was consented by our institution and performed in adequate safety cabinets (typically at least BSL2 level) with the appropriate personal protective equipment and setup to handle live human tissue. Please consult your institution to advise for a safe setup and work environment. Donated kidneys often have wedge biopsies removed, and we have not observed the presence of biopsies to significantly affect CF labeling. We first removed excess fat from the kidney to obtain a more accurate kidney weight. We were careful not to cut the renal artery or kidney. The CF dose was prepared based on kidney weight(25-mg/100-g kidney weight at a concentration of 0.5 mg/mL in phosphate-buffered saline, PBS). We typically prepared the CF solution in 50- or 60-mL syringes for manually perfusion. First, we perfused PBS through the renal artery with 120 mL of PBS. Then, we perfused the kidney with the CF solution. Then, we perfused the kidney with 120 mL of PBS to clear the kidney of remnant unbound CF. Last, we perfused the kidney with 120 mL of neutral buffered 10% formalin (~4% paraformaldehyde).

Imaging

CFE-MRI has been used to visualize CF-labeled glomeruli throughout the human kidney and identify regions of nephron loss. 3D image volumes have been acquired at field strengths of 4.7 T and higher. A quadrature volume coil was used at each field strength and was able to be tuned and matched to the load of the kidney. Dimensions of volume coils used previously had just enough space for a majority of human kidneys to fit inside (inner diameter ~ 70 mm) and an RF window that captured most of or all of the length of the kidney (~100 mm). Human kidneys were typically imaged with an isotropic resolution around 100 μm [20]. Otherwise, a similar sequence was used as outlined in section 'Kidney Preparation and Ex Vivo Imaging'. Lower field strengths typically required higher TEs (e.g. 45 ms at 4.7 T), and higher field strengths required lower TEs (e.g. 15 ms at 9.4 T) to provide contrast of individual CF-labeled glomeruli. The number of averages was adjusted for each system and hardware setup to achieve adequate SNR (~20). Other sequences have been used following to coregister other structural features of the kidney to maps of CF labeled glomeruli.

Post-processing of Nephron Features and Other Structural Features

Glomerular number and glomerular volume in the human kidney were measured by similar methods outlined in Section "Post-processing, Analysis, and Validation". CFE-MRI typically targets perfused glomeruli throughout the kidney. Thus, glomerular number measured by CFE-MRI in the human kidney has been referred to as functioning glomerular or nephron number. Cortex and medulla were also segmented for volume measurements of each in CFE-MR images. Nephron loss has been quantified by a few different methods. One way was to measure cortical volume where nephron loss was present and comparing it to total cortex volume. Glomerular density has also been measured in nearby regions where nephron loss was visible to estimate number of glomeruli lost in those regions.

The human kidney differs from many animal models (e.g. rodents and rabbits) in that human kidneys are sectioned into multiple functioning units called pyramids, whereas many animal models have only one pyramid. CFE-MRI offers the unique capability to visualize whole kidney morphology and thus segmentation of kidney pyramids [19]. Recent reports revealed that pathology is heterogeneous between pyramids, with some pyramids exhibiting significant nephron loss and other pyramids nearly no nephron loss. This offers a new method to quantify the heterogeneity of kidney morphology between individuals and the development of pathology. Other MR pulse sequences can provide additional visualization of the kidney vasculature. Recent work has quantified the branching networks of the kidney vasculature and compared branching networks between human kidneys with different morphology and pathology [52]. Together, these enable new perspectives to use multi-parametric morphology measurements to correlate with the development of human disease and pathology.

Multi-modal Imaging of Glomeruli with Positron Emission Tomography (PET) and MRI

Radioisotopes have also been conjugated to the ferritin molecule (RadioCF), so it may be visible with positron emission tomography (PET) (Fig. 21.1). PET is sensitive to contrast agents, requiring significantly reduced doses for contrast enhancement. The reduced dose required for PET is considered sub-pharmacological and increases the potential for its safe use in patients. We have shown that a PET version of CFE-MRI is feasible to image nephrons in the kidney in vivo and in human kidneys donated for research [53] (Fig. 21.3). This technology, RadioCF-PET, is sensitive to measure nephron density in the kidney and detecting regions of nephron loss.

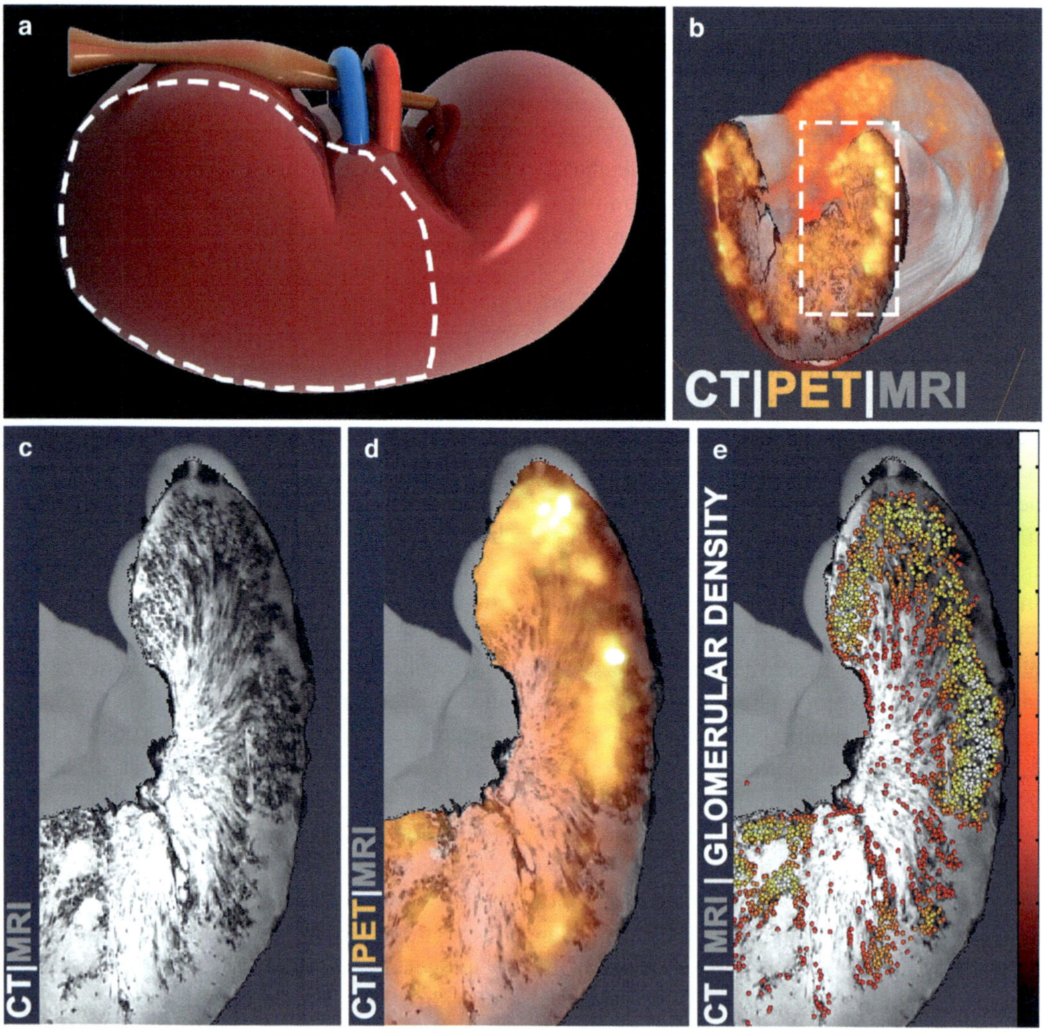

Fig. 21.3 RadioCF-PET to measure nephron mass in a perfused human kidney. (**a**, **b**) A human kidney, rejected for transplantation and consented for research received RadioCF and imaged with: PET for RadioCF enhancement; x-ray-computed tomography (CT) for localization; and CFE-MRI to verify glomerular enhancement. Three-dimensional images were co-registered. (**c–e**) RadioCF-PET revealed RadioCF accumulation in kidney cortex, which was also labeled by CFE-MRI. Color bar scale: 0–20 mm^{-3}. Adapted from Baldelomar et al. [53]

RadioCF-PET has a strong potential to translate the clinical markers of nephrons and nephron loss to aid the development of early clinical diagnostics of kidney disease.

The methods to apply RadioCF-PET in animal models are similar to CFE-MRI. Three-dimensional computed tomography (CT) was performed before 3D PET in both animal models and human kidneys. Dynamic 3D PET images were acquired for 90 min, and the standardize uptake value (SUV) was calculated at 90 min, two half-lives of the contrast agent, to correlate with nephron density. In the human kidney, RadioCF was flushed through the kidney similar as for CFE-MRI, followed by PBS to remove unbound RadioCF from the kidney. A single time-point 3D PET image was then acquired to correlate with nephron density and detect regions of nephron loss. Following PET, a larger dose of non-radioactive CF was administered to the kidney as described in Section "Preparing the Kidney" for glomerular mapping with MRI and validation of the PET signal distribution.

Conclusion

New biomarkers are needed to aid the early detection of kidney dysfunction and disease. Human nephron number and single nephron function are sensitive markers that are directly associated with kidney function. CFE-MRI has been developed for pre-clinical measurements of nephron number and single nephron GFR in animal models of human disease. CFE-MRI has also been applied to isolated human kidneys rejected for transplantation to quantify nephron number in the human kidney. CFE-MRI appears to be non-toxic at MRI detectable doses in rodents [23]. Ferritin has also been used in recent clinical trials as an antigen to enhance vaccinations [54]. We recently developed a human recombinant version of ferritin that allows us to control every step of manufacturing and minimize potential immunogenicity or toxicity in humans. Translation of imaging agents are typically less costly than therapeutic agents [55] but still require significant costs. The relatively high dose required for MRI contrast agents also require lengthy testing for safety and efficacy. However, CFE-MRI still directly impacts human health as a robust tool to study and stage nephron loss in numerous models. For example, CFE-MRI may be used in early safety and efficacy studies of new potential therapies to assess impact on kidney function at early time points before changes in the common clinical metrics such as GFR are detectable. Future efforts are also focused on using CFE-MRI to improve kidney allocation methods and improve the assessment of high-risk kidneys for transplantation that would otherwise be discarded. Other efforts are also underway to improve our understanding how nephrons are coordinated in health and disease. These measurements and more are only capable with tools such as CFE-MRI that can directly detect and map all functioning nephrons.

References

1. Luyckx VA, Brenner BM. The clinical importance of nephron mass. J Am Soc Nephrol. 2010;21(6):898–910.
2. McNamara BJ, Diouf B, Douglas-Denton RN, Hughson MD, Hoy WE, Bertram JF. A comparison of nephron number, glomerular volume and kidney weight in Senegalese Africans and African Americans. Nephrol Dial Transpl. 2010;25(5):1514–20.
3. Nyengaard JR, Bendtsen TF. Glomerular number and size in relation to age, kidney weight, and body surface in normal man. Anatomical Rec. 1992;232(2):194–201.
4. Hoy WE, Hughson MD, Singh GR, Douglas-Denton R, Bertram JF. Reduced nephron number and glomerulomegaly in Australian aborigines: a group at high risk for renal disease and hypertension. Kidney Int. 2006;70(1):104–10.
5. Hoy WE, Hughson MD, Bertram JF, Douglas-Denton R, Amann K. Nephron number, hypertension, renal disease, and renal failure. J Am Soc Nephrol. 2005;16(9):2557–64.
6. Luyckx V, Shukha K, Brenner B. Low nephron number and its clinical consequences. Rambam Maimonides Medical J. 2011;2(4):e0061.
7. Sharma A, Mucino MJ, Ronco C. Renal functional reserve and renal recovery after acute kidney injury. Nephron Clin Pract. 2014;127(1–4):94–100.
8. Denic A, Mathew J, Lerman LO, Lieske JC, Larson JJ, Alexander MP, Poggio E, Glassock RJ, Rule AD. Single-nephron glomerular Filtration rate in healthy adults. New Engl J Medicine. 2017;376(24):2349–57.
9. Denic A, Lieske JC, Chakkera HA, Poggio ED, Alexander MP, Singh P, Kremers WK, Lerman LO,

Rule AD. The substantial loss of nephrons in healthy human kidneys with aging. J Am Soc Nephrol. 2017;28(1):313.
10. Morozov D, Parvin N, Conaway M, Oxley G, Baldelomar E, Cwiek A, deRonde K, Beeman S, Charlton J, Bennett K. Estimating nephron number from biopsies: impact on clinical studies. J Am Soc Nephrol. 2022;33(1):39. https://jasn.asnjournals.org/content/early/2021/11/09/ASN.2021070998
11. Bennett KM, Zhou H, Sumner JP, Dodd SJ, Bouraoud N, Doi K, Star RA, Koretsky AP. MRI of the basement membrane using charged nanoparticles as contrast agents. Magnet Reson Med. 2008;60(3):564–74.
12. Baldelomar EJ, Charlton JR, deRonde KA, Bennett KM. In vivo measurements of kidney glomerular number and size in healthy and Os(/+) mice using MRI. Am J Physiol-Renal Physiol. 2019;317(4):F865–73.
13. Baldelomar EJ, Charlton JR, Beeman SC, Bennett KM. Measuring rat kidney glomerular number and size in vivo with MRI. Am J Physiol-renal. 2018;314(3):F399.
14. Xinpei M, Jiadi X, Honggang C. Functional nanoparticles for magnetic resonance imaging. Wiley Interdiscip Rev Nanomed Nanobiotechnol. 2016;8(6):814–41. https://doi.org/10.1002/wnan.1400.
15. Baldelomar EJ, Charlton JR, Beeman SC, Hann BD, Cullen-McEwen L, Pearl VM, Bertram JF, Wu T, Zhang M, Bennett KM. Phenotyping by magnetic resonance imaging nondestructively measures glomerular number and volume distribution in mice with and without nephron reduction. Kidney Int. 2016;89(2):498–505.
16. Charlton JR, Xu Y, Wu T, deRonde KA, Hughes JL, Dutta S, Oxley GT, Cwiek A, Cathro HP, Charlton NP, Conaway MR, Baldelomar EJ, Parvin N, Bennett KM. Magnetic resonance imaging accurately tracks kidney pathology and heterogeneity in the transition from acute kidney injury to chronic kidney disease. Kidney Int. 2020;99:173.
17. Beeman SC, Zhang M, Gubhaju L, Wu T, Bertram JF, Frakes DH, Cherry BR, Bennett KM. Measuring glomerular number and size in perfused kidneys using MRI. Am J Physiol-renal. 2011;300(6):F1454–7.
18. Charlton JR, Baldelomar EJ, deRonde KA, Cathro HP, Charlton NP, Criswell SJ, Hyatt DM, Nam S, Pearl V, Bennett KM. Nephron loss detected by MRI following neonatal acute kidney injury in rabbits. Pediatr Res. 2019;87:1185.
19. Jennifer RC, Yanzhe X, Neda P, Teresa W, Fei G, Edwin JB, Darya M, Scott CB, Jamal D, Kevin MB. Image analysis techniques to map pyramids, pyramid structure, glomerular distribution, and pathology in the intact human kidney from 3-D MRI. Am J Physiol-renal [Internet]. 2021;321(3):F293–304. https://doi.org/10.1152/ajprenal.00130.2021.
20. Beeman SC, Cullen-McEwen LA, Puelles VG, Zhang M, Wu T, Baldelomar E, Dowling J, Charlton JR, Forbes MS, Ng A, Wu QZ, Armitage JA, Egan GF, Bertram JF, Bennett KM. MRI-based glomerular morphology and pathology in whole human kidneys. Am J Physiol-Renal. 2014;306(11):F1381–90.
21. Danon D, Goldstein L, Marikovsky Y, Skutelsky E. Use of cationized ferritin as a label of negative charges on cell surfaces. J Ultra Mol Struct R. 1972;38(5–6):500–10.
22. Beeman SC, Georges JF, Bennett KM. Toxicity, biodistribution, and ex vivo MRI detection of intravenously injected cationized ferritin. Magnet Reson Med. 2012;69(3):853–61.
23. Charlton JR, Pearl VM, Denotti AR, Lee JB, Swaminathan S, Scindia YM, Charlton NP, Baldelomar EJ, Beeman SC, Bennett KM. Biocompatibility of ferritin-based nanoparticles as targeted MRI contrast agents. Nanomedicine. 2016;12(6):1735–45.
24. Parvin N, Charlton JR, Baldelomar EJ, Derakhshan J, Bennett KM. Mapping vascular and glomerular pathology in a rabbit model of acute kidney injury using MRI. Anat Rec (Hoboken). 2020;303(10):2716–28.
25. Baldelomar EJ, Charlton JR, Bennett KM. Mapping single-nephron filtration in the isolated, perfused rat kidney using magnetic resonance imaging. Am J Physiol Renal Physiol. 2022;323(5):F602–F611. https://doi.org/10.1152/ajprenal.00103.2022.
26. Gregory JAG, Daryl RAK, William AS. Whole animal perfusion fixation for rodents. J Vis Exp. 2012;65:e3564. https://www.jove.com/t/3564
27. Doty FD, Entzminger G, Kulkarni J, Pamarthy K, Staab JP. Radio frequency coil technology for small-animal MRI. NMR Biomed. 2007;20(3):304–25.
28. Insko EK, Bolinger L. Mapping of the radiofrequency field. J Magn Reson Ser A. 1993;103(1):82–5.
29. Morrell GR. A phase-sensitive method of flip angle mapping. Magnet Reson Med. 2008;60(4): 889–94.
30. Taft DR. The isolated perfused rat kidney model: a useful tool for drug discovery and development. Curr Drug Discov Technol. 2003;1(1):97–111. http://www.eurekaselect.com/91098/article
31. D. R B. The isolated perfused rat kidney. Clin Sci. 1978;55(6):513–21. https://doi.org/10.1042/cs0550513.
32. Czogalla JA, Schweda FA, Loffing JA. The mouse isolated perfused kidney technique. J Vis Exp. 2016;117:e54712.
33. Regner KR, Nilakantan V, Ryan RP, Mortensen J, White SM, Shames BD, Roman RJ. Protective effect of Lifor solution in experimental renal ischemia-reperfusion injury. J Surg Res. 2010;164(2):e291–7.
34. Alphonse N. The isolated perfused kidney: possibilities, limitations and results. Kidney Int. 1975;7(1):1–11. https://www.sciencedirect.com/science/article/pii/S0085253815314095.
35. Epstein FH, Brosnan JT, Tange JD, Ross BD. Improved function with amino acids in the isolated perfused kidney. Am J Physiol. 1982;243:F284–92. http://ajprenal.physiology.org/content/ajprenal/243/3/F284.full.pdf.

36. Rahgozar M, Guan Z, Matthias A, Gobe GC, Endre ZH. Angiotensin II facilitates autoregulation in the perfused mouse kidney: an optimized in vitro model for assessment of renal vascular and tubular function. Nephrology (Carlton). 2004;9(5):288–96.
37. Zhang M, Wu T, Beeman SC, Cullen-McEwen L, Bertram JF, Charlton JR, Baldelomar E, Bennett KM. Efficient small blob detection based on local convexity, intensity and shape information. IEEE T Med Imaging. 2016;35(4):1127–37.
38. Yanzhe X, Teresa W, Fei G, Jennifer RC, Kevin MB. Improved small blob detection in 3D images using jointly constrained deep learning and Hessian analysis. Sci Rep-uk. 2020;10(1):326. https://doi.org/10.1038/s41598-019-57223-y.
39. Zhang M, Wu T, Bennett KM. Small blob identification in medical images using regional features from optimum scale. Ieee T Bio-med Eng. 2015;62(4):1051–62.
40. Wu Lab. Mouse kidney glomeruli segmentation [Internet]. 2022. https://labs.engineering.asu.edu/wulab/resources/.
41. Hann BD, Baldelomar EJ, Charlton JR, Bennett KM. Measuring the intrarenal distribution of glomerular volumes from histological sections. Am J Physiol-renal. 2016;310(11):F1328–36.
42. Weibel ER. Stereological methods. In: Practical methods for biological morphometry, vol. 1. Cambridge: Academic Press; 1979.
43. Weibel ER. Stereological methods. In: Theoretical foundations, vol. 2. Cambridge: Academic Press; 1979.
44. Hoy WE, Douglas-Denton RN, Hughson MD, Cass A, Johnson K, Bertram JF. A stereological study of glomerular number and volume: preliminary findings in a multiracial study of kidneys at autopsy. Kidney Int. 2003;(63):S31–7.
45. Cullen-McEwen LA, Armitage JA, Nyengaard JR, Moritz KM, Bertram JF. A design-based method for estimating glomerular number in the developing kidney. Am J Physiol-renal. 2011;300(6):F1448–53.
46. Bertram JF. Analyzing renal glomeruli with the new stereology. In: International review of cytology, vol. 161. Elsevier; 1995. p. 111–72.
47. Victor GP, Alexander NC, John FB. Clearly imaging and quantifying the kidney in 3D. Kidney Int [Internet]. 2021;100(4):780–6. https://www.sciencedirect.com/science/article/pii/S0085253821005652.
48. Amann K, Nichols C, Tornig J, Schwarz U. Effect of ramipril, nifedipine, and moxonidine on glomerular morphology and podocyte structure in experimental renal failure. Nephrol Dial Transplant. 1996;11:1003–11. http://ndt.oxfordjournals.org.eres.library.manoa.hawaii.edu/content/11/6/1003.full.pdf+html.
49. Christian SH, Kerstin A, Johannes S, Barbara B, Ulrich M, Andrea H. Glomerular and renal vascular structural changes in α8 integrin-deficient mice. J Am Soc Nephrol. 2003;14(9):2288. http://jasn.asnjournals.org/content/14/9/2288.abstract.
50. Grenier N, Mendichovszky I, de Senneville BD, Roujol S, Desbarats P, Pedersen M, Wells K, Frokiaer J, Gordon I. Measurement of glomerular Filtration rate with magnetic resonance imaging: principles, limitations, and expectations. Semin Nucl Med. 2008;38(1):47–55.
51. Charlton JR, Abitbol CL. Can renal biopsy be used to estimate Total nephron number? Clin J Am Soc Nephrol. 2017;12(4):553–5.
52. Parvin N, Charlton JR, Baldelomar EJ, Derakhshan JJ, Bennett KM. Mapping vascular and glomerular pathology in a rabbit model of neonatal acute kidney injury using MRI. Anat Rec (Hoboken). 2020;303(10):2716–28.
53. Baldelomar EJ, Reichert DE, Shoghi KI, Beeman SC, Charlton JR, Strong L, Fettig N, Klaas A, Bennett KM. Mapping nephron mass in vivo using positron emission tomography. Am J Physiol. 2021;320(2):F183–92.
54. ClinicalTrials.gov. Influenza HA ferritin vaccine, alone or in prime-boost regimens with an influenza DNA vaccine in healthy adults. National Library of Medicine (US). 2000. https://clinicaltrials.gov/ct2/show/NCT03186781.
55. Nunn AD. The cost of developing imaging agents for routine clinical use. Investig Radiol. 2006;41(3):206–12.

Part III

Advanced Methods and Applications

22 CEST MRI for Monitoring Kidney Diseases

Julia Stabinska, Jochen Keupp, and Michael T. McMahon

Introduction

MRI has been actively explored in the last several decades for assessing renal function by providing several physiological information, including glomerular filtration rate, renal plasma flow, tissue oxygenation, and water diffusion. Within MRI, the developing field of chemical exchange saturation transfer (CEST) has potential to provide further functional information for diagnosing kidney diseases. The kidney is one of the most important excretory organs, clearing a variety of small organic molecules through filtration and maintaining electrolyte and water homeostasis through transport systems. Many metabolites are freely filtered across the glomerulus, while others are actively secreted or reabsorbed from the tubules. In addition, the kidney plays a crucial role in the synthesis and metabolism of amino acids that are essential for maintaining whole-body pH homeostasis. Under normal physiological conditions, the systemic acid-base equilibrium is regulated by reabsorbing bicarbonate filtered by the glomeruli and excreting acids and ammonia into the urine. As renal function declines, changes in metabolite concentrations and pH can occur via alterations in filtration, secretion, reabsorption, synthesis, and metabolism due to pathological changes in the kidney [1, 2]. In fact, serum creatinine (SCr) and cystatin C concentrations are widely used to estimate glomerular filtration rate (GFR) and remain a useful clinical tool for assessing renal function. However, creatinine estimates of GFR may not be suitable for individuals with unstable kidney function (e.g., pregnant women, patients with serious comorbid conditions, and hospitalized patients, particularly those with acute renal failure) and people with unusual muscle mass or diet [3]. Furthermore, these biomarkers give a measure of overall renal function, but they cannot distinguish the contribution of each kidney separately. SCr is both a late and unspecific marker of renal disease, observed only with marked tubular damage. Considering these limitations, novel and more accurate metabolic biomarkers for the diagnosis and monitoring of kidney disease are needed.

This book highlights the utility of a variety of MRI technologies, which can be applied to patients on clinical scanners. One of the attractive features of MR is the ability to noninvasively

J. Stabinska · M. T. McMahon (✉)
F.M. Kirby Research Center for Functional Brain Imaging, Kennedy Krieger Institute, Baltimore, MD, USA

Russell H. Morgan Department of Radiology and Radiological Science, Johns Hopkins University School of Medicine, Baltimore, MD, USA
e-mail: mcmahon@mri.jhu.edu

J. Keupp
Philips Research, Hamburg, Germany

S. D. Serai, K. Darge (eds.), *Advanced Clinical MRI of the Kidney*,
https://doi.org/10.1007/978-3-031-40169-5_22

detect and probe levels of multiple tissue metabolites, including measuring fat in the kidney, as described in Chap. 14. In fact, proton (^{1}H) and phosphorus (^{31}P) magnetic resonance spectroscopy (MRS) have been previously used to measure metabolite level changes in ischemia-reperfusion injury occurring during kidney transplantation [4–6]. Nevertheless, the clinical use of in vivo MRS is limited by its poor sensitivity, low spatial coverage, and long acquisition times. To overcome some of these limitations, CEST MRI has been developed to amplify the detection of low concentration endogenous metabolites and proteins present in biological tissues or exogenous compounds administered externally [7–9]. Both endogenous produced molecules as well as exogenously administered CEST agents have been exploited for providing functional information related to kidney diseases.

Numerous preclinical studies have demonstrated the potential of CEST imaging for detecting molecular and cellular changes associated with various renal and urinary diseases such as diabetic nephropathy [10], unilateral ureter obstruction [11], kidney fibrosis [12], sepsis-induced acute kidney injury (AKI) [13], and acute renal allograft rejection [14]. Further, because of its high sensitivity to pH changes, contrast-enhanced CEST imaging has been applied to measure renal pH values and induced pH alterations following AKI [15, 16], reperfusion ischemia [17], and chronic kidney disease [18]. The results of these studies suggest that CEST imaging offers the potential to provide additional functional information by quantifying changes in pH and metabolite levels associated with kidney disease and therefore may usefully complement the existing MRI techniques. In this chapter, we will introduce the basic concepts of CEST imaging and describe the strengths and limitations of this technology for renal CEST imaging on clinical MRI systems.

Part I: CEST MRI Physics and Acquisition Protocols

Principles of CEST Imaging

CEST is a new technique that enables the indirect detection of molecules possessing mobile protons in exchange with water. Because of this, CEST makes MRI sensitive to endogenous or exogenous molecules that possess suitable protons. The generation of contrast is based on a selective irradiation with a radiofrequency pulse at the specific absorption frequency of the exchanging proton, followed by a subsequent transfer, due to chemical exchange with bulk water, of the saturated signal. In a CEST experiment, a long radiofrequency (RF) saturation pulse or train of pulses is applied at the resonance frequency of the exchangeable solute protons, distinguished from the water resonance by the chemical shift. This results in equalization of the number of spins aligned with the magnetic field and those oriented against the magnetic field, destroying the MR signal and creating a condition known as "saturation." This saturation can be transferred to water when the labile protons on the solute pool physically exchange with the water protons. As a result, the water pool becomes partially saturated and the water magnetization decreases with the amount based on the concentration of the solute protons, exchange rate, chemical shift, saturation pulse strength, and relaxation times. This "chemical exchange saturation transfer" effect leads to a reduction in the water MR signal and can be measured using routine imaging sequences (Fig. 22.1). The exchange rate of the solute labile protons to bulk water pool protons must be slower than the chemical shift difference between them to allow sufficient RF saturation of the protons of interest. While maintaining the solute pool in saturation for a few seconds by prolonged RF irradiation, the water signal reduction accumulates over time and leads to a strong amplification in the order of 100× to 1000× as compared to direct MR detection of the solute protons.

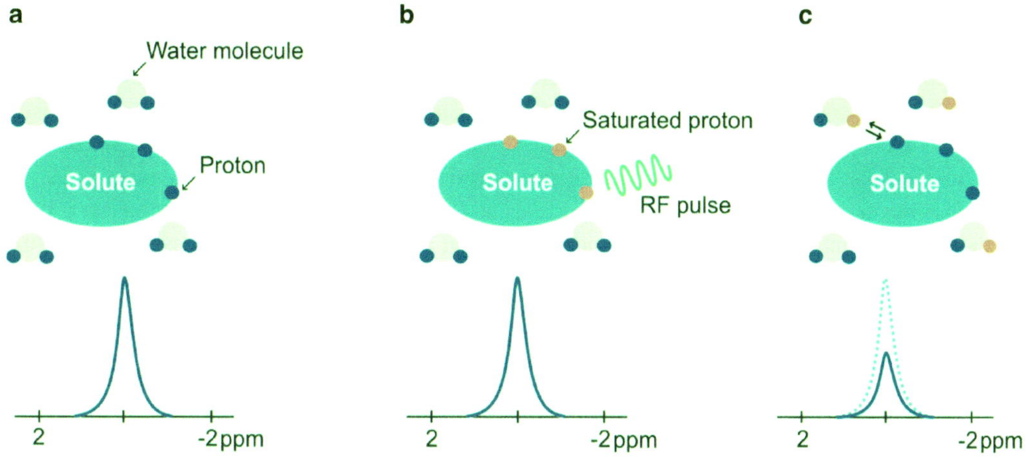

Fig. 22.1 Basic mechanism for chemical exchange saturation transfer (CEST) MRI contrast. (**a**) Endogenous or exogenous compounds with exchangeable protons (solute pool) are surrounded by water molecules (water pool); (**b**) application of a saturation RF pulse at the resonance frequency of the labile protons nulls the MRI signal of these protons; and (**c**) as the solute molecules and water exchange hydrogen atoms, the number of saturated protons in the water pool increases, causing a measurable reduction in the MRI signal.

CEST Contrast Agents

In the more than 20 years since CEST was first described [7, 19], numerous compounds have been investigated for their suitability for clinical CEST imaging, with a strong focus on endogenous metabolites and externally administrated contrast agents (exogenous agents), including a number of naturally occurring substances. CEST agents can be divided into two groups: paramagnetic CEST compounds (paraCEST) containing metallic ions that induce a large chemical shift [20–22], and diamagnetic CEST (diaCEST) molecules with chemical shifts within 6 ppm from water resonance [19, 23]. The latter group is particularly promising for clinical applications, as many diaCEST agents are well tolerated and/or biodegradable. Most endogenous diaCEST compounds contain hydroxyl (–OH), amine (–NH_2), or amide (–NH) functional groups with chemical shifts of around 0.5–1.5 ppm, 1.8–3 ppm, and ~3.5 ppm, respectively. Over the years, endogenous CEST MRI has emerged as a promising clinical tool to detect and monitor the progression of many diseases, including strokes [24, 25], cancer [26–31], neurodegenerative diseases [32, 33], and musculoskeletal disorders [34–36]. Nevertheless, as many endogenous CEST agents are present in biological tissues and organs with overlapping labile protons, the interpretation of the CEST signals from different labile protons may be challenging. In this context, a major advantage of the exogenous agents is that they can be highlighted by subtracting post-administration and pre-administration images. Another advantage is that these probes can possess larger chemical shifts, which potentially provides higher specificity than molecules that are endogenously present in tissue.

Over the past two decades, dozens of CEST-responsive agents have been designed and tested in various animal models, with many of these in clinical usage for other purposes [37–39]. Among these, the triiodobenzene contrast agents are particularly interesting (including iopamidol and ioversol), as they are routinely used for X-ray and CT examinations, and have demonstrated promise for CEST MRI-based pH mapping of kidney, bladder, and solid tumors in humans on clinical MRI scanners [40–42]. Naturally occurring D-glucose is another example of a suitable MRI agent, which can be monitored by CEST and has been shown to provide information on metabolic activity both preclinically and in humans, potentially enabling differentiation of malignant tumors from benign lesions [43–47]. Moreover, a recent preclinical study showed that glucoCEST MRI could also be used to spatially map renal glucose content and assist in determining if there is acute renal allograft rejection [14]. It is anticipated that other agents may be translated into the clinic in the near future. Interested readers are referred to several excellent reviews summarizing the development and applications of endogenous and exogenous contrast agents for CEST MRI [19, 37, 39, 48, 49].

CEST pH Imaging

One of the major strengths of CEST MRI is the ability to measure tissue pH due to the pH sensitivity of the chemical exchange between labile protons of the low-concentrated solute pool and water protons. CEST detects low concentrations of contrast agent through the application of saturation pulses on labile protons, which can have different frequency shifts, a major advantage for pH imaging, and it is important to create pH maps that are independent of agent concentration, which can be accomplished using probes with two distinct labile protons. For instance, the most widely used variant of CEST to date, amide proton transfer weighted (APTw) MRI, has emerged as a noninvasive pH-weighted imaging technique for detecting lactic acidosis during ischemic stroke [50]. A slight decrease in pH in the ischemic region leads to a decrease in exchange rate of the amide protons, and as a result, a decrease in the CEST effect at 3.5 ppm is observed. Nevertheless, the main limitation of APTw MRI for pH imaging is its relatively low sensitivity to detect small pH changes. While others have put forth alternative strategies for pH imaging using additional protons that have pH dependencies [51–53], there is still the general limitation that the endogenous CEST signal depends not only on pH but also on the concentration of the labile proton pool, so changes in the local protein concentration will affect the CEST contrast too; there is no prior knowledge on this concentration.

To overcome these limitations, exogenous pH-responsive CEST agents can be used for renal pH imaging. Contrast media are excreted primarily by glomerular filtration, ensuring a high concentration of the agent in the kidney, and hence enhancing the sensitivity of the pH measurements. Lopamidol was the first contrast agent used for CEST-based pH mapping [38]. The advantage of using this compound as a CEST agent lies in the fact that it possesses two amide groups with different chemical shifts of 4.2 and 5.5 ppm, respectively, which can be selectively saturated and which exhibit different pH responses. Thus, the ratio of the CEST contrast at these two frequencies can be calculated and used to obtain concentration-independent pH maps via a calibration curve, which has been termed ratiometric pH mapping [38]. So far, the feasibility of renal pH imaging using iopamidol has mostly been explored in preclinical studies on high magnetic field scanners [15–18]. Nevertheless, the slow/intermediate exchange rates and large chemical shifts of the two amide groups are suitable for translation of iopamidol-based renal pH mapping to a variety of patients on 3-T MRI scanners. A description of some of the initial studies in humans is provided later in this chapter.

Basic Strategies for CEST MRI Acquisition

In a basic CEST experiment, labile protons in a solute are saturated using a long RF irradiation pulse or pulse train with a duration t_{sat} and power level B_1 tuned to the labile proton offset from the water protons (chemical shift or saturation frequency offset $\Delta\omega$). Due to hardware constraints with respect to the RF amplifier duty cycle and specific absorption rate (SAR) limits, long continuous-wave RF irradiation is usually not applicable on clinical scanners, and a train of N short pulses with a duration t_{pd}, separated by delays t_{ipd}, must be used instead (Fig. 22.2a). Besides rectangular pulses, more sophisticated pulse shapes such as Gaussian, Sinc, Fermi, or spin-lock pulses can be used for CEST preparation. To increase the specificity of CEST imaging for certain functional groups, the above-

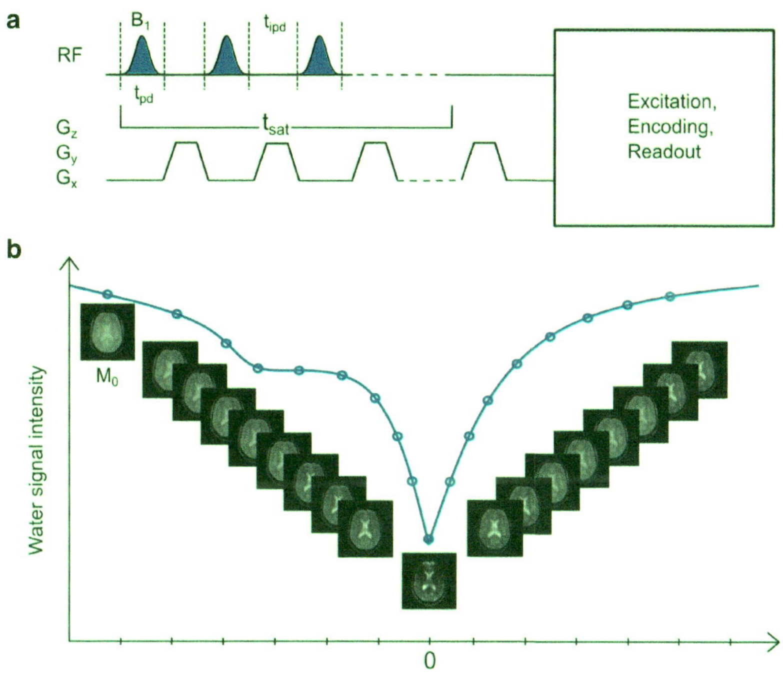

Fig. 22.2 A simplified schematic of a chemical exchange saturation transfer (CEST) pulse sequence and typical Z-spectrum. (**a**) Magnetization preparation for CEST imaging is achieved by applying a train of radio-frequency (RF) saturation pulses characterized by pulse duration, t_{pd}, interpulse delay, t_{ipd}, duty cycle (t_{pd}/t_{ipd}), and irradiation power B_1. After saturation at a frequency offset $\Delta\omega$, the prepared magnetization is measured using a fast readout sequence. (**b**) Repeating this sequence at different frequency offsets yields a set of saturated images. After normalizing these images with an unsaturated image M_0, the so-called Z-spectrum is obtained in each voxel [54]

mentioned parameters in the pre-saturation module are commonly optimized using multi-pool Bloch-McConnell simulations and in vitro experiments [55]. A more advanced option to overcome the limits on maximum pulse duration is to utilize a time-interleaved parallel transmission (pTX) technique, which uses multiple transmit RF channels to increase the duty cycle of the RF saturation pulse train to 100% over multiple seconds, thus allowing the generation of stronger CEST signals [56–58]. In fact, a preliminary study has shown that the pTx-based continuous wave RF irradiation can be advantageous for CEST-based pH mapping by maximizing the iopamidol CEST signal [59].

Similar to other MRI techniques, CEST data acquisition requires a robust readout with little image distortion, high SNR, and the shortest possible scan time. These requirements are constrained by the large number of saturation offsets (typically 6–30) needed to sufficiently sample the so-called Z-spectrum (including the CEST pools and adjacent frequencies for B_0 correction) and the long saturation time (in the order of seconds) used to achieve a high labeling efficiency. In a typical CEST experiment, the CEST sequence is repeated at different offsets within a specific range to collect a series of images. After normalizing the images acquired after pre-saturation with an unsaturated image M_0, the Z-spectrum in each voxel is obtained (Fig. 22.2b). While prolonged data collection might be acceptable when examining motionless regions such as the brain, pelvis, spine, or extremities, reducing acquisition time is crucial to limit motion artifacts in moving organs such as the heart, kidney, or liver. Along with accelerated acquisitions, specific motion compensation methods may be required for renal CEST imaging, covered in the following section, e.g., guided breathing. Furthermore, high temporal resolution is required to detect rapid CEST signal changes during the first glomerular passage of contrast medium to maximize the sensitivity of pH mapping. To speed up CEST acquisition, 2D single-shot sequences are usually used, including echo planar imaging (EPI), turbo spin-echo (TSE), gradient echo (GRE), gradient and spin-echo (GRASE), and fast imaging with steady-state precession (FISP) [60]. Generally, GRE and EPI CEST can achieve a shorter acquisition time than TSE CEST, but typically offer lower SNR efficiency and are more susceptible to B_0-field inhomogeneity artifacts that are common in body applications. Because multi-slice CEST acquisition typically suffers from contrast differences between different slices resulting from the time-dependent saturation loss, 3D acquisition is preferred for volumetric CEST imaging. More advanced methods now provide more sophisticated sampling schemes, such as 3D radial or spiral acquisitions. A substantial acceleration of 3D CEST acquisition can be achieved using advanced data sampling patterns [61, 62], the keyhole technique [63], and compressed sensing reconstruction [64].

Additional Considerations

Acquisition Strategies to Account for Motion

For CEST MRI protocols, kidney images are acquired over a relatively long period (up to several minutes), which makes this technique particularly susceptible to motion artifacts from a variety of sources including respiratory, cardiac, gastrointestinal, and voluntary movements. Because the in vivo CEST signals are relatively small, typically even 1–2% of motion-related signal fluctuations can create large errors in the contrast maps [65]. Therefore, motion correction and co-registration are essential steps in CEST MRI post-processing.

One of the most commonly used acquisition-based correction methods in renal MRI is respiratory triggering. However, the combination of a typical RF irradiation module with a respiratory trigger is not straightforward, as the length of the CEST saturation module usually exceeds a single breathing period. This issue has been addressed by Keupp et al., who proposed a technique in which pulsed RF saturation can be applied over multiple breathing cycles and data acquisition is placed in the end-expiratory phase [66]. If pTx is used for RF irradiation, an additional waiting time with no RF saturation is introduced in some of the breathing periods after acquisition to allow high-power saturation while maintaining SAR levels below the limits [59]. Despite its relatively high robustness to the breathing-related motion, respiratory triggering might significantly prolong the scan time and has reduced temporal resolution; this limits the utility of this method for monitoring changes in signal due to exogenous CEST agents in the vascular and tubular compartments of the kidney.

Another interesting approach that has previously been used to prospectively minimize the respiratory motion in renal CEST acquisition is a guided (timed) breathing technique [67, 68], which utilizes differences in noises produced during the image acquisition (the buzzing noise) and CEST saturation period. Subjects are asked to hold their breath for the acquisition and take the next breath after the completion of data collection. In contrast to multiple long breath-holds approach, this breathing strategy does not require high respiratory capacity as the repetition time of a CEST sequence is usually in the order of few seconds (~6 s), which is consistent with a comfortable respiration rate. Recently, a novel approach based on the use of interleaved volumetric EPI navigators (vNavs) to perform real-time motion correction for CEST has been proposed, but has not yet been tested for body applications on clinical scanners [69]. None of these acquisition-based techniques are sufficient for fully correcting motion, so post-processing techniques have also been developed to correct motion in CEST acquisition [70, 71]. At this time there is still active work needed to improve motion handling for CEST imaging.

Acquisition Strategies to Account for B_0 and B_1 Field Inhomogeneity

Similar to other chemical shift-based methods, CEST MRI is susceptible to static magnetic field inhomogeneity. In addition to image distortions, local B_0 shifts cause an additional frequency offset in each voxel, leading to errors in CEST quantification. Compared with the brain applications, abdominal CEST MRI is particularly heavily affected by the B_0 inhomogeneity arising from differences in magnetic susceptibility between air, soft tissues, and bones. Furthermore, B_0 inhomogeneity may vary over time induced by physiological motion. Accurate correction of the B_0 shifts is, therefore, essential for reliable CEST measurements in the body. The water-shift maps can be obtained using a water-shift referencing method (WASSR) [72] or fitted from a densely-sampled Z-spectrum. Another promising approach that has recently been applied to correct CEST images from the breast [73] and kidney [68] is the multi-point Dixon method, which uses data acquired using a multi-echo GRE sequence (with three or more echoes) to create B_0 maps. If CEST and B_0 information can be obtained from the same sequence in a similar manner as in the Dixon methods, accuracy of B_0 corrections is increased and remains robust in case of shift in the frequency references (e.g., by repeated frequency calibration) or dynamic changes of inhomogeneity.

The homogeneity of the RF transmit field is another important parameter that affects the quality of the CEST contrast. To achieve maximum CEST contrast, the saturation labeling efficiency must be optimized. In general, higher exchange rates require higher B_1 amplitudes which in turn amplify the direct water saturation (called the spillover effect). B_1 inhomogeneity can result in an increase or decrease in the applied RF power, leading to either a reduction in the labeling efficiency or an increase in spillover, and thus inaccuracies in CEST quantification. B_1 homogeneity can be improved by pTx methods. Remaining B_1 issues can be captured by B_1 mapping methods including, e.g., the double-angle approach [74], the Bloch-Siegert shift method [75], and the WASABI technique that allows simultaneous water shift and B_1 mapping [76]. Because of the non-linear and tissue type–dependent change of CEST signals with B_1, correction remains a challenge for post-processing.

Acquisition Strategies to Account for Fat

One of the main challenges with renal CEST MRI is the presence of fat signals originating from the perirenal fat surrounding the kidneys, and the renal sinus fat is located around the renal hilum. Fat can affect in vivo CEST imaging in two ways: First, the inherent differences in the resonance frequencies of fat and water protons cause chemical shift artifacts, potentially confounding image interpretation; second, it complicates the appearance of the Z-spectra and thus may lead to erroneous CEST effects [77]. In fact, the results of several CEST studies in the human breast [73] and on kidney transplants [78] indicate that in particular the APT signal at 3.5 ppm strongly depends on TE and fat fraction. Several techniques enabling the correction of fat-induced artifacts are available, including chemical-shift based approaches (SPAIR, SPIR, STIR), section-selective water-excitation, the use of a novel normalization of CEST data [79], and Dixon-based water-fat separation [80]. Most conventional fat suppression techniques via RF pulses are not sufficient for CEST, as fat signals need to be reduced to a level well below 1%. Dixon-based techniques appear to be particularly promising for breast and renal CEST MRI [73, 78]. In Dixon-based CEST imaging, the multi-point Dixon post-processing is used to obtain water-only images from the CEST images acquired at different echo times. These water-only images are then used to calculate fat-free CEST effects as shown in Fig. 22.3 [73]. Another potential advantage of the CEST-Dixon approach is that it provides a perfectly co-registered B_0 map, which can be utilized for the B_0 correction of the CEST data.

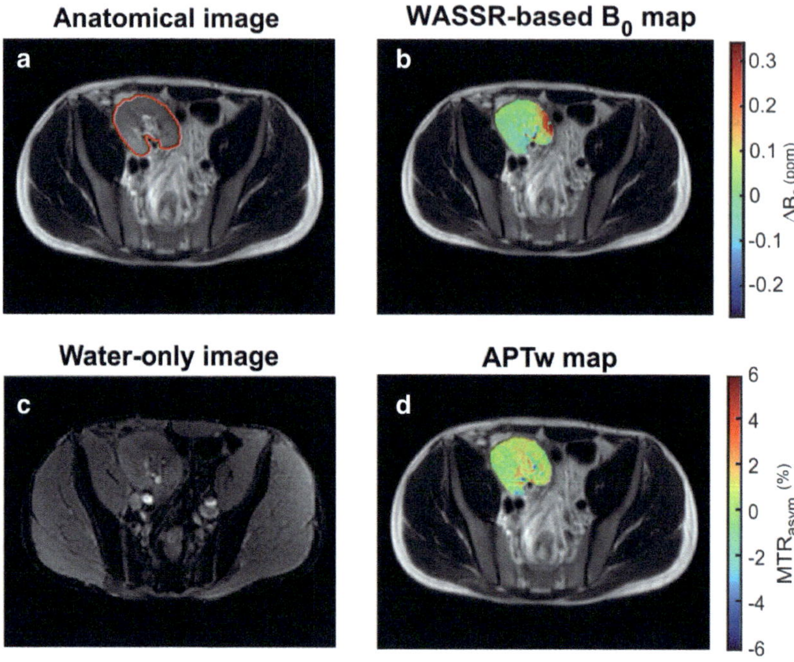

Fig. 22.3 Exemplary T2-weighted anatomical image of the lower abdomen with a segmented kidney, a B_0 map generated using the water saturation shift referencing (WASSR) approach, a water-only image obtained using the 2-pt Dixon water-fat decomposition method, and the corresponding amide proton transfer-weighted (APTw) map. (**a**) The renal transplant placed in the right iliac fossa is clearly visible in the T2w image; (**b**) the B_0 map of the renal allograft shows B_0-field variations in the range between −0.1 ppm and 0.4 ppm. The quality of the (**c**) water-only image is good with only a few water-fat swaps at the subcutaneous fat-abdominal muscle interface, which do not affect the (**d**) APT quantification in the renal graft. Adapted with permission from Stabinska et al. [78]

Part II: Post-processing and Data Analysis Methods

Z-spectra Analysis

Saturation transfer pathways in biological tissues are very complex, making the quantification and interpretation of in vivo Z-spectra challenging. Besides the CEST effects from metabolites or exogenous CEST agents, semi-solid macromolecular magnetization transfer, direct water saturation (spillover effect), and exchange-relayed nuclear Overhauser effects (NOEs) are typically observed in the in vivo Z-spectrum. The magnetization transfer ratio (MTR) can be calculated as:

$$\mathrm{MTR} = \frac{S_0 - S_{\mathrm{sat}}(+\Delta\omega)}{S_0}$$

where $+\Delta\omega$ is the frequency offset of the solute pool, S_{sat} is the signal intensity measured after applying RF saturation pulses, and S_0 refers to the signal intensity that is obtained either without pre-saturation pulse or when the saturation pulse is applied far from the water resonance (≥20 ppm). The confounding effects of spillover and concomitant magnetization transfer can be partially eliminated by using a reference scan that has no contribution from exchange processes. Thus, to quantify the CEST effects, the asymmetry of magnetization transfer ratio ($\mathrm{MTR_{asym}}$) is obtained as follows:

$$\mathrm{MTR}_{\mathrm{asym}} = \frac{S_{\mathrm{sat}}(-\Delta\omega)}{S_0} - \frac{S_{\mathrm{sat}}(+\Delta\omega)}{S_0}$$

where $S_{\mathrm{sat}}(-\Delta\omega)$ is the signal intensity measured after the saturation pulses at the opposite side of the water resonance relative to the frequency offset of the solute pool $+\Delta\omega$.

Other advanced methods to isolate pure CEST effects include multi-pool Lorentzian fitting [81], Lorentzian difference [25], the extrapolated semisolid MT model reference (EMR) approach [82], or multi-pool Bloch McConnell fitting [83]. For exogenous agent studies, Z-spectral analysis is not always necessary, as the pre-contrast image can be subtracted from the post-contrast image to extract the amount of signal loss associated with the CEST contrast agent. The amount of saturation frequencies that can be collected based on motion and acquisition time considerations will impact which of these methods is chosen.

pH Mapping Using Ratiometric Analysis

For pH mapping, the ratio of two $\mathrm{MTR_{asym}}$values obtained using one of the above-mentioned methods can be utilized to determine a concentration-independent metric, R_{ST}.

For CEST-responsive agents with more than one labile proton group separated by a large chemical shift, a ratiometric analysis of two CEST effects measured using the same RF irradiation power level can be calculated as:

$$R_{\mathrm{ST}} = \frac{\mathrm{MTR_{asym}}(\delta_1)}{\mathrm{MTR_{asym}}(\delta_2)}.$$

These can also be calculated using the ratio of MTR at δ_1 and δ_2 instead. Alternatively, the ratio of CEST effects at the same chemical shift obtained under different RF power levels can be used:

$$R_{\mathrm{ST}} = \frac{\mathrm{MTR_{asym}}(B_{1a})}{\mathrm{MTR_{asym}}(B_{1b})}.$$

However, when CEST MRI is performed at lower magnetic field strengths (B_0 <7 T), the conventional ratiometric analysis may be susceptible to the confounding concomitant saturation transfer effects and direct water saturation. To resolve the overlapping CEST effects and extend the range of pH detection, a generalized approach combining the use of the multipool Lorentzian model and mixing both RF power level and chemical shift for the ratiometric analysis has been proposed [84]:

$$R_{\mathrm{ST}} = \frac{\mathrm{MTR_{asym}}(\delta_1, B_{1a})}{\mathrm{MTR_{asym}}(\delta_2,\ B_{1b})}.$$

This generalized ratiometric analysis of resolved CEST effects extends the pH detection range of iopamidol from 5.5–7.0 to 5.5–7.5 at a sub-high magnetic field of 4.7 T. This is done by taking the ratio of the CEST effect at 5.5 ppm measured under B_1 of 2.0 μT to that at 4.2 ppm obtained with B_1 of 1.0 μT.

To determine the relation between the R_{ST} value and pH, a calibration curve needs to be established in a phantom experiment. For this purpose, z-spectra of iopamidol samples, dissolved in phosphate-buffered saline or human blood serum solution [18] and titrated to physiologically relevant pH values, are acquired under different experimental conditions. Next, the pH calibration curve is obtained using a polynomial fitting of R_{ST} values as a function of pH. The same calibration equation can be subsequently applied to measure pH in the kidney.

Part III: Results and Clinical Applications

Endogenous CEST MRI of the Kidney

In the kidney, CEST contrast can originate from different metabolites in blood, urine, and cellular and interstitial components. Urea is the most abundant solute in the urine that also happens to be an excellent natural CEST agent as it poses two C-bound amine groups with exchangeable protons. As early as 1998, Guivel-Sharen et al. identified urea as a major contributor to the kidney/urine chemical exchange at ca. 1 ppm in ex vivo tissue samples [8]. Two years later, Dagher et al. demonstrated for the first time the feasibility of endogenous CEST MRI by examining the kidneys of healthy subjects on a clinical 1.5-T scanner [85]. They observed variable saturation differences of 5–25% peaking at around 1.56 ppm in normal renal parenchyma and around 15% in urine samples. Over a decade later, Vinogradov et al. demonstrated urea-weighted CEST maps of the kidneys at 3 T, showing higher medullary urea CEST signal in "hydrated" healthy volunteers compared with "dehydrated" subjects. This observation may reflect either a decrease in urinary pH or an increase in urea concentration following food/water uptake [86] and therefore requires further clarification. In a systematic in vitro study, Stabinska et al. characterized the proton exchange properties of urea using both water-exchange (WEX) NMR spectroscopy and CEST and showed that in the physiologically relevant pH range urea protons undergo slow exchange with water protons, producing relatively low CEST contrast especially as pH becomes neutral [87]. Besides urea, other abundant kidney metabolites such as creatinine, creatine, glutamine, glutamate, and alanine showed pH- and concentration-dependent CEST effects under physiological conditions at 3 T, which may potentially overlap with the urea signal in vivo [87]. More recently, endogenous CEST MRI was employed to measure in vivo CEST effects in renal transplant recipients on a clinical 3-T scanner. In line with prior research, the highest MTR_{asym} values were measured at around 1 ppm, followed by the effects at ~2 ppm and ~3.5 ppm that can be attributed to hydroxyl (and urea), amine, and amide protons, respectively. Further, preliminary data collected in a renal cell carcinoma patient suggest that CEST-mDixon method shows promise in detecting tumor necrosis [68]. It will be interesting to see if these signals may be good markers for progression in kidney disease or if they can be used to detect injury.

Exogenous pH Imaging for Abdominal Applications

Despite encouraging results from many preclinical studies, to date, only a few publications have explored the utility of CEST-based pH mapping on clinical scanners. The feasibility of this technique on a 3-T MRI system was first demonstrated for measuring pH in the kidneys of a rat [66] and healthy human subjects [59, 88]. Using the multi-cycle respiratory trigger and alternating pTX approach explained above (Fig. 22.4) and a 19-offset acquisition scheme, relatively high CEST effects at 4.2 and 5.5 ppm (up to 20%) were measured in the renal pelvis between 7 and 20 min after iopamidol injection [59]. Lower contrast was observed in the medulla but was still sufficient in some areas to generate pixel-based pH maps (Fig. 22.5). The potential of iopamidol-enhanced CEST MRI to provide in vivo renal pH maps at 3 T was later confirmed by McMahon and colleagues (as shown in Fig. 22.6) using a 5-saturation offset method to reduce the acquisition time substantially [42]. As can be seen, using this approach at around 3 min after injection, a more uniform contrast can be observed in the kidney, which is known to be the nephrogenic phase from multi-phase spiral CT studies using iodinated contrast [89]. Further, Muller-Lutz et al. validated the accuracy of this technique by comparing CEST-based pH values obtained in the bladder with urinary pH values measured using pH electrode [40]. All of these studies sug-

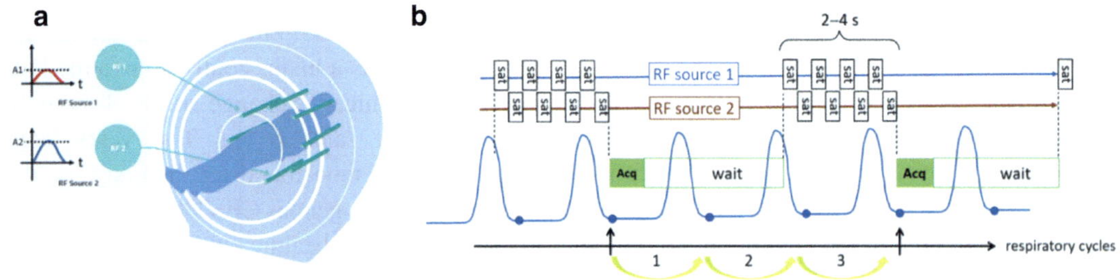

Fig. 22.4 Alternated parallel transmission (pTx) may be used via the MR system's dual channel body coil for 100% duty cycle RF saturation while the RF sources 1 and 2 operate at 50%. (**a**) The RF amplitudes A1/A2 are tuned to improve B_1 homogeneity. An acquisition scheme for renal CEST combining pTx saturation with respiratory triggering over multiple respiratory cycles is shown in (**b**) Acquisition is triggered during end expiration for every third cycle (as an example), followed by a waiting period for cooldown and alternated RF saturation continued over different respiratory phases

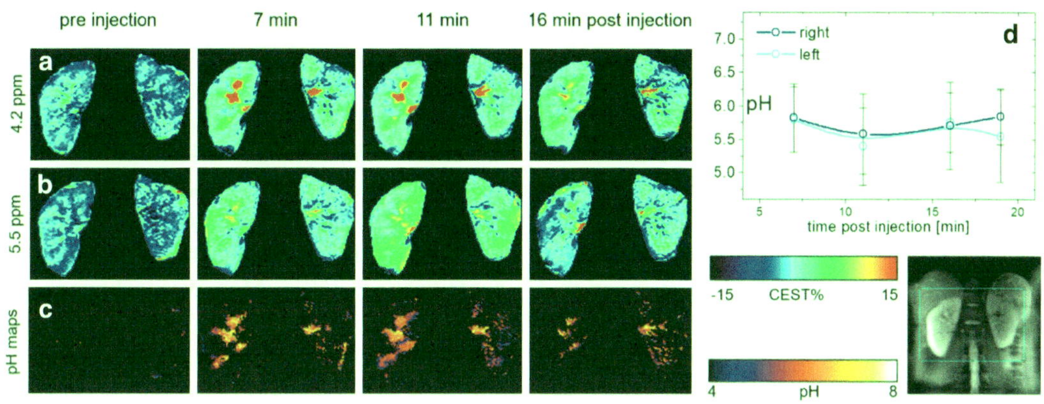

Fig. 22.5 Renal chemical exchange saturation transfer (CEST) pH mapping in a human volunteer at 3T over a time course of 20 min after iopamidol injection. (**a**, **b**) Time series of CEST maps precontrast and postcontrast injection at the 4.2 ppm/5.5 ppm amide pool of iopamidol; (**c**) ratiometric pH maps using both CEST signals for concentration independent pH assessment; (**d**) ROI-based analysis of the pH time dependence post iopamidol injection in the left and right kidney. Adapted with permission from Dimitrov et al. [59]

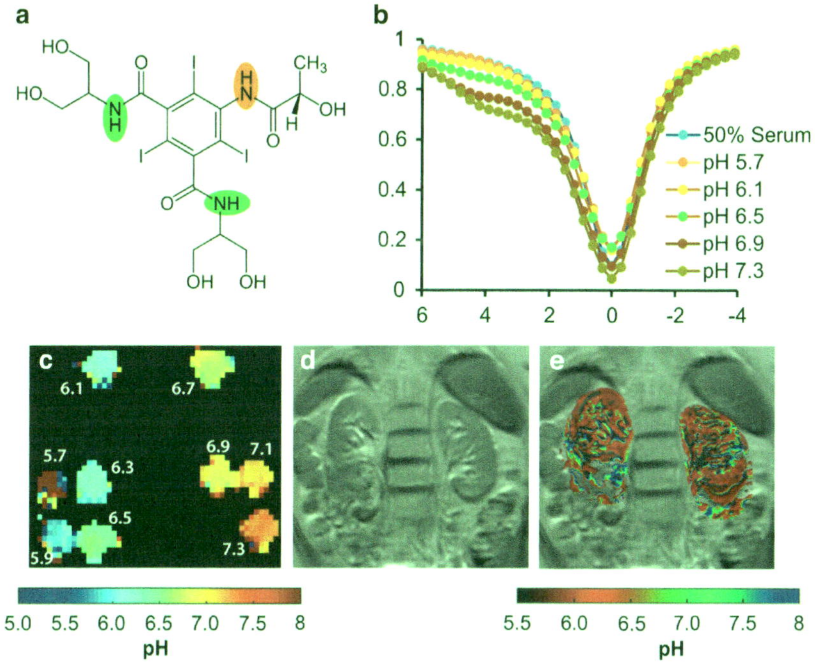

Fig. 22.6 Example of ratiometric measurement of pH using 25 mM iopamidol at 3T. (**a**) Iopamidol structure; (**b**) CEST Z-spectra measured in a phantom at pH = 5.7, 6.1, 6.5, 6.9, and 7.3 acquired at 63 offsets between −4 and 6 ppm and B_1 = 2 μT; (**c**) corresponding pH maps; (**d**) T2w image of the abdomen of a healthy human subject; (**e**) pH map of the kidneys after injection of iopamidol. CEST data were acquired for 18.9 min using B_1 = 2 μT, t_{sat} = 2 s, B_1 = 1.5 μT, and TR = 6 s, at repeated offsets of 20,000, 6.1, 5.6, 4.6, and 4.1 ppm, respectively. This set of offsets was necessary to partially compensate for the B_0-field inhomogeneity across the kidneys. CEST contrast at 4.6 and 5.6 ppm was eventually used for pH calculation. Adapted with permission from Bo et al. [42]

gest that iopamidol CEST-based pH mapping is feasible on clinical 3-T systems in the physiological pH range between 5.6 and 7.3 and for iopamidol concentrations >20 mM.

Another important application of the CEST-based pH imaging is in measuring tumor pH using iodinated contrast agents, which due to their hydrophilic chemical structure remain confined outside cells after administration and thus can be used to map extracellular pH (pH_e) and monitor tumor acidosis. Recently, Kyle et al. evaluated the clinical potential of acidoCEST MRI protocol to assess pHe in a patient with metastatic ovarian cancer at 3 T [41]. The average pH_e value of three adjacent tumors was 6.58, while the average pH in the kidney was 6.73. In another study, dual-power CEST MRI using ioversol was performed on a 3-T clinical scanner to determine pH_e in patients with liver tumors. The results of this study showed more acidic pH_e values (6.66 ± 0.19) in hepatic carcinoma and physiologically neutral pH_e (7.34 ± 0.09) in benign hemangioma.

Limitations and Future Perspectives

As indicated by the growing number of papers in this field, CEST MRI is a rapidly developing technique with enormous potential to assess (patho-)physiological changes in the concentrations of metabolites, intracellular, or extracellular pH and to depict perfusion. Nevertheless, there are still some challenges that need to be addressed before this method can be routinely used in clinical settings. Since the measured CEST effect depends not only on the microenvironmental properties but also on acquisition parameters, it is not always possible to compare the results obtained at different sites or to reproduce a CEST experiment. Standardization of CEST imaging sequences and post-processing schemes across all sites for multicenter studies is therefore required to provide clinically relevant measures and identify potential "killer applications" [90]. Other important limitations in the clinical use of CEST MRI, especially in the abdomen, are the relatively long scan times and sensitivity of CEST signal to motion artifacts, B_0- and B_1-field inhomogeneities, and confounding effects from fat signals. Hence, faster MRI acquisition techniques and advanced post-processing methods need to be further developed to allow rapid MRI measurements and robust CEST quantification [60]. Moreover, although in endogenous CEST imaging MR contrast is generated without the need for injection, which is attractive for renal applications, the lack of specificity or clear link between the observed CEST signals and renal function pose additional challenges to the adoption of this technique. More research is needed to establish the relationship between the CEST values and traditional histology characteristics and/or blood and urine biomarkers. Finally, for exogenous CEST studies, while iodinated contrast agents are generally considered safe and have been widely used for X-ray and CT examinations for decades, there are some concerns regarding their potential nephrotoxicity in patients with renal diseases. Therefore, there is increasing interest in developing novel non-iodinated contrast agents with reduced toxicity risk for the kidney [91, 92]. Despite all the current limitations, we believe that CEST imaging is well suited to provide valuable spatially localized information on renal function based on its sensitivity to changes in concentration of metabolites, clearance of administered CEST agents, and pH. This additional information could potentially improve assessment of renal diseases and pathologies compared with commonly used imaging techniques such as ultrasound, computed tomography, and renal scintigraphy and could also complement other MRI techniques described in this book.

Acknowledgements Many thanks to Silvio Aimé, A. Dean Sherry, Dario Livio Longo, Elena Vinogradov, Ivan Dimitrov, Edwin Heijman, and Sander Langereis for the fruitful collaboration on kidney CEST and iopamidol-based pH mapping. We would also like to acknowledge our funding, NIH R01DK121847 and P41EB024495.

References

1. Hood VL, Tannen RL. protection of acid–base balance by pH regulation of acid production. N Engl J Med. 1998;339(12):819–26. https://doi.org/10.1056/NEJM199809173391207.
2. Rhee EP. A systems-level view of renal metabolomics. Semin Nephrol. 2018;38(2):142–50. https://doi.org/10.1016/j.semnephrol.2018.01.005.
3. National Institute of Diabetes and Digestive and Kidney Diseases. Estimating glomerular filtration rate. Accessed 4 Apr 2022. https://www.niddk.nih.gov/health-information/professionals/clinical-tools-patient-management/kidney-disease/laboratory-evaluation/glomerular-filtration-rate/estimating.
4. Bretan PNJ, Baldwin N, Novick AC, et al. Pretransplant assessment of renal viability by phosphorus-31 magnetic resonance spectroscopy. Clinical experience in 40 recipient patients. Transplantation. 1989;48(1):48–53.
5. Hauet T, Goujon JM, Tallineau C, Carretier M, Eugene M. Early evaluation of renal reperfusion injury after prolonged cold storage using proton nuclear magnetic resonance spectroscopy. Br J Surg. 1999;86(11):1401–9. https://doi.org/10.1046/j.1365-2168.1999.01233.x.
6. Delphine B, Franois S, Thierry H. Magnetic resonance spectroscopy (MRS) in kidney transplantation: interest and perspectives. In: Kim DH, editor. Magnetic resonance spectroscopy. Rijeka: InTech; 2012. https://doi.org/10.5772/32661.
7. Wolff SD, Balaban RS. Magnetization transfer contrast (MTC) and tissue water proton relaxation in vivo. Magn Reson Med. 1989;10(1):135–44. https://doi.org/10.1002/mrm.1910100113.
8. Guivel-Scharen V, Sinnwell T, Wolff SD, Balaban RS. Detection of proton chemical exchange between metabolites and water in biological tissues. J Magn Reson. 1998;133(1):36–45. https://doi.org/10.1006/jmre.1998.1440.
9. McMahon MT, Gilad AA, JWM B, van Zijl PCM. Chemical exchange saturation transfer imaging: advances and applications. Oxfordshire: Routledge & CRC Press; 2017. Accessed 10 Dec 2021. https://www.routledge.com/Chemical-Exchange-Saturation-Transfer-Imaging-Advances-and-Applications/McMahon-Gilad-Bulte-Zijl/p/book/9789814745703.
10. Wang F, Kopylov D, Zu Z, et al. Mapping murine diabetic kidney disease using chemical exchange saturation transfer MRI. Magn Reson Med. 2016;76(5):1531–41. https://doi.org/10.1002/mrm.26045.
11. Wang F, Takahashi K, Li H, et al. Assessment of unilateral ureter obstruction with multi-parametric MRI. Magn Reson Med. 2018;79(4):2216–27. https://doi.org/10.1002/mrm.26849.
12. Li A, Xu C, Liang P, et al. Role of chemical exchange saturation transfer and magnetization transfer MRI in detecting metabolic and structural changes of renal fibrosis in an animal model at 3T. Korean J Radiol. 2020;21(5):588–97. https://doi.org/10.3348/kjr.2019.0646.
13. Liu J, Han Z, Chen G, et al. CEST MRI of sepsis-induced acute kidney injury. NMR Biomed. 2018;31(8):e3942. https://doi.org/10.1002/nbm.3942.
14. Kentrup D, Bovenkamp P, Busch A, et al. GlucoCEST magnetic resonance imaging in vivo may be diagnostic of acute renal allograft rejection. Kidney Int. 2017;92(3):757–64. https://doi.org/10.1016/j.kint.2017.04.015.
15. Longo DL, Busato A, Lanzardo S, Antico F, Aime S. Imaging the pH evolution of an acute kidney injury model by means of iopamidol, a MRI-CEST pH-responsive contrast agent. Magn Reson Med. 2013;70(3):859–64. https://doi.org/10.1002/mrm.24513.
16. Irrera P, Consolino L, Cutrin JC, Zöllner FG, Longo DL. Dual assessment of kidney perfusion and pH by exploiting a dynamic CEST-MRI approach in an acute kidney ischemia–reperfusion injury murine model. NMR Biomed. 2020;33(6):e4287. https://doi.org/10.1002/nbm.4287.
17. Longo DL, Cutrin JC, Michelotti F, Irrera P, Aime S. Noninvasive evaluation of renal pH homeostasis after ischemia reperfusion injury by CEST-MRI. NMR Biomed. 2017;30(7):e3720. https://doi.org/10.1002/nbm.3720.
18. Pavuluri K, Manoli I, Pass A, et al. Noninvasive monitoring of chronic kidney disease using pH and perfusion imaging. Sci Adv. 2019;5(8):eaaw8357. https://doi.org/10.1126/sciadv.aaw8357.
19. Ward KM, Aletras AH, Balaban RS. A new class of contrast agents for MRI based on proton chemical exchange dependent saturation transfer (CEST). J Magn Reson. 2000;143(1):79–87. https://doi.org/10.1006/jmre.1999.1956.
20. Zhang S, Winter P, Wu K, Sherry AD. A novel europium(III)-based MRI contrast agent. J Am Chem Soc. 2001;123(7):1517–8. https://doi.org/10.1021/ja005820q.
21. Aime S, Barge A, Delli Castelli D, et al. Paramagnetic lanthanide(III) complexes as pH-sensitive chemical exchange saturation transfer (CEST) contrast agents for MRI applications. Magn Reson Med. 2002;47(4):639–48. https://doi.org/10.1002/mrm.10106.
22. Sherry AD, Castelli DD, Aime S. Prospects and limitations of paramagnetic chemical exchange saturation transfer agents serving as biological reporters in vivo. NMR Biomed. 2023;36(6):e4698. https://doi.org/10.1002/nbm.4698.
23. Goffeney N, Bulte JWM, Duyn J, Bryant LH, van Zijl PCM. Sensitive NMR detection of cationic-polymer-based gene delivery systems using saturation transfer via proton exchange. J Am Chem Soc. 2001;123(35):8628–9. https://doi.org/10.1021/ja0158455.
24. Zhou J, Payen JF, Wilson DA, Traystman RJ, van Zijl PCM. Using the amide proton signals of intracellular

proteins and peptides to detect pH effects in MRI. Nat Med. 2003;9(8):1085–90. https://doi.org/10.1038/nm907.
25. Tietze A, Blicher J, Mikkelsen IK, et al. Assessment of ischemic penumbra in human hyperacute stroke patients using amide proton transfer (APT) chemical exchange saturation transfer (CEST) MRI. NMR Biomed. 2014;27(2):163–74. https://doi.org/10.1002/nbm.3048.
26. Regnery S, Adeberg S, Dreher C, et al. Chemical exchange saturation transfer MRI serves as predictor of early progression in glioblastoma patients. Oncotarget. 2018;9(47):28772–83. https://doi.org/10.18632/oncotarget.25594.
27. Paech D, Dreher C, Regnery S, et al. Relaxation-compensated amide proton transfer (APT) MRI signal intensity is associated with survival and progression in high-grade glioma patients. Eur Radiol. 2019;29(9):4957–67. https://doi.org/10.1007/s00330-019-06066-2.
28. Park JE, Kim HS, Park SY, Jung SC, Kim JH, Heo HY. Identification of early response to anti-Angiogenic therapy in recurrent glioblastoma: amide proton transfer–weighted and perfusion-weighted MRI compared with diffusion-weighted MRI. Radiology. 2020;295(2):397–406. https://doi.org/10.1148/radiol.2020191376.
29. Takayama Y, Nishie A, Togao O, et al. Amide proton transfer MR imaging of Endometrioid endometrial adenocarcinoma: association with histologic grade. Radiology. 2018;286(3):909–17. https://doi.org/10.1148/radiol.2017170349.
30. Jia G, Abaza R, Williams JD, et al. Amide proton transfer MR imaging of prostate cancer: a preliminary study. J Magn Reson Imaging. 2011;33(3):647–54. https://doi.org/10.1002/jmri.22480.
31. Chen W, Li L, Yan Z, et al. Three-dimension amide proton transfer MRI of rectal adenocarcinoma: correlation with pathologic prognostic factors and comparison with diffusion kurtosis imaging. Eur Radiol. 2021;31(5):3286–96. https://doi.org/10.1007/s00330-020-07397-1.
32. Li C, Peng S, Wang R, et al. Chemical exchange saturation transfer MR imaging of Parkinson's disease at 3 tesla. Eur Radiol. 2014;24(10):2631–9. https://doi.org/10.1007/s00330-014-3241-7.
33. Oh JH, Choi BG, Rhee HY, et al. Added value of chemical exchange-dependent saturation transfer MRI for the diagnosis of dementia. Korean J Radiol. 2021;22(5):770–81. https://doi.org/10.3348/kjr.2020.0700.
34. Schmitt B, Zbýň Š, Stelzeneder D, et al. Cartilage quality assessment by using glycosaminoglycan chemical exchange saturation transfer and 23Na MR imaging at 7 T. Radiology. 2011;260:257. https://doi.org/10.1148/radiol.11101841.
35. Kumar D, Nanga RPR, Thakuri D, et al. Recovery kinetics of Creatine in mild plantar flexion exercise using 3D Creatine chemical exchange saturation transfer (3D-CrCEST) imaging at 7T. Magn Reson Med. 2021;85(2):802–17. https://doi.org/10.1002/mrm.28463.
36. Abrar DB, Schleich C, Radke KL, et al. Detection of early cartilage degeneration in the tibiotalar joint using 3 T gagCEST imaging: a feasibility study. MAGMA. 2021;34(2):249–60. https://doi.org/10.1007/s10334-020-00868-y.
37. Chen Z, Han Z, Liu G. Repurposing clinical agents for chemical exchange saturation transfer magnetic resonance imaging: current status and future perspectives. Pharmaceuticals (Basel). 2020;14(1):11. https://doi.org/10.3390/ph14010011.
38. Longo DL, Dastrù W, Digilio G, et al. Iopamidol as a responsive MRI-chemical exchange saturation transfer contrast agent for pH mapping of kidneys: in vivo studies in mice at 7 T. Magn Reson Med. 2011;65(1):202–11. https://doi.org/10.1002/mrm.22608.
39. Longo DL, Carella A, Corrado A, et al. A snapshot of the vast array of diamagnetic CEST MRI contrast agents. NMR Biomed. 2023;36(6):e4715. https://doi.org/10.1002/nbm.4715.
40. Müller-Lutz A, Khalil N, Schmitt B, et al. Pilot study of Iopamidol-based quantitative pH imaging on a clinical 3T MR scanner. Magn Reson Mater Phy. 2014;27(6):477–85. https://doi.org/10.1007/s10334-014-0433-8.
41. Jones KM, Randtke EA, Yoshimaru ES, et al. Clinical translation of tumor acidosis measurements with AcidoCEST MRI. Mol Imaging Biol. 2017;19(4):617–25. https://doi.org/10.1007/s11307-016-1029-7.
42. Bo S, Sedaghat F, Pavuluri K, et al. Dynamic contrast enhanced-MR CEST urography: an emerging tool in the diagnosis and management of upper urinary tract obstruction. Tomography. 2021;7(1):80–94. https://doi.org/10.3390/tomography7010008.
43. Chan KWY, McMahon MT, Kato Y, et al. Natural D-glucose as a biodegradable MRI contrast agent for detecting cancer. Magn Reson Med. 2012;68(6):1764–73. https://doi.org/10.1002/mrm.24520.
44. Herz K, Lindig T, Deshmane A, et al. T1ρ-based dynamic glucose-enhanced (DGEρ) MRI at 3 T: method development and early clinical experience in the human brain. Magn Reson Med. 2019;82(5):1832–47. https://doi.org/10.1002/mrm.27857.
45. Sehgal AA, Li Y, Lal B, et al. CEST MRI of 3-O-methyl-D-glucose uptake and accumulation in brain tumors. Magn Reson Med. 2019;81(3):1993–2000. https://doi.org/10.1002/mrm.27489.
46. Xu X, Sehgal AA, Yadav NN, et al. D-glucose weighted chemical exchange saturation transfer (glucoCEST)-based dynamic glucose enhanced (DGE) MRI at 3T: early experience in healthy volunteers and brain tumor patients. Magn Reson Med. 2020;84(1):247–62. https://doi.org/10.1002/mrm.28124.
47. Kim M, Torrealdea F, Adeleke S, et al. Challenges in glucoCEST MR body imaging at 3 tesla. Quant Imaging Med Surg. 2019;9(10):1628640–1640.
48. Sherry AD, Woods M. Chemical exchange saturation transfer contrast agents for magnetic

resonance imaging. Annu Rev Biomed Eng. 2008;10:391–411. https://doi.org/10.1146/annurev.bioeng.9.060906.151929.
49. Kogan F, Hariharan H, Reddy R. Chemical exchange saturation transfer (CEST) imaging: description of technique and potential clinical applications. Curr Radiol Rep. 2013;1(2):102–14. https://doi.org/10.1007/s40134-013-0010-3.
50. Wang M, Hong X, Chang CF, et al. Simultaneous detection and separation of hyperacute intracerebral hemorrhage and cerebral ischemia using amide proton transfer MRI. Magn Reson Med. 2015;74(1):42–50. https://doi.org/10.1002/mrm.25690.
51. McVicar N, Li AX, Gonçalves DF, et al. Quantitative tissue pH measurement during cerebral ischemia using amine and amide concentration-independent detection (AACID) with MRI. J Cereb Blood Flow Metab. 2014;34(4):690–8. https://doi.org/10.1038/jcbfm.2014.12.
52. Cui J, Afzal A, Zu Z. Comparative evaluation of polynomial and Lorentzian lineshape-fitted amine CEST imaging in acute ischemic stroke. Magn Reson Med. 2022;87(2):837–49. https://doi.org/10.1002/mrm.29030.
53. Sun PZ, Xiao G, Zhou IY, Guo Y, Wu R. A method for accurate pH mapping with chemical exchange saturation transfer (CEST) MRI. Contrast Media Mol Imaging. 2016;11(3):195–202. https://doi.org/10.1002/cmmi.1680.
54. Zaiss M, Bachert P. Chemical exchange saturation transfer (CEST) and Z-spectroscopy in vivo: a review of theoretical approaches and methods. Phys Med Biol. 2013;58(22):R221–69. https://doi.org/10.1088/0031-9155/58/22/R221.
55. Zaiss M, Anemone A, Goerke S, et al. Quantification of hydroxyl exchange of D-glucose at physiological conditions for optimization of glucoCEST MRI at 3, 7 and 9.4 tesla. NMR Biomed. 2019;32(9):e4113. https://doi.org/10.1002/nbm.4113.
56. Zhu H, Keupp J, Blakeley J, Blair L, Schar M, Barker PB. Interleaved parallel transmission saturation scheme for 3d amide proton transfer imaging of brain tumors at 3 Tesla. 2012.
57. Togao O, Yoshiura T, Keupp J, et al. Amide proton transfer imaging of adult diffuse gliomas: correlation with histopathological grades. Neuro-Oncology. 2014;16(3):441–8. https://doi.org/10.1093/neuonc/not158.
58. Togao O, Keupp J, Hiwatashi A, et al. Amide proton transfer imaging of brain tumors using a self-corrected 3D fast spin-echo dixon method: comparison with separate B0 correction. Magn Reson Med. 2017;77(6):2272–9. https://doi.org/10.1002/mrm.26322.
59. Dimitrov IE, Takahashi M, Sagiyama K, Sherry AD, Keupp J. In vivo human kidney pH mapping at 3T using time-interleaved parallel RF transmission CEST. In Proceedings of the 20th Annual Meeting of ISMRM. 2012.
60. Zhang Y, Zu T, Liu R, Zhou J. Acquisition sequences and reconstruction methods for fast chemical exchange saturation transfer imaging. NMR Biomed. 2023;36(6):e4699. https://doi.org/10.1002/nbm.4699.
61. Zaiss M, Ehses P, Scheffler K. Snapshot-CEST: optimizing spiral-centric-reordered gradient echo acquisition for fast and robust 3D CEST MRI at 9.4 T. NMR Biomed. 2018;31(4):e3879. https://doi.org/10.1002/nbm.3879.
62. Sui R, Chen L, Li Y, et al. Whole-brain amide CEST imaging at 3T with a steady-state radial MRI acquisition. Magn Reson Med. 2021;86(2):893–906. https://doi.org/10.1002/mrm.28770.
63. Varma G, Lenkinski RE, Vinogradov E. Keyhole chemical exchange saturation transfer. Magn Reson Med. 2012;68(4):1228–33. https://doi.org/10.1002/mrm.23310.
64. Heo HY, Zhang Y, Lee DH, Jiang S, Zhao X, Zhou J. Accelerating chemical exchange saturation transfer (CEST) MRI by combining compressed sensing and sensitivity encoding techniques. Magn Reson Med. 2017;77(2):779–86. https://doi.org/10.1002/mrm.26141.
65. Zaiss M, Herz K, Deshmane A, et al. Possible artifacts in dynamic CEST MRI due to motion and field alterations. J Magn Reson. 2019;298:16–22. https://doi.org/10.1016/j.jmr.2018.11.002.
66. Keupp J, Heijman E, Langereis S, et al. Respiratory triggered Chemical Exchange Saturation Transfer MRI for pH Mapping in the Kidneys at 3T. In: Proceedings of the 19th Annual Meeting of ISMRM. 2011;1.
67. Robson PM, Madhuranthakam AJ, Dai W, Pedrosa I, Rofsky NM, Alsop DC. Strategies for reducing respiratory motion artifacts in renal perfusion imaging with arterial spin labeling. Magn Reson Med. 2009;61(6):1374–87. https://doi.org/10.1002/mrm.21960.
68. Zhang S, Li, B, Greer J, Madhuranthakam A, Keupp J, Dimitrov I. Toward CEST MRI of renal masses: protocol optimization and first preliminary data. In: Proceedings of the Joint Annual Meeting ISMRM-ESMRMB. 2018.
69. Poblador Rodriguez E, Moser P, Auno S, et al. Real-time motion and retrospective coil sensitivity correction for CEST using volumetric navigators (vNavs) at 7T. Magn Reson Med. 2021;85(4):1909–23. https://doi.org/10.1002/mrm.28555.
70. Bie C, Liang Y, Zhang L, et al. Motion correction of chemical exchange saturation transfer MRI series using robust principal component analysis (RPCA) and PCA. Quant Imaging Med Surg. 2019;9(10):1697713–1713.
71. Wech T, Köstler H. Robust motion correction in CEST imaging exploiting low-rank approximation of the z-spectrum. Magn Reson Med. 2018;80(5):1979–88. https://doi.org/10.1002/mrm.27206.
72. Kim M, Gillen J, Landman BA, Zhou J, van Zijl PCM. Water saturation shift referencing (WASSR) for chemical exchange saturation transfer (CEST) experiments. Magn Reson Med. 2009;61(6):1441–50. https://doi.org/10.1002/mrm.21873.

73. Zhang S, Seiler S, Wang X, et al. CEST-Dixon for human breast lesion characterization at 3 T: a preliminary study. Magn Reson Med. 2018;80(3):895–903. https://doi.org/10.1002/mrm.27079.
74. Cunningham CH, Pauly JM, Nayak KS. Saturated double-angle method for rapid B1+ mapping. Magn Reson Med. 2006;55(6):1326–33. https://doi.org/10.1002/mrm.20896.
75. Sacolick LI, Wiesinger F, Hancu I, Vogel MW. B1 mapping by Bloch-Siegert shift. Magn Reson Med. 2010;63(5):1315–22. https://doi.org/10.1002/mrm.22357.
76. Schuenke P, Windschuh J, Roeloffs V, Ladd ME, Bachert P, Zaiss M. Simultaneous mapping of water shift and B1(WASABI)—application to field-inhomogeneity correction of CEST MRI data. Magn Reson Med. 2017;77(2):571–80. https://doi.org/10.1002/mrm.26133.
77. Zhang S, Keupp J, Wang X, et al. Z-spectrum appearance and interpretation in the presence of fat: influence of acquisition parameters. Magn Reson Med. 2018;79(5):2731–7. https://doi.org/10.1002/mrm.26900.
78. Stabinska J, Müller-Lutz A, Wittsack HJ, et al. Two point Dixon-based chemical exchange saturation transfer (CEST) MRI in renal transplant patients on 3 T. Magn Reson Imaging. 2022;90:61–9. https://doi.org/10.1016/j.mri.2022.04.004.
79. Zimmermann F, Korzowski A, Breitling J, et al. A novel normalization for amide proton transfer CEST MRI to correct for fat signal–induced artifacts: application to human breast cancer imaging. Magn Reson Med. 2020;83(3):920–34. https://doi.org/10.1002/mrm.27983.
80. Dixon WT. Simple proton spectroscopic imaging. Radiology. 1984;153(1):189–94. https://doi.org/10.1148/radiology.153.1.6089263.
81. Zhou IY, Lu D, Ji Y, et al. Determination of multipool contributions to endogenous amide proton transfer effects in global ischemia with high spectral resolution in vivo chemical exchange saturation transfer MRI. Magn Reson Med. 2019;81(1):645–52. https://doi.org/10.1002/mrm.27385.
82. Heo HY, Zhang Y, Jiang S, Lee DH, Zhou J. Quantitative assessment of amide proton transfer (APT) and nuclear Overhauser enhancement (NOE) imaging with extrapolated semi-solid magnetization transfer reference (EMR) signals: II. Comparison of three EMR models and application to human brain glioma at 3 T. Magn Reson Med. 2016;75(4):1630–9. https://doi.org/10.1002/mrm.25795.
83. Woessner DE, Zhang S, Merritt ME, Sherry AD. Numerical solution of the Bloch equations provides insights into the optimum design of PARACEST agents for MRI. Magn Reson Med. 2005;53(4):790–9. https://doi.org/10.1002/mrm.20408.
84. Wu Y, Zhou IY, Igarashi T, Longo DL, Aime S, Sun PZ. A generalized Ratiometric chemical exchange saturation transfer (CEST) MRI approach for mapping renal pH using Iopamidol. Magn Reson Med. 2018;79(3):1553–8. https://doi.org/10.1002/mrm.26817.
85. Dagher AP, Aletras A, Choyke P, Balaban RS. Imaging of urea using chemical exchange-dependent saturation transfer at 1.5T. J Magn Reson Imaging. 2000;12(5):745–8. https://doi.org/10.1002/1522--2586(200011)12:5<745::aid-jmri12>3.0.co;2-h.
86. Vinogradov E, Liu Z, Madhuranthakam AJ, et al. Endogenous urea CEST (urCEST) for MRI monitoring of kidney function. In: Proceedings of the 23th Annual Meeting and Exhibition of ISMRM. 2015.
87. Stabinska J, Neudecker P, Ljimani A, Wittsack HJ, Lanzman RS, Müller-Lutz A. Proton exchange in aqueous urea solutions measured by water-exchange (WEX) NMR spectroscopy and chemical exchange saturation transfer (CEST) imaging in vitro. Magn Reson Med. 2019;82(3):935–47. https://doi.org/10.1002/mrm.27778.
88. Keupp J, Dimitrov I, Langereis S, Togao O, Takahashi M, Sherry AD. Non-invasive CEST-MRI Measurement of pH in the Human Kidneys using an Approved CT Contrast Agent. In: In Proceedings of the 19th Annual Meeting of ISMRM. 2011.
89. Fishman EK, Jeffrey RB Jr. Spiral CT: principles, techniques and clinical applications. Philadelphia: Lippincott Williams & Wilkins; 1998.
90. Herz K, Mueller S, Perlman O, et al. Pulseq-CEST: towards multi-site multi-vendor compatibility and reproducibility of CEST experiments using an open-source sequence standard. Magn Reson Med. 2021;86(4):1845–58. https://doi.org/10.1002/mrm.28825.
91. Chan KWY, Liu G, Song X, et al. MRI-detectable pH nanosensors incorporated into hydrogels for in vivo sensing of transplanted-cell viability. Nat Mater. 2013;12(3):268–75. https://doi.org/10.1038/nmat3525.
92. Yang X, Song X, Banerjee SR, et al. Developing imidazoles as CEST MRI pH sensors. Contrast Media Mol Imaging. 2016;11(4):304–12. https://doi.org/10.1002/cmmi.1693.

Renal Sodium ^{23}Na-MRI for Clinical Applications

23

Rachelle Crescenzi and Valentina Kon

Abbreviations

^{1}H	Proton, or hydrogen-1
^{23}Na	Endogenous sodium-23
ADC	Apparent diffusion coefficient
B_0	Primary magnetic field
B_1	Applied magnetic field
BOLD	Blood oxygenation level-dependent
CKD	Chronic kidney disease
cm	Centimeter
CMG	Corticomedullary gradient
CSF	Cerebrospinal fluid
DA-3DPR	Density-adapted 3D projection reconstruction
DDAVP	Desmopressin, antidiuretic
FA	Flip angle
FOV	Field of view
GRE	Gradient echo
h	Hour
Hz, MHz	Hertz, mega-Hertz
kg	Kilogram
M, mm	Meter, millimeter
min	Minute
mmol/L, mM	Millimoles per liter
mOsm	Milliosmole
MRI	Magnetic resonance imaging
ms	Millisecond
NaCl	Sodium chloride
NR	Not reported
NSA	Number of signal acquisitions
RF	Radiofrequency
SNR	Signal-to-noise ratio
T, mT	Tesla, milli-Tesla
T_1	Longitudinal relaxation time
T_2	Transverse relaxation time (or with inhomogeneous relaxation time T2*, or relaxation rate R2*)
TE	Echo time
TORO	Transmit-only, receive-only
TR	Repetition time
TSC	Tissue sodium content
Tx/Rx	Transmit/receive
UTE	Ultra-short echo time
γ	Gyromagnetic ratio
ω	Larmor resonant frequency

R. Crescenzi (✉)
Radiology and Radiological Sciences, Vanderbilt University Medical Center, Nashville, TN, USA

Vanderbilt University Institute of Imaging Science, Vanderbilt University Medical Center, Nashville, TN, USA

Biomedical Engineering, Vanderbilt University, Nashville, TN, USA
e-mail: rachelle.crescenzi@vumc.org

V. Kon
Department of Pediatrics, Vanderbilt University Medical Center, Nashville, TN, USA

S. D. Serai, K. Darge (eds.), *Advanced Clinical MRI of the Kidney*,
https://doi.org/10.1007/978-3-031-40169-5_23

Introduction

Conventional proton ^{1}H magnetic resonance imaging (MRI) has been successfully adapted for clinical use in the kidneys where total kidney size has achieved biomarker status. However, often the information from conventional MRI cannot provide direct biochemical markers necessary to follow changes in tissue viability in disease or upon treatment. A fact often overlooked is that sodium ^{23}Na yields the second strongest nuclear magnetic resonance (NMR) signal among all nuclei present in biological tissues. The NMR-active isotope of sodium is ^{23}Na with close to 100% natural abundance. Sodium ^{23}Na is also the second most abundant magnetic nuclei in the body and can be probed by noninvasive multi-nuclear MRI to provide complementary information about tissue sodium in a quantitative and non-invasive manner. Imaging ^{23}Na requires specific technology modifications from conventional imaging, as well as physiologic considerations for sodium handling in the body [1, 2]. The kidneys play a central role in regulating sodium circulation, participating directly in salvage and excretion of sodium [3]. Prior to the development of noninvasive ^{23}Na-MRI of tissue sodium, assessment of sodium handling relied on measurements of plasma sodium concentration (which does not necessarily reflect total body sodium), estimation of extracellular volume status, cumbersome urinary collections to quantify sodium excretion, or predictive equations from spot urines. Imaging technology, specifically the standardization of ^{23}Na-MRI at clinical field strength 3 Tesla (T), offers the possibility for noninvasive in vivo quantification of tissue sodium for clinical applications. In recent years, clinically feasible sodium MRI in the extremities has led to new discoveries in the role of tissue sodium in cardiovascular, neurological, oncological, autoimmune, and metabolic diseases of impaired sodium handling [4]. We outline the latest methods for image acquisition, analysis, and clinical applications of sodium ^{23}Na-MRI in the human kidneys in health and disease.

The earliest examples of renal sodium ^{23}Na-MRI in humans were performed as a multi-organ approach. In 1988, Ra et al. demonstrated the feasibility of renal sodium MRI, although the available technology generated only low resolution sodium images with mostly homogeneous contrast throughout both kidneys [5]. There was early interest in a multi-organ approach to sodium imaging, where Granot demonstrated feasible imaging of tissue sodium contrast with custom coils in the brain, kidneys, and heart [6]. In 2006, Maril et al. demonstrated a three-dimensional coronal gradient echo sequence at 3-T MRI that provided sufficient signal-to-noise ratio (SNR) to show that tissue sodium increases from the renal cortex to the medulla (Fig. 23.1) [7]. This study also demonstrated that a 12-h water deprivation increases the corticomedullary gradient (CMG) in tissue sodium by 25%. We will briefly discuss this physiology before outlining the developments in renal sodium MRI technology which followed these early discoveries.

Kidney Handling of Sodium

The kidneys maintain nearly constant blood plasma sodium and osmolality. This is achieved through glomerular filtration followed by tubular reabsorption and secretion of sodium, which involves the maintenance of an osmotic gradient that increases progressively from the outer cortex to the tip of the inner medulla. The cortical tissue is isotonic to the plasma, while the inner medullary tip is hypertonic to the plasma. In humans, renal medulla osmolality can achieve 1200 mOsm/kg, i.e., ~four times the normal plasma osmolality of ~290 mOsm/kg [8]. Approximately half of the tonicity generating the corticomedullary gradient (CMG) is due to NaCl, which is established by a number of sodium transporters (e.g., Na-K-ATPase, Na-H exchanger, and Na-K-2Cl cotransporter) and aquaporin which increase the interstitial renal sodium concentration. The rest of the CMG is due to urea.

Sodium reabsorption occurs in almost all parts of the nephron but is most important in the medulla. The CMG becomes steeper during conditions of volume depletion and antidiuresis and decreases during settings of volume expansion

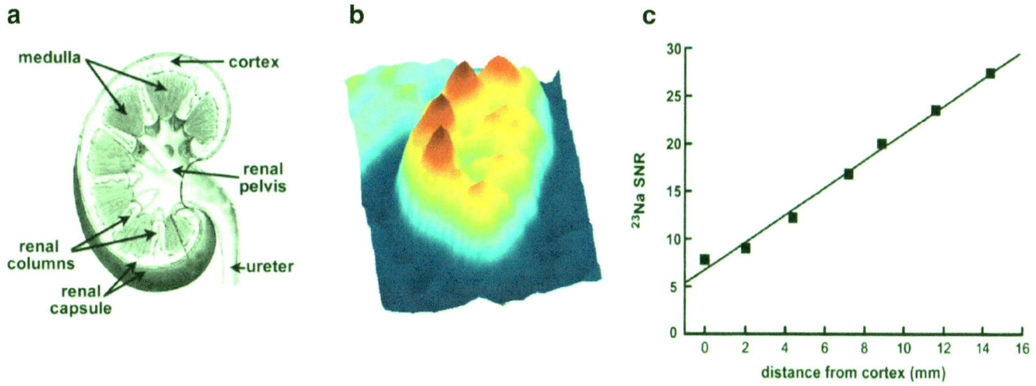

Fig. 23.1 Diagram of renal anatomy (**a**) and ^{23}Na-MRI signal topography of tissue sodium content in the human kidney (**b**) reveal a gradient from the renal cortex in the direction of each medullary pyramid. This gradient can be quantified by measuring sodium signal-to-noise ratio as a function of distance from the cortex (**c**). Reprinted with kind permission from Maril et al. 2006, original Figure 2-3 [7]

and diuresis [9]. Urinary concentration and dilution occur primarily in the renal medulla where the vasa recta, loops of Henle, and the collecting ducts participate in the countercurrent and co-current exchange of water and sodium [10]. In the outer medulla, the osmotic gradient is generated by the active reabsorption of NaCl from the thick ascending limbs of Henle's loop. The source of the gradient in the inner medulla remains undetermined and may involve the passive diffusion of NaCl into the inner medullary interstitium from the ascending thin limbs of Henle's loop [11].

Since creation and maintenance of the sodium CMG reflect key kidney functions produced by the active reabsorption of sodium in the medulla, it has been proposed as a potential imaging biomarker of tubular function [12–14]. ^{23}Na-MRI has demonstrated sensitivity for the sodium CMG and gives information on the spatial distribution of sodium in kidney tissue. Thus, as a noninvasive imaging technique, MRI-derived sodium CMG is being used to investigate kidney function in allografts, pharmaceutical modulation of tubular function, and could possibly monitor changes in tubular integrity during a variety of kidney as well as non-kidney diseases [15]. Renal sodium MRI shows promise to become an additional tool for the standard estimation of glomerular filtration rate to assess kidney function and may play an important role in new clinical discoveries.

MRI Physics and Acquisition Protocols

^{23}Na has a nuclear spin of 3/2 and hence exhibits a quadrupolar interaction. The NMR sensitivity of sodium is 9.2% of the proton sensitivity, and given a much lower biological concentration, the SNR yielded from sodium imaging is 3000–20,000 lower than conventional proton MRI [16]. The majority of current sodium MRI applications can be understood without much sophisticated theory beyond assuming the study of a nucleus with very short transverse relaxation time (T_2) and low SNR. On the other hand, contrast and quantification can in many situations be significantly affected by the underlying spin dynamics which are governed either by a residual or fluctuating quadrupolar interaction, which leads to line splitting in the former, and to biexponential relaxation in the latter case. In tissues, a complex mix of the two cases often persists, including the confounding factors of magnetic field inhomogeneities and exchange. Taking full stock of all underlying phenomena and the information available from advanced methods can allow one to extract further tissue parameters and provide opportunities for new imaging contrast. The essential elements of a sodium ^{23}Na-MRI experiment to quantify renal tissue sodium content (TSC) in the human body include (1) scanner hardware for ^{23}Na signal transmission and reception (Tx/Rx), (2) radiofrequency (RF) pulse sequence design for image acquisition and reconstruction, (3) image calibration with sodium standards, and (4) quantitation of physiologic renal sodium metrics. The unique magnetic properties of endogenous sodium ^{23}Na must be considered for each element of the experiment: quadrupolar nuclei with spin 3/2, fast bi-exponential T_2, and low SNR relative to conventional proton ^{1}H imaging.

Scanner Hardware

For the implementation of ^{23}Na MRI, the MR scanner needs to be equipped with specialized transmit and receive radiofrequency coils tuned to the resonance frequency of sodium nuclei at the respective field strength. A scanner equipped for sodium MRI will have a signal pre-amplifier that performs in the range of sodium resonance and ability to integrate multi-nuclear RF coils. Endogenous sodium ^{23}Na has a gyromagnetic ratio $\gamma(^{23}\text{Na})$ = 11.262 MHz/T, giving a Larmor resonant frequency at 3-T field strength $\omega(^{23}\text{Na})$ = 33.8 MHz. Its Larmor frequency is approximately 5% larger than that of ^{13}C and approximately 26% of the proton frequency [16]. Conventional amplifiers may not cover this range, and typically, a broadband high-power RF amplifier (i.e., 4 kW at multi-nuclear frequencies) is necessary to turn on during the sodium MRI experiment. Communication between the amplifier and scanner console may require a Tx/Rx switch specific for multi-nuclear applications. Gradient strength should also be sufficient to achieve minimum echo time sequences (i.e., gradient systems with 40-mT/m maximum amplitude and slew rate of 200 mT/m/ms) [17]. As vendors develop whole-body clinical field strength 3-T MRI scanners with multi-nuclear capabilities, the limiting hardware towards clinical application will be the availability of multi-nuclear RF coils [18]. Currently, the multi-nuclear coils for sodium imaging are not supplied by the vendors, and they need to be custom ordered from a third-party company, which requires additional design, time, and expense.

Sodium ^{23}Na signal transmission and reception for renal imaging will require a dedicated RF coil. Whether custom or commercial built, one must consider if a single- or dual-tuned coil is necessary for the desired application. If a proton body coil is available such as on 3-T scanners, a single-tuned sodium-only quadrature coil is preferred because it provides half the transmission power and twice the receive signal, with overall less interference from a proton-decoupling circuit [7]. When working on high-field 7-T+ scanners, a proton body coil may be absent and therefore a dual-tuned ^{1}H/^{23}Na coil is necessary for anatomical localization in the proton channel and sodium imaging in an identical field-of-view (FOV). Vendor-specific instructions should be available to enable the scanner to recognize the multi-nuclear RF coil channels.

Various multi-nuclear RF coil designs have been implemented for renal sodium MRI and most often aim to image the kidneys in the coronal axis [18]. A volume birdcage design offers full FOV coverage of both kidneys and a circularly polarized RF field for relatively homogeneous field profiles. However, design challenges will have to accommodate wide or long body habitus for adult renal imaging [17]. Surface coils in linear, quadrature, or Helmholtz modes are most commonly used for adult renal imaging [18]. Early implementations of renal sodium MRI employed two-loop quadrature sodium-only Tx/Rx coils (18–25 cm diameter) [5, 7]. More recently, commercial 8-element single-tuned coils and custom dual-tuned multi-element coils have improved the feasibility of renal sodium MRI [17, 19–21].

Runtime considerations: Checking the primary magnetic field B_0 and Tx/Rx magnetic field B_1 inhomogeneities on the direct sodium signal is often prohibited by low SNR and available scan time. A dual flip-angle (FA) sodium B_1 map (4-min total acquisition) has been implemented with a non-Cartesian readout for brain sodium

MRI and may also benefit renal sodium MRI [22]. For dual-tuned ^{1}H/^{23}Na coils, a separate proton B_0 and B_1 map can be acquired and a linear adjustment for sodium nuclei assumed. For surface Tx/Rx coils, B_1 sensitivity profiles may also require compensation from a reference scan. If a non-deformable sodium-only volume coil is used at 3 T, it is often sufficient to perform sodium B_0 and B_1 adjustments in real time as follows.

First, it is important to measure the offset frequency for the given sample and coil combination (i.e., for every subject) and adjust the ^{23}Na resonant frequency. This can be performed using single voxel spectroscopy covering the sample and all sodium standards. Be sure to turn off water suppression in the spectroscopy exam and post-processing. Measure the resonant frequency (approximately 33.8 MHz at 3.0 T) and adjust the offset frequency in the acquisition protocol on the order of Hz (i.e., 1150 ± 10 Hz). Shimming of the B_0 field is performed on the proton channel and assumed to improve the sodium signal. Calibration of sodium B_1 Tx/Rx power should be performed for a representative sample during the initial coil setup on the scanner. This is typically performed using single voxel spectroscopy with an array of FA (0–270°), and the reference B_1 for a 90° pulse identified in coil files for the particular coil and anatomical location. Specific instructions should be made available from the coil engineer or scanner vendor. Still, if time permits, fine adjustments in sodium B_1 can be made with B_1 calibration on each individual subject using multi-FA ^{23}Na spectroscopy.

Image Acquisition and Reconstruction

The acquisition RF pulse sequence protocol used for a sodium MRI experiment requires overcoming the low SNR and fast relaxation times T_1 and T_2 of sodium ^{23}Na nuclei. The T_2 long component was measured to be 20.5 ± 1.7 ms in 6 healthy adult kidneys at 3-T MRI, and at high-field 7-T MRI, the reported T_2 long component in the cortex was 17.9 ± 0.8 ms and in the medulla 20.6 ± 1.0 ms [23, 24]. Another estimation may be derived from animal kidney imaging at similar field strength that yields ^{23}Na relaxation times: T_1 = 34 ms, T_2 short = 2.2 ms, and T_2 long = 20.4 ms [25]. Therefore, the goal of the pulse sequence is to achieve short echo times TE < T_2 short and relatively long repetition times TR ≈4 × T_1 to maximize SNR and reduce T_1/T_2-weighted contrast that may confound absolute tissue sodium quantification. To overcome the low sensitivity of ^{23}Na MRI, SNR is gained by imaging at lower spatial resolution and signal averaging for a number of minutes compared with seconds typically used for ^{1}H MRI. The linear proportionality of the ^{23}Na NMR signal to the spin density then allows for the absolute quantification of TSC on the basis of a known concentration reference phantom placed within the scanner.

Early examples of human renal sodium MRI utilized 3D Cartesian gradient echo (GRE) imaging with partial Fourier encoding to achieve TR/TE = 30/1.8 ms [7, 19]. Image reconstruction entailed applying a Fermi filter to the raw data prior to Fourier transform and heterodyne reconstruction. These methods suffered from anisotropic image resolution (38 × 38 × 24 cm^3) and low SNR. Renal sodium MRI at high-field 7 T employed a 3D GRE sequence and multi-echo array of 2.64–60.42 ms [24].

While some scanners may support gradient strengths and slew rates fast enough to achieve sub-millisecond TE with a Cartesian GRE readout, most often non-Cartesian ultra-short echo time (UTE) acquisition techniques are necessary for in vivo sodium MRI. UTE incorporates a short excitation pulse and non-Cartesian radial trajectory GRE read out. Excitation pulse length may be shortened by using half-pulses, and the RF bandwidth increased to achieve minimal TE, while considering a trade-off in SNR and limits of the transmit power on clinical scanners. The density-adapted 3D projection reconstruction (DA-3DPR) method has been most commonly used for renal sodium MRI at 3 T [26]. With the DA-3DPR sequence, a sub-millisecond TE = 0.55 and isotropic resolution of 5 mm^3 in 16 min was achieved [20, 21, 23, 27–30]. A spiral 3D UTE acquisition achieved TR/TE = 100/0.27 ms and isotropic resolution of 3 mm^3 [17]. Image reconstruction employs 3D Kaiser-Bessel re-gridding and Hanning filtering of the raw signal. Isotropic acquisition allows for coronal image reconstructions along the CMG axis, and this custom strategy should aid standardization of sodium quantification in the kidneys [27].

Runtime considerations: Non-Cartesian imaging may be technically challenging if not already implemented for proton acquisitions on the scanner. Concerns for non-ideal gradient trajectories often require specialized image reconstruction offline. For instance, UTE image quality improves when reconstructed based upon measured readout trajectories and has been implemented for quantitative imaging of short-T_2 bone water that typically suffers from low SNR analogous to short-T_2 of sodium [31–33]. Additionally, rapid imaging schemes have special considerations of the point spread function that is the effective image resolution [34]. Often noise filters are applied to raw data to increase SNR, at the cost of the point spread function, and this tradeoff will impact the initial choice of image resolution [15]. As an alternative to post-acquisition techniques to improve SNR, sample density weighting or spectrally weighted image acquisitions have demonstrated improved SNR for sodium MRI [35, 36]. Double half-pulses may be used for UTE excitation to reduce eddy current gradient distortions [37]. Excellent theoretical work presents simulated parametrizations for radial and density-adapted non-Cartesian trajectories to optimize image quality (full-width half maximum of the point spread function and SNR) and should continue to be pursued for renal sodium imaging applications [38–41].

Sodium Standards

Standard sodium solutions are placed in the image FOV to calibrate the ^{23}Na-weighted signal intensity and produce a quantitative map of tissue sodium content (TSC). Although sometimes referred to as sodium concentration [^{23}Na], when the metric is derived in tissue from MRI we will use the term "TSC". The ^{23}Na sodium-weighted signal intensity in each voxel will represent the average sodium density in the underlying tissue, from free and bound sodium in the intra-cellular and extra-cellular pools and is weighted by T_1/T_2 relaxation factors. The range of concentrations of sodium standards should cover the range expected in the tissue of interest. In the largest study of healthy adults to date, the average TSC in the healthy human kidney cortex was 58 ± 17 mmol/L (range: 27–63 mmol/L) and 99 ± 18 mmol/L in the medulla (range: 126–187 mmol/L) [23]. Therefore, ideally at least 2 sodium standards with a linear concentration over this range would be placed in the FOV for image calibration. In practice, quantitative renal sodium MRI reports utilize a 0.6% NaCl in 2–4% agarose gel in a 50-mL plastic conical tube [21, 42]. Alternative methods place a sodium standard on each coil element as fiduciary markers for coil placement, with concentration up to 0.9% NaCl (153 mM/L) in 2% agarose [17]. It is common practice to use saline solutions for quantitative extremity sodium MRI protocols [43]. Agarose and saline solution phantoms produced similar sodium signal intensity when tested for renal applications (Fig. 23.2a) [20].

Calibration may also be accomplished using an internal standard in a tissue with consistent sodium concentration. For renal applications, this is often the cerebrospinal fluid (CSF) included in the FOV. CSF sodium content was found to be repeatable after water loading but varies depending on level in the spine [20, 27]. CSF may be a viable internal standard to check image quality and assist with signal standardization between individuals if assessed in a consistent anatomical location.

A separate calibration phantom is often necessary to monitor coil integrity and scan quality or calibrate multi-nuclear coils. Sodium phantoms for this purpose should cover the entire FOV with a similar coil filling factor as the torso (e.g., 335 × 325 × 160 mm^3) and have sodium concentrations in the expected physiologic range (e.g., 60 mmol/L NaCl) [7, 20].

Runtime considerations: Standards should be placed equidistant from any coil elements to avoid local B_1 inhomogeneity, generally 1–2 cm from a coil rung or capacitor. The placement of

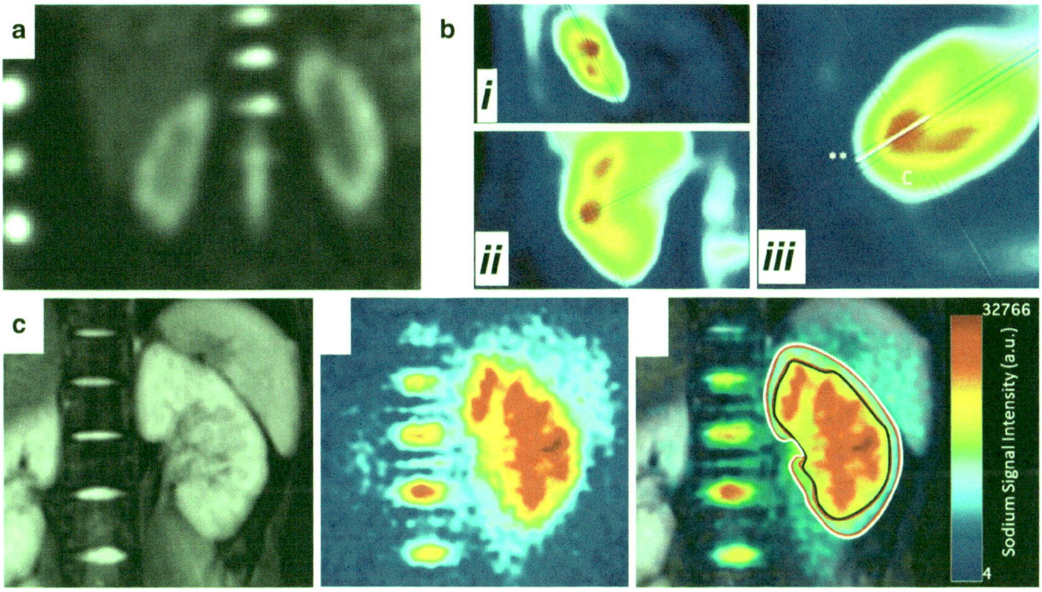

Fig. 23.2 (**a**) Sodium-weighted 3-T MRI with three sodium standards in the field of view (top to bottom: 0.9%NaCl in 2% agarose, 0.6%NaCl in 2% agarose, and 0.9%NaCl solution). (**b**) Selection of custom-angled orthogonal image reconstruction planes displayed for (i) sagittal, (ii) coronal, and (iii) axial slices, where the coronal axis aligns with the long axis of the kidney. The sodium corticomedullary gradient profile is measured from the cortex to the medulla (marked by **). (**c**) T_2-weighted 3-T MRI of the human kidney, corresponding sodium-weighted MRI, and fused image showing segmentations of the cortex (outer layer) and medulla (inner layer). Reprinted with kind permission from Haneder et al. Radiology 2011, original Figure 3 [20]; Haneder et al. Acad Radiol 2013, original Figure 1 [27]; Akbari et al. Radiology 2022, original Figure 2 [42]

sodium phantoms should also be standardized, such that the phantoms are the same size tube and oriented symmetrically in the image FOV, giving rise to at least 4 voxels in their cross-sectional area and an identical volume of solution for all concentrations; this is sufficient for quantification of sodium signal at a known concentration from a standard volume. Methods for preparation of sodium standards have been previously provided [44].

Post-processing and Data Analysis

Quantitative Sodium MRI in the Human Kidney

Renal sodium MRI in the human kidney collected in a standardized manner can provide quantitative image contrast sensitive to the CMG in TSC. The following methods outline how a quantitative parameter map is derived from sodium-weighted MRI.

Image processing begins with a choice of the slice profile during image reconstruction of an isotropic acquisition. The coronal slice that includes the thickest part of the renal cortex and greatest number of visible medullary pyramids is preferable [30]. The slice should also contain the sodium standards. The absolute quantification of sodium CMG slope will depend on the angulation of coronal image reconstruction, whether at a custom angle oriented with the long-axis of the kidney or non-angulated (Fig. 23.2b). Regardless of angulation, a similar trend of sodium CMG under water-load conditions is measured from both image orientations [27].

Next, the sodium-weighted image signal intensity is calibrated to known sodium concentration in the reference phantoms. A linear calibration curve can be generated from the mean ^{23}Na signal intensity measured in (1) a region of noise void of tissue, and either (2) the sodium standard(s), or (3) an internal standard region such as CSF. The calibration curve is applied voxel-wise to map ^{23}Na signal intensity to known concentrations and generate a TSC map. This approach has been outlined with use of one reference phantom with correction for T_1/T_2 relaxation factors in the phantom and tissue by Haneder et al. 2011 [20].

Physiologic metrics can be derived from the renal TSC map including renal cortex TSC, medullary TSC, and TSC-derived CMG. Regions of interest can be segmented from anatomical T_2 - weighted imaging in an identical FOV as sodium MRI, noting excellent recent examples of layered segmentations from the renal cortex to medulla (Fig. 23.2c) [14, 42]. SNR is quantified in regions of interest or voxel-wise and may also be used to calculate the SNR-derived CMG [24, 42]. Whether using metrics TSC or SNR, the CMG is often measured pixel-by-pixel along a profile through the cortex and a medullary pyramid, approximately 20 mm in length [20, 23, 27]. The TSC-derived or SNR-derived CMG is often reported as the slope along this profile or plotted as a function of distance from the cortex.

Runtime considerations: Sources of variability in renal sodium measurements should be considered before, during, and after the experiment. Among 50 healthy volunteers, renal sodium quantification was found to be quite variable in the cortex and medulla [23]. There may be image quantification and physiologic factors that need further standardization to improve accuracy of absolute renal TSC. Standardized imaging of tissue sodium relies on a stable coil setup and sodium standards. See methods described by Haneder et al. 2013 for image analysis strategies when sodium standards are not apparent in the reconstructed slice [27]. Image post-processing for relaxation compensation of the sodium signal should improve accuracy of absolute TSC quantification, especially if sodium relaxometry is expected to differ between the cortex vs. medulla [24]. However, this strategy relies on knowledge of the fundamental parameters for sodium T_1/T_2 in the human kidneys, which are not well established in disease states and are time consuming to measure per subject [45]. Physiologic factors that could influence absolute quantification are water loading, water deprivation, diuresis, fasting, and subsequent time prior to kidney imaging. Indeed, dynamic renal sodium imaging after water loading (15-mL water per kg body weight within 15 min) in fasting individuals revealed reduced CMG between 1 and 2 h after water loading, and increased CMG approaching baseline after 2 h 45 min, indicating the importance of standardized hydration status [42]. Additional physiologic recommendations by the PARENCHIMA network for functional renal MRI assessments may be applicable for renal sodium quantification as well [46].

Summary and Technical Future Directions

Table 23.1 summarizes specific exam parameters and clinical applications of renal sodium ^{23}Na-MRI. In summary, technical concepts for renal sodium ^{23}Na-MRI experimentation are:

1. The RF amplifier must accept a broad-band frequency range; coil Tx/Rx circuits must be tuned for ^{23}Na Larmor resonance frequency (33.8 MHz on a 3.0-T magnet); fine adjustments for resonance frequency (on the order of Hz) and B_1 power may be required for each sample and should be checked with ^{23}Na MR spectroscopy.
2. Minimum TE (<T2short ~ 2 ms) and sufficiently long TR (3–5 times the T_1 ~34 ms) must be achieved by the RF pulse sequence design to maximize SNR and reduce T_1/T_2 relaxation dependence of ^{23}Na signal contrast.
3. Standard sodium concentrations may be incorporated in the FOV to calibrate sodium-weighted MRI signal intensity to known concentrations and quantify TSC maps.
4. Image analysis of TSC and SNR in the cortex and medulla is used to assess the CMG, with relevance to fundamental renal physiology and disease.

Table 23.1 Renal sodium ^{23}Na MRI acquisition and analysis protocols for clinical applications

Citation	Clinical application	Subjects (number enrolled)	Field (T)	RF coil design	Pulse sequence	TR/TE (ms)	Slice orientation; spatial resolution	NSA; scan-time (min)	Sodium standards	Physiologic conditions	Imaging metrics
Ra et al. MRM 1988 [5]	Multi-organ sodium MRI	Healthy ($n = 1$)	1.5 T	Custom two loops, 25 cm diameter and height	3D spin-echo FID planar-projection imaging	95/14 ms	Spherical image recon. in 3 orthogonal planes with diameter 25 cm, matrix 128 × 128	6 NSA; 50 min	NR	NR	Observation
Granot, Radiology 1988 [6]	Multi-organ sodium MRI	Healthy ($n = 1$)	2 T	Custom planar square (9 × 9 cm) Tx/Rx surface coil	3D GRE with volumetric non-slice selective RF excitation	84/6.4 ms	Coronal; 3–4 mm^2, 15 mm slice thickness	32 NSA; 30 min	NR	NR	Observation
Maril et al. MRM 2006 [7]	Feasibility of 3-T renal sodium MRI in healthy kidney	Healthy ($n = 6$)	3 T	Custom single-tuned ^{23}Na quadrature surface coil (2 loops, 18 cm diameter)	3D GRE with partial Fourier echo and non-slice selective RF excitation	30/1.8 ms	Unilateral coronal; 3 × 3 × 15 mm^3	24 NSA; 25 min	B1 calibration phantom: 60 mmol/L, 20 L volume	Water deprivation (12 h)	SNR-CMG; number of medullary pyramids
Rosen, Lenkinski. Acad Radiol 2009 [19]	Kidney transplantation	Patient with end-stage hypertensive nephropathy with kidney transplantation ($n = 1$)	3 T	Commercial sodium surface coil rectangular	3D GRE with partial Fourier echo and non-slice selective RF excitation	30/1.8 ms	Unilateral sagittal; 3 × 3 × 15 mm^3	24 NSA; 25 min	NR	NR	SNR-CMG; number of medullary pyramids
Haneder, et al. Radiology 2011 [20]	Healthy kidney before and after water loading	Healthy ($n = 14$)	3 T	Commercial single-tuned ^{23}Na Rx 8-element coil	3D GRE UTE density-adapted radial; excitation pulse length = 1 ms; 8000 projections; FA = 85°; FOV = 320 × 320 mm^2	120/0.55 ms	Bilateral coronal; 5 × 5 × 5 mm^3	16 min	Phantom in FOV: 0.6% NaCl with 2% agarose in conical tube[a]	Baseline scan (abstained from water for 6 h); water loaded scan (30 min after drinking 1 L water)	TSC-CMG; TSC in CSF; TSC maps corrected for T1 and T2 weighting
Haneder et al. Strahlenther Onkol 2012 [21]	Kidney damage by radiotherapy for gastric cancer	Patients with gastric cancer irradiated ($n = 4$)	3 T	[b]	[b]	[b]	[b]	[b]	[b]	NR	TSC-CMG; proton T2* and ADC

(continued)

Table 23.1 (continued)

Citation	Clinical application	Subjects (number enrolled)	Field (T)	RF coil design	Pulse sequence	TR/TE (ms)	Slice orientation; spatial resolution	NSA; scan-time (min)	Sodium standards	Physiologic conditions	Imaging metrics
Haneder et al. Magn Reson Mater Phy 2013 [23]	Sodium and multi-parametric MRI reference values in healthy kidney	Healthy ($n = 50$)	3 T	[b]	[b]	[b]	[b]	[b]	[b]	No preparation	Sodium T1/ T2*long; TSC-CMG; proton T2* and ADC
Haneder et al. Acad Radiol 2013 [27]	Healthy kidney before and after water loading	Healthy ($n = 14$)[c]	3 T	[b]	[b]	[b]	[b]	[b]	[b]	Before and 30 min after water load	Angled and non-angled TSC-CMG; TSC in CSF
Haneder et al. Magma 2014 [28]	Effects of desmopressin in patients with central diabetes insipidus	Patients with central diabetes insipidus ($n = 4$)	3 T	[b]	[b]	[b]	[b]	[b]	[b]	Before and after desmopressin	TSC-CMG; TSC in CSF
Moon et al. Eur Radiol 2014 [17]	Kidney transplantation	Patients with kidney transplantation ($n = 3$ normal, $n = 3$ rejected); healthy ($n = 6$)	3 T	Dual-tuned 1H/23Na Tx/ Rx quadrature saddle-shape; flexible surface coil 30-channel 1H, 2-channel ^{23}Na; chosen for best fit on the torso	3D UTE spiral; excitation pulse length = 500–900 μs; FA = 90°	100/0.27–0.5 ms	Unilateral coronal, 3 × 3 × 3 mm^3	27 min	4 or 5 sodium phantoms to mark the surface coils (4% agar, 153 mM/L NaCl)	Abstain from water (4 h before scan)	SNR, TSC-CMG, reproducibility
Haneder et al. Eur Radiol 2014 [24]	Feasibility of 7 T renal sodium MRI	Healthy ($n = 8$)	7 T	Commercial single-tuned 23Na Tx/Rx 6-channel spine-array coil	3D Cartesian spoiled GRE with variable TE; FOV = 256 × 256 mm^2, 24 slices; bandwidth = 30–60 Hz/pixel	49/4.19; multi-echo: 75/2.64–60.42 ms	Coronal; 4 × 4 × 5 mm^3; multi-echo: 4 × 4 × 15 mm^3	42 min; multi-echo: 47 min	Reference scan phantom: 36 × 53 × 30 cm^3, rectangular plastic box, saline solution	Abstain from water (1 h before scan)	Sodium T2*long; SNR; SNR-CMG

Haneder et al. Strahlentherapie und Onkologie 2015 [29]	Kidney damage by radiochemotherapy for gastric cancer	Patients after radiochemotherapy (n = 13); healthy (n = 5)	3 T	Dual-tuned Tx/Rx array 1H/23Na coil	[b]	[b]	[b]	[b]	[b]	Water load (intravenous, solution: 500-mL 0.9% NaCl)	TSC-CMG; proton ADC and renal volume
Budjan et al. In Vivo 2016 [30]	Renal denervation in humans with resistant hypertension; Symplicity HTN3 clinical trial	Patients undergoing renal denervation (n = 2)	3 T	Commercial dual-tuned 1H/23Na Tx/Rx array	[b]	[b]	[b]	[b]	NR	Abstain from water (4 h before scan); scanned at same time per day	SNR-CMG; proton ADC; assessed from intervention −1, 1, 30, and 90 days
Grist et al. Kidney Int 2020 [14]	Multi-site study of renal sodium dynamics	Healthy (n = 6 per site, 2 sites)	3 T[d]	NR	NR	NR	Unilateral coronal	NR	4% agar phantoms with similar T1 as whole kidney	Water load baseline scan (500 mL before scan); diuresis scan 30 min after furosemide (0.5 mg/kg)	TSC-CMG from layered segmentations
Akbari et al. Radiology 2022 [42]	Chronic kidney disease (CKD)	Patients with CKD (n = 5); healthy (n = 10)	3 T	Custom single-tuned ^{23}Na butterfly surface coil (2-loop, 18-cm diameter)	3D GRE UTE density-adapted radial; excitation pulse length = 528 μsec; 377 projections; FA = 60°; FOV = 36 × 36 cm^2, 3D slab thickness 3 cm	50/0.65 ms	Unilateral coronal; 3 × 3 mm^2	50 NSA; 15 min	NR	Before and 1 h after water load (15 mL water per kg body weight); furosemide and spironolactone in CKD	SNR-CMG from ROI segmentations; assessed from intervention 0, 1 hr, 1 hr 35min, 1hr 10min, 2hr 45min

Abbreviations: *T* Tesla, *RF* radiofrequency, *NR* not reported, *NSA* number of signal acquisitions, *GRE* gradient echo, *UTE* ultra-short echo time, *SNR* signal to noise ratio, *TSC* tissue sodium content, *CMG* corticomedullary gradient, *ADC* apparent diffusion coefficient, *T2** transverse relaxation time, *CSF* cerebrospinal fluid, *h* hour, *min* minute, *FOV* field of view

[a] Other phantoms used include reference scan phantom: 335 × 325 × 160 mm^3, rectangular plastic box, 0.6% NaCl solution without agarose; concentration phantoms in FOV: [0.9%, 0.6%]NaCl with 2% agarose, and 0.9% NaCl solution in conical tubes.

[b] protocol parameter as described by Haneder et al. Radiology 2011.

[c] data was reanalyzed from Haneder et al. Radiology 2011.

[d] ^{23}NaMRI methods not reported but assumed acquisition at 3 T.

Promising new developments in imaging technology may enhance renal sodium MRI. Dedicated coil designs with phased arrays combined with compressed sense imaging hold potential to improve SNR and would have widespread applications in the kidneys using abdominal fittings [15]. For instance, the TORO (transmit-only, receive-only) system has multiple transmit channels and improves B_1 homogeneity using a dual-resonance system [47, 48]. Interleaved scanning for simultaneous proton and sodium MRI/MRS would provide exciting opportunities for measurement of functional (i.e., perfusion and diffusion) and sodium renal temporal dynamics, but remains technically challenging [49]. Development of a rapid scan for renal sodium relaxometry would improve the accuracy of subsequent biomarker assessment, assist with biexponential ^{23}Na signal interpretation, and could provide information about disease states such as renal cysts, fibrosis, or inflammation [50]. Multi-nuclear applications are logical developments for high-field systems and have already begun to be implemented for renal sodium MRI at 7 T [24, 51]. In the following section, we discuss findings from clinical applications of renal sodium MRI in human health and disease.

Clinical Applications

Renal Sodium MRI in Healthy Individuals

The kidneys are essential in regulating homeostatic functions in the body such as extra-cellular fluid volume, acid–base equilibrium (pH), electrolyte concentrations, and blood pressure (via maintaining salt and water balance). This role depends tightly on the regulation of extra-cellular sodium in the kidney, which maintains a concentration gradient from the cortex to the medulla (i.e. the CMG). Thus, renal function is tightly dependent on this CMG and mapping this gradient with sodium MRI could help assess kidney impairments. Human kidney tissue sodium MRI was observed in early investigations of multinuclear ^{23}Na MRI and revealed a CMG in 2006 [5–7]. The first clinical application of renal sodium MRI at 3 T demonstrated that a 12-h water deprivation increases the sodium CMG by 25% [7]. A study by Haneder et al. 2011 acquired baseline imaging after a 6-h water deprivation [20]. This was followed by ingestion of 1 L of water and a second ^{23}Na MRI acquisition. Water loading reduced the cortical sodium from 63.5 ± 9.3 to 48.6 ± 5.3 mmol/L and medullary sodium from 108.0 ± 10.9 to 81.9 ± 10.1 mmol/L. While both cortical and medullary sodium decreased, the sodium CMG was not substantially affected. In 2013, Haneder et al. demonstrated high spatial resolution isotropic imaging and a standardized quantification protocol for image-based TSC measurement in the human kidney [27]. This methodology was subsequently performed to assess renal sodium CMG in a variety of applications.

Sodium CMG has a wide variation between individuals. In the largest study to date of renal ^{23}Na MRI in healthy adults, the average TSC reported in the kidney cortex was 58 ± 17 mmol/L (range: 27–63 mmol/L) and in the medulla was 99 ± 18 mmol/L (range: 126–187 mmol/L) [23]. There was no correlation between renal TSC and age, gender, body mass index, estimated glomerular filtration rate, or serum sodium [23]. Multiparametric assessment in this study included blood oxygenation level-dependent (BOLD) ^{1}H MRI to measure renal R2* and diffusion weighted ^{1}H MRI to measure apparent diffusion coefficient (ADC); neither correlated with renal sodium nor displayed a gradient from the cortex to medulla, demonstrating the unique information provided by renal sodium assessment. These studies demonstrated the potential for noninvasive evaluation of renal TSC as well as the sodium CMG in response to water deprivation and water loading.

Complementing these findings, another study of patients with central diabetes insipidus (expected to have normal kidney morphology and function) illustrated the capacity of ^{23}Na MRI to capture a physiological renal response. Administration of intranasal desmopressin (DDAVP) to the patients with central diabetes insipidus resulted in 17% reduction in TSC. The mean TSC increased along the CMG from the cortex (pre-DDAVP 38.0 ± 6.3 mmol/L vs. post-

DDAVP 30.7 ± 3.5 mmol/L) to the medulla (pre-DDAVP 71.6 ± 14.8 mmol/L vs. post-DDAVP 59.7 ± 10.8 mmol/L) [28]. Recently, ^{23}Na MRI performed in healthy volunteers demonstrated a correlation between the sodium CMG and urinary osmolality ($r^2 = 0.22$, $p < 0.001$) [42]. These results confirm that the sodium CMG can reflect urine concentrating ability.

Renal Sodium MRI of Kidney Transplantation

One of the earliest clinical applications of renal sodium MRI in a disease setting evaluated SNR along the CMG and the number of medullary pyramids apparent on sodium-weighted contrast in a patient with a transplanted kidney [19]. Another evaluation was undertaken in patients with transplanted kidneys using standardized ^{23}Na-MRI and showed significant reduction in TSC in the transplanted kidneys (153.5 ± 11.9 mM) compared to TSC in native kidneys of healthy controls (192.9 ± 9.6 mM) [17]. The sodium CMG was also lower in the transplanted kidney (8.9 ± 1.5 mM/mm) compared to CMG in healthy kidneys (10.5 ± 0.9 mM/mm). This is notable as a possible alternative diagnostic method to assess renal transplant function. Furthermore, a noninvasive imaging method to diagnose graft dysfunction is highly preferred to reduce complications and increase the reliability of renal function screening as well as in implementing early therapeutic intervention [52]. Although no significant difference in sodium levels or corticomedullary sodium gradient was detected between transplanted patients with acute rejection versus kidneys without allograft rejection, the authors note a limited sample size (3 of the 6 transplant patients had biopsy-proven renal allograft rejection).

Renal Sodium MRI of Hypertension

Hypertension impairs the renal regulation of sodium handling that favors more avid sodium reabsorption along the length of the nephron that, at least in part, has been linked to heightened activity of the renal sympathetic nervous system. Renal denervation in animals decreases tubular sodium reabsorption and lessens renin secretion by the juxtamedullary apparatus expected to lower systemic blood pressure. These considerations form the basis for renal denervation as a treatment in patients refractory to conventional medical antihypertension therapies. Budjan et al. studied patients with therapy resistant-hypertension and performed sodium imaging of the kidneys to assess the effect of renal denervation therapy [30]. No changes were found in renal total sodium content or sodium SNR-CMG at 1, 30, or 90 days following the renal denervation. As in kidney transplantation applications, the major limitation is the low number of patients in the study.

Renal Sodium MRI of Kidney Damage and Chronic Kidney Disease

In recent years, ^{23}Na MRI of the kidneys has been applied to patients with several types of kidney injury as well as extrarenal diseases that impair kidney function, e.g., congestive heart failure. Haneder et al. combined ^{23}Na MRI and functional ^{1}H MRI to assess the damage of kidneys exposed to radiotherapy in patients undergoing treatment for gastric cancer [21, 29]. Irradiation exposure of the upper pole of the kidney caused changes in the functional ^{1}H MRI that were consistent with reduced cell density and tissue oxygenation [21]. ^{23}Na MRI showed loss of the sodium CMG in a manner dependent on radiation dose, confirming that this metric may be an early marker of kidney damage [29]. In patients with CKD from cardiorenal syndrome, a study correlating the sodium CMG and urinary osmolality was performed after water-loading [42]. The sodium CMG was lower in participants with CKD (1.35 ± 0.11) compared with healthy individuals (1.55 ± 0.11) before water loading [42]. The findings are consistent with diminished ability to concentrate urine in patients with cardiorenal syndrome because of reduced tubular function. The study highlights that among the developing field of multi-parametric renal MRI, ^{23}Na MRI provides unique functional information about tubular integrity. Indeed, the ongoing clinical trial NCT05014178 will measure the corticomedullary sodium gradient in various kidney diseases.

Sodium MRI of Extremity Skin and Muscle in Patients with Kidney Disease

^{23}Na MRI consistently shows sodium accumulation in the skin and muscle of patients with a variety of acute and chronic kidney diseases. Skin and muscle accumulation of sodium is most dramatic in patients with end-stage kidney disease requiring dialysis, although high skin and muscle sodium occurs in CKD patients not yet on dialysis and is associated with greater age, male sex, body mass index, systolic blood pressure, and left ventricular hypertrophy [53–55]. As in kidneys, ^{23}Na MRI captures changes in the extrarenal sodium stores in skin and muscle. For example, dialysis treatment reduces muscle and, to some extent, skin sodium levels. Interestingly, although patients with acute kidney injury showed higher calf muscle and skin sodium accumulation, in contrast to end-stage kidney disease, dialysis treatment did not reduce muscle or skin sodium after 4–5 treatments. Even without reduced kidney function, hypertension has been linked to excessive skin and muscle sodium accumulation [56].

Conclusion

^{23}Na MRI is a powerful technique that can noninvasively measure tissue sodium, map the distribution of sodium in the kidney, and monitor changes in the corticomedullary sodium gradient, which provides a marker of the regulation of extracellular sodium concentration. Renal sodium concentration is affected by physiologic conditions (e.g., water deprivation, water loading, and diuresis). Moreover, studies indicate that pathophysiologic conditions (e.g., kidney transplantation, radiotherapy damage, and CKD) reduce the sodium CMG that may reflect impairment in tubular function and even tissue viability. This capacity to capture nephron function is unique to ^{23}Na MRI and, therefore, along with functional ^{1}H MRI studies of tissue oxygenation, perfusion, and diffusion, ^{23}Na MRI enables non-invasive clinical characterization of relevant kidney functions and structure.

Acknowledgments The authors receive grant support from the National Institutes of Health (NIH 1P01HL116263; 1R01HL155523; 1R01HL157378) and the American Heart Association (AHA 18CDA34110297, 19IPLOI34760518).

Disclosures The authors have nothing to disclose.

References

1. Ouwerkerk R. Sodium magnetic resonance imaging: from research to clinical use. J Am Coll Radiol. 2007;4(10):739–41.
2. Madelin G, Lee JS, Regatte RR, Jerschow A. Sodium MRI: methods and applications. Prog Nucl Magn Reson Spectrosc. 2014;79:14–47.
3. Pitts RF. Physiology of the kidney and body fluids; an introductory text, vol. xi. Chicago: Year Book Medical Publishers; 1974. p. 315.
4. Martin K, Tan SJ, Toussaint ND. Magnetic resonance imaging determination of tissue sodium in patients with chronic kidney disease. Nephrology (Carlton). 2022;27(2):117–25.
5. Ra JB, Hilal SK, Oh CH, Mun IK. In vivo magnetic resonance imaging of sodium in the human body. Magn Reson Med. 1988;7(1):11–22.
6. Granot J. Sodium imaging of human body organs and extremities in vivo. Radiology. 1988;167(2):547–50.
7. Maril N, Rosen Y, Reynolds GH, Ivanishev A, Ngo L, Lenkinski RE. Sodium MRI of the human kidney at 3 tesla. Magn Reson Med. 2006;56(6):1229–34.
8. Knepper MA. Measurement of osmolality in kidney slices using vapor pressure osmometry. Kidney Int. 1982;21(4):653–5.
9. Jamison RL, Oliver RE. Disorders of urinary concentration and dilution. Am J Med. 1982;72(2):308–22.
10. Lemley KV, Kriz W. Cycles and separations: the histotopography of the urinary concentrating process. Kidney Int. 1987;31(2):538–48.
11. Rocha AS, Kokko JP. Sodium chloride and water transport in the medullary thick ascending limb of Henle. Evidence for active chloride transport. J Clin Invest. 1973;52(3):612–23.
12. Berry MR, Mathews RJ, Ferdinand JR, et al. Renal sodium gradient orchestrates a dynamic antibacterial defense zone. Cell. 2017;170(5):860–874 e819.

13. Aw M, Armstrong TM, Nawata CM, et al. Body mass-specific Na(+)-K(+)-ATPase activity in the medullary thick ascending limb: implications for species-dependent urine concentrating mechanisms. Am J Phys Regul Integr Comp Phys. 2018;314(4):R563–73.
14. Grist JT, Riemer F, Hansen ESS, et al. Visualization of sodium dynamics in the kidney by magnetic resonance imaging in a multi-site study. Kidney Int. 2020;98(5):1174–8.
15. Zollner FG, Konstandin S, Lommen J, et al. Quantitative sodium MRI of kidney. NMR Biomed. 2016;29(2):197–205.
16. Madelin G, Regatte RR. Biomedical applications of sodium MRI in vivo. J Magn Reson Imaging. 2013;38(3):511–29.
17. Moon CH, Furlan A, Kim J-H, Zhao T, Shapiro R, Bae KT. Quantitative sodium MR imaging of native versus transplanted kidneys using a dual-tuned proton/sodium (1H/23Na) coil: initial experience. Eur Radiol. 2014;24(6):1320–6.
18. Bangerter NK, Kaggie JD, Taylor MD, Hadley JR. Sodium MRI radiofrequency coils for body imaging. NMR Biomed. 2016;29(2):107–18.
19. Rosen YMD, Lenkinski REP. Sodium MRI of a human transplanted kidney. Acad Radiol. 2009;16(7):886–9.
20. Haneder S, Konstandin S, Morelli JN, et al. Quantitative and qualitative (23)Na MR imaging of the human kidneys at 3 T: before and after a water load. Radiology. 2011;260(3):857–65.
21. Haneder S, Michaely HJ, Schoenberg SO, et al. Assessment of renal function after conformal radiotherapy and intensity-modulated radiotherapy by functional 1H-MRI and 23Na-MRI. Strahlenther Onkol. 2012;188(12):1146–54.
22. Madelin G, Kline R, Walvick R, Regatte RR. A method for estimating intracellular sodium concentration and extracellular volume fraction in brain in vivo using sodium magnetic resonance imaging. Sci Rep. 2014;4:4763.
23. Haneder S, Kettnaker P, Konstandin S, et al. Quantitative in vivo Na-23 MR imaging of the healthy human kidney: determination of physiological ranges at 3.0T with comparison to DWI and BOLD. Magn Reson Mater Phy. 2013;26(6):501–9.
24. Haneder S, Juras V, Michaely HJ, et al. In vivo sodium (23Na) imaging of the human kidneys at 7T: preliminary results. Eur Radiol. 2014;24:494–501.
25. Maril N, Margalit R, Mispelter J, Degani H. Functional sodium magnetic resonance imaging of the intact rat kidney. Kidney Int. 2004;65(3):927–35.
26. Nagel AM, Laun FB, Weber MA, Matthies C, Semmler W, Schad LR. Sodium MRI using a density-adapted 3D radial acquisition technique. Magn Reson Med. 2009;62(6):1565–73.
27. Haneder S, Konstandin S, Morelli JN, Schad LR, Schoenberg SO, Michaely HJ. Assessment of the renal corticomedullary (23)Na gradient using isotropic data sets. Acad Radiol. 2013;20(4):407–13.
28. Haneder S, Michaely HJ, Konstandin S, et al. 3T renal (23)Na-MRI: effects of desmopressin in patients with central diabetes insipidus. MAGMA. 2014;27(1):47–52.
29. Haneder S, Budjan JM, Schoenberg SO, et al. Dose-dependent changes in renal (1)H–/(23)Na MRI after adjuvant radiochemotherapy for gastric cancer. Strahlenther Onkol. 2015;191(4):356.
30. Budjan J, Benck U, Lammert A, et al. Renal denervation in patients with resistant hypertension-assessment by 3T renal 23Na-MRI: preliminary results. In Vivo. 2016;30(5):657–62.
31. Manhard MK, Horch RA, Harkins KD, Gochberg DF, Nyman JS, Does MD. Validation of quantitative bound- and pore-water imaging in cortical bone. Magn Reson Med. 2014;71(6):2166–71.
32. Manhard MK, Harkins KD, Gochberg DF, Nyman JS, Does MD. 30-second bound and pore water concentration mapping of cortical bone using 2D UTE with optimized half-pulses. Magn Reson Med. 2017;77(3):945–50.
33. Kronthaler S, Rahmer J, Bornert P, et al. Trajectory correction based on the gradient impulse response function improves high-resolution UTE imaging of the musculoskeletal system. Magn Reson Med. 2021;85(4):2001–15.
34. Robson MD, Gore JC, Constable RT. Measurement of the point spread function in MRI using constant time imaging. Magn Reson Med. 1997;38(5):733–40.
35. Stobbe R, Beaulieu C. Advantage of sampling density weighted apodization over postacquisition filtering apodization for sodium MRI of the human brain. Magn Reson Med. 2008;60(4):981–6.
36. Boada FE, Shen GX, Chang SY, Thulborn KR. Spectrally weighted twisted projection imaging: reducing T2 signal attenuation effects in fast three-dimensional sodium imaging. Magn Reson Med. 1997;38(6):1022–8.
37. Josan S, Pauly JM, Daniel BL, Pauly KB. Double half RF pulses for reduced sensitivity to eddy currents in UTE imaging. Magn Reson Med. 2009;61(5):1083–9.
38. Gurney PT, Hargreaves BA, Nishimura DG. Design and analysis of a practical 3D cones trajectory. Magn Reson Med. 2006;55(3):575–82.
39. Konstandin S, Nagel AM. Performance of sampling density-weighted and postfiltered density-adapted projection reconstruction in sodium magnetic resonance imaging. Magn Reson Med. 2013;69(2):495–502.
40. Bydder M, Ali F, Saucedo A, et al. A study of 3D radial density adapted trajectories for sodium imaging. Magn Reson Imaging. 2021;83:89–95.
41. Polak P, Schulte RF, Noseworthy MD. An approach to evaluation of the point-spread function for (23) Na magnetic resonance imaging. NMR Biomed. 2022;35(2):e4627.
42. Akbari A, Lemoine S, Salerno F, et al. Functional sodium MRI helps to measure Corticomedullary sodium content in Normal and diseased human kidneys. Radiology. 2022;303(2):384–9.

43. Kopp C, Linz P, Wachsmuth L, et al. (23)Na magnetic resonance imaging of tissue sodium. Hypertension. 2012;59(1):167–72.
44. Grist JT, Hansen ES, Zollner FG, Laustsen C. Sodium ((23)Na) MRI of the kidney: experimental protocol. Methods Mol Biol. 2021;2216:473–80.
45. Boada FE, Christensen JD, Huanghellinger FR, Reese TG, Thulborn KR. Quantitative in-vivo tissue sodium concentration maps—the effects of Biexponential relaxation. Magn Reson Med. 1994;32(2):219–23.
46. Mendichovszky I, Pullens P, Dekkers I, et al. Technical recommendations for clinical translation of renal MRI: a consensus project of the cooperation in science and technology action parenchima. MAGMA. 2020;33(1):131–40.
47. Barberi EA, Gati JS, Rutt BK, Menon RS. A transmit-only/receive-only (TORO) RF system for high-field MRI/MRS applications. Magn Reson Med. 2000;43(2):284–9.
48. Wetterling F, Corteville DM, Kalayciyan R, et al. Whole body sodium MRI at 3T using an asymmetric birdcage resonator and short echo time sequence: first images of a male volunteer. Phys Med Biol. 2012;57(14):4555–67.
49. Lopez Kolkovsky AL, Carlier PG, Marty B, Meyerspeer M. Interleaved and simultaneous multi-nuclear magnetic resonance in vivo. Review of principles, applications and potential. NMR Biomed. 2022;35:e4735.
50. Alhulail AA, Xia P, Shen X, et al. Fast in vivo (23) Na imaging and T 2^* mapping using accelerated 2D-FID UTE magnetic resonance spectroscopic imaging at 3 T: proof of concept and reliability study. Magn Reson Med. 2021;85(4):1783–94.
51. de Boer A, Hoogduin JM, Blankestijn PJ, et al. 7 T renal MRI: challenges and promises. MAGMA. 2016;29(3):417–33.
52. Schutter R, Lantinga VA, Borra RJH, Moers C. MRI for diagnosis of post-renal transplant complications: current state-of-the-art and future perspectives. MAGMA. 2020;33(1):49–61.
53. Dahlmann A, Dorfelt K, Eicher F, et al. Magnetic resonance-determined sodium removal from tissue stores in hemodialysis patients. Kidney Int. 2015;87(2):434–41.
54. Schneider MP, Raff U, Kopp C, et al. Skin sodium concentration correlates with left ventricular hypertrophy in CKD. J Am Soc Nephrol. 2017;28:1867.
55. Sahinoz M, Tintara S, Deger SM, et al. Tissue sodium stores in peritoneal dialysis and hemodialysis patients determined by 23-sodium magnetic resonance imaging. Nephrol Dial Transplant. 2020;36:1307.
56. Kopp C, Linz P, Dahlmann A, et al. 23Na magnetic resonance imaging-determined tissue sodium in healthy subjects and hypertensive patients. Hypertension. 2013;61(3):635–40.

24 Hyperpolarized ^{13}C Renal Magnetic Resonance Imaging: Practical Considerations for Clinical Use

Renal Hyperpolarized ^{13}C MRI

Nikolaj Bøgh and Christoffer Laustsen

MRI Physics and Acquisition Protocols

Basic Concepts Behind d-DNP Hyperpolarized ^{13}C MRI

Transient enhancement of nuclear magnetism beyond thermal equilibrium is referred to as hyperpolarization, which greatly increases the magnetic resonance (MR) signal. In hyperpolarized carbon-13 magnetic resonance imaging (MRI), carbon-13 enriched molecules are hyperpolarized using dissolution dynamic nuclear polarization (d-DNP). The method achieves liquid-state polarization of up to five orders of magnitude over thermal state polarization [1, 2]. After administration of the hyperpolarized molecule, a transiently high signal can be imaged. In contrast to gadolinium-based contrast agents, which generate contrast by modulating tissue relaxation, hyperpolarized agents are the signal source themselves. This resamples that of the radioactive tracers seen in positron emission tomography (PET) without relying on ionizing radiation. Additionally, the hyperpolarized agent and its metabolites can be detected separately owing to the chemical shift effect.

Hyperpolarized substrates for human use are produced using commercially available equipment (SPINlab®, GE Healthcare) [1]. A sample consisting of an isotope-enriched substrate, typically [1-^{13}C]pyruvate, and a stable organic free radical (electron paramagnetic agent or EPA), is packaged aseptically in a sterile container (the pharmacy kit) and subsequently placed in a strong magnetic field (5 T) at very low temperatures (0.8 K). The sample is then irradiated with microwaves at a specific frequency, defined by the EPA and the ^{13}C-molecule, to transfer the high polarization from the electron spins to the ^{13}C spins. After ~2 h, the solid sample is rapidly dissolved into a liquid with superheated water. The liquid is received in a power injector syringe and buffered. Once dissolved, the polarization of the sample starts to decay toward thermal equilibrium. The depolarization is determined by the longitudinal relaxation time of the ^{13}C spin in the liquid state (typically 60–70 s). The syringe is quickly transferred to the MRI scanner for intravenous injection and imaging (Fig. 24.1).

Renal Functional and Metabolic Investigations Using ^{13}C-Pyruvate MRI

Currently, the only approved tracer in humans is pyruvate labeled either at the first ([1-^{13}C]pyruvate) or second ([2-^{13}C]pyruvate) position. The

N. Bøgh · C. Laustsen (✉)
Department of Clinical Medicine, Aarhus University, Aarhus, Denmark
e-mail: cl@clin.au.dk

S. D. Serai, K. Darge (eds.), *Advanced Clinical MRI of the Kidney*,
https://doi.org/10.1007/978-3-031-40169-5_24

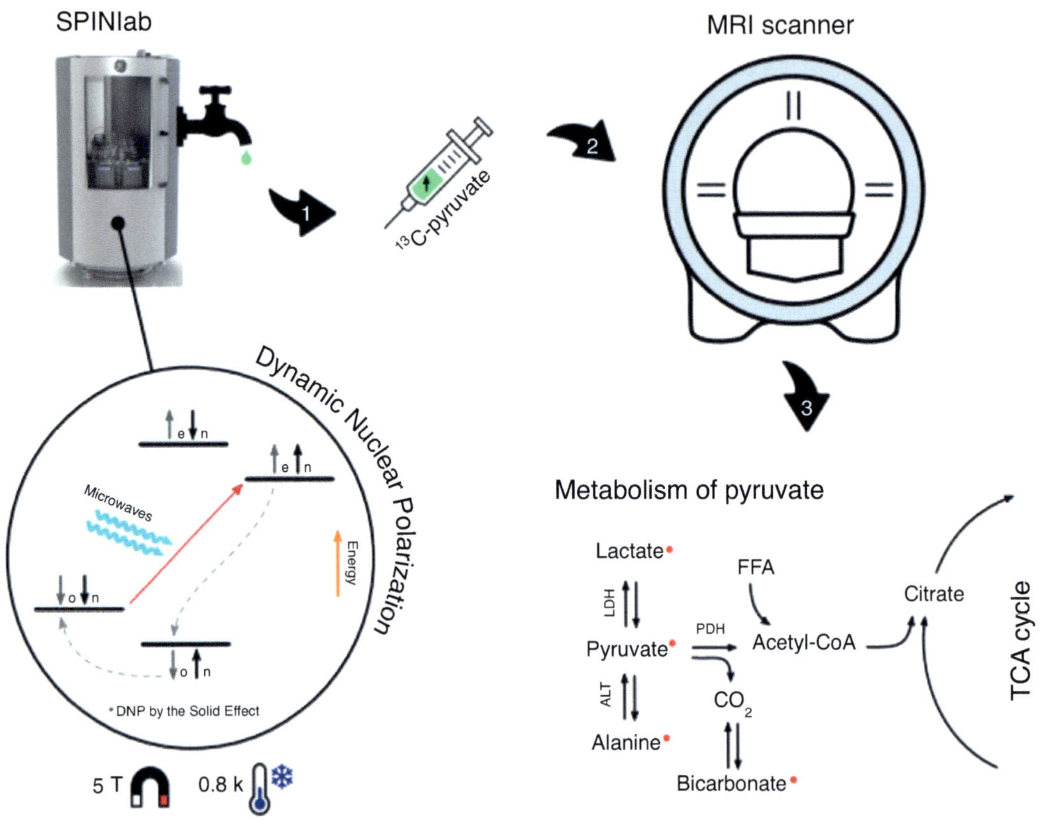

Fig. 24.1 Hyperpolarized MRI is performed using ^{13}C-enriched molecules with augmented polarization and thus the MR-signal. Hyperpolarization for clinical use is carried out in the SPINlab system by dynamic nuclear polarization. Then, the hyperpolarized molecule is dissolved and injected intravenously for *in vivo* detection. In the case of [1-^{13}C]pyruvate, estimates from perfusion and metabolism can be derived from separate signals of pyruvate and its downstream metabolites. *The illustration is courtesy of Christian Ø. Mariager and reproduced under the Creative Commons CC BY license [32]*

former is used the most and is the focus of this chapter.

Hyperpolarized [1-^{13}C]pyruvate offers many possibilities for investigations of renal function and metabolism. Using this tracer, dynamic images of the delivery, uptake, and metabolism of [1-^{13}C]pyruvate into its products [1-^{13}C]lactate, [1-^{13}C]alanine, and $^{13}CO_2$/^{13}C-bicarbonate can be obtained. The experiment spans five dimensions (three spatial, one temporal, and one spectral), providing vast information that presents a unique challenge and opportunity. Kidney vasculature and perfusion can be visualized from the pyruvate signal over time, while the metabolic breakdown from pyruvate (171 ppm) into lactate (183 ppm), alanine (176 ppm), and bicarbonate (160 ppm) can be obtained using spectral information.

Pyruvate is a key metabolite at the intersection of glycolysis and mitochondrial glucose oxidation. It is metabolized to lactate, alanine, acetyl-CoA, and CO_2 + bicarbonate by lactate dehydrogenase (LDH), alanine aminotransferase (ALT), and pyruvate dehydrogenase (PDH), respectively. The spectral separation of pyruvate, lactate, alanine, and bicarbonate is sufficient to perform separate quantification. Pyruvate hydrate is formed in solution and observable using spectroscopic approaches, but it is metabolically inert and usually not considered or even acquired. Using dynamic metabolite signals, conversion between pyruvate and metabolites can be estimated as ratios or kinetic modeling of apparent rate constants. These quantities must be understood in the context of the experiment, that is, a sub-minute acquisition of the first pass of a large dose of pyruvate. For instance, reduced perfusion causes decreased tracer delivery as well as ischemia with higher LDH flux and slower lactate removal. The lactate-to-pyruvate ratio or its model-based equivalent (k_{PL}) reflects all of these and not merely the flux through the LDH. Generally speaking, the ratios and rate constants reflect pyruvate delivery and uptake, tissue cellularity, activities of LDH, PDH, and ALT, as well as endogenous pool sizes of the metabolites, cofactors for conversion, such as $NADH/NAD^+$, and the relaxation properties between metabolites and their interactions with pathophysiology. For example, a low bicarbonate signal is often observed in the kidneys. This does not necessarily indicate low rates of oxidative metabolism compared to glycolysis, but likely simply reflects the small pool size. Understanding the influence of different pathological phenomena on metabolic quantities, for example, using other MRI techniques, is an important area of research for unleashing the potential of hyperpolarized MRI.

Practical Considerations for Hyperpolarized ^{13}C MRI Kidney Exams

The use of hyperpolarized [1-^{13}C]pyruvate in clinical trials is rapidly expanding. More than 600 examinations have been performed worldwide. Before initiating trials, researchers must consider hyperpolarized [1-^{13}C]pyruvate as an investigational medicinal product. Regulatory approval must be secured, and special requirements for manufacturing and monitoring must be in place. The Cancer Imaging Program under the National Cancer Institute maintains and shares an investigator's brochure and investigational medicinal product dossier for use in these processes. In addition to approvals, the following specialized equipment is required:

1. Clinical hyperpolarizer
2. Multi-nuclear ready clinical scanner
3. ^{13}C transmit and receive coils for abdominal imaging
4. Pharmacy facilities for compounding the drug
5. Power injector

When performing clinical examinations, it is imperative to consider quality assurance and proper workflow. The compounding of the products and filling of the pharmacy kit follows different guidelines at different sites. These are not described here, but researchers should be aware that proper arrangements are made to ensure the quality of the filled pharmacy kit. In addition, the MR equipment warrants some attention. The SPINlab polarizer requires regular service and calibrations of microwave power and frequency. The polarization levels (solid-state or liquid) should be monitored so that deviations can be handled. The external quality-control module should be calibrated and serviced regularly. Lastly, the scanner and coil setup should undergo regular quality assurance on ^{13}C-enriched thermal phantoms.

The low abundance and thermal polarization of ^{13}C, as well as the non-recoverable magnetization loss from the hyperpolarized probes, prohibit extensive preparatory and pre-scanning procedures. Therefore, care must be taken during the preparatory steps of an exam. First, it is paramount that the radio frequency (RF) coils are working and positioned correctly. For this purpose, quality assurance should be employed as described above. Furthermore, the phantoms can be used as fiducial markers and to assure signal when the patient is in the scanner. The ^{13}C power can often be calibrated on a suitably loaded ^{13}C phantom prior to the exams and kept constant across all patients.[6] However, care must be taken when calibrating the center frequency using phantoms as these typically lie outside the area of interest. Thus, their B_1 position is likely to be very different and the frequency may be shifted compared to the region of interest. Therefore, we suggest using the ^{1}H-water frequency from the region of interest as a reference for the ^{13}C-frequency [3]. During this process, we also recommend obtaining a B_0 field map to ensure proper shim. Finally, obtaining a coil sensitivity map is desirable for post-processing when using multi-element receiver coils or acceleration methods. Rigid coils can be acquired using phantoms [4]. However, rigid coils are impractical for abdominal imaging. Instead, we suggest using acceleration methods that do not require sensitivity profiles [5]. For coil combinations, the need for a coil profile can be circumvented by using the pyruvate signal as a pseudo-sensitivity map. Of note, power and frequency calibrations can be performed directly on the ^{13}C signals initially during the acquisition of the hyperpolarized tracer. This further allows estimation of the B_1^+ field, potentially improving quantifications over larger fields of view or when using inhomogeneous transmit coils. However, this is technically challenging and currently requires third-party software, making it a non-standard practice in the field.

Many different imaging sequences have been used in renal applications [6]. Currently, we recommend the use of spectral-spatial excitation followed by a fast readout using either echo planar imaging (EPI) or spirals (Fig. 24.2). We favor spirals, as the EPI readout is typically associated with a longer echo-time, which might result in signal loss. The spirals are also less sensitive to movement artifacts such as from breathing. Spectral-spatial excitation allows for different flip angles as well as temporal and spatial resolutions on different resonances (pyruvate vs. metabolites). For renal applications, we currently recommend a 1 s resolution on pyruvate and a 3 s resolution on metabolites, with a high flip (60–90°) on the metabolites and a low flip (5–10°) on pyruvate. In-plane resolutions of 1–1.5 cm^2 and 1.5–2 cm^2 for pyruvate and metabolites, respectively, and a slice thickness of 2–3 cm, are good starting points. It is currently unclear if 3D encoding provides substantial signal gains over 2D multi-slice approaches in ^{13}C MRI [7]. The acquisition should be started for full temporal dynamics, which typically corresponds to the end-of-injection period and one minute onwards.

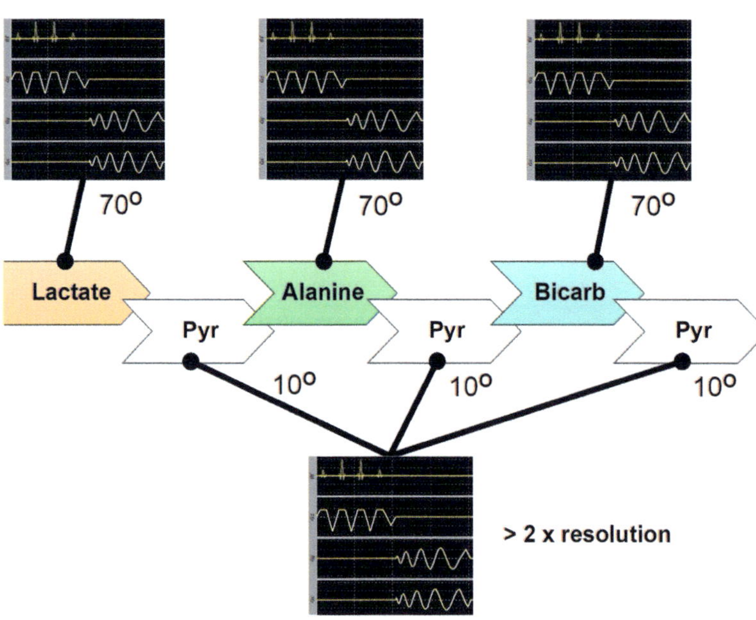

Fig. 24.2 Our recommendation for kidney examinations with hyperpolarized [1-^{13}C]pyruvate is to use spectral-spatial excitation with spiral readouts. This allows the researcher to capture the entire temporal dynamics and use different flip angles as well as spatial and temporal resolutions. Hereby, the higher signal-to-noise ratio on pyruvate can utilized to better account for perfusion and partial volume effects near the vasculature while the metabolites are captured under SNR optimal conditions. As little spectral information is obtained, care must be taken during the scan preparation, which is further described in the text

After imaging, a spectrum should be obtained to confirm the correct prescription of the center frequency.

It is important to acquire anatomical images that can serve as a reference for the ^{13}C data. This approach depends on the available hardware and the desired proton protocol. If $^{1}H/^{13}C$ coils are used, all images may be acquired without changing the coils. If a change is required, an anatomical reference image should be acquired using the built-in body coil before moving the patient. This can be used for subsequent registration. For functional and anatomical images, we suggest using consensus-based multiparametric protocols [8–10].

Post-Processing and Data Analysis

The nature of the data warrants careful consideration for post-processing, analysis, and interpretation. The signal decays rapidly from depolarization by relaxation and excitation. Furthermore, pyruvate and its metabolites undergo several biological processes. As such, any quantification represents a complex set of interactions, all of which represent ongoing research and development efforts. Here, we suggest a few simple and relatively robust methods suitable for clinical translation.

The reconstruction of images from raw data is dependent on the sequence employed. EPI data are phase-corrected and Fourier transformed. Non-Cartesian spiral data must be gridded prior to the Fourier transformation. Appropriate filters are used to reduce the noise and other artifacts. Frameworks for reconstruction are usually provided by the scanner vendors. For multi-channel acquisitions, we recommend coil combination with singular value decomposition or use of the summed pyruvate signal for estimation of individual coil weights, as this optimizes the signal-to-noise ratio and maintains phase information and noise distribution [11]. Lastly, acceleration methods require additional steps in reconstruction that are not covered here, as these are under active research and are not routinely used for human imaging.

For quantification, the sum over time of the individual resonances ([1-^{13}C]pyruvate, [1-^{13}C]lactate, [1-^{13}C]alanine, and ^{13}C-bicarbonate) can be used directly in many cases, providing reasonable coil uniformity or correction. Simple normalization to muscle or total kidney signals allows comparison between patients. Furthermore, the ratios between a metabolite and pyruvate provide a measure of conversion (Fig. 24.3). Under a set of assumptions, these correlate with the apparent forward rate constants of the relevant enzymes (PDH, LDH, or ALT). In extension, the ratios between the metabolites represent a convenient measure of relative metabolic conversion and metabolic reprogramming. These model-free quantities are prone to changes in timing, bolus, and flip angles and therefore require that the same imaging protocol is used throughout a trial [12]. If this is fulfilled, the simplicity and easy interpretation of model-free approaches are compelling in a clinical setting.

Several advanced model-based methods have been proposed for quantification. Perfusion or delivery of [1-^{13}C]pyruvate can be estimated both quantitatively and semi-quantitatively using the principles of dynamic contrast-enhanced MRI. Thus, time-to-peak, mean transit time, first-order moment, blood volume, and blood flow can be estimated [13]. However, one must be careful in interpreting these due to pyruvate metabolization, thus breaking a central assumption in perfusion-weighted imaging using intravascular tracers. As such, the perfusion estimates carry a metabolic component that is not currently well described. In addition to perfusion, the apparent rate constants of LDH, PDH, and ALT can be modeled using a two-site metabolic exchange model, which further accounts for the relaxation rates and flip angles. This approach is widely used, and routines for fitting are freely available in the hyperpolarized MRI toolbox currently provided by the University of California, San Francisco [12]. It is unresolved if the more complicated model-based approaches provide significant advantages over model-free approaches, and thus we suggest using the simplest metrics as a minimum.

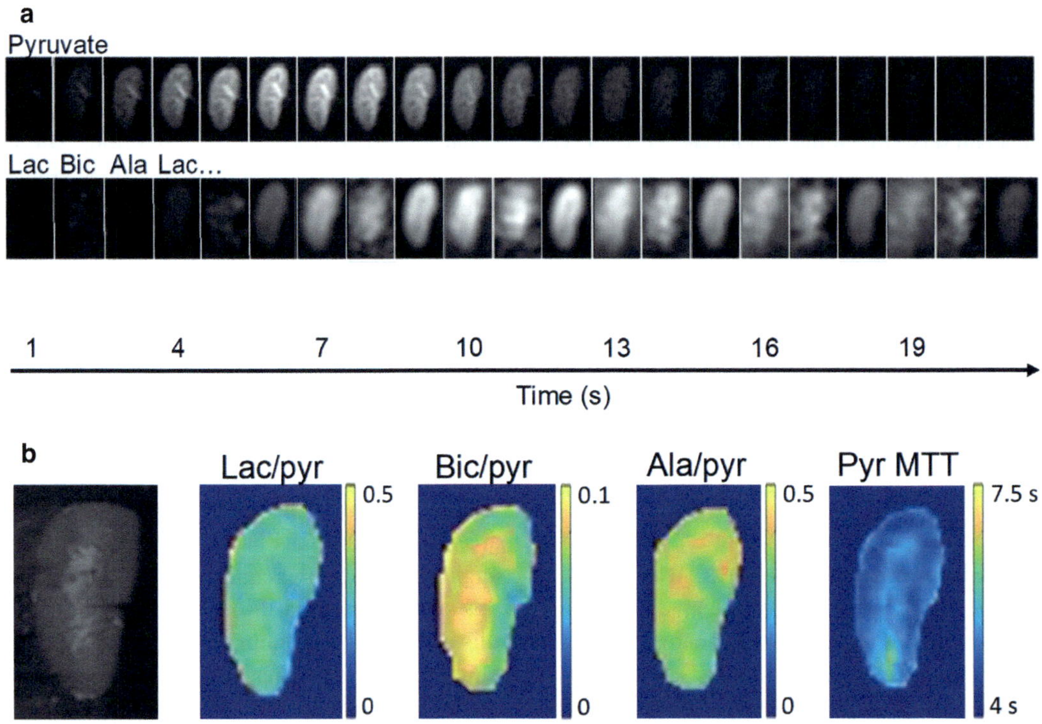

Fig. 24.3 Data examples from a pig experiment following the protocol suggested in this chapter (**a**). Pyruvate and its metabolites lactate (lac), bicarbonate (bic) and alanine (ala) were imaged following injection of hyperpolarized [1-^{13}C]pyruvate. MRI was performed with spectral-spatial excitation with a 10° flip angle on pyruvate and 70° flip angle on metabolites. A spiral readout was employed over a 34 × 34 cm field-of-view for a 2 cm slice thickness. Pyruvate and metabolites were acquired with 90 × 90 and 40 × 40 matrix sizes, respectively. The entire temporal dynamics were captured at 1 s time resolution for pyruvate, while the metabolites were acquired interleaved at 3 s time resolution. This allows quantification (**b**) of metabolism as the ratios of metabolites to pyruvate, as well as estimation of pyruvate delivery by calculation of the pyruvate mean transit time (MTT)

For research purposes, the data can be analyzed using regions-of-interest (ROIs). The optimal approach is based on the research question. ROIs can be drawn in the cortex, medulla, the entire kidney, or in focal disease. However, one must be careful and consider partial volume effects, especially with the slice thickness being currently used, and partial volume effect correction may prove to be an important fool for the future. Alternatively, a semi-automated layer-based approach can be used. Regardless of the analysis performed, care must be taken when selecting the appropriate constraints for data quality. We suggest using an SNR >3 for both pyruvate and metabolites. Furthermore, an error criterion should be employed when using model-based estimates. Here, a hard threshold or a fraction of the fitted parameter can be used [14].

Clinical Applications

Hyperpolarized [1-^{13}C]pyruvate MRI is an emerging modality for clinical use; but thus far, limited applications have been demonstrated in patients [2]. We will highlight the most promising renal applications based on preclinical literature. Hyperpolarized [1-^{13}C]pyruvate has very promising applications for renal cancer since the metabolic pattern associated with renal cell carcinoma (RCC) is distinct compared to non-cancerous tissue and different tumor subtypes may have distinct, targetable metabolic phenotypes [15]. Preclinical and translational studies suggest that hyperpolarized pyruvate MRI can detect this metabolic phenotype in RCC [16, 17] and other cancers [18]. Furthermore, pyruvate to lactate conversion seems to be a marker of aggressiveness and treatment response in several solid tumors [19–22]. As such, this technology may allow for metabolic imaging of kidney cancer that PET is unable to perform. The only registered clinical trial is investigating renal cancer (NCT04258462).

Another potential application of hyperpolarized [1-^{13}C]pyruvate MRI is for diagnosing chronic kidney disease (CKD). The metabolic profile might serve as an earlier biomarker of renal decline and can thus be used as a sensitive prognostic marker. Diabetes is an inherently metabolic disease and is the most common cause of CKD. Moreover, a particular amount of preclinical work has dealt with diabetes-induced changes in renal metabolism and progression into diabetic nephropathy. Prolonged hyperglycemia is associated with a profound renal metabolic shift toward lactate production, which is a direct consequence of toxic glucose metabolic pathways [23]. This change can be monitored using hyperpolarized [1-^{13}C]pyruvate [24], and therapeutic interventions targeting toxic pathways may be assessed [25]. Another interesting case is the possibility of imaging the underlying need for amino acids for the production of fibrosis [26]. It is important to note that the use of hyperpolarized MRI is limited to perfused tissue; thus, this technology is less applicable for severe CKD and vascular diseases.

Lastly, early and accurate detection of acute kidney injury (AKI) is an unresolved clinical need, as the current standard for estimating kidney function from plasma creatinine is not sensitive in the early stages. Preclinical studies have demonstrated changes in metabolism and pyruvate perfusion in AKI [27, 28]. These studies have been performed in rodent models of ischemia reperfusion, which does not fully reflect the common pre-renal etiologies of human AKI. To our knowledge, intrinsic AKI, such as nephritis or glomerulonephritis, has not been investigated using hyperpolarized [1-^{13}C]pyruvate, but hyperpolarized pyruvate has been shown to be sensitive to inflammation in other organs [29]. Notably, hyperpolarized [1,4-$^{13}C_2$] fumarate enables the assessment of necrosis in AKI [30, 31].

In conclusion, hyperpolarized MRI may be a useful clinical tool for a number of indications. Cancerous disease is currently the most promising as well as the most elucidated application of this technology. Ongoing clinical trials will inform the clinical utility of this technology. In addition, CKD patients, especially those belonging to specific subpopulations, represent an intriguing avenue of research. Studying the use of hyperpolarized MRI for more acute indications may be currently impractical. Regardless of the disease, more preclinical and translational work is needed to inform larger trials and identify future clinical use of hyperpolarized MRI.

Notes

1. Microwave irradiation is applied near the EPR frequency corresponding to this magnetic field (~140 GHz), with a typical power of ~20 mW.
2. Power and frequency sweeps may be performed separately from human examinations at regular intervals depending on the exam frequency. If lower than the expected polarization is achieved, calibrations should always be considered.
3. The QC module measures pH, residual EPA, pyruvate concentration, volume, temperature, and polarization before injection.
4. This may include SNR tests, noise assessment, and assessment of uniformity or individual channel performance depending on the coil.
5. A typical phantom for B_1^+ calibration, SNR test, etc., is 8M ^{13}C urea in 90% H_2O/10% Glycerol w/3 mL/mL gadolinium-based contrast agent (OmniScan). 488 mg of ^{13}C Urea dissolved in 900 mL of solvent (1.26 g Glycerol: 9.00 g Water: 30 μL OmniScan).

6. As the ^{13}C frequency is four times lower than the ^{1}H frequency, it is significantly less impacted by the load.

Acknowledgments The authors would like to acknowledge the PARENCHIMA initiative "MRI Biomarkers for CKD" (CA16103), a community-driven Action of the European Cooperation in Science and Technology (COST) program of the European Union.

References

1. Ardenkjaer-Larsen JH, Fridlund B, Gram A, Hansson G, Hansson L, Lerche MH, Servin R, Thaning M, Golman K. Increase in signal-to-noise ratio of > 10,000 times in liquid-state NMR. Proc Natl Acad Sci U S A. 2003;100:10,158–63.
2. Wang ZJ, Ohliger MA, Larson PEZ, Gordon JW, Bok RA, Slater J, Villanueva-Meyer JE, Hess CP, Kurhanewicz J, Vigneron DB. Hyperpolarized ^{13}C MRI: state of the art and future directions. Radiology. 2019;291:273–84.
3. Grist JT, Hansen ESS, Sánchez-Heredia JD, et al. Creating a clinical platform for carbon-13 studies using the sodium-23 and proton resonances. Magn Reson Med. 2020;84:1817–27.
4. Hansen RB, Sánchez-Heredia JD, Bøgh N, Hansen ESS, Laustsen C, Hanson LG, Ardenkjaer-Larsen JH. Coil profile estimation strategies for parallel imaging with hyperpolarized ^{13}C MRI. Magn Reson Med. 2019;82:2104–17.
5. Gordon JW, Hansen RB, Shin PJ, Feng Y, Vigneron DB, Larson PEZ. 3D hyperpolarized C-13 EPI with calibrationless parallel imaging. J Magn Reson. 2018;289:92–9.
6. Gordon JW, Chen HY, Dwork N, Tang S, Larson PEZ. Fast imaging for hyperpolarized MR metabolic imaging. J Magn Reson Imaging. 2020:686–702.
7. Wild JM, Woodhouse N, Paley MNJ, Fichele S, Said Z, Kasuboski L, van Beek EJR. Comparison between 2D and 3D gradient-echo sequences for MRI of human lung ventilation with hyperpolarized ^{3}He. Magn Reson Med. 2004;52:673–8.
8. Bane O, Mendichovszky IA, Milani B, et al. Consensus-based technical recommendations for clinical translation of renal BOLD MRI. Magn Reson Mater Physiol. 2020;33:199–215.
9. Dekkers IA, de Boer A, Sharma K, et al. Consensus-based technical recommendations for clinical translation of renal T1 and T2 mapping MRI. MAGMA. 2020;33:163–76.
10. Nery F, Buchanan CE, Harteveld AA, et al. Consensus-based technical recommendations for clinical translation of renal ASL MRI. Magn Reson Mater Phys. 2020;33:141–61.
11. Zhu Z, Zhu X, Ohliger MA, et al. Coil combination methods for multi-channel hyperpolarized ^{13}C imaging data from human studies. J Magn Reson. 2019;301:73–9.
12. Larson PEZ, Chen H-Y, Gordon JW, et al. Investigation of analysis methods for hyperpolarized 13C-pyruvate metabolic MRI in prostate cancer patients. NMR Biomed. 2018;31:e3997.
13. Johansson E, Månsson S, Wirestam R, Svensson J, Petersson JS, Golman K, Ståhlberg F. Cerebral perfusion assessment by bolus tracking using hyperpolarized ^{13}C. Magn Reson Med. 2004;51:464–72.
14. Mammoli D, Gordon J, Autry A, et al. Kinetic modeling of hyperpolarized carbon-13 pyruvate metabolism in the human brain. IEEE Trans Med Imaging. 2019;39:320–7.
15. Rathmell WK, Rathmell JC, Linehan WM. Metabolic pathways in kidney cancer: current therapies and future directions. J Clin Oncol. 2018;36:3540–6.
16. Ahamed F, Van Criekinge M, Wang ZJ, Kurhanewicz J, Larson P, Sriram R. Modeling hyperpolarized lactate signal dynamics in cells, patient-derived tissue slice cultures and murine models. NMR Biomed. 2021;34:e4467.
17. Tran M, Latifoltojar A, Neves JB, et al. First-in-human in vivo non-invasive assessment of intra-tumoral metabolic heterogeneity in renal cell carcinoma. BJR Case Rep. 2019;5:20190003. https://doi.org/10/ggsdwc
18. Kurhanewicz J, Vigneron DB, Ardenkjaer-Larsen JH, et al. Hyperpolarized ^{13}C MRI: path to clinical translation in oncology. Neoplasia. 2019;21:1–16.
19. Aggarwal R, Vigneron DB, Kurhanewicz J. Hyperpolarized 1-[^{13}C]-pyruvate magnetic resonance imaging detects an early metabolic response to androgen ablation therapy in prostate cancer. Eur Urol. 2017;72:1028–9.
20. Granlund KL, Tee SS, Vargas HA, et al. Hyperpolarized MRI of human prostate cancer reveals increased lactate with tumor grade driven by monocarboxylate transporter 1. Cell Metab. 2019;31:105–14.
21. Woitek R, McLean MA, Gill AB, et al. Hyperpolarized ^{13} C MRI of tumor metabolism demonstrates early metabolic response to neoadjuvant chemotherapy in breast cancer. Radiol Imaging Cancer. 2020;2:e200017.
22. Gallagher FA, Woitek R, McLean MA, et al. Imaging breast cancer using hyperpolarized carbon-13 MRI. Proc Natl Acad Sci U S A. 2020;117:2092–8.
23. Zhang G, Darshi M, Sharma K. The Warburg effect in diabetic kidney disease. Semin Nephrol. 2018;38:111–20.
24. Laustsen C, Østergaard JA, Lauritzen MH, Nørregaard R, Bowen S, Søgaard LV, Flyvbjerg A, Pedersen M, Ardenkjær-Larsen JH. Assessment of early diabetic renal changes with hyperpolarized [1-^{13}C]pyruvate. Metab Res Rev. 2013;29:125–9.
25. Qi W, Keenan HA, Li Q, et al. Pyruvate kinase M2 activation may protect against the progression of dia-

betic glomerular pathology and mitochondrial dysfunction. Nat Med. 2017;23:753–62.
26. Nielsen PM, Mariager CØ, Mølmer M, Sparding N, Genovese F, Karsdal MA, Nørregaard R, Bertelsen LB, Laustsen C. Hyperpolarized [1-^{13}C] alanine production: A novel imaging biomarker of renal fibrosis. Magn Reson Med. 2020;84:2063–73.
27. Baligand C, Qin H, True-Yasaki A, et al. Hyperpolarized ^{13}C magnetic resonance evaluation of renal ischemia reperfusion injury in a murine model. NMR Biomed. 2017;30. https://doi.org/10/gbnnsz
28. Nielsen PM, Laustsen C, Bertelsen LB, Qi H, Mikkelsen E, Kristensen ML, Nørregaard R, Stødkilde-Jorgensen H. In situ lactate dehydrogenase activity: a novel renal cortical imaging biomarker of tubular injury? Am J Physiol Ren Physiol. 2017;312:F465–73.
29. Anderson S, Grist JT, Lewis A, Tyler DJ Hyperpolarized ^{13}C magnetic resonance imaging for noninvasive assessment of tissue inflammation. NMR Biomed 2020:e4460
30. Clatworthy MR, Kettunen MI, Hu DE, et al. Magnetic resonance imaging with hyperpolarized [1,4-^{13}C2]fumarate allows detection of early renal acute tubular necrosis. Proc Natl Acad Sci U S A. 2012;109:13,374–9.
31. Nielsen PM, Eldirdiri A, Bertelsen LB, Jørgensen HS, Ardenkjaer-Larsen JH, Laustsen C. Fumarase activity: an in vivo and in vitro biomarker for acute kidney injury. Sci Rep. 2017;7:40812.
32. Vaeggemose MF, Schulte R, Laustsen C. Comprehensive literature review of hyperpolarized carbon-13 MRI: the road to clinical application. Metabolites. 2021;11:219.

25 Bridging the Gap Between Imaging and Biopsy

Mohana Sopanahalli Narasimhamurthy
and Menaka Ambarishan

Introduction

The kidneys are retroperitoneal organs located on either side of the vertebral column and closely related to many surrounding organs, namely the liver, diaphragm, pleura, stomach, omentum, and muscles [1]. In addition, numerous developmental anomalies, such as ectopic or horseshoe-shaped kidneys, necessitate prerequisite imaging techniques to map and obtain kidney tissue for microscopic examination [2]. Nephrologists and interventional radiologists routinely plan the needle tract before the procedure using various imaging modalities (ultrasound (US), computed tomography (CT), or magnetic resonance imaging (MRI) [3]. The mapping of the needle tract helps navigate during the biopsy procedure and decreases the potential complications. Renal tissue thus obtained under imaging guidance is examined under light microscopy, immunofluorescence, and electron microscopy, whose findings generate an integrated diagnosis. This chapter discusses the indications, essential requirements for a successful renal biopsy, common lesions, limitations, and contraindications in routine practice.

Kidney biopsies are primarily performed for medical renal diseases than surgical mass lesions [4, 5]. Clinical indications for kidney biopsy are outlined in Table 25.1.

Two types of kidney biopsies are routinely performed:

1. **Nontargeted biopsies (NTB)**: Primarily used to evaluate acute kidney injury, distinguish various types of chronic diffuse parenchymal renal diseases, and evaluate transplanted kidneys [4, 6].
2. **Targeted biopsies (TB):** Evaluation of small renal masses and high-risk surgical patients to establish a tissue diagnosis of malignancy to consider the chances of significant surgery. Another scenario is to get a tissue diagnosis

Table 25.1 Indications for kidney biopsy

• Unexplained renal failure
• Acute nephritic syndrome
• Nephrotic syndrome
• Isolated non nephrotic proteinuria
• Isolated glomerular hematuria
• Connective-tissue diseases (e.g., systemic lupus erythematosus)
• Renal transplant rejection
• Renal transplant dysfunction
• Renal masses (primary or metastatic)

M. S. Narasimhamurthy (✉)
Department of Pathology, University of Pennsylvania Health System, Philadelphia, PA, USA
e-mail: Mohana.SopanahalliNarasimhamurthy@Pennmedicine.upenn.edu

M. Ambarishan
North Tyneside General Hospital, Newcastle-upon Tyne, UK

S. D. Serai, K. Darge (eds.), *Advanced Clinical MRI of the Kidney*,
https://doi.org/10.1007/978-3-031-40169-5_25

for further management in a patient with an unresectable renal tumor [7, 8].

Below are the different approaches employed to perform the kidney biopsy in the order of decreasing frequency [9, 10].

- Percutaneous
- Laparoscopic
- Transvenous
- Open surgical approach

Percutaneous Renal Biopsy Procedure

Paul Iverson and Claus Brun pioneered the percutaneous renal biopsy technique and published their findings in a seminal paper in 1951 [11]. They found that only 50% of the tissue obtained was adequate for diagnosis. However, the diagnostic yield dramatically improved to 96% using the Vim-Silverman needle in the Kark and Muehrcke series of 50 cases in 1954 [12]. Since then, nephrologists have increasingly performed the biopsy. The introduction of a spring-loaded, automated cutting-needle biopsy gun with ultrasound guidance in the early 1990s has improved the diagnostic specimen yield [13, 14]. In our institution, we use 16- or 18-gauge needles with a trend toward minimizing bleeding complications with smaller needles. The average internal diameter of an 18-gauge needle is 400 μm, slightly larger than the intact normal glomeruli, which average 200–250 μm in diameter [9]. On many occasions, it leads to fragmented glomeruli. Hence, the ideal gauge would be 16 gauge with an internal diameter of 600–700 μm in adults [9, 15]. The ideal needle provides intact glomeruli with minimal bleeding complications.

Nephrologists place the mildly sedated patients on the bed in a prone position and localize the left kidney's lower pole under ultrasound guidance, the preferred site for the biopsy [16]. Sometimes body habitus requires a supine anterolateral position for the biopsy procedure. Under universal aseptic precautions, 2% lidocaine, the local anesthetic agent, infiltrates the skin at the previously designated point. Then, a stab incision is made to ease the passage of the biopsy needle at an angle of 70 degrees to the skin under USG. As the needle approaches the renal capsule, the patient holds a breath so that the lower pole of the kidney rests just under the biopsy needle (Fig. 25.1). As the biopsy needle touches the renal capsule, the needle is fired by releasing the trigger mechanism. The needle is withdrawn, and the contents are pushed into the saline plates. The pathologist on site examines the fresh cores to ensure the presence of glomeruli using dissecting microscope (Fig. 25.2). The pre-procedure dialogue between the biopsy-performing nephrologist and the pathologist providing diagnostic interpretation is invaluable. It sets the adequacy criteria for the amount of tissue needed for the various laboratory tests based on the clinical indication and requirements including, immunofluorescence, electron microscopy, flow cytometry, culture & sensitivity, and cytogenetics.

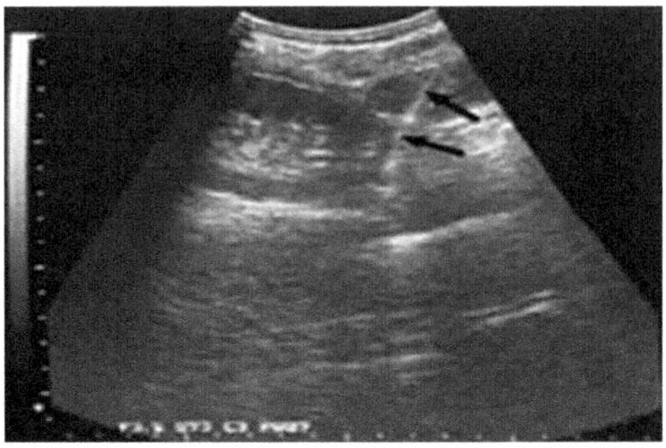

Fig. 25.1 Renal biopsy imaging. An ultrasound scan shows the needle entering the lower pole of the left kidney

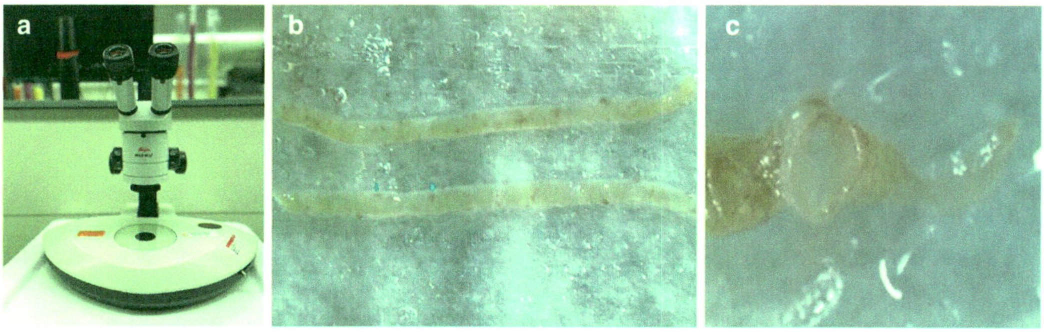

Fig. 25.2 Dissecting microscope used to inspect the core biopsy at the site of the procedure (**a**), Two cores of renal biopsies with arrow showing the glomerulus (**b**) and large caliber artery obtained during the biopsy procedure which resulted in immediate bleeding (**c**)

Other Renal Biopsy Techniques

Percutaneous biopsy is the most commonly employed technique to obtain kidney tissue. Transvenous and laparoscopic methods are alternate approaches employed under particular circumstances when the percutaneous approach is contraindicated, such as in bleeding diathesis [17–20]. Transvenous renal biopsy is performed via jugular vein placement of a catheter into the renal vein, usually in the setting of medical renal biopsies [21]. Further detailed discussion on the equipment and technique are beyond the scope of this chapter.

Personnel

A team of clinicians and nurses working in tandem to optimize the patient outcome by educating them about the rationale for the procedure in comparison to the imaging and anticipated management options for theoretical complications.

The renal biopsy procedure involves sedation and vital signs monitoring by nurses trained in conscious sedation, a nurse anesthetist, or an anesthesiologist. A radiology technologist assists with the equipment. A cytotechnologist or pathologist assesses the adequacy of specimens (rapid on-site evaluation (ROSE)) and ensures that samples are placed in the appropriate preservatives for the subsequent laboratory tests that best address the clinical scenario [10].

Tissue Sample Preparation

Once the tissue core is obtained, the pathologist on site receives the specimen. The specimen should be handled carefully, avoiding squeezing and compression. Many institutions use wooden sticks instead of forceps to minimize tissue injury. The pathologist examines the tissue core specimen under a dissecting microscope to ensure that the renal cortex and medulla are present (Fig. 25.2). Additional needle passes depend on the necessity for immunofluorescence and electron microscopy examination. If insufficient tissue is obtained, additional needle passes are made. However, any pass more than four times increases the post-biopsy complications. On completion of the biopsy procedure, dressing is applied to the incised skin, and the patient is rolled directly into the bed for observation.

Biopsy Adequacy

- Assess adequacy at the site of the procedure using a dissecting microscope. An adequate sample typically contains cortex and medulla with 10–15 glomeruli. Yoshinari demonstrated that each 1 cm length of an 18 g specimen of the renal cortex averaged over 11 glomeruli [22]. Then renal cores are triaged and divided into three pieces, as shown in Fig. 25.3.

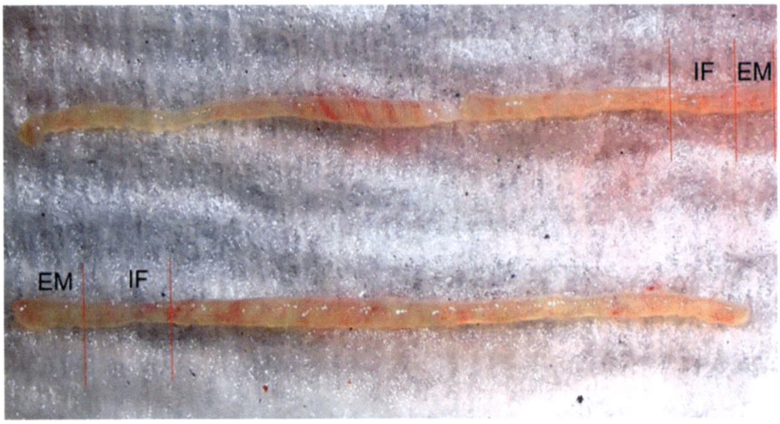

Fig. 25.3 The triaging of the core biopsies for electron microscopy (EM) and immunofluorescence (IF) as shown

Fragmented, triaged core tissues are placed in the appropriate fixatives.

- Formalin for light microscopy
- Normal saline for immunofluorescence
- Glutaraldehyde for electron microscopy

The following glomeruli meet the adequacy criteria for interpretation by different methods to generate an integrative diagnosis in various clinical scenarios.

- 6 glomeruli in native kidney
- 2–5 glomeruli for immunofluorescence
- 1-glomeruli for electron microscopy
- 10 glomeruli for renal allograft evaluation

Microscopic Examination

Light microscopy usually on day one with the examination of hematoxylin and eosin (H&E) stained histological sections invariably accompanied by PAS, Jones (methenamine silver), trichrome special stains (Fig. 25.4)

Generalizations About Glomerular Diseases

- A distinctive pattern of injury may be associated with many diseases, for example, MPGN pattern can be seen in C3 glomerulopathy, SLE, IgA nephropathy, HCV, etc.
- One disease may produce different patterns of injury (SLE, IgA nephropathy, FSGS)
- Renal histology is "specific" in only a few diseases (Anti-GBM disease, Alport disease)

Immunofluorescence (IF on day 2): Fresh tissue is snap frozen and cut 2–4 um thick sections using a cryostat. Routinely, we use the following antigen panel IgG, IgA, IgM, C1q, C3, albumin, fibrinogen (k and Y light chains) for diagnosis. The slides are then examined under a high-power fluorescent microscope for deposits, localization, intensity, and staining pattern as described below and as shown in Fig. 25.5.

Interpretation:

- Deposits vs non-specific staining (e.g., areas of necrosis)
- Location—mesangium, GMB, tubular BM, vessels
- Pattern—granular (fine, coarse) or linear
- Intensity—0–3 or 4+

Note: some diseases can only be diagnosed by IF—IgA nephropathy.

Electron Microscopy: Tissue fixed in glutaraldehyde is cut 1 μm thin section and stained with toluidine blue [9]. The sections are reviewed to find the appropriate glomerulus and other structures for ultrastructural findings. Photomicrographs at various magnifications are taken to view glomerular architecture, which includes capillary loops and mesangial regions (Fig. 25.6). It usually

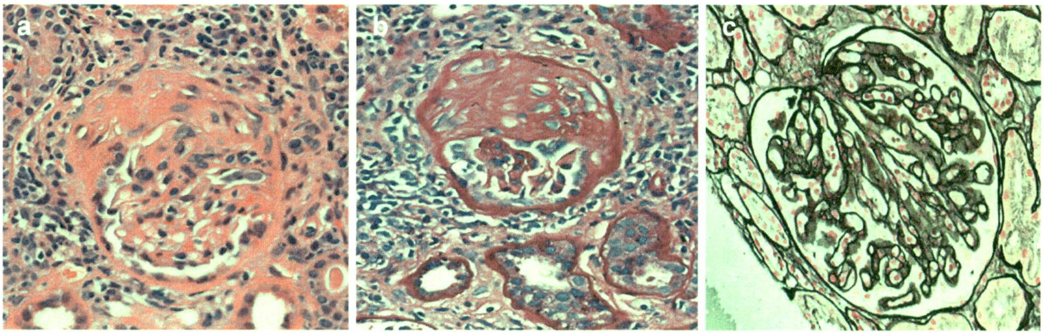

Fig. 25.4 H& E section (magnification 200×) shows crescent and increased mesangial cellularity (**a**), PAS highlights the same crescent and also basement membrane thickening (**b**). Jones stain the basement membrane (**c**)

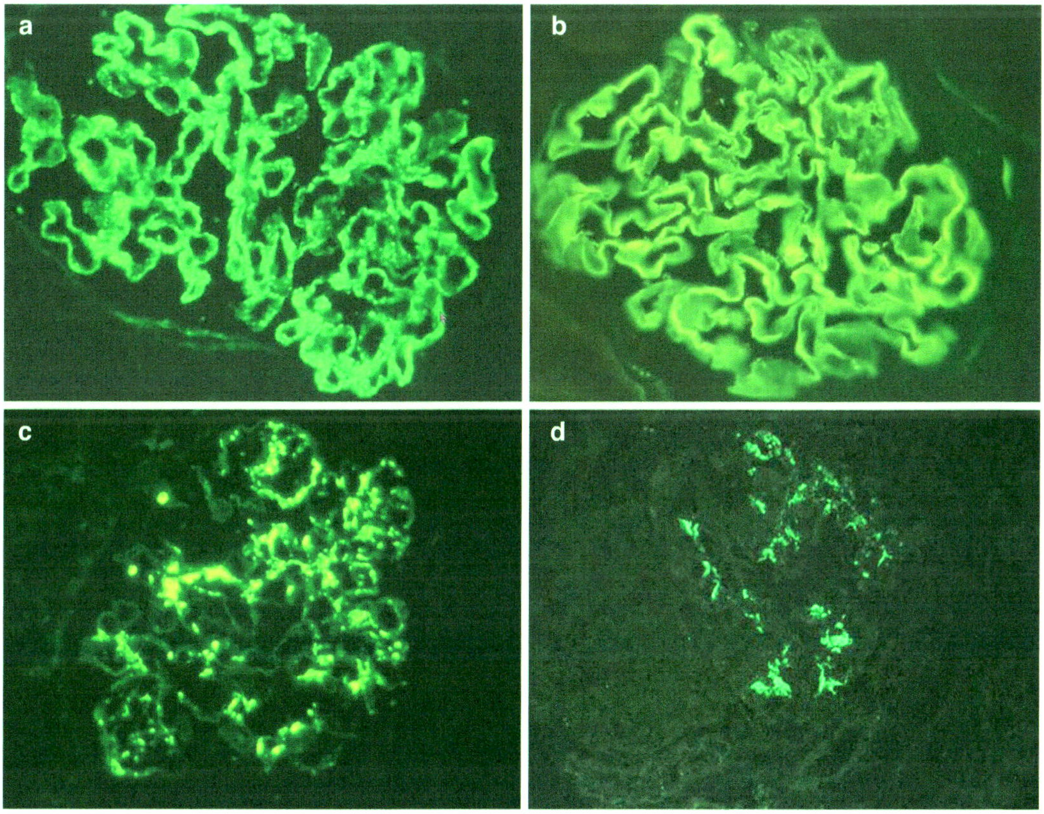

Fig. 25.5 Immunofluorescence staining patterns. (**a**) linear basement membrane staining, (**b**) diffuse membranous type, (**c**) granular staining, (**d**)mesangial deposits

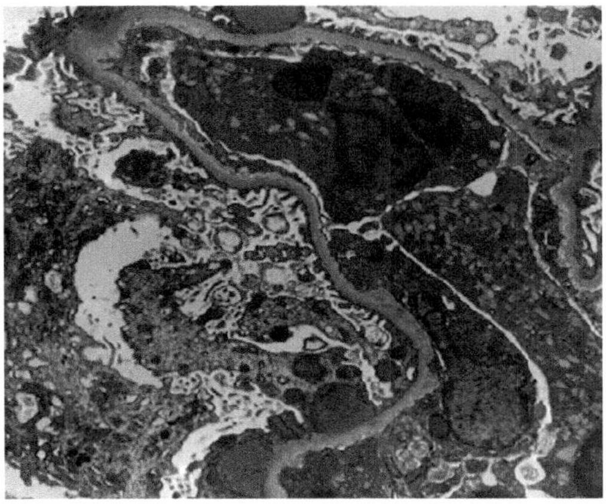

Fig. 25.6 Electron microscopy shows subepithelial deposits

takes 5–7 days for the preparation and interpretation.

Renal Transplant Biopsy

The renal biopsy is the gold standard for assessing the transplanted kidneys [23]. The renal biopsy procedure is performed under three scenarios in the field of kidney transplant [24–26]. They are as follows:

- To assess the suitability of a donor's kidney
- Allograft evaluation
- Transplant protocols to detect subclinical rejections [27]

The transplanted kidneys are in the anterior abdominal wall. Under ultrasound guidance, the biopsy is performed using a spring-loaded, automated cutting-needle biopsy gun. In most patients, a renal transplant biopsy is performed to identify the cause of acute graft dysfunction (Fig. 25.7). If the vascular rejection is suspected, a snap-frozen sample for C4d immunostaining should also be obtained, although some laboratories can detect C4d on formalin-fixed material.

Targeted Biopsy

According to World Health Organization, kidney cancer is the seventh most common cancer in men and the tenth among women [28]. Traditionally, abdominal imaging studies provide high diagnostic accuracy for renal masses, reducing the need for core biopsy for histological diagnosis prior to surgery. However, tremendous advances in imaging have increased the detection of small renal masses, thus identifying renal cell carcinoma (RCC) at the initial stage, constituting up to 15% of small renal masses [29]. Small renal masses require needle core biopsy to establish the histological diagnosis to guide active surveillance strategies, cryosurgery, radiofrequency, and ablation strategies.

Many factors help to differentiate between benign and malignant masses and thus raising suspicion for biopsy requirement [30, 31]. Contrast CT or MRI studies and contrast subtraction technology help confidently ascertain the enhancement of renal masses. A non-enhancing mass without fat can be renal cell carcinoma (RCC) or oncocytoma, both being in the differential diagnosis. The presence of mesenchymal fat in addition to the variable mixture of blood vessels, and smooth muscles favors angiomyolipoma (AML) [32, 33]. The Bosniak measured the cystic lesions based on medical imaging appearance and estimated the risk of primary renal carcinoma in partially cystic renal lesions [34]. Based on the Bosniak observations, category 2F and category 3 lesions are considered indeterminate for malignancy [35]. Infiltrative renal mass without macroscopic fat that retains a normal bean shape without risk factors for urinary tract infection should raise suspicion for non-renal cell carcinomas like lymphoma or urothelial carcinoma [36].

When the imaging is equivocal for renal mass, and the patient has renal insufficiency, the current guidelines recommend that a biopsy is more beneficial and appropriate than a non-contrast MRI or CT. The contrast is deemed too risky for

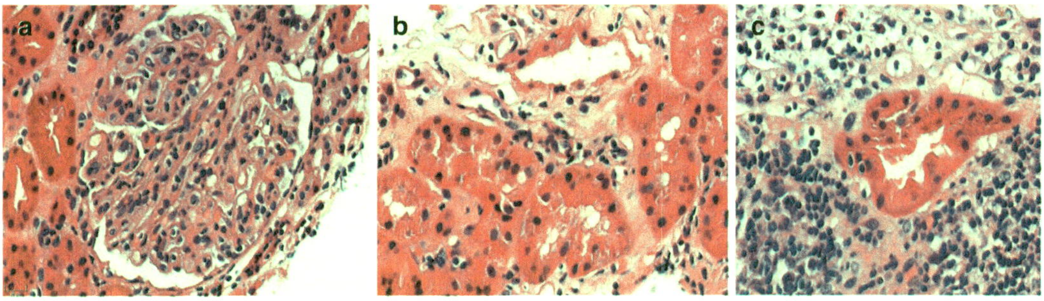

Fig. 25.7 Various patterns of injury seen in transplant rejection biopsies

intravenous (IV) infusion for an assessment by a nephrologist. Studies have shown that needle tract seeding is controversial [37–39]. Some imaging findings preclude resorting to renal mass biopsy. They are (1) a complex cyst with evidence of hemorrhage, inspissated fluid resembling solid tissue. However, contrast subtraction imaging technology assists in getting clarity on the true nature of these conditions. (2) Small lesions (<2 cm) sometimes lead to pseudo enhancement raising a concern. Depending on other factors, surveillance with repeat imaging is appropriate, given the small lesion size in these situations.

The targeted biopsies (TB) have high sensitivity and specificity with a high positive predictive value in accurately diagnosing renal masses. However, in a systematic review, Patel et al. demonstrated that the targeted biopsies have a significant nondiagnostic rate and negative predictive value [31]. Histologic subtyping of various renal cell carcinoma (e.g., clear cell, papillary, or chromophobic subtypes) on renal biopsy is 95% accurate. However, this subtyping does not alter the management as per NCCN guidelines when imaging workup suggests malignancy [40]. When imaging workup is indeterminate, studies have shown the biopsy was valuable and could have avoided at least 26% of surgical interventions. However, the converse point is that about 75% of patients in the study population underwent "unnecessary" biopsies and could have proceeded straight to surgical resection [41–43].

Contraindications: Biopsies should be delayed when the risks of hemorrhage outweigh the benefits of a tissue diagnosis. SIR recommends a platelet count of 50,000/mL and an International Normalized Ratio (INR) of 1.5–1.8 at the renal biopsy procedure [44]. Extreme hypertension also worsens hemorrhagic risks [45]. The contraindications are listed in Table 25.2.

Table 25.2 Absolute and relative contraindications

Absolute	Relative
Patient refusal	Uncooperative patient
Bleeding diathesis	Solitary native kidney
Uncontrolled severe hypertension	Small sized kidney
	Azotemia Anatomical abnormalities Skin infection Hemostasis altering drugs Pregnancy Urinary tract infections Obesity

Complications: Renal biopsy is a safe procedure. The complications have dramatically decreased with the increasing usage of spring-loaded biopsy guns with ultrasound guidance. Rarely, the following complications have been observed [46, 47].

- Gross hematuria (0.5%)
- Clinically significant renal hematoma (4.9%)
- Hemorrhage requiring transfusion (0.4%)
- Clinically significant pain (1.2%)
- Pneumothorax (0.6%)
- Loss of life (<0.1%)

Limitations

The nondiagnostic rate of first targeted biopsy is approximately greater than or equal to 10% [48]. Targeted biopsies in a small subset of patients can miss combined tumors such as benign oncocytoma and concurrent RCC. The accuracy of Fuhrman histologic grading in core biopsies is variable with a range of 50–75% [49]. The AUA guidelines comment on this fact as indicating that the accuracy of histologic grading is "variable" [29]. It has been shown that nontargeted biopsy (NTB) resulted in change of the pre-biopsy clinical diagnosis in 44% of cases and therapy in 31% of cases. With this, one study inferred that NTB was unnecessary in about 70% of cases [10].

Conclusion

Renal biopsies are excellent at achieving a diagnosis without complication. Its role in establishing the correct diagnosis, especially in renal parenchymal diseases, is undeniable; however, its ability to alter patient outcomes is minimal if the patients are not selected carefully. The 2016 AUA guidelines state that biopsy usually is not indicated for a solid tumor in the setting of (1) young or healthy patients who are unwilling to accept the uncertainties associated with (biopsy) or (2) older or frail patients who will be managed conservatively independent of renal mass biopsy findings.

References

1. Soriano RM, Penfold D, Leslie SW. Anatomy, abdomen and pelvis, kidneys. In: StatPearls [Internet]. Treasure Island (FL): StatPearls Publishing; 2022 [cited 2022 Oct 26]. http://www.ncbi.nlm.nih.gov/books/NBK482385/
2. Ramanathan S, Kumar D, Khanna M, Al Heidous M, Sheikh A, Virmani V, et al. Multi-modality imaging review of congenital abnormalities of kidney and upper urinary tract. World J Radiol. 2016;8(2):132–41.
3. Emelianova D, Prikis M, Morris CS, Gibson PC, Solomon R, Scriver G, et al. The evolution of performing a kidney biopsy: a single center experience comparing native and transplant kidney biopsies performed by interventional radiologists and nephrologists. BMC Nephrol. 2022;23(1):226.
4. Uppot RN, Harisinghani MG, Gervais DA. Imaging-guided percutaneous renal biopsy: rationale and approach. AJR Am J Roentgenol. 2010;194(6):1443–9.
5. Bandari J, Fuller TW, Turner Ii RM, D'Agostino LA. Renal biopsy for medical renal disease: indications and contraindications. Can J Urol. 2016;23(1):8121–6.
6. Yang L, Bonventre JV. Diagnosis and clinical evaluation of acute kidney injury. In: Comprehensive clinical nephrology [Internet]. Elsevier; 2010 [cited 2022 Oct 26]. p. 821–9. https://linkinghub.elsevier.com/retrieve/pii/B978032305876600068X
7. Richard PO, Martin L, Lavallée LT, Violette PD, Komisarenko M, Evans AJ, et al. Identifying the use and barriers to the adoption of renal tumour biopsy in the management of small renal masses. Can Urol Assoc J. 2018;12(8):260–6.
8. Pagnini F, Cervi E, Maestroni U, Agostini A, Borgheresi A, Piacentino F, et al. Imaging guided percutaneous renal biopsy: do it or not? Acta Biomed. 2020;91(8-S):81–8.
9. Walker PD. The renal biopsy. Arch Pathol Lab Med. 2009;133(2):181–8.
10. Young M, Leslie SW. Renal biopsy. In: StatPearls [Internet]. Treasure Island (FL): StatPearls Publishing; 2022 [cited 2022 Oct 26]. http://www.ncbi.nlm.nih.gov/books/NBK470275/
11. Iversen P, Brun C. Aspiration biopsy of the kidney. Am J Med. 1951;11(3):324–30.
12. Kark Robert M, Muehrcke Robert C. Biopsy of kidney in prone position. Lancet. 1954;263(6821):1047–9.
13. Preda A, Van Dijk LC, Van Oostaijen JA, Pattynama PMT. Complication rate and diagnostic yield of 515 consecutive ultrasound-guided biopsies of renal allografts and native kidneys using a 14-gauge Biopty gun. Eur Radiol. 2003;13(3):527–30.
14. Ori Y, Neuman H, Chagnac A, Siegal A, Tobar A, Itkin M, et al. Using the automated biopsy gun with real-time ultrasound for native renal biopsy. Isr Med Assoc J. 2002;4(9):698–701.
15. Sekulic M, Crary GS. Kidney biopsy yield: an examination of influencing factors. Am J Surg Pathol. 2017;41(7):961–72.
16. Granata A, Distefano G, Pesce F, Battaglia Y, Suavo Bulzis P, Venturini M, et al. Performing an ultrasound-guided percutaneous needle kidney biopsy: an up-to-date procedural review. Diagnostics (Basel). 2021;11(12):2186.
17. Stiles KP, Yuan CM, Chung EM, Lyon RD, Lane JD, Abbott KC. Renal biopsy in high-risk patients with medical diseases of the kidney. Am J Kidney Dis. 2000;36(2):419–33.
18. Sam R, Leehey DJ, Picken MM, Borge MA, Yetter EM, Ing TS, et al. Transjugular renal biopsy in patients with liver disease. Am J Kidney Dis. 2001;37(6):1144–51.

19. Abbott KC, Musio FM, Chung EM, Lomis NN, Lane JD, Yuan CM. Transjugular renal biopsy in high-risk patients: an American case series. BMC Nephrol. 2002;3(1):5.
20. Fine DM, Arepally A, Hofmann LV, Mankowitz SG, Atta MG. Diagnostic utility and safety of transjugular kidney biopsy in the obese patient. Nephrol Dial Transplant. 2004;19(7):1798–802.
21. Rathod KR, Popat BA, Pandey A, Jamale TE, Hase NK, Deshmukh HL. Safety and effectiveness of transjugular renal biopsy: a single center study. Indian J Nephrol. 2017;27(2):118–23.
22. Yoshinari M, Suzuki R, Watanabe K, Katoh T, Watanabe T. How long is enough: length of renal needle biopsy specimen for histological diagnosis. Am J Nephrol. 2002;22(4):402.
23. Ahmad I. Biopsy of the transplanted kidney. Semin Intervent Radiol. 2004;21(4):275–81.
24. Williams WW, Taheri D, Tolkoff-Rubin N, Colvin RB. Clinical role of the renal transplant biopsy. Nat Rev Nephrol. 2012;8(2):110–21.
25. Colvin RB, et al. Diagnostic pathology: kidney diseases. Salt Lake City: Amirsys; 2011.
26. Colvin RB, Nickeleit V. In: Heptinstall's pathology of the kidney. Jennette JC, Olson JL, Schwartz MM, Silva FG, editors. Vol. 2. Lippincott-Raven; Philadelphia, pp. 1347–1490; 2006.
27. Lim M, Park BK, Lee KW, Park JB, Kim KD, Yang J, et al. Two-week protocol biopsy in renal allograft: feasibility, safety, and outcomes. J Clin Med. 2022;11(3):785.
28. Raspollini MR, Moch H, Tan PH, Mahul B. Amin Samra Turajlic Chapter III: Tumours of the kidney: WHO Classification of Tumours Editorial Board. Urinary and male genital tumours. Lyon (France): International Agency for Research on Cancer; 2022. (WHO classification of tumours series, 5th ed.; vol. 8). https://publications.iarc.fr. In.
29. American Urological Association 2015. Quality oncology guidelines. AUA Guideline J Urol 2013 [cited 2021];190:419. https://www.auanet.org/guidelines/guidelines/oncology-guidelines.
30. Sanchez A, Feldman AS, Hakimi AA. Current management of small renal masses, including patient selection, renal tumor biopsy, active surveillance, and thermal ablation. J Clin Oncol. 2018;36(36):3591–600.
31. Patel HD, Johnson MH, Pierorazio PM, Sozio SM, Sharma R, Iyoha E, et al. Diagnostic accuracy and risks of biopsy in the diagnosis of a renal mass suspicious for localized renal cell carcinoma: systematic review of the literature. J Urol. 2016;195(5):1340–7.
32. Razik A, Goyal A, Sharma R, Kandasamy D, Seth A, Das P, et al. MR texture analysis in differentiating renal cell carcinoma from lipid-poor angiomyolipoma and oncocytoma. Br J Radiol. 2020;93(1114):20200569.
33. Li H, Li A, Zhu H, Hu Y, Li J, Xia L, et al. Whole-tumor quantitative apparent diffusion coefficient histogram and texture analysis to differentiation of minimal fat angiomyolipoma from clear cell renal cell carcinoma. Acad Radiol. 2019;26(5):632–9.
34. Bosniak MA. The current radiological approach to renal cysts. Radiology. 1986;158(1):1–10.
35. Gillingham N, Chandarana H, Kamath A, Shaish H, Hindman N. Bosniak IIF and III renal cysts: can apparent diffusion coefficient-derived texture features discriminate between malignant and benign IIF and III cysts? J Comput Assist Tomogr. 2019;43(3):485–92.
36. Raza SA, Sohaib SA, Sahdev A, Bharwani N, Heenan S, Verma H, et al. Centrally infiltrating renal masses on CT: differentiating intrarenal transitional cell carcinoma from centrally located renal cell carcinoma. Am J Roentgenol. 2012;198(4):846–53.
37. Herts BR, Baker ME. The current role of percutaneous biopsy in the evaluation of renal masses. Semin Urol Oncol. 1995;13(4):254–61.
38. Smith EH. Complications of percutaneous abdominal fine-needle biopsy. Review. Radiology. 1991;178(1):253–8.
39. Renshaw AA, Powell A, Caso J, Gould EW. Needle track seeding in renal mass biopsies. Cancer Cytopathol. 2019;127(6):358–61.
40. Motzer RJ, Jonasch E, Boyle S, Carlo MI, Manley B, Agarwal N, et al. NCCN guidelines insights: kidney cancer, version 1.2021. J Natl Compr Canc Netw. 2020;18(9):1160–70.
41. Sahni VA, Silverman SG. Biopsy of renal masses: when and why. Cancer Imaging. 2009;6(9):44–55.
42. Li G, Cuilleron M, Gentil-Perret A, Tostain J. Characteristics of image-detected solid renal masses: implication for optimal treatment. Int J Urol. 2004;11(2):63–7.
43. Beland MD, Mayo-Smith WW, Dupuy DE, Cronan JJ, DeLellis RA. Diagnostic yield of 58 consecutive imaging-guided biopsies of solid renal masses: should we biopsy all that are indeterminate? AJR Am J Roentgenol. 2007;188(3):792–7.
44. Brachemi S, Bollée G. Renal biopsy practice: What is the gold standard? World J Nephrol. 2014;3(4):287–94.
45. Kriegshauser JS, Patel MD, Young SW, Chen F, Eversman WG, Chang YHH. Risk of bleeding after native renal biopsy as a function of preprocedural systolic and diastolic blood pressure. J Vasc Interv Radiol. 2015;26(2):206–12.
46. Bakdash K, Schramm KM, Annam A, Brown M, Kondo K, Lindquist JD. Complications of percutaneous renal biopsy. Semin Intervent Radiol. 2019;36(2):97–103.
47. Whittier WL, Korbet SM. Timing of complications in percutaneous renal biopsy. J Am Soc Nephrol. 2004;15(1):142–7.
48. Maturen KE, Nghiem HV, Caoili EM, Higgins EG, Wolf JS, Wood DP. Renal mass core biopsy: accuracy and impact on clinical management. AJR Am J Roentgenol. 2007;188(2):563–70.
49. Millet I, Curros F, Serre I, Taourel P, Thuret R. Can renal biopsy accurately predict histological subtype and Fuhrman grade of renal cell carcinoma? J Urol. 2012;188(5):1690–4.

Renal Modeling and 3D Printing

26

Elizabeth Silvestro, Susan J. Back,
and Suraj D. Serai

Introduction

Additive manufacturing and 3-dimensional (3D) printing have positively impacted clinical care by aiding surgical planning, implant design, and training models. Despite the relatively high manufacturing expense, models aid communication between doctors, patients, and parents of pediatric patients. Comparisons between 3D printed models of normal and abnormal anatomy have also been used to educate trainees and patients. Application of personalized 3D renal models has proved to be clinically useful and has positively impacted patient care. The relative ease of osseous segmentation on imaging led to early applications for maxillofacial and orthopedic surgeries [1]. Recently, advances in medical imaging and the availability and decreasing cost of 3D printing and materials have allowed exploration of modeling and printing for soft tissue applications. The most examined role of renal modeling has been in nephron sparing surgery (NSS), where both printed and holographic models have been used to support patient counseling, surgical planning, and physician education in both pediatric and adult practice [1–10]. Most of the contemporary medical imaging is based on combinations of two-dimensional images. For performing a partial nephrectomy, it is of utmost importance to identify the exact tumor location to minimize unnecessary dissection and bleeding. However, even experienced surgeons sometimes encounter problems identifying the renal tumor, particularly in small endophytic tumors. Patient's position is another deteriorating factor; as most of the renal surgery is performed in the flank position, the location of kidney tends to be rotated compared with the orientation of preoperative imaging studies. 3D renal models can help surgeons establish the surgical plan and can also be useful education materials for medical students. While most publications to date describe using computed tomography for image acquisition, magnetic resonance (MR) imaging is advantageous to avoid radiation and potentially avoid intravenous contrast in patients with compromised renal function. In our experience, anatomy from each modality can be segmented and combined into a single model when clinically relevant. Future work may focus on modeling with materials that more closely simulate human tissue, virtual reality applications, and shifting from manual to automated or semiautomated segmentation. Here we describe our approach to MR image acquisition, segmentation, and model creation, which can serve as a basis for current and future modeling applications.

E. Silvestro · S. J. Back · S. D. Serai (✉)
Children's Hospital of Philadelphia, University of Pennsylvania, Philadelphia, PA, USA
e-mail: SILVESTRO@chop.edu; BackS@chop.edu; serais@chop.edu

S. D. Serai, K. Darge (eds.), *Advanced Clinical MRI of the Kidney*,
https://doi.org/10.1007/978-3-031-40169-5_26

MRI Acquisition Protocols

Imaging sequences for 3D modeling are added to our renal mass MR protocol.

Our image acquisition method includes an isotropic voxel proton density-weighted (PD) 3D fast spin-echo (FSE) sequence and post-gadolinium dynamic 3D T1-weighted volume interpolated breath-hold examination (VIBE). High-resolution isotropic volumetric data provide optimal results to avoid partial-volume effects through-plane thick slice. This allows the data to be reformatted into additional planes to better view regions of interest and to generate views that correspond to other acquired sequences, if desired. The acquired MR images' quality dictates the final quality of the printed 3D model. High spatial resolution with respiratory motion corrections and high temporal resolution (in cardiac and respiratory motion-affected studies) are critical requirements for 3D modeling and printing applications. The true resolution of an image is not simply determined by the acquisition matrix; rather, it depends on blurring artifacts as well. Artifacts must be recognized and accounted for by the person segmenting the data or, ideally, eliminated or corrected for during the MR acquisition. While relatively motionless anatomies such as brain, spine, and extremities can be exquisitely imaged by MRI, motion in pelvis and kidney anatomies and in restless/pediatric patients is one of the most common and problematic sources of artifacts, creating ghosting and blurring that severely hinders segmentation. Motion often becomes more problematic with higher resolution acquisitions, and a balance must be found between the desire for smaller voxels and the need to minimize motion artifacts. In general, a clinically superior diagnostic MRI study will yield optimal 3D printing quality. Multiphase coronal gadolinium-enhanced images are obtained to delineate the renal vasculature, tumors, and urinary collecting system during contrast excretion.

Post-Processing and Data Analysis Methods

The pathway to realizing patient-specific anatomical parts involves a two-stage process: the design and manufacturing phases. While image quality from clinical standard of care acquisition is sufficient for 3D printing, final product realization requires financial resources and a trained workforce. The creation of anatomic 3D printed models is an integrated collaborative process between the radiologist, surgeon, and segmenting technologist or engineer. Each provides a key insight necessary for accurate and valuable models. The following section will cover the modeling process from imaging to printing (Fig. 26.1).

Anatomy and Segmentation

Once the imaging is complete, a radiologist works with the engineer or 3D technologist to select the sequence or sequences that best capture the anatomy of interest and a general base series. The first step in the workflow is to convert medical imaging data in digital imaging and communications in medicine (DICOM) format to a meshed surface file such as a standard tessellation language (STL) file. This requires a segmentation step, where structures of interest are designated to be included in the model and superfluous surrounding structures are excluded. The images for segmentation can include selections across a variety of sequences and those that change across time lapses or contrast enhancement. Our practice includes creating a selection of key diagnostic image captures annotated with series and slice numbers. This preparatory document is often shared with the surgical team. The next step involves image segmentation, which can be achieved using multiple techniques including thresholding, auto contouring, region growing, and manual segmentation. The segmentation of anatomy should be completed using a program ideal for 3D print modeling, such as Materialise

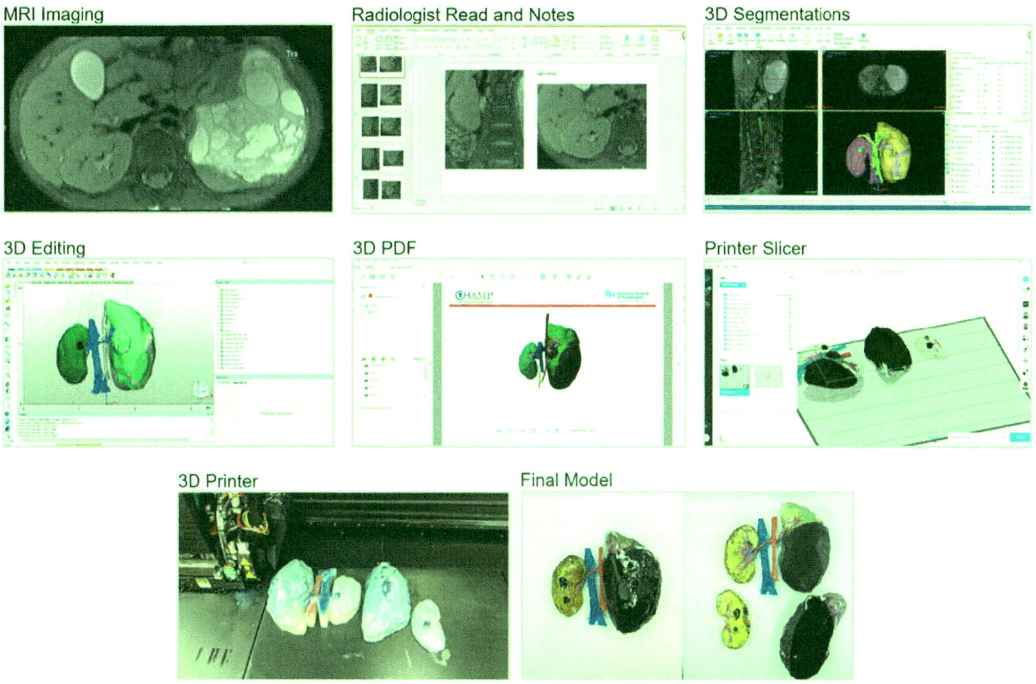

Fig. 26.1 Visual walkthrough of steps to create 3D printed model from MRI imaging of the kidney for surgical planning. Steps (from top left): MR imaging optimized for modeling, reading, and interpretation by a radiologist with notes documented in slide deck, 3D segmentation of ROI in Materialise Mimics, 3D Editing in Materialise 3-Matic, virtual model sharing in 3D PDF for review, preparing of models in Printers Slicer Program, printing and cleaning of the model, and delivering the final model to the surgical team

Mimics (https://www.materialise.com/en/healthcare/mimics-innovation-suite/mimics) or 3D Slicer (https://www.slicer.org/). Region growing, the most common method, connects all pixels or voxels of similar intensity within the stack of images in preparation for creating a 3D volume. Region growing may be performed with manual seeding, in which the operator selects a particular image intensity manually or with an automated algorithm. Each of the areas of interest should be segmented in the ideal series for the anatomy or pathology and can then be overlaid on the base series to combine. Generally, the kidney and tumor are segmented from the isotropic PD sequence, and the vascular and collecting systems are molded from time lapsed post-gadolinium series. Small modifications can be made to adjust for motion in the base series.

In the case that sequences are not captured at the same scan time (e.g., patients required repositioning during the examination or images are from different study dates or modalities), modifications can be made. An unrelated consistent body region, such as a vertebra, is segmented from each scan set and used to resize and reorient the anatomy of interest. After the anatomy is aligned using the unrelated region, it can be removed. In this scenario, the altered anatomy should be noted by varied color on the model to indicate the change and the surgeons should be notified of the merger and adjustment. Post segmentation, the DICOM data are converted into STL files for 3D printing.

Clinical Review of Segmentation

Once the general segmentation is completed, the next step is to review the anatomy with the radiologist to confirm the clinical accuracy and anatomic representation. Key aspects to review include the anatomic contours, interconnections, and confirmation of any adjustments made to the models. The radiologist reviews both the segmentation and the 3D renderings of the model. We utilize an interactive 3D portable document format (PDF) file. 3D PDFs allow the user to view and work with the model using common readers such as Adobe or other PDF viewers, which is beneficial for sharing the virtual file with other team members. This allows the surgeon or clinicians to express preferences about the anatomic depiction and confirm if a printed model is needed or if they prefer to use the interactive virtual model for its own features. 3D virtual models allow the user to move, rotate, and hide aspects of the model to gain additional anatomic perspectives.

Printing Design and Considerations

3D printing applications are helpful for clinical evaluation, preoperative planning, patient and trainee education, and simulation. Printing design is an important consideration to ensure that the virtual model will translate to a physical model that is usable and represents the intended areas of interest. Feature size, resolution, weight, and usability are all key aspects. Feature size and resolution inform what is possible to fabricate and the realism of the model; they are dictated by the printing machines available and could lead to variation in the models. The weight of the model and its parts may require additional support posts to hold it together and prevent it from breaking. If the model is intended to have the kidney suspended in a vertical orientation and connected to the vascular system, it may be necessary to add a support post below the kidney or to the thicker sections of the vascular system (e.g., aorta or inferior vena cava). This post will prevent the smaller renal arteries and veins from acting like a cantilever.

Finally, considering the usability—how the model will be held, moved, and understood—while planning a print is key to ensuring the additive value of the model. Some models are used to simulate surgery, warranting consideration of material selection, and the ability to cut or suture the material. The 3D printing process typically consists of depositing material layer-by-layer in a semiliquid, liquid, or powder form and solidifying the material using light energy (e.g., UV or laser), an electron beam, chemical binders, or by heating and cooling it to solidify at room temperature. The printer's resolution and material constraints dictate the cost of the printers and their applications. In general, 3D printed resolutions are in the range of 30–200 microns, which is much higher than the image data, and any variation from the printable file to the physical model is negligible. Multi-material machines offer the potential to print with various colors and material compositions (e.g., different hardness, texture, and plastic types). If possible, it is useful to create a standard color-coding practice for consistency across models and improved understanding. A simple example is black for tumors, green for kidney, and red for arteries. On a single material machine, it is possible to paint or label regions to achieve the same end. Using transparent materials on the outer aspect of the model (e.g., renal parenchyma) can improve visualization of internal components such as intrusion of a tumor on the collection system or blood supply. Additionally, it can be advantageous to create parts that open to offer unique views. We often create a renal model that can be opened along the oblique coronal plane of the kidney to view the tumor relationship to the urinary collecting system and vasculature. These openable models should include small posts to allow parts to be connected and easily separated either by snap fits (like children's building block pieces) or magnets (which need to be kept away from MRI).

Quality Control and Storage

Quality control (QC) and assurance is essential in providing accurate models. Machine maintenance and testing is critical to keep equipment in the ideal condition. The QC process includes measurement assessment throughout the process and at key intervals including at imaging and after segmentation and printing.

Storage can be a challenge with the unique file formats including printing files (stereolithography STL or object file OBJ), 3D PDFs, and segmentation files. If it is not possible to store all aspects in the radiology picture archiving and communication system (PACS) or other standard system, it is best to set up an alternative secure system for storage to preserve the printing and segmentation files. This allows for later review and long-term assessment if needed.

Clinical Applications

One of the most widespread medical applications of 3D printing to date is the creation of patient-specific anatomical 3D models for presurgical planning. The clinical applications section will detail the 3D printing applications from MRI in clinical scenarios. We include several clinical examples of imaging and modeling where this technology has made a clinical impact at our tertiary care children's hospital.

Patient 1: A 5-year-old girl with history of bilateral Wilms tumors underwent prior chemotherapy, left nephrectomy, and right kidney exploration. She had disease recurrence with a large tumor in the central aspect of her solitary right kidney. After restarting chemotherapy, presurgical magnetic resonance imaging was performed. A 3D model was created to demonstrate the relationship between the lesion, urinary collecting system, and vasculature and to plan for partial nephrectomy (Fig. 26.2).

Patient 2: A 4-year-old girl with a palpable abdominal mass was diagnosed with bilateral Wilms tumors after undergoing abdominal MRI. She received 6 weeks of chemotherapy with interval decrease in size of her tumors. After 12 total weeks of chemotherapy, a preoperative MRI showed continued decrease in size of the tumors. A presurgical planning 3D model was created to depict the relationship of the tumors to the collecting system and vasculature (Fig. 26.3). She then underwent staged partial nephrectomies of each kidney.

Patient 3: A 12-year-old girl with caudal regression syndrome with imperforate anus, neurogenic bowel, and bladder. Magnetic resonance imaging was obtained of her abdomen and pelvis to evaluate her urogenital and bowel anatomy. Her horseshoe shaped kidney and dilated right ureter with ectopic insertion were included in her 3D PDF document (Fig. 26.4).

Patient 4: An 11-month-old girl presented with a palpable abdominal mass. Her abdominal ultrasound showed a large complex cystic mass arising from the right kidney. Magnetic

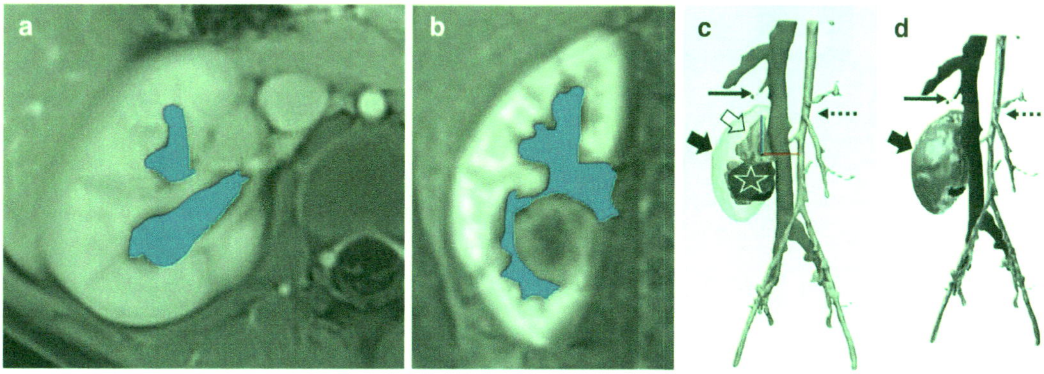

Fig. 26.2 A 5-year-old girl with recurrent Wilms tumor in a solitary kidney. (**a**) Axial T1 CAIPIRINHA-VIBE and (**b**) coronal 3D VIBE both post-gadolinium administration is annotated during pre-modeling review of the images. The blue regions are the renal urinary collecting system. In (**b**) the relationship between the tumor (star) and the collecting system (blue region) is depicted. 3D renderings of the segmented anatomy in (**c**) transparent and (**d**) solid renderings. The aorta (dashed thin arrow), inferior vena cava (solid thin arrow), kidney (solid thick arrow), tumor (star), and renal collecting system (open thick arrow) are depicted. Note that the tumor and renal collecting system are visible when the kidney parenchyma is made transparent (**c**)

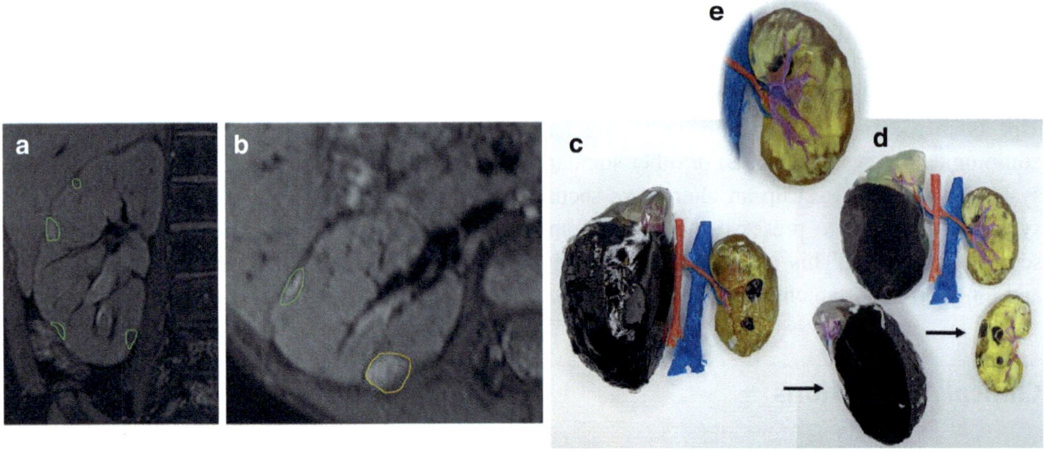

Fig. 26.3 A 4-year-old girl with bilateral Wilms tumors kidney modeling done for presurgical planning of staged partial nephrectomies. (**a**) Coronal isovoxel proton density-weighted SPACE sequence with fat suppression and (**b**) axial reformat of the right kidney showing annotations made during anatomic segmentation. Lesions with imaging features of nephrogenic rests (green outline) were distinguished from those with imaging features of Wilms tumor (yellow outline). (**c**) 3D printed model of both kidneys. The kidneys were printed using a transparent material for the parenchyma so the tumor (black), collecting system (hollow cavity), and vasculature (red, blue, and purple) could be visualized from the exterior of the model. The large left renal tumor (black) takes up most of the kidney while smaller tumors are seen in the right kidney (black) as well as nephrogenic rests (light gray). (**d**) For an additional vantage point, the model can be bivalved, here along the coronal oblique axis of each kidney with half of each kidney removed (arrows) to better examine the structural relationships. (**e**) Magnified view of the right kidney. Multiple small vessels in the central aspect of the kidney could not be definitively resolved as arteries or veins. To depict the presence of these vessels, a purple material was used. *Red = aorta/arteries; blue = inferior vena cava/veins*

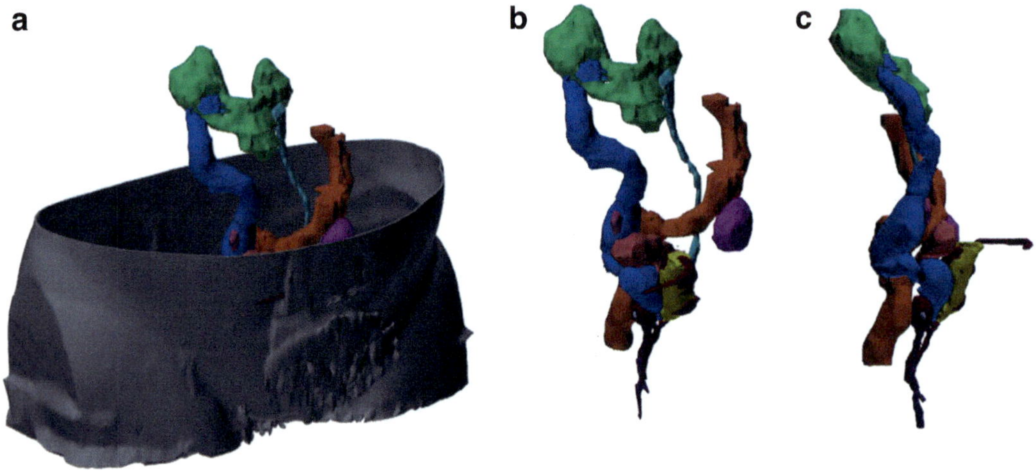

Fig. 26.4 A 12-year-old girl with caudal regression syndrome and complex genitourinary anatomy. Modeling done for presurgical planning. (**a**) Her horseshoe kidney (green) and dilated and tortuous right ureter (blue) are depicted on the PDF version of the model. The gray structure is a surface rendering of her pelvic wall. With the body surface removed and the model rotation of the anatomy, isometric (**b**) and right (**c**), the ectopic insertion of the right ureter is seen on the bladder (yellow)

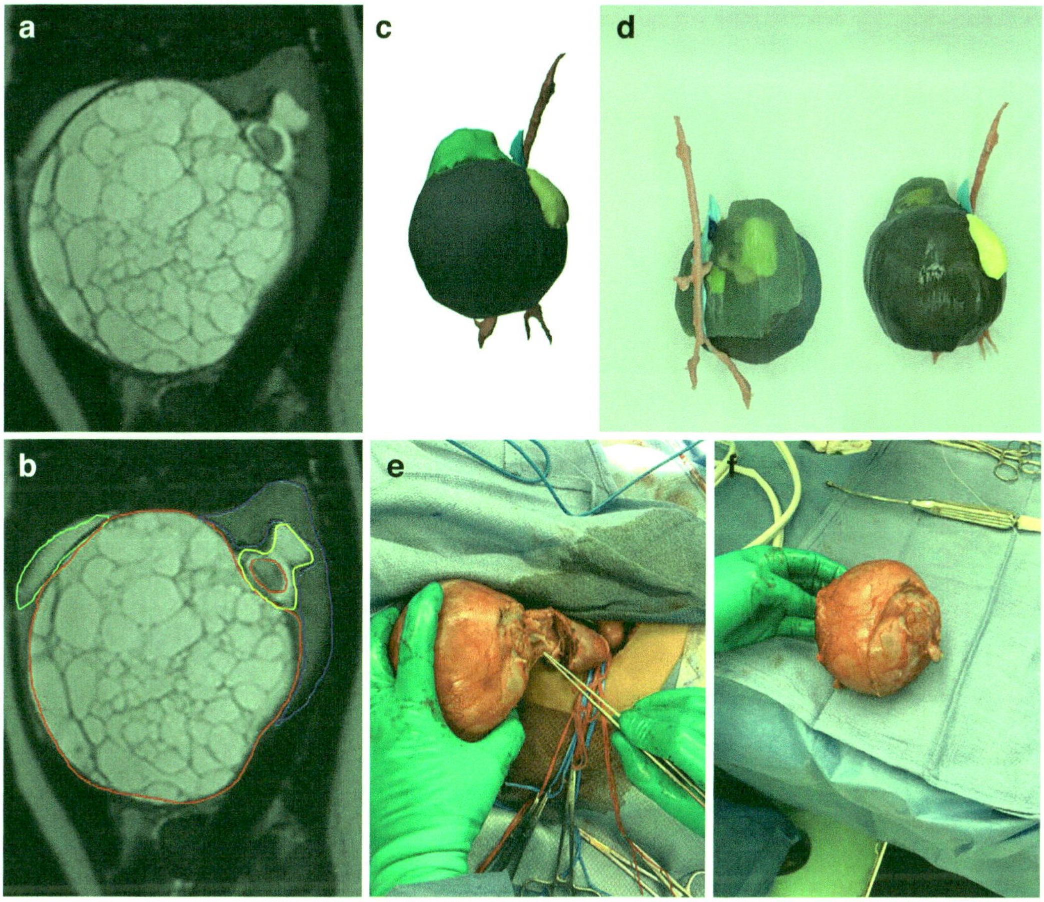

Fig. 26.5 An 11-month-old girl with cystic nephroma. Presurgical planning for partial nephrectomy. Sagittal T2 HASTE image with fat suppression of the right kidney without (**a**) and with (**b**) imaging annotation during anatomic segmentation planning. The large cystic tumor (red outline) occupies a large portion of the kidney compressing the renal parenchyma (purple outline). The gallbladder (green outline) draped over the tumor and was included in the segmentation planning to distinguish it from the cystic mass. A portion of the tumor extends into the renal collecting system (yellow outline). (**c**) 3D PDF of the right kidney and tumor. (**d**) 3D printed model viewed from the anterior and posterior aspects. *Red = aorta/arteries; blue = inferior vena cava/veins; black = tumor; yellowish green = urinary collecting system; yellow = gall bladder.* (**e**) Intraoperative photo during right kidney dissection. Surgical instrument depicting point where the tumor extended into the renal collecting system. (**f**) Tumor specimen following resection

resonance imaging was obtained for further characterization and preoperative planning (Fig. 26.5). She underwent a partial nephrectomy with surgical pathology confirming a cystic nephroma.

Patient 5: An 11-year-old girl with history of autosomal recessive polycystic kidney disease underwent renal transplant with resection of her native kidneys. The transplant graft was positioned in her right upper quadrant. She developed a renal cell carcinoma in the transplanted kidney. Multi-disciplinary team discussion included the possibility of a percutaneous cryoablation. Imaging was obtained, and a pre-procedural model was created. The body wall and bowel were important structures to consider in the model to plan for a possible percutaneous approach. Her anatomy was segmented from an abdominal magnetic resonance exam as well as from chest computed tomography (Fig. 26.6).

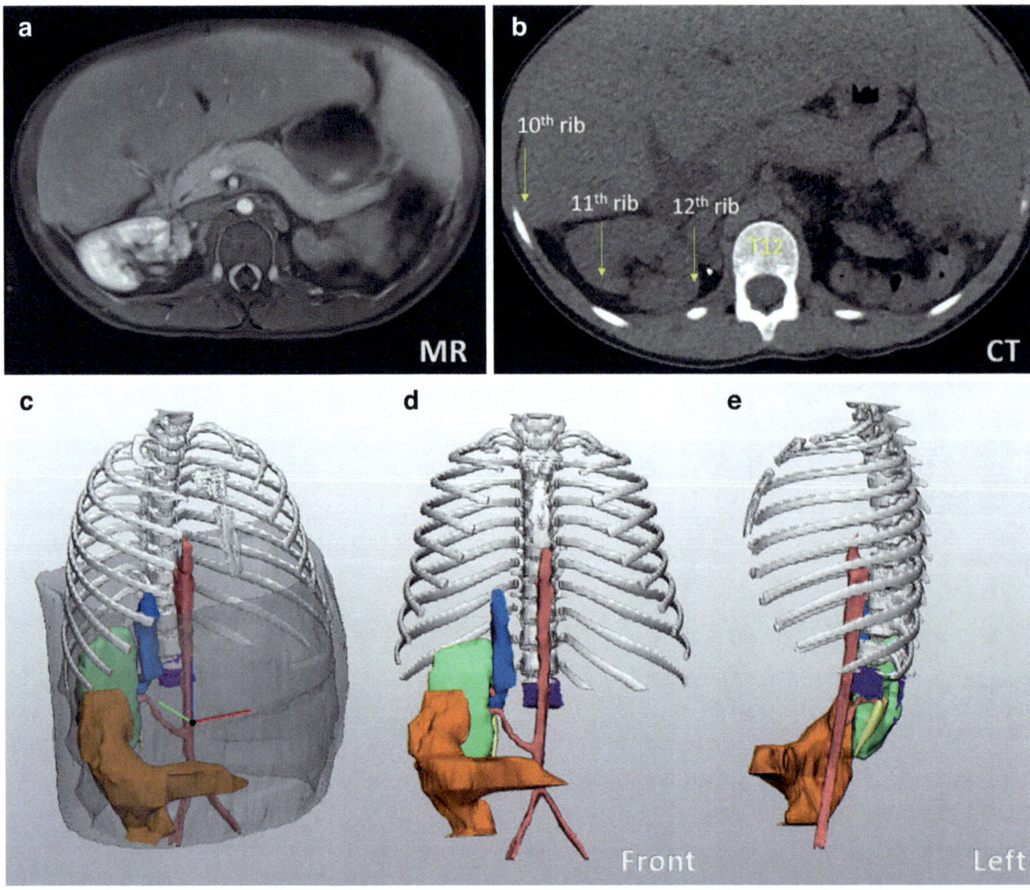

Fig. 26.6 An 11-year-old girl with renal cell carcinoma in a right upper quadrant transplant kidney. (**a**) Axial STAR VIBE post-contrast image obtained during a magnetic resonance imaging (MRI) examination of the abdomen for preoperative planning. (**b**) Axial non-contrast chest computed tomography (CT) image where the osseous anatomy is identified in preparation for 3D modeling. A vertebral body from the upper abdomen was used to modify and combine anatomic structures between MRI and CT. Images from the dynamic PDF of the chest and body wall showing the anatomic depictions in an anterior oblique plane (**c**) with the body wall present (translucent gray structure), (**d**) frontal view, and (**e**) left lateral views with the body wall removed. The overlapping vertebral body that was used to align the studies is purple. *Orange = bowel; green = kidney; blue = inferior vena cava/veins*

Future Directions

3D modeling and printing of these models are invaluable tools not only in surgical planning, but also in trainee, parent, and patient education. The future of 3D modeling and printing for applications in kidney imaging is expected to expand in new directions. New MRI sequences for fast and motion-robust isotropic imaging will widen the scope of applications. Two hurdles in using the technology are high infrastructure and operating costs. The emergence of low-cost printers with high-resolution printing capability over the last few years has made it possible for low budget labs to flourish, but high software costs are still unavoidable. Since 3D printing in medical applications is a relatively new and small area of specialization, trained personnel with the desired skill sets are lacking. Also, structured training programs are needed to focus on merging image post-processing for 3D modeling and printing. However, the growth of artificial intelligence and deep-learning applications in radiological image processing will lead to more automated segmentation, promising to reduce subjective human factor discrepancies. The development of materials for 3D printing is a potential area for the focus of industry and academic research. Most of the currently available materials for 3D printing, initially developed for industry, are being adapted to the medical field. Therefore, the properties are close to but not the same as those of human body tissues. Patient-specific 3D printing models and devices need to evolve from a visualization and surgical planning tool to a functional tool that simulates the human body in form and physiological and pathological conditions. Collaborative research between industry and end users will drive 3D modeling and printing evolution, ultimately leading to the availability of materials simulating the physical and mechanical properties of human organs.

References

1. Lee H, Nguyen NH, Hwang SI, et al. Personalized 3D kidney model produced by rapid prototyping method and its usefulness in clinical applications. Int Braz J Urol. 2018;44:952–7.
2. Silberstein JL, Maddox MM, Dorsey P, et al. Physical models of renal malignancies using standard cross-sectional imaging and 3-dimensional printers: a pilot study. Urology. 2014;84:268–72.
3. Bernhard JC, Isotani S, Matsugasumi T, et al. Personalized 3D printed model of kidney and tumor anatomy: a useful tool for patient education. World J Urol. 2016;34:337–45.
4. Golab A, Smektala T, Kaczmarek K, et al. Laparoscopic partial nephrectomy supported by training involving personalized silicone replica poured in three-dimensional printed casting Mold. J Laparoendosc Adv Surg Tech A. 2017;27:420–2.
5. Wake N, Rude T, Kang SK, et al. 3D printed renal cancer models derived from MRI data: application in pre-surgical planning. Abdom Radiol (NY). 2017;42:1501–9.
6. Wellens LM, Meulstee J, van de Ven CP, et al. Comparison of 3-dimensional and augmented reality kidney models with conventional imaging data in the preoperative assessment of children with Wilms tumors. JAMA Netw Open. 2019;2:e192633.
7. Checcucci E, De Cillis S, Porpiglia F. 3D-printed models and virtual reality as new tools for image-guided robot-assisted nephron-sparing surgery: a systematic review of the newest evidences. Curr Opin Urol. 2020;30:55–64.
8. Chaussy Y, Vieille L, Lacroix E, et al. 3D reconstruction of Wilms' tumor and kidneys in children: variability, usefulness and constraints. J Pediatr Urol. 2020;16:830 e831–8.
9. Checcucci E, Amparore D, Pecoraro A, et al. 3D mixed reality holograms for preoperative surgical planning of nephron-sparing surgery: evaluation of surgeons' perception. Minerva Urol Nephrol. 2021;73:367–75.
10. Gurung PMS, Melnyk R, Holler T, et al. Application of IRIS three-dimensional anatomical models as preoperative surgical planning tools in the management of localized renal masses. J Endourol. 2021;35:383–9.

27 Radiomics and Texture Analysis

Adarsh Ghosh and Suraj D. Serai

Introduction

Conventional assessment of medical images by radiologists does not use much of the latent pixel-based information. The term "radiomics" refers to the extraction of this latent data from clinical images using mathematical analysis of pixels, thereby providing quantitative information [1–4]. Radiomics is an emerging field, which attempts to extract data from imaging to provide information beyond what can be achieved from human imaging interpretation alone. The radiomics approach quantitatively evaluates image heterogeneity, removing some subjectivity in image analysis [4]. The plethora of quantitative features extracted from these images are used in conjunction with various machine learning and artificial intelligence techniques to predict clinical- or patient-based outcomes like a response to therapy or tumor genotypes [5, 6]. The heterogeneity of the grayscale pixel values in the tumor image reflects the tumor's genotypic or phenotypic variations[7, 8]. Radiomics aims to optimize precision medicine. The parameters frequently used in radiomics literature are texture, shape, and morphometry of the tumor. Since imaging is a vital component of any clinical workup, radiomics has had broad utility when applied to routine point-of-care images.

Using radiomics, entire tumors can be evaluated through imaging, overcoming the blind spots associated with a biopsy-based evaluation, in which only a small part of the tumor is sampled [9–11]. While radiomics has been used extensively in oncology, it has also been used in other diseases to predict treatment outcomes or pathologies non-invasively. Renal tumors encompass a heterogeneous disease spectrum, which confounds patient management and treatment. MRI provides rich imaging data sets because of the multiple image contrast mechanisms available with this technique. These datasets offer a unique opportunity to implement radiomic analysis. Radiomics may provide detail beyond what can be achieved from human interpretation. Understanding what new technologies offer will allow radiologists to play a greater role in caring for patients with renal pathologies. This chapter presents the typical workflow needed for radiomics analysis, followed by a discussion of the current applications in renal MRI.

Steps of a Radiomics Project

A typical radiomics workflow comprises five parts: image acquisition, image segmentation, image processing, feature extraction, and feature selection and modeling.

A. Ghosh · S. D. Serai (✉)
Children's Hospital of Philadelphia, University of Pennsylvania, Philadelphia, PA, USA
e-mail: serais@chop.edu

S. D. Serai, K. Darge (eds.), *Advanced Clinical MRI of the Kidney*,
https://doi.org/10.1007/978-3-031-40169-5_27

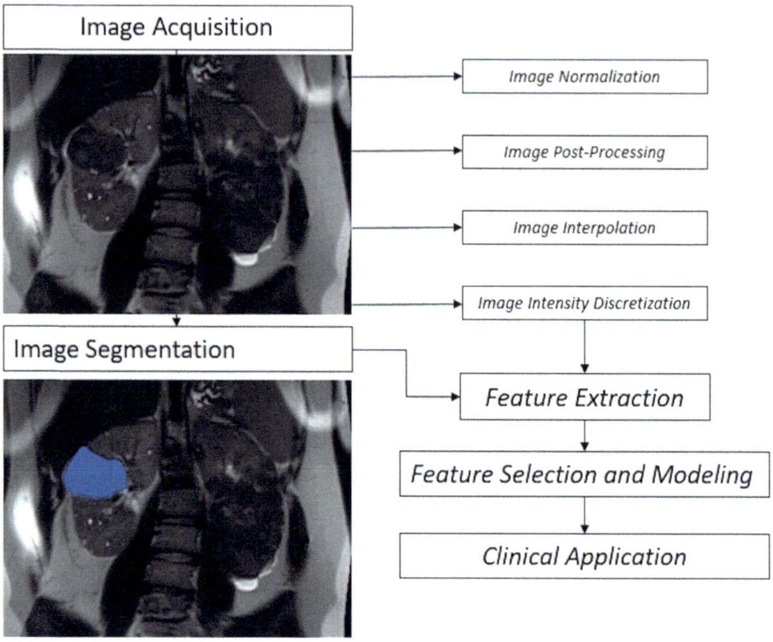

Fig. 27.1 A schematic illustration of the steps involved in radiomics analysis. After image acquisition and segmentation, radiomic features are extracted and statistical or deep learning models are generated to predict clinical outcomes of interest

The Image Biomarker Standardization Initiative has provided detailed descriptions of the steps involved in such an analysis (Fig. 27.1) [12].

Image Acquisition

Radiomics can be used with a wide range of imaging modalities, including MRI [13, 14], ultrasound [15], and computed tomography [16]. The information obtained from these imaging modalities can be used separately or combined to help solve various clinical problems. Wide variations in image acquisition and reconstruction protocols affect the consistency of the radiomics features obtained from different data sets. This means that the generalizability of multi-institutional radiomics studies is limited. Radiomics-specific phantoms with known features have value for protocol optimization and image processing to mitigate the effects of scanner and vendor variability associated with radiomics analysis [17–19].

Image Segmentation: Identification of the Region of Interest

Delineating the pathology in the images is one of the most important steps in radiomics. Typically, manual or semiautomatic segmentation techniques have been used, with recent trends weighing in toward the use of automated deep learning algorithms [20]. No single segmentation technique is considered the gold standard, as each method has limitations. Manual segmentation is very time-consuming, especially when working with 3D datasets, and is prone to inter- and intra-observer variability [21]. Studies recommend evaluating the reproducibility of radiomic features between segmentations done by different observers and using only the reproducible features. Since manual segmentation is tedious, especially when done by multiple observers, semiautomatic algorithm-based segmentation such as edge detection and thresholding [22, 23] have also been used. The basic premise is that such segmentations might be less time-consuming or more reproducible.

Image Processing

After image acquisition, the vendor software usually post-processes MR images to enhance image quality or account for image noise. Post-processing can affect the radiomic parameters obtained, which should be kept in mind when designing a radiomics pipeline to ensure uniformity in the post-processing steps applied [12].

Image Interpolation

Radiomics features are dependent on the size of image voxels from which they are derived. Since MR images are often acquired with asymmetric voxel sizes, interpolation to isotropic voxel spacing is needed to ensure rotationally invariant images. This is an important step to ensure that the radiomics features are less dependent on image acquisition parameters and hardware. No fixed protocols are prescribed for the standards used for interpolation. Up-sampling images to smaller voxel size result in the imputation of synthetic data, while down-sampling to a larger voxel size results in loss of information [12, 22]. Though the details of the algorithms used are beyond the scope of this discussion, their basic premise is to impute the values of interpolated voxels based on calculations carried out on the original neighboring voxels. Image intensities thus interpolated may require rounding off. Once the image is interpolated, the segmentation should be interpolated as well to ensure that the segmentation continues to represent a meaningful part of the image. In addition, the coordinate system used to interpolate the image must be aligned to the coordinate system of the original images to ensure the reproducibility of the radiomic features.

Image Normalization

Unlike CT scans, pixels in MR images have no absolute values associated with them. To ensure generalizability, image normalization is carried out by intensity filtering for MR images [12, 22]. The mean and standard deviation of all pixel values in a region of interest (ROI) are determined, and pixels with intensity values beyond three standard deviations from the mean are removed. Additionally, the intensity values of the pixels can be normalized using the following formula [23]:

$$\text{Normalized intensity} = \frac{\begin{array}{c}\text{Intensity} - \text{mean of all}\\ \text{intensity in image}\end{array}}{\begin{array}{c}\text{Standard deviation}\\ \text{of all intensity}\end{array}}.$$

Image Intensity Discretization

Gray value discretization involves grouping ("binning") pixels according to intensity values to facilitate the calculation of higher-order features (Fig. 27.2) [24]. The three parameters considered in the image discretization process include [12, 22] (a) *Range*—the range of pixel intensities in each image, (b) *Bin Number*—the number of groups into which the range of pixel intensities are subdivided, and (c) *Bin Width*—the size of the groups into which each pixel is grouped. For a given range of pixel intensities in an image, the three above parameters are correlated by the formula $\text{Bin Width} = \frac{\text{Intensity Range}}{\text{Number of Bins}}$. Fixed bin numbers help normalize MRI data in particular because intensity in MRI data is arbitrary and varies from scanner to scanner. There is no single specific bin number recommended in the literature, with some studies showing that the optimal bin number can vary according to the image acquisition parameters and MR sequence under evaluation.

Feature Extraction

Mathematical formulae are used to extract several radiomic features from images. The Image Biomarker Standardization Initiative guidelines define the formulae [12, 22] used to extract these features (Table 27.1). Very briefly, histogram-

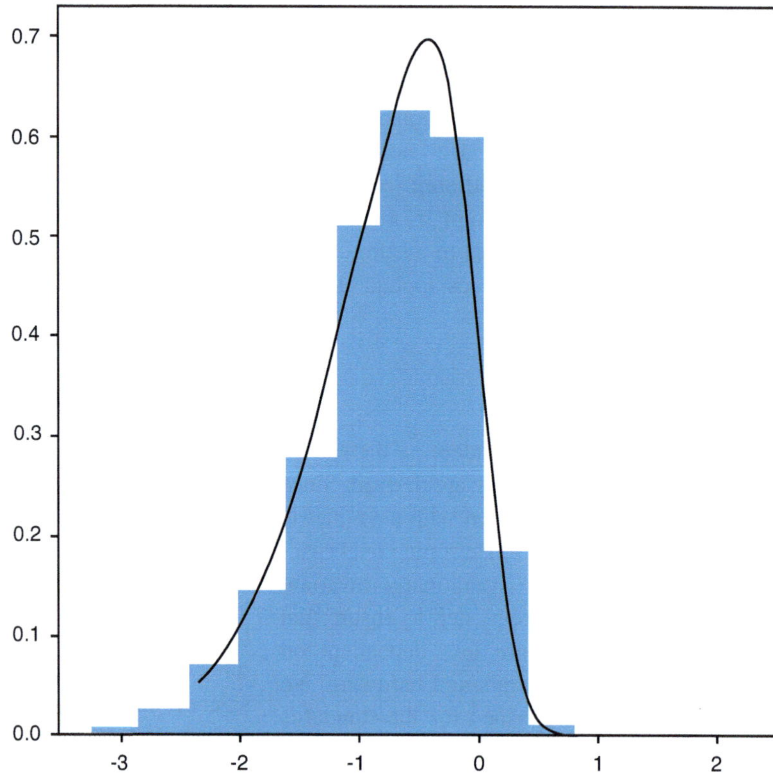

Fig. 27.2 Image intensity discretization. Original data (black line) and a generic discretized version (blue histogram)

Table 27.1 A list of features which can be used in the radiomics pipeline

Gray Level Size Zone Matrix (GLSZM) Features	Large area low gray level emphasis, zone variance, large area high gray level emphasis, zone entropy, small area high gray level emphasis, small area low gray level emphasis, high gray level zone emphasis, size zone non uniformity, gray level non uniformity normalized, small area emphasis, zone percentage, size zone non uniformity normalized, low gray level zone emphasis, gray level non uniformity, gray level variance, large area emphasis
First-order Features	Maximum, Uniformity, Robust Mean Absolute Deviation, Minimum, Total Energy, Median, 90 Percentile, Root Mean Squared, Range, 10 Percentile, Energy, Mean Absolute Deviation, Variance, Skewness, Mean, Entropy, Kurtosis, Interquartile Range
Gray Level Run Length Matrix (GLRLM) Features	Short Run Emphasis, High gray Level Run Emphasis, Short Run Low gray Level Emphasis, Long Run High gray Level Emphasis, Short Run High gray Level Emphasis, Run Percentage, gray Level Non Uniformity Normalized, Low gray Level Run Emphasis, Run Entropy, Run Variance, Long Run Low gray Level Emphasis, Run Length Non Uniformity, gray Level Non Uniformity, gray Level Variance, Run Length Non Uniformity Normalized, Long Run Emphasis
Neighboring gray Tone Difference Matrix (NGTDM) Features	Busyness, Coarseness, Contrast, Complexity, Strength
Gray Level Co-occurrence Matrix (GLCM) Features	Difference Variance, Contrast, Imc1, Difference Average, Joint Energy, Maximum Probability, Idn, Idmn, Correlation, MCC, Inverse Variance, Difference Entropy, Idm, Joint Entropy, Sum Average, Cluster Tendency, Cluster Prominence, Cluster Shade, Autocorrelation, Sum Squares, Sum Entropy, Id, Joint Average, Imc2
Gray Level Dependence Matrix (GLDM) Features	Small Dependence Emphasis, Small Dependence High gray Level Emphasis, Dependence nonuniformity, Large Dependence Low gray Level Emphasis, Large Dependence High gray Level Emphasis, High gray Level Emphasis, Dependence Entropy, Small Dependence Low gray Level Emphasis, Dependence nonuniformity Normalized, Dependence Variance, Large Dependence Emphasis, gray Level Non Uniformity, gray Level Variance, Low gray Level Emphasis

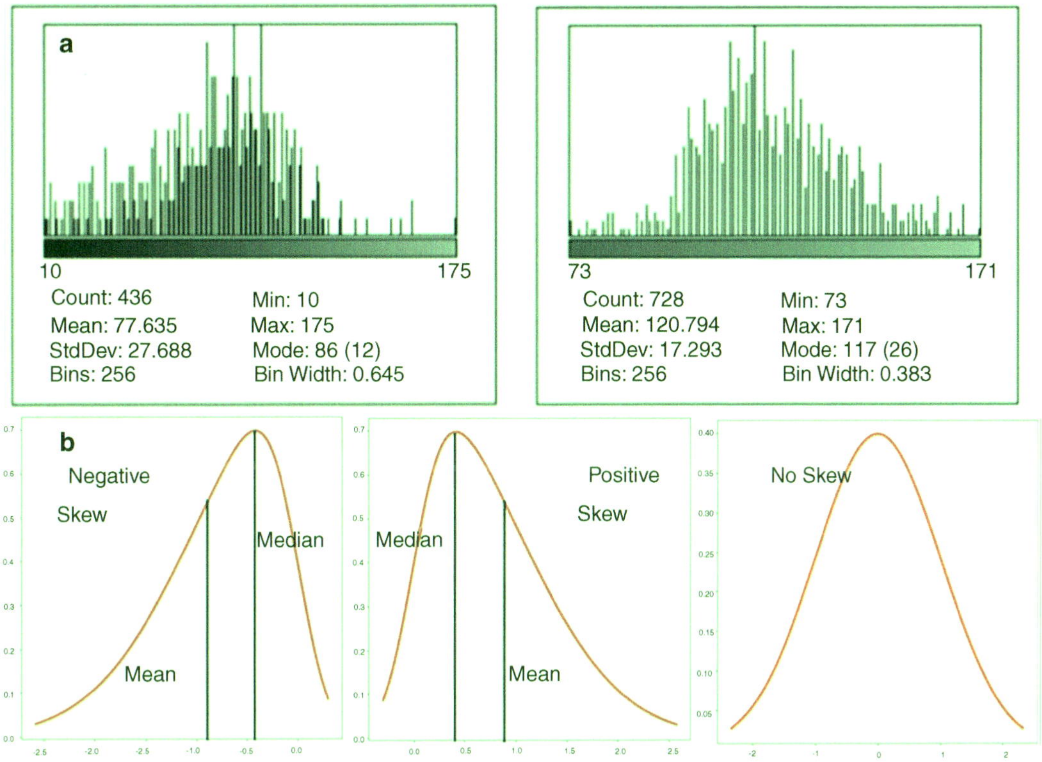

Fig. 27.3 (**a**, **b**) Examples of pixel histogram obtained from tumors in each region of interest demonstrating the frequency and distribution of pixel attenuation values. The histogram on the left (**a**) is demonstrating a negative skew, while the other histogram (**b**) demonstrates a relatively normal distribution. Examples of negatively and positively skewed histograms and a normally distributed histogram are shown separately

based statistical features evaluate the features summarizing the pixel intensities in each image, discounting the spatial distribution of these gray levels (Fig. 27.3). Higher-order features like gray level run length matrix metrics and gray level size zone matrix metrics utilize the value of pixel intensities and consider their spatial distribution. Transform-based features extract the global periodicity of the gray levels in the image. In addition to the above features, several filters like wavelet and Gaussian-based filters are applied to images to help extract a greater number of radiomics features [25].

Feature Selection and Modeling

Consequent to using multiple image filtration algorithms and second-order texture parameters, several hundred features are usually obtained for each case in a study. Not all of the derived features are informative, and some of them represent noise. Therefore, if all the generated features are used to predict the outcome of choice, there is a high likelihood of overfitting the prediction model, which means the model cannot be generalized to external images [26]. To build statistical or machine learning models, reducing the number of features used is paramount, a process called feature selection. Many methods exist for feature selection and dimension reduction, which have been described in several research papers [27]. Some radiomics features are highly dependent on the volumes of the ROI they are derived from, and the differences in the ROI between observers can result in non-reproducibility. The first step of feature selection usually involves screening out these non-reproducible features using the interclass correlation coefficient. The most relevant features for the outcome of interest are selected using various approaches like random forest algorithm, LASSO regression, knock of filters, recursive feature elimination, or stepwise feature selection.

Additionally, radiomics features may be highly correlated, and the inclusion of interrelated features into machine learning models reduces generalizability. Unsupervised clustering is sometimes used to identify clusters of correlated features, and usually, only one feature per correlated cluster is selected. Many machine learning models such as logistic regression, random forests, LASSO regression, support-vector Machines, and Naïve Bayes have been used to predict the outcome of interest. Splitting the data into training and test set is typical; at this point, all feature selection and model training steps should be applied solely to the training set to ensure that the feature selection steps do not cause data leakage into the test set.

Radiomics as Applied to Renal Magnetic Resonance Imaging

Radiomics for the Identification of Renal Masses

Evaluation and management of renal masses detected incidentally on imaging are challenging. Preoperative diagnosis of the malignant potential of an incidental lesion is heavily dependent on imaging. Several medical and surgical society guidelines recommend multiphasic cross-sectional scans to confirm the suspicion of malignancy [28]. For lesions identified as benign, management is conservative. Renal mass biopsy (RMB) is often recommended when clinical and imaging diagnoses are uncertain. However, RMB is associated with a significant negative predictive value. In a systematic review by Patel et al., 37% of clinically high-risk lesions deemed benign on RMB turned out to be malignant on excision [29]. Because indeterminate incidental masses can be treated either by active surveillance or invasive procedures like partial or radical nephrectomy, radiomics-guided virtual imaging biopsy of these renal tumors can provide additional insights for decision-making. While a simple cyst can be easily identified on MR scans, follow-up is often required for more complex cysts to identify potential malignancy (Fig. 27.4). However, the transition to malignancy is not via increased size but by developing complex septae in the preexisting cyst. Radiomics-based evaluation can help identify such suspicious cysts, which subsequently develop malignancy on follow-up. In a study of 27 Bosniak IIF and III cysts, several first-order histogram parameters of baseline ADC maps differed in the 7 lesions, which on follow-up turned out to be malignant [30].

The presence of fat in a solid renal mass is often considered characteristic of angiomyolipoma (AML), a lesion composed of variable amounts of mesenchymal adipose tissue, blood vessels, and muscles; however, the presence of fat is not a foolproof marker. Fat can be present in dedifferentiated renal cell carcinomas (RCCs), and over 5% of AMLs are considered fat-poor. Because CT is often the first-line modality used to evaluate renal masses, several studies have utilized CT- and MR-based radiomics to differentiate AML from malignant renal lesions (Fig. 27.5). A study of 54 masses demonstrated a high-class separation capacity with an AUC of >0.8 in differentiating RCC from fat-poor AML and oncocytomas using MR texture analysis of multiphasic contrast-enhanced MR, T2-weighted images, and diffusion-weighted imaging (DWI) [31]. Using whole tumor histogram ADC maps, a study of 27 fat-poor AMLs and 113 clear cell RCCs showed that fat-poor AML had significantly lower histogram parameters than clear cell renal cell carcinoma (ccRCC) with 90th percentile of ADC providing 78% sensitivity and 81.5% specificity [32]. Additional studies have extrapolated histogram analysis to intravoxel incoherent motion imaging, and the mean, standard deviation of diffusivity, and skewness of the perfusion fraction could differentiate ccRCC from fat-poor AML while kurtosis could differentiate oncocytomas from ccRCC [33].

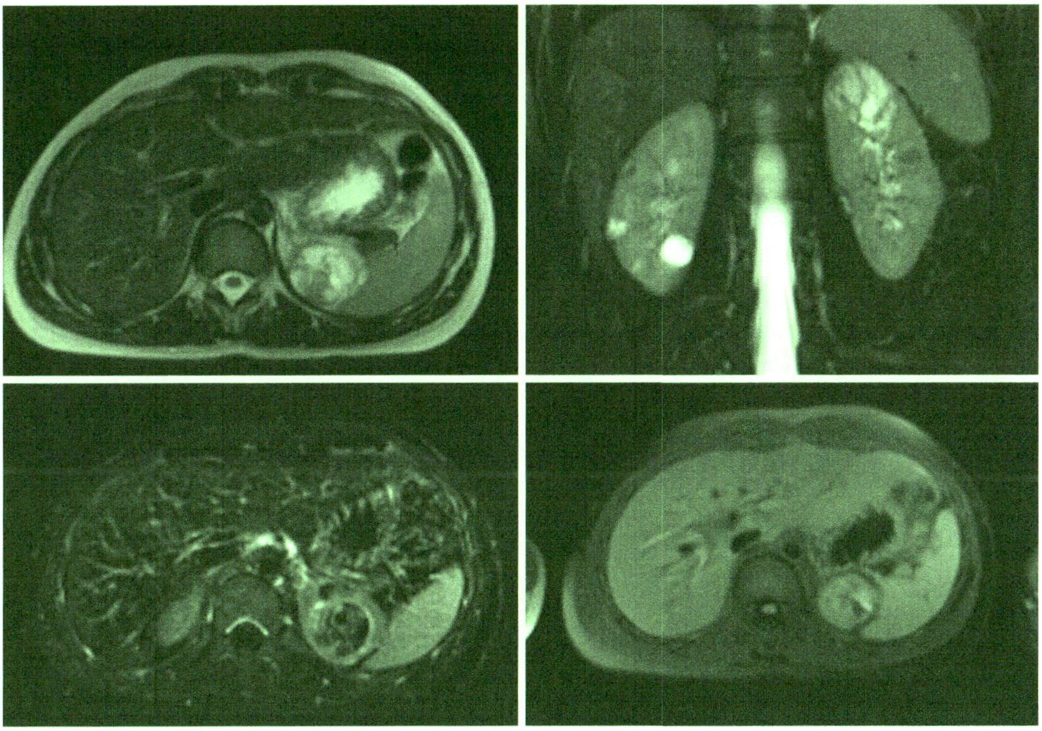

Fig. 27.4 A 15-year-old male undergoing surveillance for evaluation of suspicious cystic renal lesions. The partially exophytic complex solid and cystic lesion with intrinsic foci of T1 hyperintensity within the upper pole of the left kidney demonstrates increased in size and cystic changes. In view of the increase in complexity of the lesion, the patient underwent percutaneous biopsy, and the lesion was found to be renal cell carcinoma. Radiomics can be used to identify renal cysts that go on to develop malignancies in lieu of serial follow-up or biopsy

Radiomics and Characterization of Renal Cell Carcinoma Biology

Patients with RCCs larger than 7 cm undergo radical nephrectomies with a potential curative intent. Still, for lesions smaller than 4 cm, management decisions are often affected by multiple patient and tumor-specific factors [34]. For example, in patients with co-morbidities or lesions less than 3 cm, the tumor grade, the extent of tumor necrosis, and subtype of RCC are important determinants of therapy and patient outcome. Clear cell RCC, rarer variants like collecting duct or renal medullary carcinoma, or tumors with sarcomatoid or rhabdoid transformation have poor outcomes. Similarly, tumors categorized as Fuhrman's grade 1 have an 86% survival rate of 5 years compared to 46% in grades 3–4. Because a limited volume of tumor can be sampled in a needle biopsy, percutaneous biopsies may not accurately sample the heterogeneity characteristic of RCCs. This is exemplified by an upward revision of nuclear grade on >40% of surgically removed tumors compared to the grade determined on biopsy [35]. Radiomics could identify such regions of high nuclear grade, or dedifferentiation/ transformations on imaging, thus enabling targeted biopsy. Or, radiomics could be used to provide an imaging-based prediction of tumor grade and subtype. For example, papillary RCCs are known to be hypointense on T2-weighted images with less intense contrast enhancement than ccRCC [36]. Radiomics has been shown to quantify the differences between ccRCC and pRCC as greater textural heterogeneity on multiphasic contrast-enhanced and T2-weighted MRI images with AUCs >0.8 [37]. Additionally, radiomics has a role in predicting the stage, size, grade, and necrosis score (SSIGN) in ccRCC [38]. Studies have also evaluated the

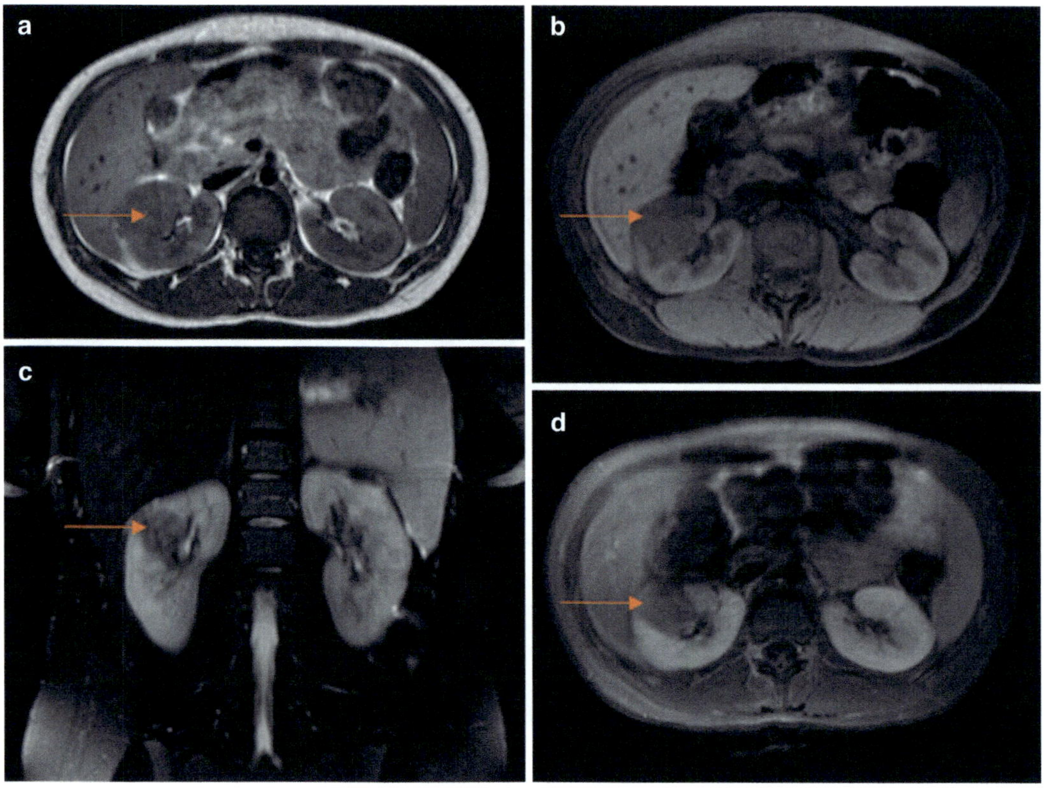

Fig. 27.5 A 15-year-old female with a mass in the upper pole of the right kidney extending into the interpolar. (**a**) The lesion is isointense to renal cortex on T1, (**b**) with decreased signal intensity on T2 and (**c** and **d**) slightly hypointense to the renal cortex on T1 with fat saturation. The mass is lobulate, heterogeneous, and abuts the renal pelvis. There is no definite enhancement or evidence of macroscopic fat. Because of interval increase in size of the lesion, the patient underwent right partial nephrectomy, and the pathology was suggestive of angiomyolipoma with predominant vascular component. Radiomics can help differentiate fat-poor angiomyolipoma from other malignant pathologies and could have obviated the need for partial nephrectomy

role of multiphasic DCE MRI-based radiomic features in identifying nuclear grade in ccRCC [39] and tumor subtypes in pRCC [40].

The development of microarray technology has allowed the identification of specific molecular pathways associated with RCC pathogenesis, which has accelerated the development of targeted therapies. Not only is each subtype of RCC associated with specific somatic mutations, but they may also be associated with hereditary syndromes. Tumor markers potentially associated with poorer outcomes in RCC include human B7 homolog 1 and 4, low levels of carbonic anhydrase IX, high levels of the proliferation marker Ki-67, and hypoxia-inducible factor (HIF)-1 alpha expression, among several other genotypes. Yin et al. evaluated the associations between tumor vascularity, vascular endothelial growth factor expression, and PET/MRI radiomic signatures in ccRCC. Radiomics features extracted from DCE-MRI provided a stronger radiomic correlation to micro-vascular density than to markers of VEFG expression [41]. While biopsy-based genotyping remains the gold standard, imaging-based radiomics can provide preoperative whole tumor genotyping, circumventing the limitations of the tumor sampled during a percutaneous biopsy [42].

Radiomics in the Treatment Assessment of Renal Cell Carcinoma

There has been a paradigm shift in the therapeutic management of locally advanced RCC, with multiple therapies now targeting the molecular pathways that drive disease progression. Checkpoint inhibition of cell cycle with immunotherapy targeting either the programmed cell death receptor 1 pathway and/or cytotoxic T lymphocyte-associated antigen 4 (ipilimumab) is useful in clear cell RCC, as have anti-angiogenic therapies (sunitinib, pazopanib, cabozantinib) targeting the vascular endothelial growth factor pathway [36]. Changes in the size of the tumor in response to chemotherapy (RECIST 1.1) have been used as predictors of disease response; however, these may not reflect the changes seen in response to targeted molecular therapies. In a study of 201 patients, optimal radiomics features from multiparametric MRI were used to predict distant synchronous metastasis in patients with ccRCC with an AUC of greater than 0.8 [43]. Similar to studies in CT imaging [44], a pilot study using fluoro-thymidine F-18 PET and MRI-derived radiomics features was able to quantify treatment-related changes in patients with advanced metastatic RCC undergoing sunitinib therapy [45]. Radiomics may provide insights into treatment response before radiologically visible changes are observed, providing direction to further therapy and optimizing precision medicine.

Applications in Chronic Renal Diseases

Chronic Kidney Disease (CKD) is associated with progressive decline in glomerular function over time, culminating in end-stage renal disease (ESRD). Many factors interplay to cause renal damage, and biochemical markers poorly indicate the rate of decline in renal function. While eGFR determined by serum creatinine has been used extensively as an indicator of renal decline, its applicability has several limitations. For example, the serum creatinine-based eGFR calculation is affected by several other disease and physiological states. Further, a decline in nephron mass is not always reflected in eGFR. The kidneys compensate for the loss of nephron mass by hyperfiltration and increased solute and water reabsorption in the remaining nephrons. Repeated biopsies cannot be used to monitor the changes in renal perfusion, hypoxia, fibrosis, and inflammation. Instead, radiomics-based evaluation of MRI images has been used to provide proxy markers of the underlying pathology that causes renal function decline. In a study of ischemic reperfusion renal injury (IRI) in rabbits, researchers found a significant correlation between histopathological findings of IRI at different durations of ischemia and radiomic parameters obtained from T2-weighted, susceptibility-weighted (SWI) images and blood oxygen level-dependent (BOLD) MRI images [46]. Similar evaluations have also been conducted in humans. Though such applications of radiomics are very promising, human experimentation remains limited by the utilization of serum creatinine-based eGFR or similar biochemical markers [47] as the gold standard rather than histopathological gold standards. Radiomics parameters obtained from DWI, BOLD, and SWI could differentiate patients with eGFR <30, 30–80, and >80 mL/min/1.73 m^2. Albuminuria and microalbuminuria are often used to monitor the progression of diabetic kidney disease. However, patients with advanced diabetic nephropathy may have normal urinary albumin. A diffusion tensor imaging-based radiomic score differentiated healthy volunteers from diabetic patients with micro-normo-albuminuria with an AUC of 0.8 [48].

Evaluation of Renal Pathology

Percutaneous renal biopsies are often used to monitor progression and therapeutic response in many renal diseases, including renal allograft dysfunction and a gamut of nephrotic and nephritic syndromes. Because of the invasive nature of biopsies, radiomics has been evaluated as an alternative to predicting changes in renal pathology. BOLD MRI quantifies deoxygenated blood in tissues and is a marker of perfusion. Preliminary analysis of BOLD MRI radiomics detected four groups of pathological patterns [49] in lupus nephritis. Similarly, a small pilot study has detected a correlation of eGFR in transplant kidneys with radiomics parameters obtained from T2-weighted images [50].

Limitation of Radiomics and Future Directions

Though promising, radiomics research is plagued by the lack of standardization, methodological variability, and poor reproducibility. Different authors use different algorithms to acquire the radiomics parameters. The methodologies used for feature selection and machine learning algorithm development vary significantly among researchers. Radiomics parameters obtained from one scanner might not be generalizable to images acquired on different scanners, further limiting the validity and generalizability of such studies. Most radiomics research is carried out on retrospectively collected data, and prospective studies validating the role of radiomics in clinical research are generally lacking. The limitations of radiomics research can be summarized as follows.

Variability in image acquisition and image post-processing: Radiomics features are affected by the variations in scanner field, scanner software, matrix size, field of view, acceleration techniques, and contrast MR image acquisition [51–54]. Phantom studies have evaluated the effect of acquisition parameters on MR-derived radiomics features, and future studies need to address how differences in acquisition protocols affect radiomics research.

Causality: Radiomics research aims to find imaging-based predictors of genotypic or phenotypic outcomes. However, because of the mathematical nature of the parameters obtained, there is no understanding of what the radiomics features represent biologically. Currently, most studies attempt to find a correlation between the parameters of interest and the radiomics features, but this should not be mistaken for causation.

Variability of algorithms used for radiomics feature generation: There are numerous software available to generate radiomics features. Studies have shown that while first-order parameters are reproducible between the software, the second-order texture parameters show moderate to poor reproducibility. ISBI standards [12] have described the methodology of extracting radiomics features, and radiomics researchers should strive to meet these standards in order to ensure generalizability of the radiomics features calculated [55].

Conclusion

Radiomics and texture analysis provide excellent insight into the genotypes and phenotypes of diseases. While the field continues to grow, researchers have identified several limitations associated with the generalizability and reproducibility of radiomics, and further research should be directed to address these limitations. Since imaging plays a pivotal role in clinical practice, ongoing research will help its translation into clinical practice.

References

1. Neisius U, El-Rewaidy H, Nakamori S, Rodriguez J, Manning WJ, Nezafat R. Radiomic analysis of myocardial native T1 imaging discriminates between hypertensive heart disease and hypertrophic cardiomyopathy. JACC Cardiovasc Imaging. 2019;12(10):1946–54.
2. Castellano G, Bonilha L, Li LM, Cendes F. Texture analysis of medical images. Clin Radiol. 2004;59(12):1061–9.
3. Tourassi GD. Journey toward computer-aided diagnosis: role of image texture analysis. Radiology. 1999;213(2):317–20.
4. Gillies RJ, Kinahan PE, Hricak H. Radiomics: images are more than pictures, they are data. Radiology. 2016;278(2):563–77.
5. Li H, El Naqa I, Rong Y. Current status of radiomics for cancer management: challenges versus opportunities for clinical practice. J Appl Clin Med Phys. 2020;21(7):7–10.

6. Lambin P, Leijenaar RTH, Deist TM, Peerlings J, de Jong EEC, van Timmeren J, et al. Radiomics: the bridge between medical imaging and personalized medicine. Nat Rev Clin Oncol. 2017;14(12):749–62.
7. van Timmeren JE, Cester D, Tanadini-Lang S, Alkadhi H, Baessler B. Radiomics in medical imaging-"how-to" guide and critical reflection. Insights Imaging. 2020;11(1):91.
8. Aerts HJWL, Velazquez ER, Leijenaar RTH, Parmar C, Grossmann P, Carvalho S, et al. Decoding tumour phenotype by noninvasive imaging using a quantitative radiomics approach. Nat Commun. 2014;5:4006.
9. Nguyen PL, Schultz D, Renshaw AA, Vollmer RT, Welch WR, Cote K, et al. The impact of pathology review on treatment recommendations for patients with adenocarcinoma of the prostate. Urol Oncol. 2004;22(4):295–9.
10. Staradub VL, Messenger KA, Hao N, Wiley EL, Morrow M. Changes in breast cancer therapy because of pathology second opinions. Ann Surg Oncol. 2002;9(10):982–7.
11. Kronz JD, Westra WH, Epstein JI. Mandatory second opinion surgical pathology at a large referral hospital. Cancer. 1999;86(11):2426–35.
12. The image biomarker standardisation initiative—IBSI 0.0.1dev documentation [Internet]. [cited 2021 Sep 20]. https://ibsi.readthedocs.io/en/latest/
13. de Leon AD, Kapur P, Pedrosa I. Radiomics in kidney cancer: MR imaging. Magn Reson Imaging Clin N Am. 2019;27(1):1–13.
14. Thomas JV, Abou Elkassem AM, Ganeshan B, Smith AD. MR imaging texture analysis in the abdomen and pelvis. Magn Reson Imaging Clin N Am. 2020;28(3):447–56.
15. Zhang L, Chen Z, Feng L, Guo L, Liu D, Hai J, et al. Preliminary study on the application of renal ultrasonography radiomics in the classification of glomerulopathy. BMC Med Imaging. 2021;21(1):115.
16. Lubner MG, Smith AD, Sandrasegaran K, Sahani DV, Pickhardt PJ. CT texture analysis: definitions, applications, biologic correlates, and challenges. Radiographics. 2017;37(5):1483–503.
17. Nordstrom RJ. The quantitative imaging network in precision medicine. Tomography. 2016;2(4):239–41.
18. Mackin D, Fave X, Zhang L, Fried D, Yang J, Taylor B, et al. Measuring computed tomography scanner variability of radiomics features. Investig Radiol. 2015;50(11):757–65.
19. Shafiq-Ul-Hassan M, Latifi K, Zhang G, Ullah G, Gillies R, Moros E. Voxel size and gray level normalization of CT radiomic features in lung cancer. Sci Rep. 2018;8(1):10545.
20. Ronneberger O, Fischer P, Brox T. U-net: convolutional networks for biomedical image segmentation. In: Navab N, Hornegger J, Wells WM, Frangi AF, editors. Medical image computing and computer-assisted intervention (MICCAI). Cham: Springer International Publishing; 2015. p. 234–41.
21. Parmar C, Rios Velazquez E, Leijenaar R, Jermoumi M, Carvalho S, Mak RH, et al. Robust radiomics feature quantification using semiautomatic volumetric segmentation. PLoS One. 2014;9(7):e102107.
22. Zwanenburg A, Vallières M, Abdalah MA, Aerts HJWL, Andrearczyk V, Apte A, et al. The image biomarker standardization initiative: standardized quantitative radiomics for high-throughput image-based phenotyping. Radiology. 2020;295(2):328–38.
23. Collewet G, Strzelecki M, Mariette F. Influence of MRI acquisition protocols and image intensity normalization methods on texture classification. Magn Reson Imaging. 2004;22(1):81–91.
24. Yip SSF, Aerts HJWL. Applications and limitations of radiomics. Phys Med Biol. 2016;61(13):R150–66.
25. Welcome to pyradiomics documentation!—pyradiomics v3.0.1.post4+gad5b2de documentation [Internet]. [cited 2021 Sep 20]. https://pyradiomics.readthedocs.io/en/latest/
26. Varghese BA, Cen SY, Hwang DH, Duddalwar VA. Texture analysis of imaging: what radiologists need to know. AJR Am J Roentgenol. 2019;212(3):520–8.
27. Parmar C, Grossmann P, Bussink J, Lambin P, Aerts HJWL. Machine learning methods for quantitative radiomic biomarkers. Sci Rep. 2015;5:13,087.
28. Sanchez A, Feldman AS, Hakimi AA. Current management of small renal masses, including patient selection, renal tumor biopsy, active surveillance, and thermal ablation. J Clin Oncol. 2018;36(36):3591–600.
29. Patel HD, Johnson MH, Pierorazio PM, Sozio SM, Sharma R, Iyoha E, et al. Diagnostic accuracy and risks of biopsy in the diagnosis of a renal mass suspicious for localized renal cell carcinoma: systematic review of the literature. J Urol. 2016;195(5):1340–7.
30. Gillingham N, Chandarana H, Kamath A, Shaish H, Hindman N. Bosniak IIF and III renal cysts: can apparent diffusion coefficient-derived texture features discriminate between malignant and benign IIF and III cysts? J Comput Assist Tomogr. 2019;43(3):485–92.
31. Razik A, Goyal A, Sharma R, Kandasamy D, Seth A, Das P, et al. MR texture analysis in differentiating renal cell carcinoma from lipid-poor angiomyolipoma and oncocytoma. Br J Radiol. 2020;93(1114):20200569.
32. Li H, Li A, Zhu H, Hu Y, Li J, Xia L, et al. Whole-tumor quantitative apparent diffusion coefficient histogram and texture analysis to differentiation of minimal fat angiomyolipoma from clear cell renal cell carcinoma. Acad Radiol. 2019;26(5):632–9.
33. Gaing B, Sigmund EE, Huang WC, Babb JS, Parikh NS, Stoffel D, et al. Subtype differentiation of renal tumors using voxel-based histogram analysis of intravoxel incoherent motion parameters. Investig Radiol. 2015;50(3):144–52.
34. Campbell S, Uzzo RG, Allaf ME, Bass EB, Cadeddu JA, Chang A, et al. Renal mass and localized renal cancer: AUA guideline. J Urol. 2017;198(3):520–9.
35. Abel EJ, Carrasco A, Culp SH, Matin SF, Tamboli P, Tannir NM, et al. Limitations of preoperative biopsy in patients with metastatic renal cell carcinoma: comparison to surgical pathology in 405 cases. BJU Int. 2012;110(11):1742–6.

36. Shinagare AB, Krajewski KM, Braschi-Amirfarzan M, Ramaiya NH. Advanced renal cell carcinoma: role of the radiologist in the era of precision medicine. Radiology. 2017;284(2):333–51.
37. Wang W, Cao K, Jin S, Zhu X, Ding J, Peng W. Differentiation of renal cell carcinoma subtypes through MRI-based radiomics analysis. Eur Radiol. 2020;30(10):5738–47.
38. Choi JW, Hu R, Zhao Y, Purkayastha S, Wu J, McGirr AJ, et al. Preoperative prediction of the stage, size, grade, and necrosis score in clear cell renal cell carcinoma using MRI-based radiomics. Abdom Radiol (NY). 2021;46(6):2656–64.
39. Dwivedi DK, Xi Y, Kapur P, Madhuranthakam AJ, Lewis MA, Udayakumar D, et al. Magnetic resonance imaging radiomics analyses for prediction of high-grade histology and necrosis in clear cell renal cell carcinoma: preliminary experience. Clin Genitourin Cancer. 2021;19(1):12–21.e1.
40. Vendrami CL, Velichko YS, Miller FH, Chatterjee A, Villavicencio CP, Yaghmai V, et al. Differentiation of papillary renal cell carcinoma subtypes on MRI: qualitative and texture analysis. AJR Am J Roentgenol. 2018;211(6):1234–45.
41. Yin Q, Hung S-C, Wang L, Lin W, Fielding JR, Rathmell WK, et al. Associations between tumor vascularity, vascular endothelial growth factor expression and PET/MRI radiomic signatures in primary clear-cell-renal-cell-carcinoma: proof-of-concept study. Sci Rep. 2017;7:43,356.
42. Wang W, Ding J, Li Y, Wang C, Zhou L, Zhu H, et al. Magnetic resonance imaging and computed tomography characteristics of renal cell carcinoma associated with Xp11.2 translocation/TFE3 gene fusion. PLoS One. 2014;9(6):e99990.
43. Bai X, Huang Q, Zuo P, Zhang X, Yuan J, Zhang X, et al. MRI radiomics-based nomogram for individualised prediction of synchronous distant metastasis in patients with clear cell renal cell carcinoma. Eur Radiol. 2021;31(2):1029–42.
44. Goh V, Ganeshan B, Nathan P, Juttla JK, Vinayan A, Miles KA. Assessment of response to tyrosine kinase inhibitors in metastatic renal cell cancer: CT texture as a predictive biomarker. Radiology. 2011;261(1):165–71.
45. Antunes J, Viswanath S, Rusu M, Valls L, Hoimes C, Avril N, et al. Radiomics analysis on FLT-PET/MRI for characterization of early treatment response in renal cell carcinoma: a proof-of-concept study. Transl Oncol. 2016;9(2):155–62.
46. Pan L, Chen J, Zha T, Zou L, Zhang J, Jin P, et al. Evaluation of renal ischemia-reperfusion injury by magnetic resonance imaging texture analysis: An experimental study. Magn Reson Med. 2021;85(1):346–56.
47. Zhang G, Liu Y, Sun H, Xu L, Sun J, An J, et al. Texture analysis based on quantitative magnetic resonance imaging to assess kidney function: a preliminary study. Quant Imaging Med Surg. 2021;11(4):1256–70.
48. Deng Y, Yang B-R, Luo J-W, Du G-X, Luo L-P. DTI-based radiomics signature for the detection of early diabetic kidney damage. Abdom Radiol (NY). 2020;45(8):2526–31.
49. Shi H, Jia J, Li D, Wei L, Shang W, Zheng Z. Blood oxygen level-dependent magnetic resonance imaging for detecting pathological patterns in patients with lupus nephritis: a preliminary study using gray-level co-occurrence matrix analysis. J Int Med Res. 2018;46(1):204–18.
50. Grzywińska M, Jankowska M, Banach-Ambroziak E, Szurowska E, Dębska-Ślizień A. Computation of the texture features on T2-weighted images as a novel method to assess the function of the transplanted kidney: primary research. Transplant Proc. 2020;52(7):2062–6.
51. Baeßler B, Weiss K, Pinto Dos Santos D. Robustness and reproducibility of radiomics in magnetic resonance imaging: a phantom study. Investig Radiol. 2019;54(4):221–8.
52. Bianchini L, Botta F, Origgi D, Rizzo S, Mariani M, Summers P, et al. PETER PHAN: an MRI phantom for the optimisation of radiomic studies of the female pelvis. Phys Med. 2020;71:71–81.
53. Fiset S, Welch ML, Weiss J, Pintilie M, Conway JL, Milosevic M, et al. Repeatability and reproducibility of MRI-based radiomic features in cervical cancer. Radiother Oncol. 2019;135:107–14.
54. Yang F, Dogan N, Stoyanova R, Ford JC. Evaluation of radiomic texture feature error due to MRI acquisition and reconstruction: a simulation study utilizing ground truth. Phys Med. 2018;50:26–36.
55. Bologna M, Corino V, Mainardi L. Technical note: virtual phantom analyses for preprocessing evaluation and detection of a robust feature set for MRI-radiomics of the brain. Med Phys. 2019;46(11):5116–23.

28 The Role of Artificial Intelligence in Automated Data Analysis of the Kidney

Adriana V. Gregory and Timothy L. Kline

Introduction

Artificial intelligence (AI) is no longer considered science fiction. AI technology has rapidly become part of our daily lives operating behind countless applications, in many cases free of cost, making it accessible to everyone. The presence of AI is almost pervasive, from voice recognition (i.e., voice command virtual assistants such as Google and Siri), image recognition (i.e., face and object recognition features on cell phones and photo applications or cars with lane detection or self-driving capabilities), text recognition (such as editors that offer grammar assistance), forecast prediction, to recommendation-based subscriptions and more. However, the use of AI in other fields like medical imaging is taking longer to be fully realized. Expectations for the performance of any method that will be implemented clinically are very high as it will have implications on patient care. This divergence can be seen when comparing visual performance of segmentation programs designed for natural images (for example, crudely outlining objects on a city street) vs. the very stringent requirements of exact object boundary definition defining organs or tumors on medical images.

The top performance of AI models can only be achieved through large quantities of data (i.e., hundreds to thousands of examples). In radiology, the number of images available for a specific disease or condition from a single center is usually not high enough to create a high-performing AI model. Multicenter collaborations can aid to solve this problem, but justifiable concerns regarding data privacy in healthcare stifle these efforts [1]. This is just one of the difficulties that slows down large-scale model development. In general, numerous challenges need to be addressed to have a fully functional AI model in clinical practice. Fortunately, methods such as Federated Learning have been developed, which allow models to be trained without the need for sharing data between institutions [2, 3].

AI can be broadly defined as a group of algorithms or methods that can learn, adapt, and self-correct based on experience without the need for specifically programmed instructions. Two of the major sub-fields of AI are machine learning (ML) and deep learning (DL). ML algorithms specifically learn from manually selected data features, whereas DL algorithms automatically learn the important features to build a model. The success of AI models in many imaging applications has resulted in the application of these methods in a variety of biomedical imaging settings. In kidney

A. V. Gregory
Division of Nephrology and Hypertension, Mayo Clinic, Rochester, MN, USA
e-mail: Gregory.Adriana@mayo.edu

T. L. Kline (✉)
Department of Radiology, Mayo Clinic, Rochester, MN, USA
e-mail: Kline.Timothy@mayo.edu

S. D. Serai, K. Darge (eds.), *Advanced Clinical MRI of the Kidney*,
https://doi.org/10.1007/978-3-031-40169-5_28

MR imaging, the two major tasks that have been explored by AI methods are segmentation and classification. Segmentation refers to identifying regions within an image corresponding to different structures (e.g., which voxels pertain to kidney), and classification refers to distinguishing various properties about a region (e.g., whether a tumor is benign or malignant).

In this chapter, we will review the role of AI in kidney MR imaging, highlighting historical work to put more recent developments in context. We have structured this chapter to break out the major topic areas, including segmentation, classification, augmentation, and reconstruction. We also provide an overview of the common requirements needed for implementation of an AI algorithm. Lastly, we provide insights on the current state of the art, as well as recommendations for future research in this area. Although discussed heavily, specific details and theory of ML or DL algorithms are beyond the scope of this chapter but can be found in Ref. [4, 5].

Detection and Segmentation

Detection and segmentation are processes by which labels are assigned to specific regions within an image. In the case of MR imaging of the kidneys, some examples include identifying and labeling: (i) the right and/or left kidney, (ii) abnormalities such as cysts or tumors, or (iii) other relevant structures such as vasculature, renal pelvis, adrenal glands, and so on. In the case of segmentation, this process allows for measurement of region properties such as overall size/volume, contrast/image intensity, as well as radiomic features. In general, the segmentation of kidneys on medical images provides valuable prognostic and diagnostic information in the assessment of healthy and diseased kidneys.

Kidney volumetry is one of the most widely used imaging biomarkers that requires 3D image segmentation and is useful in many clinical management settings, including evaluating the progression of different renal diseases. For example, larger kidney volumes in polycystic kidney disease (PKD) are associated with lower kidney function [6], whereas smaller than normal kidney volumes can be related to kidney atrophy [7]. Recent studies on the presence and characteristics of cysts, renal tumors, and changes of the renal cortex, renal medulla, and collecting system have given insight into physiological changes of the kidneys and their relationship with renal function [8–12]. Additionally, the 3D segmentations can be used in preoperative settings to facilitate augmented reality or the generation of 3D printed models for surgical planning and staff training. Figure 28.1 shows the potential to evaluate and plan the surgical removal of a renal tumor using segmentation to visualize the tumor and surrounding structures in 3D.

Manual segmentation is the process of an expert human segmenter labeling the images by hand. Although it is thought to be the most accurate method for measuring region properties (e.g., volume), manual annotation of 3D images is a tedious and time-consuming task that cannot be easily integrated into clinical practice. Moreover, it requires considerable staff training to minimize the inter and intra reader variability.

Several methods have been developed to provide more efficient and accurate ways to segment the renal structures of interest in cross-sectional imaging. For a long time, traditional computer vision (i.e., methods that follow specifically programmed instructions) was the mainstream approach to automate the segmentation process. Methods such as active shape models [13], level set [14–16], graph cut [17], region growing [18], thresholding [19, 20], edge detection [21], and atlases [22], to name just a few, were used alone or in combination with minimal human interaction to provide accurate segmentations. However, these methods suffer from low generalizability, meaning that the programmed algorithm works well only for a subset of images.

One of the main difficulties in creating approaches that generalize well is the prevalence of different image artifacts on MR imaging, since the performance of these algorithms largely depends on the quality of the images. MR image artifacts can be caused by different sources that

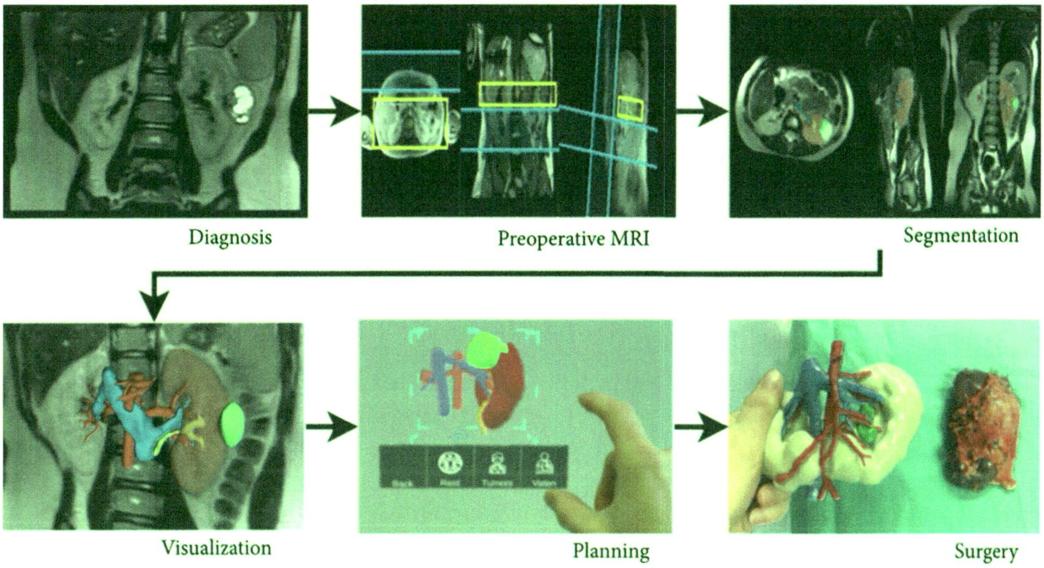

Fig. 28.1 Schematic of a 3D tumor visualization workflow. Reprinted from "MRI-Based 3-Dimensional Visualization Workflow for the Preoperative Planning of Nephron-Sparing Surgery in Wilms' Tumor Surgery: A Pilot Study" by Fitski, M., J. W. Meulstee, et al., 2020, Journal of Healthcare Engineering, 2020, no pagination

could be related to the human physiology, like patient movement (e.g., breathing) or to vascular pulsation which can cause blurring or ghosting artifacts, or to the physics of MR imaging like field inhomogeneity artifacts that cause image distortions, shading, spectral saturation errors, and reduction of the signal-to-noise ratio (SNR). Computer vision algorithms that rely on edge information are impacted mostly from human physiology related artifacts, whereas algorithms that depend on patterns and intensities are affected by inherent MR physical or hardware artifacts.

More recently, research on medical image segmentation has shifted toward machine learning (ML) methods, as they have provided significant advances for image detection and segmentation tasks, particularly with artificial neural networks in the form of convolutional neural networks (CNNs). Although not a specifically new idea, the ability to train large networks (thanks to ever-increasing computational power mostly afforded by graphics processing units (GPUs)), with access to large numbers of training examples, has been realized only in the last decade or so in the area of medical image processing. The main difference between ML-based and traditional computer vision-based algorithms is that ML-based algorithms do not rely on a specific sequence of pre-programmed instructions. Instead, they use large quantities of data and allow the computer program to learn from the data. This inductive approach has been shown to provide better generalization of the algorithms as it is noted in the works described in the next sections.

Machine Learning-Based Segmentation

In kidney MR imaging segmentation, the introduction of AI/ML algorithms began as an additional step to traditional computer vision algorithms to further identify or refine the segmented internal renal compartments (Fig. 28.2). Clustering ML algorithms were one of the most applied methods, particularly on dynamic contrast-enhanced (DCE) MR images. These algorithms, as their name indicates, can cluster

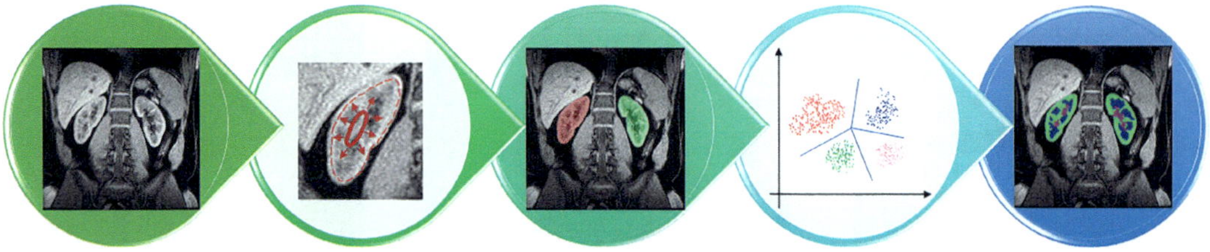

Fig. 28.2 Kidney segmentation overview. First the kidneys are segmented using a computer vision approach. Next, each voxel is classified as renal cortex, renal medulla, or collecting system using a machine learning algorithm

different voxels based on their similarity, thus, hyperintense (bright) and hypointense (dark) voxels can be segmented as two different groups. In 2009, K-means was the first implemented clustering method for the differentiation of the renal cortex from the renal medulla on DCE-MR imaging, followed by a few other similar studies reporting segmentation accuracies above 88% [23–25]. Another clustering algorithm used for kidney parenchyma, cortex, and medulla segmentation was fuzzy clustering, in which voxels are assigned a probability score of belonging to a certain cluster. This algorithm provided better results due to the higher performance when the borders between structures were not well defined [26–28].

Other more sophisticated classifiers like support vector machine (SVM), a supervised machine learning algorithm that creates a hyperplane by maximizing the margin between the data points to determine the different classes, were implemented by Gloger et al. to segment the kidney parenchyma achieving a Dice score of 0.91 [29]. The random forest classifier, which constructs ensembles of decision trees, also was tested in combination with the GrabCut algorithm to segment the renal cortex, medulla and collecting system with a mean F1-score of 0.93 [30]. Figure 28.3a depicts a general ML-based segmentation algorithm pipeline. Although these studies provided higher segmentation accuracy, some AI/ML methods still rely heavily on image intensity information. Note that the automation of tumor segmentation at this point in MR imaging had not been realized, likely due to the wide range of tumor intensity and textural presentations.

Deep Learning-Based Detection and Segmentation

In deep learning, the main network architecture is based on convolutional neural networks. These networks contain multiple layers that are used to extract and learn the most important image features to perform the segmentation task. Currently, deep learning models offer state-of-the-art accuracy for multiple medical imaging segmentation problems. Figure 28.3b illustrates a deep learning segmentation algorithm pipeline. In MR imaging, the first deep learning algorithm used for the task of fully automating kidney segmentations was published in 2017 by Kline et al. [31]. This algorithm was trained to segment kidneys from patients affected by autosomal dominant polycystic kidney disease (ADPKD) using an ensemble approach with the U-net convolutional neural network architecture [32]. In 2018, several other studies using deep learning were published for the segmentation of MR abdominal imaging. The study by Haghighi et al. focused on the detection of kidneys using a bounding box approach to predict the kidney location [33], while other studies focused on the segmentation of kidneys and other abdominal organs using the U-net architecture with Dice scores ranging from 0.76 to 0.96 [34–39]. A probabilistic segmentation and image distribution matching generative adversarial network (GAN) showed similar results to supervised approaches in normal kidney segmentation with an average Dice score of 0.90 [40]. Later, a multi-to-binary network proposed by Zhao et al. to segment normal kidney parenchyma reached a Dice score of 0.87 and 0.91 on T1-dual and T2-spir MR images, respectively [41]. The nnU-net

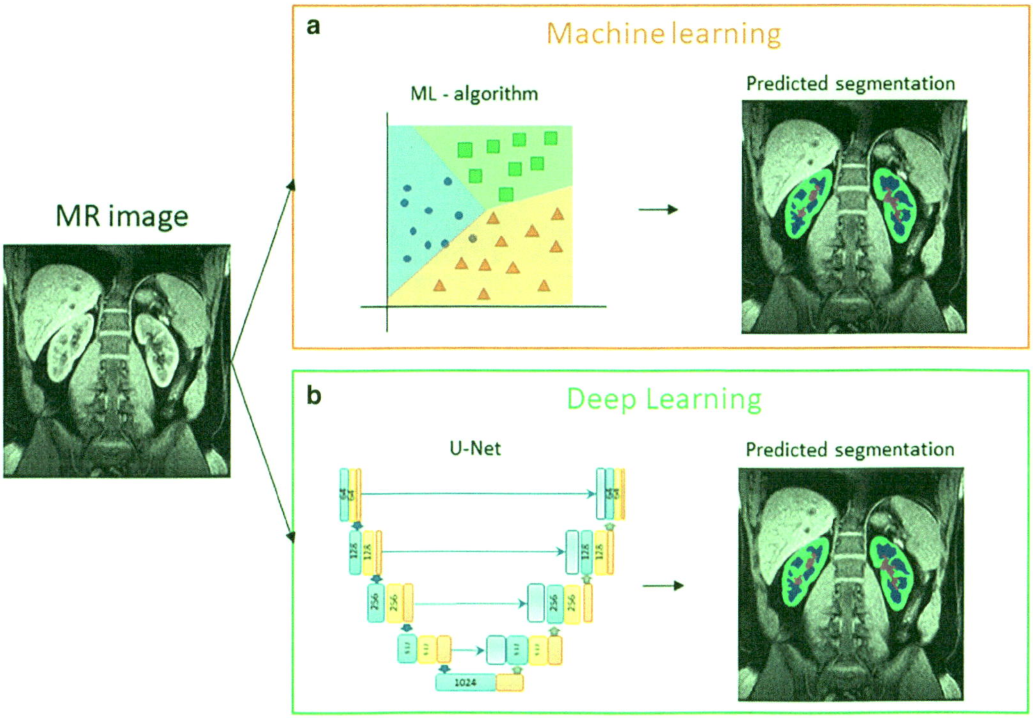

Fig. 28.3 Illustration of AI-based pipelines for kidney cortex, medulla, and collecting system segmentation. The input image is a coronal abdominal MR image. (**a**) ML-based segmentation pipeline. Each voxel is segmented based on its intensity information. Some ML methods include clustering algorithms, SVM, decision trees, and random forests. (**b**) DL-based segmentation. The U-Net architecture is the most used algorithm to perform segmentations tasks

architecture was trained using the T1-weighted images from the UK Biobank and the German National Cohort data sets to predict kidney parenchyma achieving an average Dice score of 0.97 [42]. Other study assessed the performance of multiple CNN architectures with similar configurations to segment ADPKD kidneys reaching a mean accuracy of up to 0.88 [43]. Among other kidney pathologies, a study focused on the comparison of the U-net performance in healthy and CKD patients using T2-weighted MR images, the model showed high accuracy in the two cohorts with an average Dice score of 0.93 [44].

The U-net model also showed promising results in the segmentation of kidney compartments [45], and semantic segmentation of cysts in ADPKD [46], as well as a study that allowed for instance-level cyst segmentations by reformulating the instance-based segmentation task into a semantic task using a unique edge-core approach [47]. Results from the automated approach are shown in Fig. 28.4.

To date, the only study attempting to segment kidney tumors in MR imaging was by Muller et al., who performed an extensive study to define the reference standard segmentation of Wilms' tumor. In addition, they tested multiple computer vision and AI/ML approaches from Chan-Vase active contour and entropy rate superpixel segmentation to K-means clustering, SVM, random forests, and the U-net architecture [48]. The study highlights the difficulty in defining the tumor reference standard segmentations as they observed large interobserver variability among five human raters.

The use of ML and DL methods to segment medical images has changed dramatically how these problems are approached. Fully automated

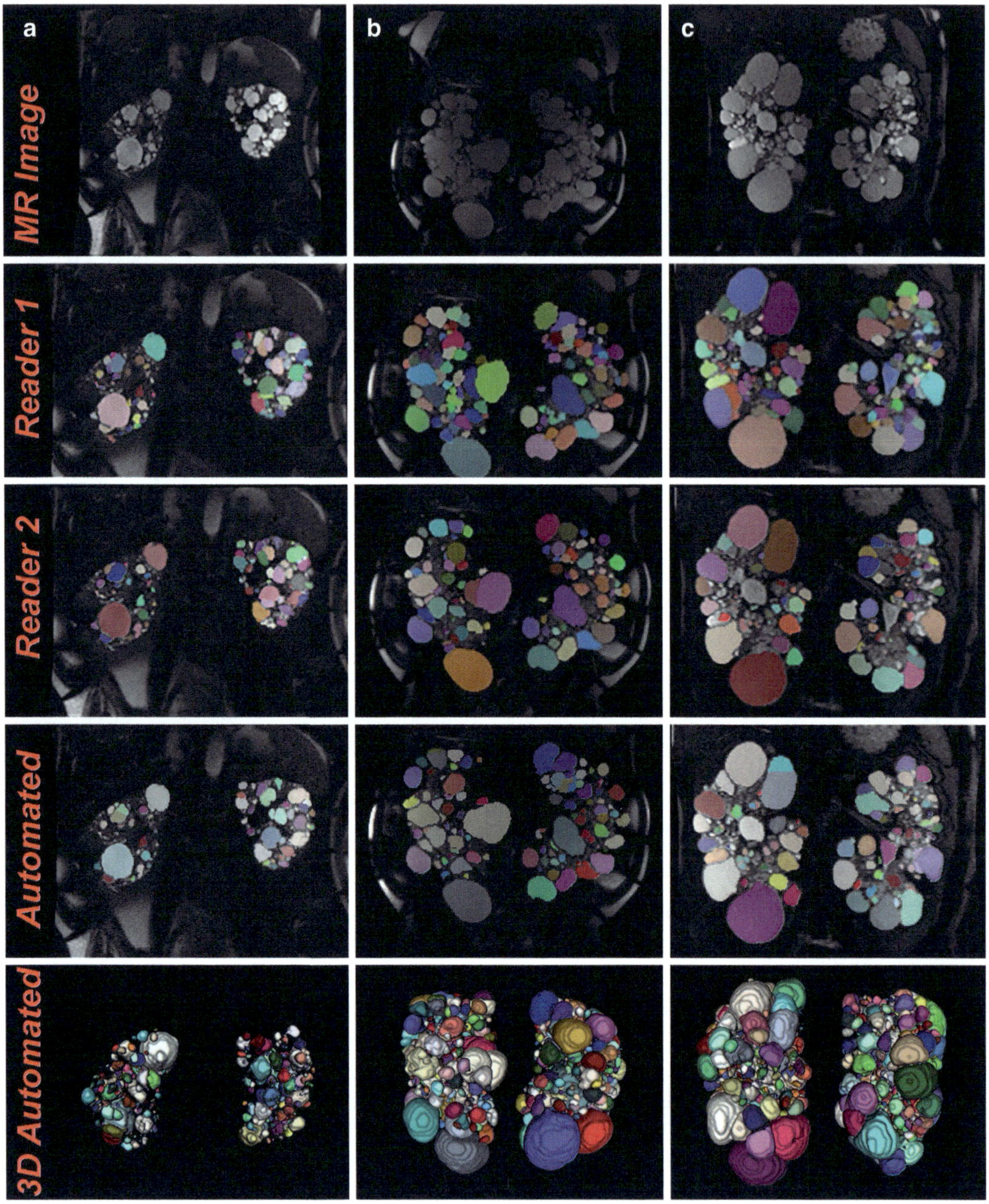

Fig. 28.4 Fully automated instance-level segmentation of cysts in ADPKD. Segmentation comparison between the automated method and 2 human readers in a (**a**) moderate and (**b**, **c**) two severely affected patients. Reprinted from "Semantic Instance Segmentation of Kidney Cysts in MR Images: A Fully Automated 3D Approach Developed Through Active Learning" By Gregory, A.V., Anaam D. A., et al., 2021, Journal of Digital Imaging, pp. 1–15

segmentation algorithms not only help to significantly reduce the annotation time but also better suited for clinical implementation. An important consideration currently is the number of representative cases with expert annotations needed to successfully train these algorithms.

Performance Metrics in Detection and Segmentation Tasks

Some of the most widely used functions to evaluate the accuracy of the segmentations (given the reference standard segmentation and the segmentation to be evaluated) are as follows: (i) the Dice coefficient (defined as two times the overlap divided by the total number of voxels in both images), (ii) the Jaccard index (defined as the intersection of both images divided by the union of both images), (iii) the Hausdorff distance (defined as the maximum distance between the two contours), (iv) volume similarity (defined as the difference in calculated volumes, often presented in absolute measurements, as well as in percentages), (v) the F1-score (defined as the harmonic mean between precision and recall).

Unbalanced Dataset Handling

In segmentation, class imbalance occurs when voxels corresponding to a label are far more numerous than the voxels of a different label. Trained segmentation algorithms using images with imbalanced labels have the tendency to predict mainly the majority label. One way to minimize this effect is by using an appropriate loss function. The Tversky loss function can increase the predicted segmentation accuracy by penalizing the false negative voxels. It is defined as:

$$\text{Tversky loss} = 1 - \frac{\text{TP}}{\text{TP} + \alpha\text{FN} + \beta\text{FP}}$$

where TP is true positive, FN is false negate, FP is false positive, and α and β are the coefficients to penalize FNs and FPs, where $\alpha > \beta$ and $\alpha + \beta = 1$.

Classification

In radiology, the classification of observations presented on the medical images is one of the most important steps for clinical decision-making. Visually recognizing characteristics that could help differentiate different pathologies, such as benign from malignant tumors, is not a trivial task. Since the digitalization of medical images and the exponential growth of computing power, there has been a lot of interest in extracting high-dimensional quantitative information from images. The extraction and collection of these quantitative parameters are known as radiomics. Radiomic data can then be used to create new enhanced classification models to improve current diagnosis, prognosis, and therapy response prediction algorithms.

MR imaging can provide excellent quality three-dimensional anatomical images with high soft-tissue contrast. Contrast is a very important aspect in clinical imaging since it makes possible the identification and classification of abnormalities within the body. The different configuration of parameters in MR imaging can produce sequences with different contrasts. In kidney imaging, T1-weighted sequences can show renal corticomedullary differentiation where the renal cortex has slightly higher signal (brighter) compared to the medulla. Hemorrhagic, proteinaceous, and other complex renal cysts have a high intensity signal on T1-weighted images; on the other hand, simple cysts have high intensity signals on T2-weighted images. Simple cysts presenting septations, low intensity nodularity or content in T2-weighted images can be associated with malignancy. In renal tumor imaging, T1- and T2-weighted images are useful for a comprehensive tumor characterization. Multiparametric MR imaging also plays a large role showing different renal features, dynamic contrast-enhanced MR imaging, and diffusion weighted imaging are becoming standard sequences acquired routinely in renal imaging protocols.

Radiomic features quantitatively characterize the tissue gray-scale pattern beyond what is visually seen by the human eye on the images. These include (i) intensity statistical features—based on the histogram distribution, such as the mean, median, minimum, and maximum intensities, skewness, kurtosis, entropy, etc. (ii) Shape-based features, such as the maximum diameter, perimeter, volume, surface area, sphericity, etc. (iii) Descriptors related to the neighboring voxels (textural features), such as the gray-level cooccurrence matrix features. (iv) Fractal features, such as the fractal dimension. The calculation of these features is performed through data characterization algorithms. One of the most comprehensive open-source toolboxes to extract radiomic features is pyradiomics [49] which has been developed adhering to the IBSI standard.

Machine learning classifiers are data-driven algorithms that can self-generate models without the need for programming specific instructions. In machine learning, radiomic features and the patient's relevant clinical information are considered the attribute values that describe the outcome (i.e., diagnosis, prognosis, or therapy response). Outcomes are expressed as labels and can be dichotomous (i.e., acute kidney transplant rejection vs non-rejection) for classification problems, or a polychotomous (i.e., stages of chronic kidney disease) for classification or to predict a value from a range.

MR images often have the presence of noise and artifacts that can affect the textural patterns of tissues. Image normalization before feature extraction has been shown to reduce classification errors due to these heterogeneities. It has been proposed that the recommended normalization parameters for MR images be 1–99% normalization with 256 intensity levels [50]. Additionally, datasets that suffer from technical biases or systematic differences can benefit from toolboxes like ComBat to correct these effects [51].

Radiomics and Machine Learning-Based Classification

Initial classification studies focused on the discriminative value of textural features in MR imaging mainly for the differentiation of renal tumors (Fig. 28.5). In a study by Chandarana et al., it was found that histogram analysis of the whole lesion enhancement and histogram distribution parameters such as kurtosis and skewness were able to differentiate between clear cell and papillary renal cell carcinoma (RCC) [52]. Doshi et al. tried to differentiate between type 1 and 2 papillary RCCs where mean entropy was found to be significantly different between the 2 types of papillary RCC on contrast-enhanced nephrographic phase images and apparent diffusion coefficient maps [53]. Another study that looked at differentiating type 1 from type 2 papillary RCC concluded that the combination of quantitative textural features and qualitative parameters is necessary to achieve the best prediction accuracy [54]. Kierans et al. evaluated the textural features to discriminate low-stage from high-stage clear cell RCC, concluding that skewness, kurtosis, correlation, sum of squares, and sum of variance can help differentiate the tumor stage on apparent diffusion coefficient image maps [55]. A study looking into early treatment response of metastatic RCC in PET/MR suggested that texture analysis might be able to show early functional and structural RCC response to cytostatic treatment [56]. Furthermore, a strong correlation between spaciotemporal features from DCE-MR imaging and RCC tumor microvascular density was reported by Yin et al. [57]. Later studies on the discrimination of benign and malignant renal tumors found that histogram and textural features from multiphasic contrast-enhanced MR images using random forest classifiers can help differentiate not only benign from malignant masses but also RCC subtypes [58, 59].

Li et al. specifically evaluated the diagnostic value of texture analysis for differentiating minimal fat angiomyolipoma and clear cell RCC and found that histogram percentiles and skewness were the best predictors in DWI [60]. A study evaluating texture features on ADC maps and T2-weighted images to detect caval wall invasion in RCC showed that tumor thrombus volume and entropy were among the most prominent features associated with invasion [61]. Newer textural features such as the high gray-level run emphasis and high gray-level zone emphasis were able to discriminate RCC subtypes on T1-weighted, T2-weighted, and enhanced T1-weighted images in the corticomedullary phase [62].

As the number of extracted radiomic features started to increase over time from tens to hundreds of parameters, recent studies have incorporated better ways to perform feature selection: the least absolute shrinkage and selection operator

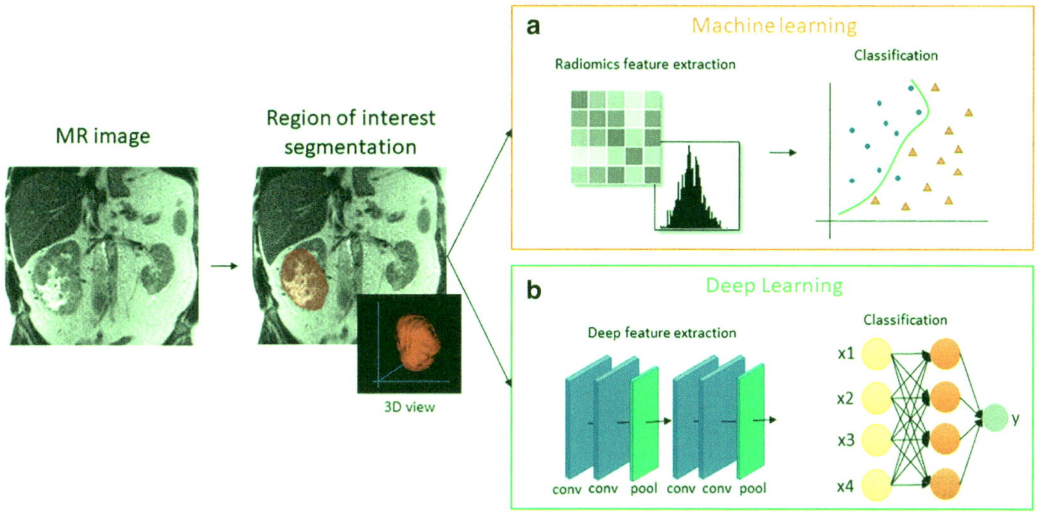

Fig. 28.5 Illustration of AI-based pipelines for renal tumor characterization. In this example, the input image is a coronal abdominal MR image. Next, the renal tumor is segmented manually or by semiautomated or fully automated methods. (**a**) ML-based radiomics pipeline. Radiomic features are extracted from the segmented region, then a ML-based classification algorithm such as k-nearest neighbor, support vector machine or random forest is used to create the classification model. (**b**) DL-based feature extraction and classification. Deep feature extraction is performed from segmented patches or the entire image using a deep convolutional neural network. The extracted features are then used to train a deep neural network classification algorithm

(LASSO), minimum redundancy maximum relevance (MRMR) method, as well as principal component analysis (PCA) are some of the methods used for feature reduction/selection (i.e., to reduce the number of features used to develop the ML models as a method to reduce overfitting). Then machine learning classifiers are applied to the selected features such as clustering, random forests, logistic regression, or support vector machines (Fig. 28.5a).

Some recent studies, testing different classifiers [63], found that random forest has good performance in the differentiation of benign and malignant renal lesions [64, 65]. In clear cell RCC tumor grade classification, multivariable logistic regression, random forests, and the tree-based pipeline optimization tool were found to satisfactorily distinguish between low-grade and high-grade clear cell RCC [66–71].

Other studies focused on the repeatability of textural features. The study by Becker et al. evaluated the textural features on DWI sequences, concluding that textural features on healthy abdominal organs vary at different *b*-values, thus *b*-values should be considered when performing radiomics on DWI [72]. In a study by Ciritsis et al., principal component analysis was performed to determine the most important b-values on DWI data to discriminate abdominal organs using KNN clustering analysis [73]. Regarding multi-sequence and multi-phase analysis, a study by Cui et al. concluded that the combination of extracted features from T1-weighted, T2-weighted, corticomedullary, and nephrographic phase in MR performed better than any single sequence or phase in the differentiation of clear cell RCC grade [74].

Clustering algorithms are among the first implemented ML classification methods in kidney MR imaging. Khalifa et al. implemented the KNN clustering algorithm to differentiate kidney non-rejection from acute kidney rejection using the parameters obtained from modeling the dynamic contrast agent kinetic curves in DCE-MR imaging [75]. Among other methods, linear regression, a ML algorithm used to predict continuous values instead of classes, was implemented by Kline et al. to predict subsequent changes in kidney function (i.e., estimated glomerular filtration rate) based on T2-weighted MR textural features and relevant clinical parameters in ADPKD patients. A decision tree model was built using radiomic features from BOLD-MR images to assess the classification of lupus nephritis, showing promising results [76]. Additionally, texture features from BOLD-MR and SWI data indicated potential for assessing renal function decline at early stages [77]. A LASSO regression model was generated to assess diabetic kidney damage. In this study, the 30 best diffusion tensor imaging features were used to build an ML model resulting in an AUC = 0.88, showing that radiomics could be used to detect early diabetic kidney damage [78].

Deep Learning-Based Classification

Deep learning classifiers use deep convolutional networks to extract image features, thus only require the annotated images and the output label for model development (Fig. 28.5b). Most

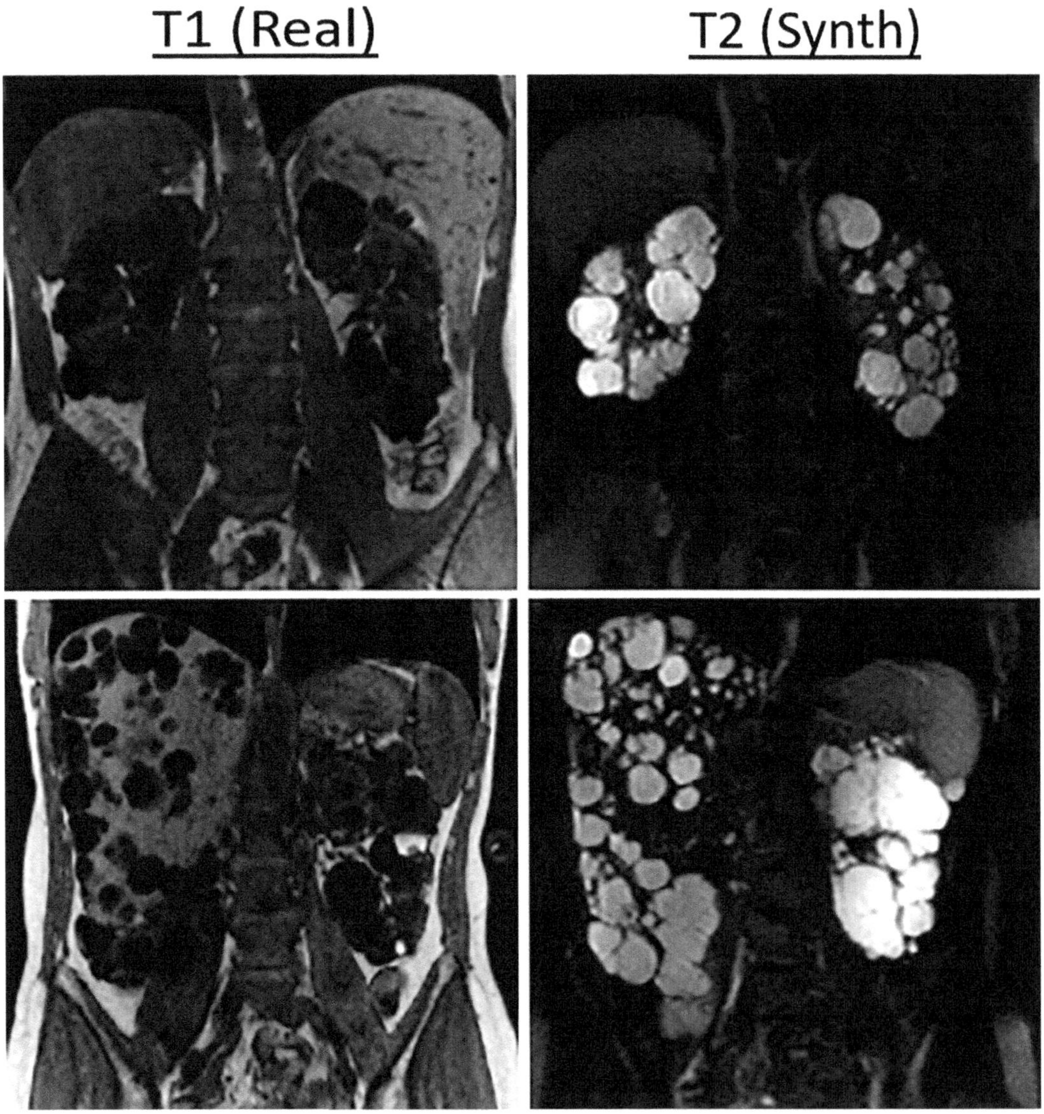

Fig. 28.6 Examples of two real T1-weighted MR images and corresponding synthesized T2-weighted MR images. Reprinted from "Segmenting new image acquisitions without labels" By Kline, T.L., 2019, IEEE 16th International Symposium on Biomedical Imaging, pp. 330–333

deep learning algorithms have been proposed for the differentiation of renal tumors in MR imaging. Soma et al. used the LeNet architecture to differentiate fat-poor angiomyolipomas from RCC subtypes using T2-weighted images; the reported accuracy on a holdout dataset was 75% [79]. Zheng et al. built a model using the ResNet architecture to distinguish clear cell RCC, chromophobe RCC, papillary RCC, and angiomyolipomas with T2-weighted fat saturated images resulting in an overall accuracy of 60.4% [80]. The combination of DWI and T2-weighted imaging to discriminate between benign and malignant renal tumors was further tested using the ResNet-18 architecture with a promising accuracy of 81.8% in a testing cohort [81]. Other deep learning studies focused on the early detection of acute transplanted kidney rejection using DWI data. The studies performed a 3D segmentation of the transplanted kidney, followed by the diffusion parameter estimation (with one study combining the ADC maps with clinical biomarkers). Then the extracted parameters were input into a CNN classifier to classify acute rejection and non-rejection kidney transplants. The studies had similar resulting accuracies of 94% and 93%, demonstrating the potential of CNN-based methods for the early detection of kidney rejection [12, 82].

Performance Metrics in Classification Tasks

The classification performance of AI models is usually evaluated by the same metrics used in clinical research studies. The sensitivity, specificity, accuracy, and the area under the receiver operating characteristic (ROC) curve (AUC) are some of the most common parameters calculated to measure the model performance. These metrics should be evaluated in a separate test set, unseen by the AI algorithm during the training process.

Other Applications

In a smaller scale, AI algorithms have been applied to solve other MR imaging tasks. In this section, we will cover the topics of image synthesis and image reconstruction.

Image Synthesis

Image synthesis is defined as the process of artificially generating new images with a predetermined style or content (i.e. Generative AI). In radiotherapy treatment planning, there has been interest in using MR abdominal imaging to generate corresponding CT images. MR images are often acquired for high soft-tissue contrast (useful for tumor visualization), and CT images are acquired for calculation of dose deposition. However, MR to CT registration is often difficult due to changes in patient position, patient motion, and different organ filling status. Two different studies used CNN networks to generate synthetic CT abdominal images from MR images. Liu et al. proposed to first generate semi-synthetic CT images (reference standard) by combining the skeletal contrast from the CT scans and the output of an intensity voxel classification algorithm to create the soft tissue and air CT contrast from MR images. Then the MR and semi-synthetic CT images were used to train a U-net network [83]. Similarly, Florkow et al. adopted the U-net architecture, in this case to predict pediatric CT images from T1- and T2-weighted MR images [84]. The CT image prediction results in both studies were acceptable to support MR-only radiotherapy treatment planning. In another study, Kline used a cycle-GAN architecture, incorporating an edge-based loss term, to synthesize different MR sequences (i.e., T2-weighted MRs from T1-weighted) (Fig. 28.6) in order to use an existing automated segmentation model on a completely different image domain [85]. Image synthesis approaches have also been used to improve segmentation model generalizability, for example, using neural style transfer as an extreme form of image augmentation [86].

Image Reconstruction

MR imaging requires long scanning times which often results in patient motion image artifacts. The reduction of acquisition time can be achieved through k-space undersampling; however, this method can produce aliasing imaging artifacts. To address this effect, Sui et al. proposed using deep neural networks to reconstruct abdominal MR images. The performance of the K-SVD algorithm was compared to the U-net architecture and a proposed RecSec cascade DL network. The DL algorithms (U-net and RecSec) showed the best reconstruction performance, with higher peak-SNR and structural similarity index measure [87].

Implementing a Deep Learning Algorithm

The increasing use of web-based open repositories has created a vast library of ML and DL project scripts and in some cases available data. Navigating the different repository structures can be overwhelming without a proper idea of the key information and resources required to implement the algorithms. In this section, a list of the main components to implement an AI project are described.

Data Availability and Data Curation

Rarely medical imaging data is available online, although, some datasets are available through image competitions (i.e., CHAOS challenge, Leanr2 Reg, KiTS challenge). Often, researchers will need to collect and curate their own image dataset. The necessary steps for data curation are but are not limited to:

- Querying the data
- Retrieving the images/data deidentification
- Image quality control
- Labeling of the images
- Label quality control

Data curation for ML and DL applications is a wide topic. Additional guidelines and recommendations specifically for medical image can be found in [88].

Downloading/Cloning Algorithms from Code Repositories

Regarding code repositories, GitHub and GitLab are two of the major project code repositories used to share algorithm implementations. The following points are the minimum required information for proper project implementation:

- System requirements
- Library requirements
- Data preprocessing steps
- Model training scripts
- Prediction generator script

Efforts are being made to standardize implementation workflow pipelines and could serve as a valuable resource when creating new repositories [89].

Discussion

In this chapter, we provided an overview of the current state of the art related to AI in kidney MR imaging, focusing on the tasks of segmentation and classification using ML and DL approaches. Each publication is unique in certain aspects: the research question, the cohort, the chosen MR sequence, and the type of ML or DL method applied. It is difficult to perform one-to-one study comparisons as all of these factors play a role in achieving different accuracy results.

The evolution of automatic segmentation of the kidney and its internal structures on MR abdominal imaging started as hand-crafted computer vision algorithms designed by researchers with significant domain knowledge that was leveraged to solve relatively narrow tasks. ML methods were then introduced as more generalizable approaches. With the advances of deep neural networks on image segmentation, the trend in recent years has shifted to developing purely DL-based algorithms. The latest studies have implemented a version of the U-Net architecture along with a few ML approaches to compare and highlight the better performance of DL algorithms. The U-Net architecture has dramatically improved the segmentation task but image preprocessing steps have been shown to provide an extra boost of performance [90]. On the other hand, transformers, although not applied to MR abdominal/pelvic imaging thus far, have shown to improve the U-Net performance when used as image encoders [91–93].

In classification, radiomics still plays a large role in tissue characterization, with histogram and textural features being the most commonly extracted parameters. Recent studies calculate hundreds to even thousands of radiomic features per image. The large data dimensionality can slow the training process and make the problems harder to solve. Appropriate feature reduction should be applied to remove redundant information without losing any important features. In the area of kidney MR imaging, DL studies in classification are still limited; thus, future studies should provide further information on the potential role of DL on kidney MR imaging classification tasks.

ML and DL algorithms are data-driven methods, meaning that the results are directly impacted by the quality of the data used to train the models. Training data that contains noise, artifacts, outliers, and errors will make the process of learning the most important data features more difficult. Researchers spend a lot of time carefully curating the reference standard images. This step usually goes unnoticed in research articles as there is not a lot of innovation or excitement about this process, but it is a key step to build a successful algorithm.

Data labeling is unquestionably the most time-consuming step that requires expert input, and in many cases, it can become a limiting factor for using all the images available to train an AI model. Notably, most studies use supervised learning models which require ample labeled data; however, less explored approaches such as few-shot learning (ML models designed to learn from small sets of examples) or zero-shot learning (ML models that learn data attributes to make inferences on sets with new classes) can be used to rapidly annotate and build larger labeled datasets. Additionally, unsupervised and self-supervised learning could aid in model generalizability as they can make inferences directly from the images and do not require labels. Moreover, federated learning allows inter-institution collaborative model development without the need of sharing patient clinical information. Federated learning can especially help in avoiding model bias as it enables model development from diverse sources.

Although AI-based models are showing highly accurate results, particularly in segmentation tasks, these models are designed to solve very specific problems. A robust model should be able to differentiate, for example, all types of benign and malignant renal tumors or segment any requested structure within the 3D image. Training generalized models is still a big challenge with AI, and the expectations of what AI can do are still very much overestimated. This misinterpretation of the capabilities of AI has caused major uncertainties on the role of AI in radiology. Even though the majority of these methods are fully automated, they still need human supervision. Outlier cases such as a rare disease or variant anatomical landmarks can result in erroneous AI results; furthermore, imaging software and hardware technologies are always evolving, trying to generate better images, these updates will result in images new to the algorithms. It is expected that an AI model will become obsolete without a proper active learning workflow, thus, frameworks for continuous learning need to be established.

The overarching goal of AI algorithm development in medical imaging is clinical implementation [94]. Currently, limited evidence is available regarding AI model integration into clinical practice. From an engineering point of view, the AI algorithm needs to be able to easily integrate with existing clinical systems without causing disruptions, and computational resources need to be allocated to meet processing demands. More importantly, an active evaluation of the AI model is necessary to identify potential sources of bias and re-training opportunities. Alongside, teams from different disciplines within the medical institution will play key roles in AI model implementation. The workforce education and AI-adoption will present other challenges. IT teams are envisioned to ensure model integration into clinical applications and store model generated data, medical imaging and data analysts will perform quality control of the AI outputs, and physicians will review and interpret the algorithm results. It is anticipated that the first AI models implemented clinically will be segmentation algorithms as the results can be visually validated, whereas classification algorithms will require a more robust generalization performance.

In summary, during the last decade, AI algorithms have made their way into radiology research with significant progress in renal MR imaging. It is natural to wonder if AI will replace radiologists in the future. Considering the current state of the art and the single-problem approach to develop these algorithms, it is highly unlikely that AI will become a stand-alone self-sustained system. Nevertheless, the question of an AI agent being capable to resemble human-level intelligence (i.e., artificial general intelligence) is still being debated. For the near future, the clinical use of AI algorithms will likely result in the development of new skills, enhanced workflows, and more time to focus on patient needs.

References

1. Price WN, Cohen IG. Privacy in the age of medical big data. Nat Med. 2019;25(1):37–43.
2. Rieke N, Hancox J, Li W, Milletari F, Roth HR, Albarqouni S, et al. The future of digital health with federated learning. NPJ Dig Med. 2020;3(1):1–7.
3. McMahan B, Moore E, Ramage D, Hampson S, y Arcas BA. Communication-efficient learning of deep networks from decentralized data. Artif Intell Stat PMLR. 2017:1273–82.
4. Géron A. Hands-on machine learning with Scikit-Learn, Keras, and TensorFlow: concepts, tools, and techniques to build intelligent systems. O'Reilly Media; 2019.
5. Goodfellow I, Bengio Y, Courville A. Deep learning. MIT press; 2016.
6. Grantham JJ, Torres VE, Chapman AB, Guay-Woodford LM, Bae KT, King BF Jr, et al. Volume progression in polycystic kidney disease. N Engl J Med. 2006;354(20):2122–30.
7. Piras D, Masala M, Delitala A, Urru SA, Curreli N, Balaci L, et al. Kidney size in relation to ageing, gender, renal function, birthweight and chronic kidney disease risk factors in a general population. Nephrol Dial Transplant. 2020;35(4):640–7.
8. Kline TL, Korfiatis P, Edwards ME, Bae KT, Yu A, Chapman AB, et al. Image texture features predict renal function decline in patients with autosomal dominant polycystic kidney disease. Kidney Int. 2017;92(5):1206–16. https://doi.org/10.1016/j.kint.2017.03.026.
9. Mazin A, Hawkins SH, Stringfield O, Dhillon J, Manley BJ, Jeong DK, et al. Identification of sarcomatoid differentiation in renal cell carcinoma by machine learning on multiparametric MRI. Sci Reports. 2021;11(1):3785. https://doi.org/10.1038/s41598-021-83271-4.
10. Uhlig J, Uhlig A, Bachanek S, Onur MR, Kinner S, Geisel D, et al. Primary renal sarcomas: imaging features and discrimination from non-sarcoma renal tumors. Eur Radiol. 2021;31:31. https://doi.org/10.1007/s00330-021-08201-4.
11. Denic A, Lieske JC, Chakkera HA, Poggio ED, Alexander MP, Singh P, et al. The substantial loss of nephrons in healthy human kidneys with aging. J Am Soc Nephrol. 2017;28(1):313–20.
12. Abdeltawab H, Shehata M, Shalaby A, Khalifa F, Mahmoud A, El-Ghar MA, et al. A novel CNN-based CAD system for early assessment of transplanted kidney dysfunction. Sci Reports. 2019;9(1):5948. https://doi.org/10.1038/s41598-019-42431-3.
13. Barstugan M, Ceylan R, Asoglu S, Cebeci H, Koplay M. Adrenal tumor segmentation method for MR images. Comput Methods Prog Biomed. 2018;164:87–100. https://doi.org/10.1016/j.cmpb.2018.07.009.
14. Li X, Li C, Liu H, Yang X. A modified level set algorithm based on point distance shape constraint for lesion and organ segmentation. Phys Med. 2019;57:123–36. https://doi.org/10.1016/j.ejmp.2018.12.032.
15. Gui L, Li C, Yang X. Medical image segmentation based on level set and isoperimetric constraint. Phys Med. 2017;42:162–73. https://doi.org/10.1016/j.ejmp.2017.09.123.
16. Bae K, Park B, Sun H, Wang J, Tao C, Chapman AB, et al. Segmentation of individual renal cysts from MR images in patients with autosomal dominant polycystic kidney disease. Clin J Am Soc Nephrol. 2013;8(7):1089–97. https://doi.org/10.2215/CJN.10561012.
17. Chen X, Bagci U. 3D automatic anatomy segmentation based on iterative graph-cut-ASM. Med Phys. 2011;38(8):4610–22.

18. Mignani R, Corsi C, De Marco M, Caiani EG, Santucci G, Cavagna E, et al. Assessment of kidney volume in polycystic kidney disease using magnetic resonance imaging without contrast medium. Am J Nephrol. 2011;33(2):176–84. https://doi.org/10.1159/000324039.
19. Will S, Martirosian P, Wurslin C, Schick F. Automated segmentation and volumetric analysis of renal cortex, medulla, and pelvis based on non-contrast-enhanced T1- and T2-weighted MR images. MAGMA. 2014;27(5):445–54. https://doi.org/10.1007/s10334-014-0429-4.
20. Seuss H, Janka R, Prummer M, Cavallaro A, Hammon R, Theis R, et al. Development and evaluation of a semi-automated segmentation tool and a modified ellipsoid formula for volumetric analysis of the kidney in non-contrast T2-weighted MR images. J Digit Imaging. 2017;30(2):244–54. https://doi.org/10.1007/s10278-016-9936-3.
21. Friedli I, Crowe LA, Viallon M, Porter DA, Martin P-Y, de Seigneux S, et al. Improvement of renal diffusion-weighted magnetic resonance imaging with readout-segmented echo-planar imaging at 3T. Magn Reson Imaging. 2015;33(6):701–8. https://doi.org/10.1016/j.mri.2015.02.023.
22. Shen J, Baum T, Cordes C, Ott B, Skurk T, Kooijman H, et al. Automatic segmentation of abdominal organs and adipose tissue compartments in water-fat MRI: application to weight-loss in obesity. Eur J Radiol. 2016;85(9):1613–21. https://doi.org/10.1016/j.ejrad.2016.06.006.
23. Zollner FG, Sance R, Rogelj P, Ledesma-Carbayo MJ, Rorvik J, Santos A, et al. Assessment of 3D DCE-MRI of the kidneys using non-rigid image registration and segmentation of voxel time courses. Comput Med Imaging Graph. 2009;33(3):171–81. https://doi.org/10.1016/j.compmedimag.2008.11.004.
24. Li S, Zollner FG, Merrem AD, Peng Y, Roervik J, Lundervold A, et al. Wavelet-based segmentation of renal compartments in DCE-MRI of human kidney: initial results in patients and healthy volunteers. Comput Med Imaging Graph. 2012;36(2):108–18. https://doi.org/10.1016/j.compmedimag.2011.06.005.
25. Yang X, Le Minh H, Tim Cheng K-T, Sung KH, Liu W. Renal compartment segmentation in DCE-MRI images. Med Image Anal. 2016;32:269–80. https://doi.org/10.1016/j.media.2016.05.006.
26. Udupa JK, Odhner D, Zhao L, Tong Y, Matsumoto MMS, Ciesielski KC, et al. Body-wide hierarchical fuzzy modeling, recognition, and delineation of anatomy in medical images. Med Image Anal. 2014;18(5):752–71. https://doi.org/10.1016/j.media.2014.04.003.
27. Feng Y, Kawrakow I, Olsen J, Parikh PJ, Noel C, Wooten O, et al. A comparative study of automatic image segmentation algorithms for target tracking in MR-IGRT. J Appl Clin Med Phys. 2016;17(2):441–60. https://doi.org/10.1120/jacmp.v17i2.5820.
28. Gloger O, Tonnies K, Laqua R, Volzke H. Fully automated renal tissue volumetry in MR volume data using prior-shape-based segmentation in subject-specific probability maps. IEEE Trans Biomed Eng. 2015;62(10):2338–51. https://doi.org/10.1109/TBME.2015.2425935.
29. Gloger O, Tonnies K, Mensel B, Volzke H. Fully automatized renal parenchyma volumetry using a support vector machine based recognition system for subject-specific probability map generation in native MR volume data. Phys Med Biol. 2015;60(22):8675–93. https://doi.org/10.1088/0031-9155/60/22/8675.
30. Yoruk U, Hargreaves BA, Vasanawala SS. Automatic renal segmentation for MR urography using 3D-GrabCut and random forests. Magn Reson Med. 2018;79(3):1696–707. https://doi.org/10.1002/mrm.26806.
31. Kline TL, Korfiatis P, Edwards ME, Blais JD, Czerwiec FS, Harris PC, et al. Performance of an artificial multi-observer deep neural network for fully automated segmentation of polycystic kidneys. J Digit Imaging. 2017;30(4):442–8. https://doi.org/10.1007/s10278-017-9978-1.
32. Ronneberger O, Fischer P, Brox T. U-net: convolutional networks for biomedical image segmentation. In: International conference on medical image computing and computer-assisted intervention. Springer; 2015. p. 234–41.
33. Haghighi M, Warfield SK, Kurugol S. Automatic renal segmentation in DCE-MRI using convolutional neural networks. Proc IEEE Int Symp Biomed Imaging. 2018;2018:1534–7. https://doi.org/10.1109/ISBI.2018.8363865.
34. Lv D, Zhuang J, Chen H, Wang J, Xu Y, Yang X, et al. Dynamic contrast-enhanced magnetic resonance images of the kidney. IEEE Eng Med Biol Mag. 2008;27(5):36–41. https://doi.org/10.1109/MEMB.2008.923949.
35. Bobo MF, Bao S, Huo Y, Yao Y, Virostko J, Plassard AJ, et al. Fully convolutional neural networks improve abdominal organ segmentation. Proc SPIE Int Soc Opt Eng. 2018:10,574. https://doi.org/10.1117/12.2293751.
36. Fu Y, Mazur TR, Wu X, Liu S, Chang X, Lu Y, et al. A novel MRI segmentation method using CNN-based correction network for MRI-guided adaptive radiotherapy. Med Phys. 2018;45(11):5129–37. https://doi.org/10.1002/mp.13221.
37. Chen Y, Ruan D, Xiao J, Wang L, Sun B, Saouaf R, et al. Fully automated multiorgan segmentation in abdominal magnetic resonance imaging with deep neural networks. Med Phys. 2020;47(10):4971–82. https://doi.org/10.1002/mp.14429.
38. Langner T, Ostling A, Maldonis L, Karlsson A, Olmo D, Lindgren D, et al. Kidney segmentation in neck-to-knee body MRI of 40,000 UK Biobank participants. Sci Rep. 2020;10(1):20,963. https://doi.org/10.1038/s41598-020-77981-4.
39. van Gastel MDA, Edwards ME, Torres VE, Erickson BJ, Gansevoort RT, Kline TL. Automatic measurement of kidney and liver volumes from MR images of patients affected by autosomal dominant polycystic

kidney disease. J Am Soc Nephrol. 2019;30(8):1514–22. https://doi.org/10.1681/ASN.2018090902.
40. Jiang J, Hu Y-C, Tyagi N, Rimner A, Lee N, Deasy JO, et al. PSIGAN: joint probabilistic segmentation and image distribution matching for unpaired cross-modality adaptation-based MRI segmentation. IEEE Trans Med Imaging. 2020;39(12):4071–84. https://doi.org/10.1109/TMI.2020.3011626.
41. Zhao X, Huang M, Li L, Qi XS, Tan S. Multi-to-binary network (MTBNet) for automated multi-organ segmentation on multi-sequence abdominal MRI images. Phys Med Biol. 2020;65(16):165013. https://doi.org/10.1088/1361-6560/ab9453.
42. Kart T, Fischer M, Kustner T, Hepp T, Bamberg F, Winzeck S, et al. Deep learning-based automated abdominal organ segmentation in the UK biobank and German National Cohort Magnetic Resonance Imaging Studies. Investig Radiol. 2021;56(6):401–8. https://doi.org/10.1097/RLI.0000000000000755.
43. Bevilacqua V, Brunetti A, Cascarano GD, Guerriero A, Pesce F, Moschetta M, et al. A comparison between two semantic deep learning frameworks for the autosomal dominant polycystic kidney disease segmentation based on magnetic resonance images. BMC Med Inf Decis Mak. 2019;19(Suppl 9):244. https://doi.org/10.1186/s12911-019-0988-4.
44. Daniel AJ, Buchanan CE, Allcock T, Scerri D, Cox EF, Prestwich BL, et al. Automated renal segmentation in healthy and chronic kidney disease subjects using a convolutional neural network. Magn Reson Med. 2021;86(2):1125–36. https://doi.org/10.1002/mrm.28768.
45. Korfiatis P, Denic A, Edwards M, Gregory A, Wright D, Mullan A, et al. Automated segmentation of kidney cortex and medulla in CT images: a multisite evaluation study. J Am Soc Nephrol. 2022;33:420–30.
46. Kline TL, Edwards ME, Fetzer J, Gregory AV, Anaam D, Metzger AJ, et al. Automatic semantic segmentation of kidney cysts in MR images of patients affected by autosomal-dominant polycystic kidney disease. Abdom Radiol. 2021;46(3):1053–61. https://doi.org/10.1007/s00261-020-02748-4.
47. Gregory AV, Anaam DA, Vercnocke AJ, Edwards ME, Torres VE, Harris PC, et al. Semantic instance segmentation of kidney cysts in MR images: a fully automated 3D approach developed through active learning. J Digit Imaging. 2021:05. https://doi.org/10.1007/s10278-021-00452-3.
48. Muller S, Farag I, Weickert J, Braun Y, Lollert A, Dobberstein J, et al. Benchmarking Wilms' tumor in multisequence MRI data: why does current clinical practice fail? Which popular segmentation algorithms perform well? J Med Imaging (Bellingham). 2019;6(3):034001. https://doi.org/10.1117/1.JMI.6.3.034001.
49. Van Griethuysen JJ, Fedorov A, Parmar C, Hosny A, Aucoin N, Narayan V, et al. Computational radiomics system to decode the radiographic phenotype. Cancer Res. 2017;77(21):e104–e7.
50. Kociolek M, Strzelecki M, Obuchowicz R. Does image normalization and intensity resolution impact texture classification? Comput Med Imaging Graph. 2020;81:101716. https://doi.org/10.1016/j.compmedimag.2020.101716.
51. Johnson WE, Li C, Rabinovic A. Adjusting batch effects in microarray expression data using empirical bayes methods. Biostatistics. 2007;8(1):118–27.
52. Chandarana H, Rosenkrantz AB, Mussi TC, Kim S, Ahmad AA, Raj SD, et al. Histogram analysis of whole-lesion enhancement in differentiating clear cell from papillary subtype of renal cell cancer. Radiology. 2012;265(3):790–8. https://doi.org/10.1148/radiol.12111281.
53. Doshi AM, Ream JM, Kierans AS, Bilbily M, Rusinek H, Huang WC, et al. Use of MRI in differentiation of papillary renal cell carcinoma subtypes: qualitative and quantitative analysis. Am J Roentgenol. 2016;206(3):566–72.
54. Vendrami CL, Velichko YS, Miller FH, Chatterjee A, Villavicencio CP, Yaghmai V, et al. Differentiation of papillary renal cell carcinoma subtypes on MRI: qualitative and texture analysis. AJR Am J Roentgenol. 2018;211(6):1234–45. https://doi.org/10.2214/AJR.17.19213.
55. Kierans AS, Rusinek H, Lee A, Shaikh MB, Triolo M, Huang WC, et al. Textural differences in apparent diffusion coefficient between low-and high-stage clear cell renal cell carcinoma. Am J Roentgenol. 2014;203(6):W637–W44.
56. Antunes J, Viswanath S, Rusu M, Valls L, Hoimes C, Avril N, et al. Radiomics analysis on FLT-PET/MRI for characterization of early treatment response in renal cell carcinoma: a proof-of-concept study. Transl Oncol. 2016;9(2):155–62. https://doi.org/10.1016/j.tranon.2016.01.008.
57. Yin Q, Hung S-C, Wang L, Lin W, Fielding JR, Rathmell WK, et al. Associations between tumor vascularity, vascular endothelial growth factor expression and PET/MRI radiomic signatures in primary clear-cell-renal-cell-carcinoma: proof-of-concept study. Sci Rep. 2017;7:43,356. https://doi.org/10.1038/srep43356.
58. Hoang UN, Mojdeh Mirmomen S, Meirelles O, Yao J, Merino M, Metwalli A, et al. Assessment of multiphasic contrast-enhanced MR textures in differentiating small renal mass subtypes. Abdom Radiol. 2018;43(12):3400–9. https://doi.org/10.1007/s00261-018-1625-x.
59. Goyal A, Razik A, Kandasamy D, Seth A, Das P, Ganeshan B, et al. Role of MR texture analysis in histological subtyping and grading of renal cell carcinoma: a preliminary study. Abdom Radiol. 2019;44(10):3336–49. https://doi.org/10.1007/s00261-019-02122-z.
60. Li H, Li A, Zhu H, Hu Y, Li J, Xia L, et al. Whole-tumor quantitative apparent diffusion coefficient histogram and texture analysis to differentiation of minimal fat angiomyolipoma from clear cell renal cell

carcinoma. Acad Radiol. 2019;26(5):632–9. https://doi.org/10.1016/j.acra.2018.06.015.
61. Alayed A, Krishna S, Breau RH, Currin S, Flood TA, Narayanasamy S, et al. Diagnostic accuracy of MRI for detecting inferior vena cava wall invasion in renal cell carcinoma tumor thrombus using quantitative and subjective analysis. AJR Am J Roentgenol. 2019;212(3):562–9. https://doi.org/10.2214/AJR.18.20209.
62. Wang W, Cao K, Jin S, Zhu X, Ding J, Peng W. Differentiation of renal cell carcinoma subtypes through MRI-based radiomics analysis. Eur Radiol. 2020;30(10):5738–47. https://doi.org/10.1007/s00330-020-06896-5.
63. Lopes Vendrami C, McCarthy RJ, Villavicencio CP, Miller FH. Predicting common solid renal tumors using machine learning models of classification of radiologist-assessed magnetic resonance characteristics. Abdom Radiol. 2020;45(9):2797–809. https://doi.org/10.1007/s00261-020-02637-w.
64. Said D, Hectors SJ, Wilck E, Rosen A, Stocker D, Bane O, et al. Characterization of solid renal neoplasms using MRI-based quantitative radiomics features. Abdom Radiol. 2020;45(9):2840–50. https://doi.org/10.1007/s00261-020-02540-4.
65. Arita Y, Yoshida S, Kwee TC, Akita H, Okuda S, Iwaita Y, et al. Diagnostic value of texture analysis of apparent diffusion coefficient maps for differentiating fat-poor angiomyolipoma from non-clear-cell renal cell carcinoma. Eur J Radiol. 2021;143:109895. https://doi.org/10.1016/j.ejrad.2021.109895.
66. Li Q, Liu Y-J, Dong D, Bai X, Huang Q-B, Guo A-T, et al. Multiparametric MRI radiomic model for preoperative predicting WHO/ISUP nuclear grade of clear cell renal cell carcinoma. J Magn Reson Imaging. 2020;52(5):1557–66. https://doi.org/10.1002/jmri.27182.
67. Purkayastha S, Zhao Y, Wu J, Hu R, McGirr A, Singh S, et al. Differentiation of low and high grade renal cell carcinoma on routine MRI with an externally validated automatic machine learning algorithm. Sci Rep. 2020;10(1):19,503. https://doi.org/10.1038/s41598-020-76132-z.
68. Stanzione A, Ricciardi C, Cuocolo R, Romeo V, Petrone J, Sarnataro M, et al. MRI radiomics for the prediction of Fuhrman grade in clear cell renal cell carcinoma: a machine learning exploratory study. J Digit Imaging. 2020;33(4):879–87. https://doi.org/10.1007/s10278-020-00336-y.
69. Choi JW, Hu R, Zhao Y, Purkayastha S, Wu J, McGirr AJ, et al. Preoperative prediction of the stage, size, grade, and necrosis score in clear cell renal cell carcinoma using MRI-based radiomics. Abdom Radiol. 2021;46(6):2656–64. https://doi.org/10.1007/s00261-020-02876-x.
70. Dwivedi DK, Xi Y, Kapur P, Madhuranthakam AJ, Lewis MA, Udayakumar D, et al. Magnetic resonance imaging radiomics analyses for prediction of high-grade histology and necrosis in clear cell renal cell carcinoma: preliminary experience. Clin Genitourin Cancer. 2021;19(1):12–21.e1. https://doi.org/10.1016/j.clgc.2020.05.011.
71. Sun J, Pan L, Zha T, Xing W, Chen J, Duan S. The role of MRI texture analysis based on susceptibility-weighted imaging in predicting Fuhrman grade of clear cell renal cell carcinoma. Acta Radiol. 2021;62(8):1104–11. https://doi.org/10.1177/0284185120951964.
72. Becker AS, Wagner MW, Wurnig MC, Boss A. Diffusion-weighted imaging of the abdomen: impact of b-values on texture analysis features. NMR Biomed. 2017;30(1):01. https://doi.org/10.1002/nbm.3669.
73. Ciritsis A, Rossi C, Wurnig MC, Phi Van V, Boss A. Intravoxel incoherent motion: model-free determination of tissue type in abdominal organs using machine learning. Investig Radiol. 2017;52(12):747–57. https://doi.org/10.1097/RLI.0000000000000400.
74. Cui E, Li Z, Ma C, Li Q, Lei Y, Lan Y, et al. Predicting the ISUP grade of clear cell renal cell carcinoma with multiparametric MR and multiphase CT radiomics. Eur Radiol. 2020;30(5):2912–21. https://doi.org/10.1007/s00330-019-06601-1.
75. Khalifa F, Abou El-Ghar M, Abdollahi B, Frieboes HB, El-Diasty T, El-Baz A. A comprehensive non-invasive framework for automated evaluation of acute renal transplant rejection using DCE-MRI. NMR Biomed. 2013;26(11):1460–70. https://doi.org/10.1002/nbm.2977.
76. Shi H, Jia J, Li D, Wei L, Shang W, Zheng Z. Blood oxygen level dependent magnetic resonance imaging for detecting pathological patterns in lupus nephritis patients: a preliminary study using a decision tree model. BMC Nephrol. 2018;19(1):33. https://doi.org/10.1186/s12882-017-0787-z.
77. Ding J, Xing Z, Jiang Z, Zhou H, Di J, Chen J, et al. Evaluation of renal dysfunction using texture analysis based on DWI, BOLD, and susceptibility-weighted imaging. Eur Radiol. 2019;29(5):2293–301. https://doi.org/10.1007/s00330-018-5911-3.
78. Deng Y, Yang B-R, Luo J-W, Du G-X, Luo L-P. DTI-based radiomics signature for the detection of early diabetic kidney damage. Abdom Radiol. 2020;45(8):2526–31. https://doi.org/10.1007/s00261-020-02576-6.
79. Soma T, Ishioka J, Tanaka H, Matsuoka Y, Saito K, Fujii Y. Potential for computer-aided diagnosis using a convolutional neural network algorithm to diagnose fat-poor angiomyolipoma in enhanced computed tomography and T2-weighted magnetic resonance imaging. Int J Urol. 2018;25(11):978–9. https://doi.org/10.1111/iju.13784.
80. Zheng Y, Wang S, Chen Y, Du H-Q. Deep learning with a convolutional neural network model to differentiate renal parenchymal tumors: a preliminary study. Abdom Radiol. 2021;46(7):3260–8. https://doi.org/10.1007/s00261-021-02981-5.
81. Xu Q, Zhu Q, Liu H, Chang L, Duan S, Dou W, et al. Differentiating benign from malignant renal tumors using T2- and diffusion-weighted images: a comparison of deep learning and radiomics models versus

assessment from radiologists. J Magn Reson Imaging. 2021;30:30. https://doi.org/10.1002/jmri.27900.
82. Shehata M, Khalifa F, Soliman A, Ghazal M, Taher F, El-Ghar MA, et al. Computer-aided diagnostic system for early detection of acute renal transplant rejection using diffusion-weighted MRI. IEEE Trans Biomed Eng. 2019;66(2):539–52. https://doi.org/10.1109/TBME.2018.2849987.
83. Liu L, Johansson A, Cao Y, Dow J, Lawrence TS, Balter JM. Abdominal synthetic CT generation from MR Dixon images using a U-net trained with 'semi-synthetic' CT data. Phys Med Biol. 2020;65(12):125001. https://doi.org/10.1088/1361-6560/ab8cd2.
84. Florkow MC, Guerreiro F, Zijlstra F, Seravalli E, Janssens GO, Maduro JH, et al. Deep learning-enabled MRI-only photon and proton therapy treatment planning for paediatric abdominal tumours. Radiother Oncol. 2020;153:220–7. https://doi.org/10.1016/j.radonc.2020.09.056.
85. Kline TL. Segmenting new image acquisitions without labels. 2019 IEEE 16th International Symposium on Biomedical Imaging (ISBI 2019): IEEE; 2019. pp. 330–3.
86. Kline TL. Improving domain generalization in segmentation models with neural style transfer. 2021 IEEE 18th International Symposium on Biomedical Imaging (ISBI): IEEE; 2021. p. 1324–8.
87. Sui B, Lv J, Tong X, Li Y, Wang C. Simultaneous image reconstruction and lesion segmentation in accelerated MRI using multi-tasking learning. Med Phys. 2021;20:20. https://doi.org/10.1002/mp.15213.
88. Willemink MJ, Koszek WA, Hardell C, Wu J, Fleischmann D, Harvey H, et al. Preparing medical imaging data for machine learning. Radiology. 2020;295(1):4–15.
89. Muller D, Kramer F. MIScnn: a framework for medical image segmentation with convolutional neural networks and deep learning. BMC Med. 2021;21(1):12. https://doi.org/10.1186/s12880-020-00543-7.
90. Isensee F, Petersen J, Klein A, Zimmerer D, Jaeger PF, Kohl S, et al. nnU-Net: Self-adapting framework for u-net-based medical image segmentation. arXiv preprint arXiv:180910486; 2018.
91. Chen J, Lu Y, Yu Q, Luo X, Adeli E, Wang Y, et al. TransUNet: Transformers make strong encoders for medical image segmentation. arXiv preprint arXiv:210204306; 2021.
92. Chang Y, Menghan H, Guangtao Z, Xiao-Ping Z. Transclaw u-net: Claw U-Net with transformers for medical image segmentation. arXiv preprint arXiv:210705188; 2021.
93. Hatamizadeh A, Tang Y, Nath V, Yang D, Myronenko A, Landman B, et al. UNETR: Transformers for 3d medical image segmentation. Proceedings of the IEEE/CVF Winter Conference on Applications of Computer Vision; 2022. pp. 574–84.
94. Potretzke TA, Korfiatis P, Blezek DJ, Edwards ME, Klug JR, Cook CJ, et al. Clinical Implementation of an Artificial Intelligence Algorithm for Magnetic Resonance–Derived Measurement of Total Kidney Volume. Mayo Clin Proc. 2023;98(5):689–700. https://doi.org/10.1016/j.mayocp.2022.12.019.

Ultra-high Field MRI of the Kidney 29

Anneloes de Boer, J. M. Hoogduin, and G. J. Metzger

Abbreviations

ASL	Arterial spin-labeling
ATP	Adenosine triphosphate
B_0	Static magnetic field
BOLD	Blood oxygenation level dependent
CE	Contrast enhanced
CKD	Chronic kidney disease
CNR	Contrast-to-noise ratio
CPMG	Carr-Purcell-Meiboom-Gill
EM	Electromagnetic
EPI	Echo planar imaging
FAIR	Flow-sensitive alternating inversion recovery
GBCA	Gadolinium-based contrast agent
GRAPPA	GeneRalized Autocalibrating Partial Parallel Acquisition
MRA	Magnetic resonance angiography
MRI	Magnetic resonance imaging
MRS	MR spectroscopy
MRSI	MR spectroscopic imaging
PCASL	Pseudo-continuous ASL
RF	Radiofrequency magnetic field
SAR	Specific absorption rate
SENSE	SENSitivity Encoding
SNR	Signal-to-noise ratio
SS-FSE	Single shot fast spin echo
TOF	Time of flight
UHF	Ultra-high field

A. de Boer · J. M. Hoogduin
Department of Radiology, University Medical Center Utrecht, Utrecht University, Utrecht, The Netherlands
e-mail: a.deboer-13@umcutrecht.nl; j.m.-hoogduin-2@umcutrecht.nl

G. J. Metzger (✉)
Center for Magnetic Resonance Research, University of Minnesota, Minneapolis, MN, USA
e-mail: gmetzger@umn.edu

Introduction

While ultra-high field (UHF) imaging is increasingly adopted in neuroscience, MRI research on 7 T and beyond in the body and kidneys is limited. However, results to date indicate that renal imaging at 7 T is not only feasible but very clearly benefits from the increased field strength, although the technical difficulties of imaging at UHF are even more pronounced in the abdomen compared to the head. In this chapter, we provide an overview of benefits and difficulties associated with renal UHF imaging, as well as a literature review on the topic, including a glimpse into the research landscape and applications on the UHF horizon.

The migration to scanners operating at increasingly high field strengths is mainly driven by the supra-linear increase in signal-to-noise-ratio (SNR). This increase can be employed in various ways—the most straightforward being an increase in spatial resolution. Alternatively, acquisition speed can be increased

S. D. Serai, K. Darge (eds.), *Advanced Clinical MRI of the Kidney*,
https://doi.org/10.1007/978-3-031-40169-5_29

by supporting increased undersampling or reduced averaging. Apart from proton imaging, however, this SNR gain is especially beneficial when imaging other, less abundant nuclei with intrinsically lower sensitivity like sodium and phosphorus [1].

One of the main challenges of proton imaging at UHF is the decrease in wavelength of the radiofrequency (RF) or electromagnetic fields. At 3 T, a Larmor frequency of 128 MHz results in a 26 cm wavelength. However, moving to 7 T the Larmor frequency increases to 298 MHz, with associated wavelength of around 11 cm, and for 10.5 T a frequency of 447 MHz and wavelength of 7.5 cm. Shorter wavelengths result in interference patterns of the electromagnetic fields causing local signal voids in case of destructive RF interferences in the transmit magnetic field (B_1+) while causing local hot spots due to the constructive interferences of the electric fields as characterized by the specific absorption rate (SAR). To address these inhomogeneities, parallel transmit hardware and RF pulse design strategies can be employed or, in the case of SAR limitations, sequence timing can be adjusted. Note however, that for nuclei other than protons, these issues are less of an issue. For phosphorus, for example, the wavelength at 7 T equals 28 cm.

Other changes at UHF benefit one acquisition technique while hindering another—or even have both advantages and disadvantages for a single application. The Blood Oxygenation Level Dependent (BOLD) effect, for example, is enhanced at UHF thanks to the increase in susceptibility effects, but this increase in susceptibility sensitivity can amplify artifacts as well, sometimes rendering BOLD images partly undiagnostic even at 3 T. Imaging at UHF is associated with an increase in T_1 and a decrease in T_2. The increase in T_1 is favorable in Arterial Spin-Labeling (ASL) applications as discussed later, but requires longer repetition times when performing T_1 mapping acquisitions, thus less time efficient. An increase in water fat shift might enhance (spectral) fat suppression, but also aggravates chemical shift artifacts [1].

Clinical Practice and Potential of Ultra-High Field Renal MRI

The clinical use of 7 T MRI currently is mostly limited to neuroimaging applications [2]. For body applications, research is focusing on technical developments and innovations to overcome the challenges posed by the increase in field strength. Several applications, however, are expected to benefit from imaging at UHF. Non-contrast enhanced angiography profits from increased spatial resolution and, for time-of-flight angiography, from an increase in contrast-to-noise ratio (CNR) of the vessel signal. This enables high-resolution angiography of the vascular tree, up to the level of the interlobar arteries running between the medullary pyramids [3]. Depiction of those vessels is challenging in conventional contrast-enhanced angiography since background enhancement limits CNR in those distal vessels. Anatomical depiction of those vessels might be of clinical use in patients suffering from renal artery stenosis, since it may identify those patients with a vessel stenosis limited to the main renal artery and therefore would benefit from an intervention. Non-contrast enhanced imaging of the renal vasculature also is relevant in kidney transplant recipients, who often suffer from vascular complications of the transplant surgery in the form of aneurysms and stenoses at the anastomosis site.

Next, in BOLD MRI, the BOLD effect is enhanced due to an increase in susceptibility effects. In the kidney, this is mostly relevant in the cortex which functions at the shoulder of the oxygen-hemoglobin dissociation curve so that changes in oxygen pressure only have limited effect on the ratio between oxygenated and deoxygenated hemoglobin. Hence, changes in cortical oxygen pressure have limited influence on the BOLD signal. At ultra-high field, this might partly be overcome by the abovementioned increase in susceptibility. Renal (cortical) oxygenation has been proven to be an important clinical marker since it is capable of predicting future decline in renal function [4].

As mentioned in the introduction, sodium and phosphorus imaging and spectroscopy strongly benefit from imaging at ultra-high fields. Physiologically, both elements are of interest in the kidney. ^{31}P spectroscopy allows the study of ATP concentrations in vivo, a molecule that provides energy to virtually all active biological processes in the human cell. Furthermore, the relative position of the inorganic phosphate peak in the ^{31}P spectrum allows calculation of the pH. In ex vivo experiments on rat kidneys, it was already shown in 1983 that diminished ATP content could be measured in kidneys exposed to simulated hemorrhagic shock as well as in kidneys perfused with an anoxic fluid [5]. Since ATP content reflects the metabolic activity of tissue, it can provide crucial information in numerous renal diseases, for example, in acute kidney injury following shock, in delayed graft function after kidney transplantation or in chronic kidney disease, the loss in kidney function which is observed in patients suffering from various conditions, including hypertension and diabetes. Remnant metabolic activity as measured by ^{31}P (spectroscopic) imaging might be able to predict recovery of renal function following acute renal damage or provide insight in the pathophysiology underlying the development of chronic kidney disease (CKD) [6].

Renal sodium imaging (^{23}Na MRI) is of interest since the kidneys play the central role in sodium homeostasis. A renal sodium image clearly shows the increasing sodium concentration toward the tip of the medullary pyramid, as expected from renal physiology. ^{23}Na MRI showed that this gradient increases after water deprivation [7], while it slightly decreases after a water load [8]. While these reports support the validity of the technique, its value might be found in studying altered sodium handling in obesity [9], hypertension [10], CKD [11], and nephrotic syndrome [12], in order to provide a better understanding of those entities.

Current State-of-the-Art in Ultra-High Field Renal MRI

Anatomical Imaging and Angiography

The clinical use of anatomical images of the kidney acquired at 7 T has mainly been studied by Umutlu et al. A series of papers covering both contrast enhanced, and native imaging of the renal anatomy and vasculature were published between 2011 and 2018 [13–17]. Regarding unenhanced T_1 weighted imaging, diagnostic quality images were obtained by conventional 2D and 3D spoiled gradient echo imaging, with fat saturation applied successfully in 2D only [13]. Alternatively, 2D opposed phase imaging could be used to optimize kidney delineation, avoiding the need of fat suppression. Hoogduin et al. applied the Dixon method for low-cost fat suppression in terms of acquisition time and SAR [1] (Fig. 29.1a). At 7 T, this method has the advantage of not requiring a SAR-intensive saturation pulse. However, for the Dixon technique to succeed sufficiently high quality B_0 shimming is

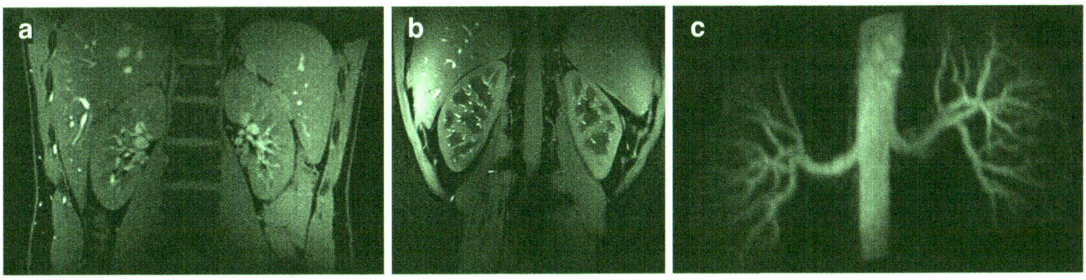

Fig. 29.1 (**a**) Anatomical coronal TFE images with Dixon reconstruction [*Modified from de Boer* et al. [1] *under the terms of Creative Commons Attribution (CC-BY) International license*]; (**b**) Coronal T_1 weighted gradient echo inversion recovery enhanced image [*Modified with permission from Metzger* et al. [19]]; (**c**) Cropped coronal MIP from healthy volunteer with a trade-off shim solution for saturation pulse, magnitude, and phase homogeneous shim for conventional pulses [*Modified with permission from Metzger* et al. [19]]

required—which Hoogduin et al. proved to be feasible at 7 T.

Alternatively, contrast agents can be used to enhance corticomedullary contrast when images are acquired in the arterial phase [14]. However, because of associated risks and uncertainties regarding gadolinium-based contrast agent (GBCA) accumulation (see Chap. 20), administration of GBCAs solely for this purpose is not recommended in the authors' opinion.

T_2 weighted imaging at 7 T is relatively challenging due to the need of large refocusing pulses and the sensitivity to field inhomogeneities. The first forces the use of extremely long repetition times to keep SAR within limits [1]. The latter can render the image undiagnostic if B_0 and B_1 shimming is insufficient [13].

Compared to T_1 and T_2 weighted anatomical imaging, the advantages of 7 T are more pronounced for the application of renal MR angiography (MRA). Vessels appear hyperintense on T_1 weighted images at 7 T, partly explained by enhanced inflow effects due to the local RF coils typically used in 7 T imaging [18]. Both GBCA enhanced and unenhanced angiography have been studied. Umutlu et al. compared time-of-flight (TOF) to regular gradient echo images obtained at 7 T and concluded that TOF MRA was superior in depicting the aorta and renal arteries. In this first study, segmental arteries were not considered; however, in a later publication by her group, Laader et al. [17] showed that TOF MRA is capable of visualizing the segmental branches of the renal arteries. Unfortunately, maximum intensity projections (MIPs) were not shown, so the ability to assess the anatomy over the full course of the artery could not be assessed. An abstract by McAteer et al. describes multi-echo TOF MRA at 3 and 7 T. Vessels as distal as the interlobar artery at 7 T could be visualized using MIPs. However, quality of the 7 T angiograms was variable, mostly due to imperfect B_1^+ shimming [3].

At lower field strengths, the TOF technique is not preferred for the renal arteries because of their course in the axial plane, which impedes the inflow effect. Metzger et al. [19] therefore employed another technique which proved to be successful at lower field strength: inflow dependent inversion recovery. An adiabatic inversion pulse was implemented before a 3D gradient echo readout with an inversion time of 1000 ms. This resulted in excellent corticomedullary contrast in the anatomical images as well as an excellent depiction of the vascular tree enabling visualization of the renal branch up to the segmental arteries (Fig. 29.1b and c). Note however that this adiabatic inversion pulse is SAR intensive at 7 T, requiring adequate SAR modeling and power monitoring. Furthermore, separate shim solutions were needed for the adiabatic inversion pulse, requiring adequate peak B_1^+, and the gradient echo readout, which requires optimal B_1^+ homogeneity.

The previously mentioned study of Laader et al. [17] compared TOF MRA to low-dose GBCA enhanced imaging. Although 2D TOF MRA was acquired in significantly lower spatial resolution compared to contrast enhanced MRA, image quality in terms of vessel delineation and contrast-to-noise ratio (CNR) were reported to be comparable. TOF MRA however was acquired in three separate breath-holds in the axial orientation, resulting in some misalignment between the slices. In patients, this will hamper the assessment of vessel continuity and stenosis between slices.

Quantitative Imaging

T1 and *T2* Measurements

The measurement of longitudinal ($R_1 = 1/T_1$) and transverse ($R_2 = 1/T_2$) relaxation rate can provide valuable information revealing insights into renal structure and function in native and transplant kidneys ([20] and references therein) as well as the needed information for optimizing results from other quantitative imaging techniques such as ASL [21]. In order to perform relaxometry, it is typical for several measurements to be needed providing images with different T_1 or T_2 weighting through which a parametric fitting is performed on a voxel-wise basis. As motion is a major consideration when imaging the native kidneys, acquiring the multiple weighted images in a single breath-hold is highly advantageous. To date, relaxometry in the kidneys at 7 T was performed by only a single group using a single shot fast spin echo (SS-FSE) readout suitable for both 7 T and lower field applications [22]. To minimize the influence of B_1^+ inhomogeneities and reduce local SAR, RF shimming was performed by optimizing the transmit phases of a 16 channel stripline array to achieve maximum average efficiency over a single kidney. For T_1 mapping, an adiabatic inversion pulse was used to address remaining RF field non-uniformities. Within a single breath-hold, 6 images were acquired with varying delay times. For T_2 mapping, a Carr-Purcell-Meiboom-Gill (CPMG) module of varying duration was inserted between the excitation and refocusing pulse of the SS-FSE sequence providing varying T_2 weightings while minimizing contributions from diffusion. To minimize the formation of stimulated echoes, spoiling gradients on either side of the refocusing pulses were employed in the preparation module. Figure 29.2 shows T_1 and T_2 maps obtained using the above strategies and (Table 29.1) provides a comparison of relaxation times measured at 3 T and 7 T using the above methods highlighting the field strength dependent differences between the medulla and cortex. The expected increase in T_1 and decrease in T_2 with increasing field strength are observed in the kidney when using the same technique at both field strengths to obtain the relaxometry results.

Blood Oxygenation Level Dependent MRI

In BOLD MRI, local differences in concentration of deoxygenated hemoglobin in blood are used to generate contrast in T_2* weighted scans. A gradient echo sequence can be used to visualize the locally induced field inhomogeneity's caused by the presence of de-oxyhemoglobin. In kidney imaging, this technique is used to obtain information on renal cortical and medullary hypoxia in various diseases [23]. The medulla is at the edge of hypoxia in a healthy kidney which leads to an increase in R_2* ($1/T_2$*) when compared to the cortex. A "challenge," like water loading or the administration of a drug-like furosemide can be used to influence the oxygen consumption of the medulla. Thus far, only two high field MR groups

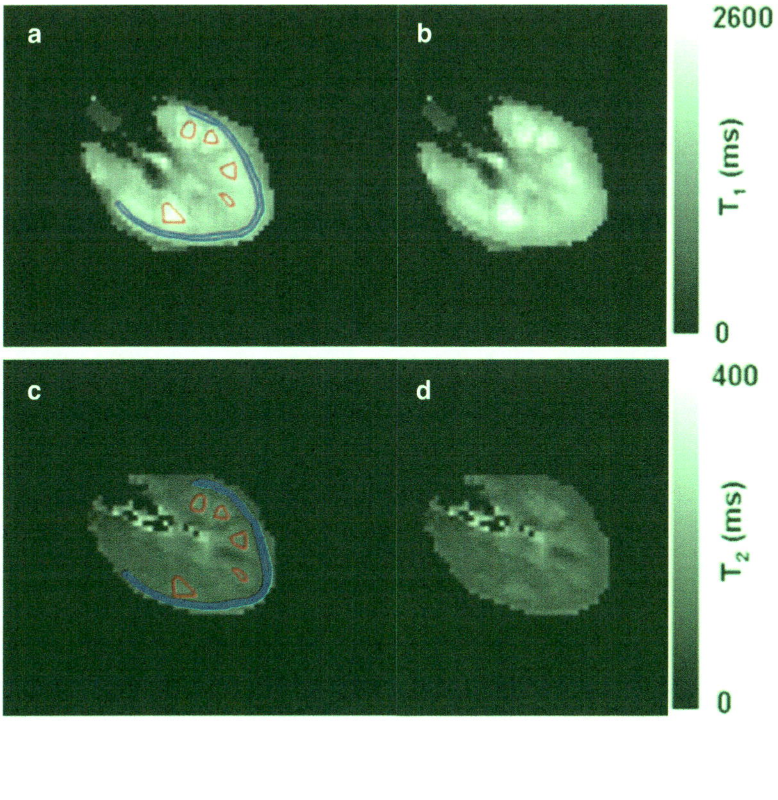

Fig. 29.2 (**a**, **b**) T_1 maps with and without ROIs for T_1 estimation; (**c**, **d**) T_1 maps with and without ROIs for T_1 estimation (all ss-FSE images were acquired at six different inversion times or effective echo times to minimize short-term SAR) [*Modified with permission from Li* et al. [22]]

have used a multi-echo readout to measure kidney T_2* values quantitatively [24, 25]. An example is shown in Fig. 29.3. Given the relative large T_2* difference between cortex and medulla, most work (including in patients, e.g., [26]) using the BOLD contrast mechanism has been performed using 3 T systems.

Arterial Spin Labeling

Perfusion imaging using ASL is an attractive approach for studying renal physiology and assessing renal diseases and is well suited for the longitudinal monitoring of renal function. In ASL, arterial blood is used as an endogenous tracer [27], which is advantageous especially in the presence of renal insufficiency where the slow clearance of exogenous contrast agent makes repeat studies difficult and raises concern for nephrogenic systemic fibrosis [28] despite reports that more stable gadolinium chelates present limited risk for patients [29]. ASL is performed by labeling blood spins with an adiabatic inversion RF pulse as in flow-sensitive alternating inversion recovery (FAIR) or in pseudo-continuous ASL (PCASL). The signal from the labeled spins which perfuse the tissue of interest decay at the rate $R_1 = 1/T_1$, thus the longer T_1 values at 7 T benefit ASL acquisitions in multiple ways. First, the longer T_1 values result in higher perfusion signal greatly benefitting this intrinsically low SNR method. Second, the persistence in the labeling at higher field allows for longer total delay times following inversion labeling, thus reducing the impact of intravascular signals, the presence of which reduces quantification reliability. For renal ASL, those longer delay times are especially beneficial in the medulla because of its lower levels of perfusion and the relatively long delay times needed for proper perfusion measurements. Medullary perfusion measurements at 1.5 or 3 T are therefore considered unre-

Table 29.1 T_1 and T_2 values on 3 and 7 T [22]

	Cortex		Medulla	
	T_1	T_2	T_1	T_2
3 T	1261 ± 68	121 ± 5	1676 ± 94	138 ± 7
7 T	1668 ± 46	109 ± 6	2095 ± 52	125 ± 5

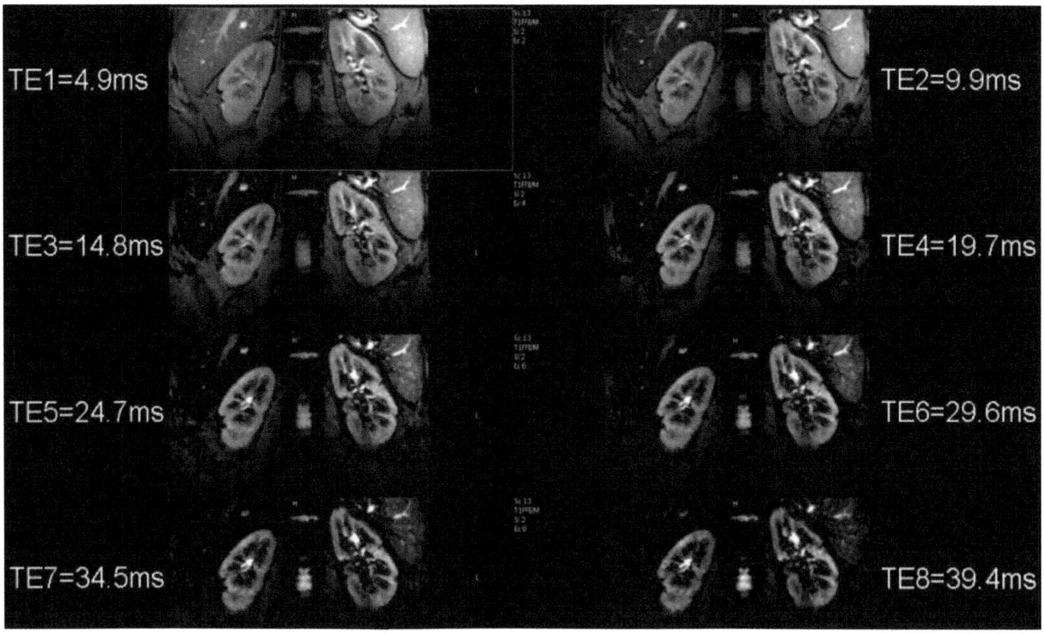

Fig. 29.3 Multi-echo gradient echo images used for calculating T_2*. Sequence details: 3 coronal slices, 1 slice per breath-hold of 15 s, resolution 1.5 × 1.5 × 5 mm^3, 20 echoes: first TE = 4.9 ms, ΔTE = 4.9 ms, water and fat in phase. Note the faster signal decrease in the medulla relative to the signal in the cortex [25].

liable [30]. When using an echo planar readout method, theoretical simulations of renal perfusion SNR efficiency are increased at 7 T even if longer repetition times are needed due to possible SAR constraints [31] (Fig. 29.4). Studies at 7 T using FAIR with a single shot echo planar imaging (EPI) readout were accomplished with no SAR issues when used in a respiratory triggered acquisition [32, 33].

Further demonstrating the benefit of increased SNR at 7 T, single breath-hold renal perfusion imaging was obtained using FAIR for spin labeling and a single shot fast spin echo (ss-FSE) readout [33]. An important considerations for this and previous 7 T renal perfusion studies was the absence of a whole body transmitter necessitating the use of local transceiver coil [34] with implications on sequence timing and the type of spin labeling deployed. First, for improved perfusion quantification, the prescribed temporal bolus width in the sequence was defined to be shorter than the temporal bolus width supported by the local RF coil as determined through multi-delay studies. Second, the limited transmit field generated by the local coil above and below the extent of the coil made it impractical to use PCASL which labels the blood in the descend-

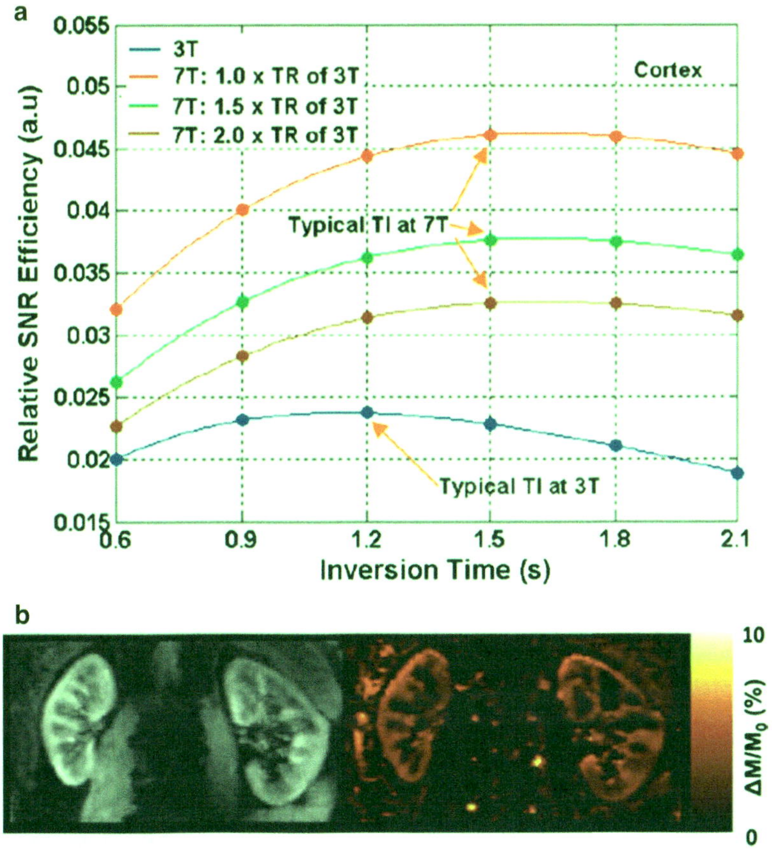

Fig. 29.4 (**a**) Theoretical simulations of renal perfusion SNR efficiencies at 3 T and 7 T for renal perfusion imaging using FAIR-EPI. TR represents repetition time, and TI represents total inversion time; (**b**) One subject's proton (left) and normalized perfusion-weighted (right) images from a respiratory triggered perfusion study using FAIR-EPI at 7 T with 2 × 2 × 5 mm^3 resolution. ΔM represents perfusion-weighted signal evaluated as the signal difference between label and control images, and M_0 the fully relaxed renal tissue signal. [*Modified from a conference proceeding by Li* et al. [31], *and reused from de Boer* et al. [1] *under the terms of Creative Commons Attribution (CC-BY) International license*]

ing aorta above the level of the kidneys where the B_1^+ fields are weak. Along with being less power-intensive, FAIR can label the spins in a region under the extent of the local coil where transmit fields of the local array are the strongest. To further improve the quality and SNR of the perfusion data, dynamically applied static B_1^+ shimming solutions were applied with different B_1^+ shimming solutions optimized to satisfy the unique requirements of each pulse in the sequence [19, 33]. Despite the use of the lower power FAIR for spin labeling and RF management strategies, high SAR needed to be managed by lengthening repetition times, using high parallel imaging reduction factors and implementing hyper-echoes for the ss-FSE readout. Figure 29.5 shows perfusion imaging results from Li et al. [21] where these strategies were implemented to measure renal perfusion in healthy controls. While the quantitative results reported were similar to previously reported 3 T studies [35], the ability to obtain this data in a single breath-hold at 7 T promises reduced motion sensitivity and increased quantification reliability capitalizing on the increased SNR, prolonged blood [36] and renal tissue [22] T_1s, and improved parallel imaging performance [34].

X-Nuclei Imaging in the Kidneys

Sodium Imaging

A healthy kidney produces around 180 L of (pre) urine a day, and in order to reduce this to the 1–2 L of urine we actually lose on a daily base, the pre-urine has to be heavily concentrated. In order to achieve this, the kidney maintains a strong sodium gradient with increasing concentration from the cortex to the tip of the medullary pyramids, where the concentrated urine enters the collecting system. Kidney failure influences this corticomedullary sodium gradient. At 7 T, this gradient was visualized at a slightly increased resolution compared to 3 T several years ago [37]. The combination of low sodium concentration in vivo, short relaxation times and intrinsically low MR sensitivity, makes sodium imaging a challenging technique even at 7 T despite its theoretical increased SNR of 2.33 relative to 3 T and the lack of B_1 inhomogeneity effects due to the longer wavelengths of this nuclei. The Larmor frequency of sodium is 78.8 MHz at 7 T, which translates to a wavelength of 45 cm in vivo. This is slightly shorter than the wavelength for protons at 1.5 T indicating that B_1 inhomogeneity effects are not an issue for sodium. However, the acquisition of sodium

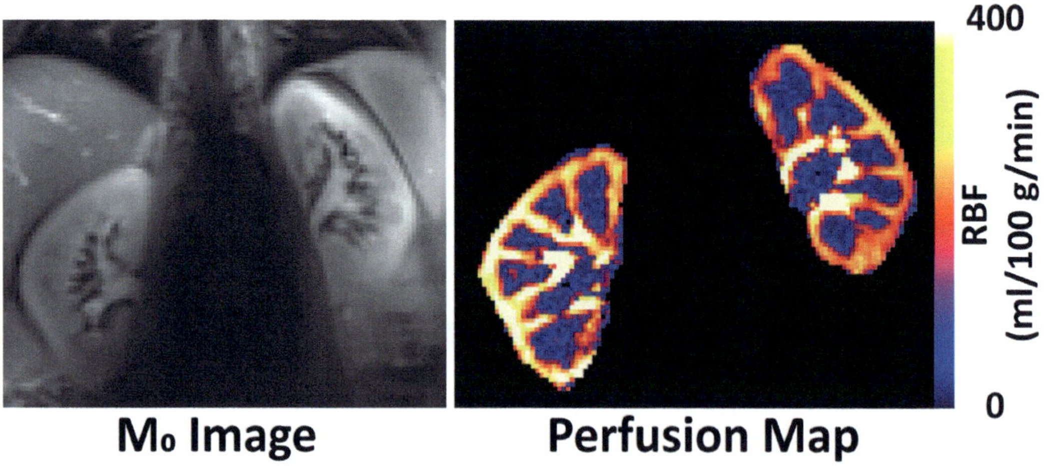

Fig. 29.5 Quantitative renal perfusion imaging using the FAIR ss-FSE study at 7 T and a single-subtraction approach from one volunteer: M0 image (left) renal blood flow map (right) [*Modified with permission from Li* et al. [21]]

images is further complicated by respiratory motion. A recent conference abstract [38] investigates the use of self-gating which sorts the acquired data into respiratory phases greatly reducing the blurring in the sodium images due to motion. Other development work includes the design of a new 8-channel proton/sodium RF coil array facilitating the benefits of combined sodium and proton studies of the kidneys [39].

Phosphorus Spectroscopy and Spectroscopic Imaging

Phosphorus (31P) magnetic resonance spectroscopy provides metabolic information which might help in assessing the physiological status of the kidneys. This was already recognized as early as 1989 [40]. At the field strength available at that time, six peaks were visible in the ^{31}P spectrum of a healthy kidney: phosphomonoesters (PMEs), phosphodiesters (PDEs), inorganic phosphorus (Pi), and gamma, alpha, and beta adenosine triphosphate (ATP). Phosphocreatine (PCr) is not expected in the kidney but can be visible in the spectrum due to partial volume effects with surrounding tissue. To obtain localized information, MR spectroscopic imaging (MRSI) can be used. Early attempts to monitor kidney allografts non-invasively at low field (1.5 T) showed that ^{31}P MRSI can distinguish the two main causes of kidney failure after transplantation [41]. Given that transplanted kidneys are close to the surface of the body and are hardly moving, ^{31}P MRSI has the potential to replace the current clinical procedure of repeated invasive biopsies to monitor allograft status. Therefore it is surprising that there are no published MRS or MRSI studies exploring the possibilities for kidney MRS(I) at 7 T. Figure 29.6

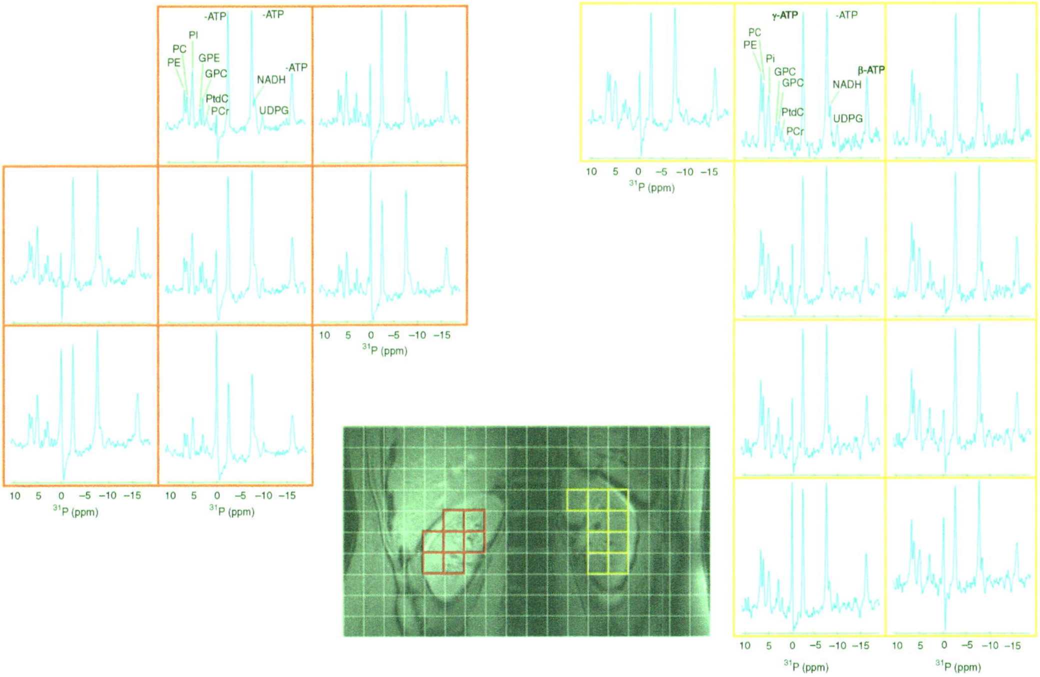

Fig. 29.6 Preliminary 31P MRSI data of a subject. The data was acquired using a phosphorus body coil for excitation and a 16 channel receive array. Phosphomonoesters (PMEs) (phosphocholine (PC) and phosphoethanolamine (PE)), phosphodiesters (PDEs) (glycerophosphocholine (GPC) and glycerophosphoethanolamine (GPE), inorganic phosphorus (Pi), gamma, alpha, and beta adenosine triphosphate (ATP) are clearly visible. Phosphocreatine (PCr) is not expected but most likely a result from partial volume effects from surrounding tissue © *J.Prompers & J.M. Hoogduin 2021 All Rights Reserved* [*courtesy J. Prompers and colleagues, University Medical Center Utrecht, Utrecht, The Netherlands*]

shows unpublished work (courtesy J. Prompers and colleagues, UMC Utrecht, Utrecht, The Netherlands) using a phosphorus body coil for RF transmission [42] in combination with a 16 channel local receive array. Given the spectral quality it is clear that it is worth investigating what ^{31}P MRSI has to offer for monitoring the kidney.

Kidney Imaging at 10.5 T

To explore the potential of imaging beyond 7 T, preliminary imaging studies throughout the human torso, including the kidney, were performed on a 10.5 T whole body MRI system in the work by He et al. [43]. While the primary goal of these studies was to gather initial safety data on human exposure to this high magnetic field, imaging acquisition was also performed to investigate RF management strategies and the ability to implement standard acquisitions to determine the extent to which expected contrasts could be obtained. Examples of T_1 weighted, fat suppressed anatomic images and inflow angiography acquisitions in a human subject are shown in Fig. 29.7. Even at this extremely high field strength, imaging over large fields of view were feasible in the human torso while the expected increase in inflow enhancement can be appreciated driven by the improved saturation of long T_1 spins in the background.

To acquire these data, RF management strategies previously used at 7 T were employed. The challenge of RF management at 10.5 T is increased compared to 7 T due to the higher resonance frequency (i.e., 448 MHz) and shorter wavelengths (i.e., ~7 cm). For the examples given in Fig. 29.7, tailored regions of interest were used to constrain RF shimming and pulse design across multiple slices similar to what has been done at 7 T [44]. For anatomic imaging, regions of interest for RF shimming encompassed the kidneys themselves. When the goal was to visualize the renal vasculature; however, the regions of interest for RF optimization included the kidneys, renal arteries, and the descending aorta. Beyond RF shimming employing phase-only solutions, magnitude shimming and multiple spoke pulses were also explored in the context of gradient echo sequences to experimentally investigate previously presented theoretical benefits of improving B_1^+ homogeneity while maintaining SAR performance [45]. The increased degrees of freedom helped address the increased B_1^+ non-uniformities at 10.5 T but also promise to further improve imaging performance at 7 T. In addition to the potential for improved anatomic resolution and non-contrast angiogra-

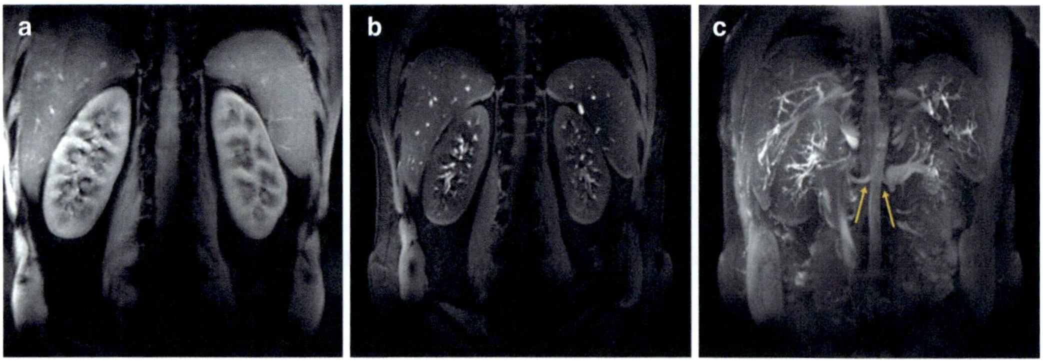

Fig. 29.7 Example of breath-hold renal images acquired with lipid suppression, including a 2D coronal anatomic GRE (**a**) and an inflow-enhanced acquisition (**b**); (**c**) MIP across the stack of images represented in (**b**) demonstrates the high inflow enhancement and background suppression afforded by the increased T1 of tissues and blood at 10.5 T. After phase-only shimming, a relatively uniform signal intensity was achieved in the oblique coronal plane over which these images were acquired. The origins of renal arteries are well visualized on the MIP image (yellow arrows), while distal arterial branches can also be appreciated [*With permission from He* et al. [43]]

phy and perfusion, the greatest benefit of 10.5 T in the study of renal function and disease may be the higher SNR afforded to non-proton imaging and spectroscopy specifically targeting sodium and phosphorus, respectively.

Challenges and Opportunities of Renal MRI at 7 T

RF Inhomogeneity

Due to the short RF wavelength at 298 MHz (~11 cm in tissue) compared to the dimensions of the human body, kidney imaging at 7 T is always hampered by some sort of inhomogeneity in the RF transmit field. An example is shown in the top row of Fig. 29.8. The most commonly used solution is based on parallel transmit: an array of transmit elements close to the body [13, 46–48], usually 8 or 16, used in combination with RF shimming [49]. By adapting the individual phases and, if needed, amplitudes, of the coil elements, RF interferences can be steered toward a region where they are less harmful, (Fig. 29.8) bottom row, note that there is now a dark band in the center of the images along the spine. Most published work on kidney imaging [13, 24, 49] has been performed by phase-only RF shimming. Although this can already provide reasonable good RF homogeneity over the two kidneys, usually, an RF void is present in the central part of the image near the spine. If this is undesirable like in non-CE MRA, multiple shim sets could be used as was shown by Metzger et al. [44]. One possible interesting avenue worth pursuing but not yet investigated for kidney imaging would be the use of something similar to "universal pulses" [50] for RF shimming. Using a "universal" shim setting for all subjects could speed up the workflow considerably by eliminating the scans that are needed to calculate the per subject optimal RF shim settings.

Going beyond RF shimming toward transmit SENSE where every sample in the RF pulse of each coil can have its own amplitude and phase is still terra incognita for kidney imaging and might not be needed given the homogeneity provided by RF shimming. This is probably, apart from the additional computational efforts needed, the reason why, for example, spokes or spiral non-selective pulses [51] have not yet been tested in kidney imaging thus far.

Yet another avenue is provided by the group of the Erwin Hahn institute. Following up on earlier attempts by Vaughan et al. [52], they managed to build a proton body coil (Fig. 29.9) driven by 32 1kW RF amplifiers [53]. In combination with the "time interleaved acquisition of modes technique [54]," which basically interleaves two RF shims (i.e., modes) and GRAPPA to reconstruct the images, they imaged the body from below the hip up to the top of the head using three stacks (stations) (Fig. 29.9), including the kidneys.

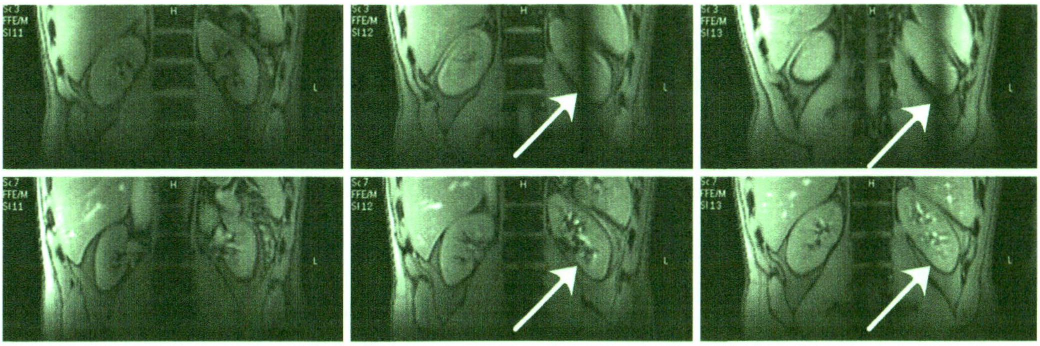

Fig. 29.8 Survey pre (upper row) and post (lower row) RF shimming. Only phase shimming was performed. Arrows: region of destructive interference in the left kidney in two of three images acquired before RF shimming, disappearing after shimming. [*From de Boer* et al. [1] *under the terms of Creative Commons Attribution (CC-BY) International license*]

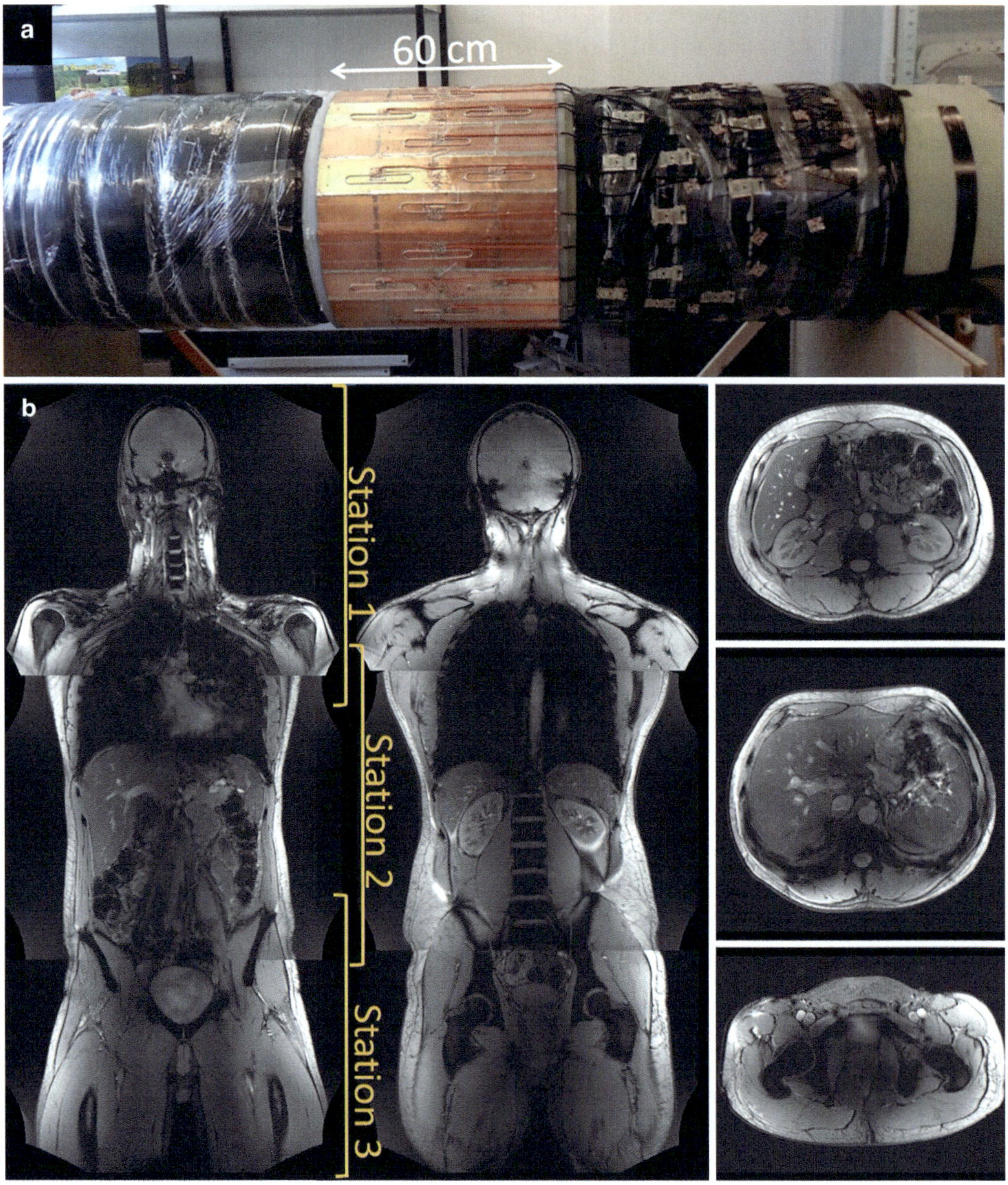

Fig. 29.9 (**a**) A 32 channel proton body coil array for 7 T [53]. (**b**) images obtained using this array in combination with the TIAMO technique [55] to reduce the RF inhomogeneity issues associated with proton imaging at 7 T [*From* Orzada et al. [53] *under the terms of Creative Commons Attribution (CC-BY) International license*]

SAR Limitations

Recent work on managing SAR in body imaging has focused on providing more human models for electromagnetic (EM) simulations [55, 56]. The workflow for this procedure is shown in Fig. 29.10. The goal of the work was to provide insights on intersubject SAR variations which are beneficial when determining the power deposition limits that are needed for safe body imaging. Unfortunately, this work focused on the pelvis [55, 56] and thus not yet applicable for the kid-

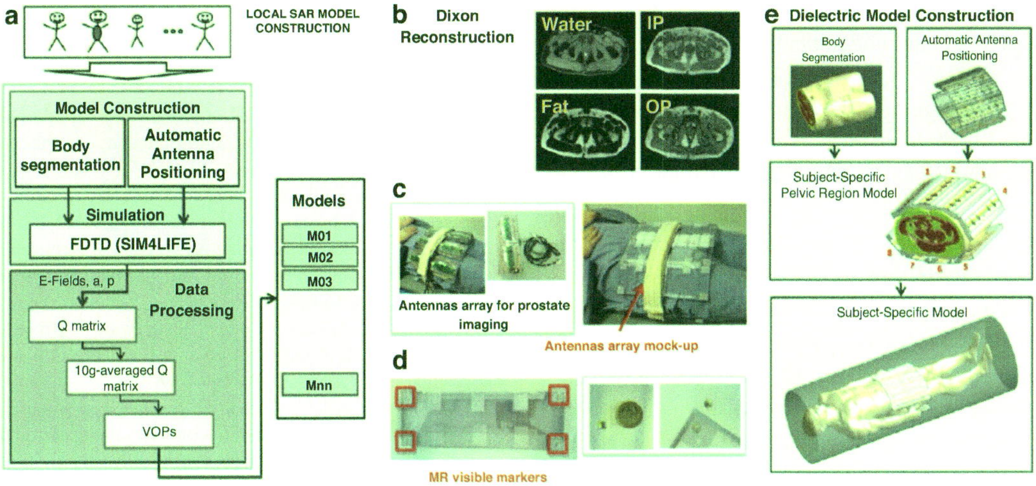

Fig. 29.10 (**a**) Workflow to obtain subject specific local SAR models. (**b**) Dixon images are acquired with mock-up antenna's in place and used for tissue segmentation in muscle, fat, cortical bone and skin. (**c**) The mock-up antenna array setup with (**d**) MR-visible markers to identify the antenna's and place them correctly in the simulation environment. (**e**) The Dixon-based segmentation and antenna placement are combined and used to create a subject-specific model, which is used in an electromagnetic simulation to calculate local SAR distribution. The procedure was performed in 23 volunteers and provides insight into variations of local SAR (both amount and location) over subjects. [*With permission from Meliadò* et al. [55]]

neys. A similar effort to develop models in the region of the kidney would be helpful in providing safe but not too stringent power limits in this anatomy.

The previous pelvic models were also used in a deep learning approach to assess SAR in individuals using measured B_1^+ amplitude and phase maps as an input and predicted local SAR distribution as an output [57]. This strategy could provide even more personalized power limits.

Availability of 7 T Scanners

At the moment, there are less than 100 MRI scanners with a field strength of 7 T or more installed in the world. Most large research hospitals have access to such a system in some way or another. Kidney imaging at these machines is still in its infancy. Given the tools that have been developed to overcome the inhomogeneity problems associated with ultra-high field MRI and the potential of non-proton spectroscopy and imaging, it is up to the research community together with radiologists and nephrologists, to explore and validate the benefits of UHF in the diagnosis and treatment monitoring of patients with kidney disease.

Conclusion and Discussion

Steady progress has been made in the field of UHF renal imaging. Angiography, functional imaging (BOLD, ASL), relaxometry, and X-nuclei imaging all have been shown to be feasible at UHF in the kidney.

Nevertheless, all work currently published has been performed in healthy volunteers. When moving to patient studies, new challenges will arise. Just like at lower field strengths, the 60 cm bore size and (sometimes) long acquisition times might prove to be an obstacle for real-life kidney patients, who are often obese and suffer from comorbidities which might impair their ability to perform breath-holds or lie still for extensive periods of time.

Although increasingly widespread, the vast majority of hospitals do not have access to a 7 T scanner even in developed countries. Its added value therefore should be found in its contribution to a better understanding of renal physiology as well as pathophysiology. Considering the ongoing ageing of our population and the ever-increasing incidence of diseases like hypertension and diabetes, which are detrimental to renal health, early detection of renal damage and development of new interventions become increasingly urgent. MRI, and UHF MRI in particular, provides us with the unique opportunity to study physiology and metabolism of the kidneys in vivo. It can be used to study subtle changes in early phase renal disease or the mechanism of action of targeted drugs and provide us with new insights in renal pathophysiology. This knowledge is crucial in the development of new therapies and interventions to slow down or even halt the progression of renal disease.

References

1. de Boer A, Hoogduin JM, Blankestijn PJ, Li X, Luijten PR, Metzger GJ, et al. 7 T renal MRI: challenges and promises. Magn Reson Mater Phy. 2016;29:417–33.
2. Barisano G, Sepehrband F, Ma S, Jann K, Cabeen R, Wang DJ, et al. Clinical 7 T MRI: are we there yet? A review about magnetic resonance imaging at ultra-high field. Br J Radiol. 2019;92:20180492.
3. McAteer JM, Doran E, Mirfin C, Glover P, Francis S, Gowland P. High resolution multi-echo time-of-flight angiography of the kidney at 3 and 7T. Proceedings of the 27th scientific meeting, International Society for Magnetic Resonance in Medicine. 2019:1914.
4. Pruijm M, Milani B, Pivin E, Podhajska A, Vogt B, Stuber M, et al. Reduced cortical oxygenation predicts a progressive decline of renal function in patients with chronic kidney disease. Kidney Int. 2018;93:932–40.
5. Rhodes RS, Jentoft JE, Barr RG, Robinson AV. 31P NMR studies of energy metabolism in perfused rat kidney. J Surg Res. 1983;35:373–82.
6. Fine LG, Norman JT. Chronic hypoxia as a mechanism of progression of chronic kidney diseases: from hypothesis to novel therapeutics. Kidney Int. 2008;74:867–72.
7. Maril N, Rosen Y, Reynolds GH, Ivanishev A, Ngo L, Lenkinski RE. Sodium MRI of the human kidney at 3 Tesla. Magn Reson Med. 2006;56:1229–34.
8. Haneder S, Konstandin S, Morelli JN, Nagel AM, Zoellner FG, Schad LR, et al. Quantitative and qualitative 23 Na MR imaging of the human kidneys at 3 T: before and after a water load. Radiology. 2011;260:857–65.
9. Than WH, Chan GC-K, Ng JK-C, Szeto C-C. The role of obesity on chronic kidney disease development, progression, and cardiovascular complications. Adv Biomarker Sci Technol. 2020;2:24–34.
10. Frame AA, Wainford RD. Mechanisms of altered renal sodium handling in age-related hypertension. Am J Physiol Renal Physiol. 2018;315:F1–6.
11. Soi V, Yee J. Sodium homeostasis in chronic kidney disease. Adv Chronic Kidney Dis. 2017;24:325–31.
12. Gupta S, Pepper RJ, Ashman N, Walsh SB. Nephrotic syndrome: oedema formation and its treatment with diuretics. Front Physiol. 2019:9.
13. Umutlu L, Orzada S, Kinner S, Maderwald S, Brote I, Bitz AK, et al. Renal imaging at 7 Tesla: preliminary results. Eur Radiol. 2011;21:841–9.
14. Umutlu L, Kraff O, Orzada S, Fischer A, Kinner S, Maderwald S, et al. Dynamic contrast-enhanced renal MRI at 7 Tesla preliminary results. Investig Radiol. 2011;46:425–33.
15. Umutlu L, Maderwald S, Kraff O, Kinner S, Schaefer LC, Wrede K, et al. New look at renal vasculature: 7 tesla nonenhanced T1-weighted FLASH imaging. J Magn Reson Imaging. 2012;36:714–21.
16. Umutlu L, Maderwald S, Kinner S, Kraff O, Bitz AK, Orzada S, et al. First-pass contrast-enhanced renal MRA at 7 Tesla: initial results. Eur Radiol. 2013;23:1059–66.
17. Laader A, Beiderwellen K, Kraff O, Maderwald S, Ladd ME, Forsting M, et al. Non-enhanced versus low-dose contrast-enhanced renal magnetic resonance angiography at 7 T: a feasibility study. Acta Radiol. 2018;59:296–304.
18. Grinstead JW, Rooney W, Laub G, editors. The origins of bright blood MPRAGE at 7 tesla and a simultaneous method for T1 imaging and non-contrast MRA. Proceedings of the 18th scientific meeting, International Society for Magnetic Resonance in Medicine; 2010. Stockholm.
19. Metzger GJ, Auerbach EJ, Akgun C, Simonson J, Bi X, Uğurbil K, et al. Dynamically applied B1 + shimming solutions for non-contrast enhanced renal angiography at 7.0 tesla. Magn Reson Med. 2013;69:114–26.
20. Wolf M, de Boer A, Sharma K, Boor P, Leiner T, Sunder-Plassmann G, et al. Magnetic resonance imaging T1- and T2-mapping to assess renal structure and function: a systematic review and statement paper. Nephrol Dial Transplant. 2018;33:ii41–50.
21. Li X, Auerbach EJ, Van de Moortele PF, Ugurbil K, Metzger GJ. Quantitative single breath-hold renal arterial spin labeling imaging at 7T. Magn Reson Med. 2018;79:815–25.
22. Li X, Bolan PJ, Ugurbil K, Metzger GJ. Measuring renal tissue relaxation times at 7 T. NMR Biomed. 2015;28:63–9.
23. Pruijm M, Mendichovszky IA, Liss P, Van der Niepen P, Textor SC, Lerman LO, et al. Renal blood oxygenation level-dependent magnetic resonance imaging to measure renal tissue oxygenation: a statement paper

and systematic review. Nephrol Dial Transplant. 2018;33:ii22–i8.

24. Brinkmann I, Darji N, Speck O, Bock M, editors. BOLD MRI of the kidneys under water loading at 7 tesla using parallel transmission and RF shimming of individual slices. Proceedings of the 22nd scientific meeting, International Society for Magnetic Resonance in Medicine; 2014. Milan.
25. Hoogduin H, Raaijmakers A, Visser F, Luijten P, editors. Initial experience with BOLD imaging of the kidneys at 7T. Proceedings of the 22nd scientific meeting, International Society for Magnetic Resonance in Medicine; 2014. Milan.
26. Vink EE, de Boer A, Hoogduin HJ, Voskuil M, Leiner T, Bots ML, et al. Renal BOLD-MRI relates to kidney function and activity of the renin-angiotensin-aldosterone system in hypertensive patients. J Hypertens. 2015;33:597–603; discussion −4.
27. Wong EC. An introduction to ASL labeling techniques. J Magn Reson Imaging. 2014;40:1–10.
28. Martino F, Amici G, Rosner M, Ronco C, Novara G. Gadolinium-based contrast media nephrotoxicity in kidney impairment: the physio-pathological conditions for the perfect murder. J Clin Med. 2021:10.
29. Weinreb JC, Rodby RA, Yee J, Wang CL, Fine D, McDonald RJ, et al. Use of intravenous gadolinium-based contrast media in patients with kidney disease: consensus statements from the American College of Radiology and the National Kidney Foundation. Radiology. 2021;298:28–35.
30. Nery F, Buchanan CE, Harteveld AA, Odudu A, Bane O, Cox EF, et al. Consensus-based technical recommendations for clinical translation of renal ASL MRI. Magn Reson Mater Phys. 2020;33:141–61.
31. Li X, Ugurbil K, Metzger G, editors. Theoretical evaluation of ultrahigh field benefits to non-contrast enhanced renal perfusion imaging using FAIR-EPI. Proceedings of the 21th scientific meeting, International Society for Magnetic Resonance in Medicine; 2013. Salt Lake City.
32. Li X, Snyder C, Van de Moortele PF, Ugurbil K, Metzger G, editors. Non-contrast enhanced human renal perfusion imaging using arterial spin llabeling at 7T: initial experience. Proceedings of the 20th scientific meeting, International Society for Magnetic Resonance in Medicine; 2012. Melbourne.
33. Li X, Snyder C, Van de Moortele PF, Ugurbil K, Metzger G, editors. Feasibility of single breath-hold renal perfusion imaging at 7T. Proceedings of the 21st scientific meeting, International Society for Magnetic Resonance in Medicine; 2013. Salt Lake City.
34. Snyder CJ, Delabarre L, Moeller S, Tian J, Akgun C, Van de Moortele PF, et al. Comparison between eight- and sixteen-channel TEM transceiver arrays for body imaging at 7 T. Magn Reson Med. 2012;67:954–64.
35. Odudu A, Nery F, Harteveld AA, Evans RG, Pendse D, Buchanan CE, et al. Arterial spin labelling MRI to measure renal perfusion: a systematic review and statement paper. Nephrol Dial Transplant. 2018;33:ii15–21.
36. Zhang X, Petersen ET, Ghariq E, De Vis JB, Webb AG, Teeuwisse WM, et al. In vivo blood T(1) measurements at 1.5 T, 3 T, and 7 T. Magn Reson Med. 2013;70:1082–6.
37. Haneder S, Juras V, Michaely HJ, Deligianni X, Bieri O, Schoenberg SO, et al. In vivo sodium (23Na) imaging of the human kidneys at 7 T: preliminary results. Eur Radiol. 2014;24:494–501.
38. Scheipers A, Lott J, Nagel A, Bachert P, Ladd M, Platt T, editors. Quantitative sodium MRI of the human kidney at 7T applying respiratory sorting. Proceedings of the 29th scientific meeting, International Society for Magnetic Resonance in Medicine; 2021. Online.
39. Boehmert L, Kuehne A, Waiczies H, Wenz D, Eigentler T, Nagel A, et al., editors. Cardiorenal sodium MRI at 7.0 tesla using an 8-channel 1H/23Na RF coil Array. Proceedings of the 27th scientific meeting, International Society for Magnetic Resonance in Medicine; 2019. Montréal.
40. Hricak H. Phosphorus-31 MRS of the kidney. Investig Radiol. 1989;24:993–6.
41. Vyhnanovská P, Dezortová M, Herynek V, Táborský P, Viklický O, Hájek M. In vivo 31P MR spectroscopy of human kidney grafts using the 2D-chemical shift imaging method. Transplant Proc. 2011;43:1570–5.
42. van Houtum Q, Welting D, Gosselink WJM, Klomp DWJ, Arteaga de Castro CS, van der Kemp WJM. Low SAR (31) P (multi-echo) spectroscopic imaging using an integrated whole-body transmit coil at 7T. NMR Biomed. 2019;32:e4178.
43. He X, Ertürk MA, Grant A, Wu X, Lagore RL, DelaBarre L, et al. First in-vivo human imaging at 10.5T: imaging the body at 447 MHz. Magn Reson Med. 2020;84:289–303.
44. Metzger GJ, Auerbach EJ, Akgun C, Simonson J, Bi X, Ugurbil K, et al. Dynamically applied B1+ shimming solutions for non-contrast enhanced renal angiography at 7.0 tesla. Magn Reson Med. 2013;69:114–26.
45. Erturk MA, Wu X, Eryaman Y, Van de Moortele PF, Auerbach EJ, Lagore RL, et al. Toward imaging the body at 10.5 tesla. Magn Reson Med. 2017;77:434–43.
46. Raaijmakers AJ, Italiaander M, Voogt IJ, Luijten PR, Hoogduin JM, Klomp DW, et al. The fractionated dipole antenna: a new antenna for body imaging at 7 tesla. Magn Reson Med. 2015;
47. Voogt IJ, Klomp D, Hoogduin H, Luttje MP, Luijten P, van den Berg CAT, et al., editors. Combined 8-channel transceiver fractionated dipole antenna array with a 16-channel loop coil receive array for body imaging at 7 tesla. Proceedings of the 23rd scientific meeting, International Society for Magnetic Resonance in medicine; 2015. Toronto.
48. Metzger GJ, van de Moortele PF, Akgun C, Snyder CJ, Moeller S, Strupp J, et al. Performance of external and internal coil configurations for prostate investigations at 7 T. Magn Reson Med. 2010;64:1625–39.
49. Metzger GJ, Snyder C, Akgun C, Vaughan T, Ugurbil K, Van De Moortele PF. Local B1 + shimming for prostate imaging with transceiver arrays at 7T based

on subject-dependent transmit phase measurements. Magn Reson Med. 2008;59:396–409.
50. Gras V, Vignaud A, Amadon A, Le Bihan D, Boulant N. Universal pulses: a new concept for calibration-free parallel transmission. Magn Reson Med. 2017;77:635–43.
51. Padormo F, Beqiri A, Hajnal JV, Malik SJ. Parallel transmission for ultrahigh-field imaging. NMR Biomed. 2016;29:1145–61.
52. Vaughan JT, Snyder CJ, Delabarre LJ, Bolan PJ, Tian J, Bolinger L, et al. Whole-body imaging at 7T: preliminary results. Magn Reson Med. 2009;61:244–8.
53. Orzada S, Solbach K, Gratz M, Brunheim S, Fiedler TM, Johst S, et al. A 32-channel parallel transmit system add-on for 7T MRI. PLoS One. 2019;14:e0222452.
54. Orzada S, Maderwald S, Poser BA, Bitz AK, Quick HH, Ladd ME. RF excitation using Time Interleaved Acquisition of Modes (TIAMO) to address B1 inhomogeneity in high-field MRI. Magn Reson Med. 2010;64:327–33.
55. Meliadò EF, van den Berg CAT, Luijten PR, Raaijmakers AJE. Intersubject specific absorption rate variability analysis through construction of 23 realistic body models for prostate imaging at 7T. Magn Reson Med. 2019;81:2106–19.
56. Steensma BR, Meliadò EF, Luijten P, Klomp DWJ, van den Berg CAT, Raaijmakers AJE. SAR and temperature distributions in a database of realistic human models for 7 T cardiac imaging. NMR Biomed. 2021;34:e4525.
57. Meliadò EF, Raaijmakers AJE, Sbrizzi A, Steensma BR, Maspero M, Savenije MHF, et al. A deep learning method for image-based subject-specific local SAR assessment. Magn Reson Med. 2020;83:695–711.

Quantification of Renal Metabolic Rate of Oxygen

30

Rajiv S. Deshpande, Michael C. Langham, and Felix W. Wehrli

Introduction

The kidneys are highly metabolically active organs that play a homeostatic role in electrolyte maintenance and fluid balance. One of the most energetically demanding tasks of the kidney is the reabsorption of filtered plasma. Sodium is a particularly important ion as its concentration gradient drives the reabsorption of several solutes. Approximately 99.5% of filtered sodium is reabsorbed by the kidney in healthy humans. This effort understandably requires a large amount of adenosine triphosphate (ATP).

During early diabetes, there is a mismatch in ATP generation and demand [1]. For instance, the diabetic milieu adversely impacts mitochondrial efficiency, thereby impairing ATP generation. This is problematic for the kidney because it must reabsorb electrolytes and molecules. Coughlan et al. studied the time course of diabetic kidney disease in a rat model and found that renal mitochondria exhibited abnormalities before tissue damage occurred. Similar findings were reported in experiments using a pig model of metabolic syndrome. The diminished supply is also exacerbated by an increase in ATP demand due to an elevated glomerular filtration rate. Kidney hyperfiltration is characteristic of the initial stages of diabetic kidney disease. This supply-demand mismatch causes an increase in renal oxygen utilization. Prior studies in an animal model of diabetes have found that the whole-kidney metabolic rate of oxygen (MRO_2) is 40-65% higher compared to controls. Increased MRO_2, by definition, consumes more oxygen, thereby decreasing its availability in kidney tissue, and results in kidney hypoxia. Renal tissue hypoxia is believed to be the common pathway of disease progression.

Noninvasive measurements of kidney hypoxia have typically been performed with T_2*-weighted magnetic resonance imaging (MRI) because the T_2* relaxation time is known to correlate with oxygenation. However, T_2* is not expressed in physiological units and may be confounded by fractional blood volume and renal hemodynamics, and the parameter is sensitive to magnetic field inhomogeneity. Given that elevated MRO_2 is the root cause of tissue hypoxia, direct quantification of renal MRO_2 expressed in absolute physiologic units may be a preferable approach.

R. S. Deshpande (✉) · M. C. Langham · F. W. Wehrli
Laboratory for Structural, Physiologic, and Functional Imaging, Department of Radiology, University of Pennsylvania, Philadelphia, PA, USA
e-mail: Rajiv.Deshpande@pennmedicine.upenn.edu; felix.wehrli@pennmedicine.upenn.edu

S. D. Serai, K. Darge (eds.), *Advanced Clinical MRI of the Kidney*,
https://doi.org/10.1007/978-3-031-40169-5_30

Quantification of Whole-Organ MRO_2

Quantification of whole-organ MRO_2 follows from conservation of mass (Fick's principle): $MRO_2 = C_{RBC} \cdot hct \cdot BFR/mass \cdot (SaO_2 - SvO_2)$, where C_{RBC} is a known constant representing the oxygen carrying capacity of red blood cells (22.02 μmol O_2/mL RBC [2]), hct is hematocrit, BFR is blood flow rate in the feeding arteries normalized by kidney mass (mL/min/100 g tissue), SaO_2 is arterial oxygenation level in the feeding artery, and SvO_2 is venous oxygenation level in the draining vein (expressed as percent of full O_2 saturation). Hematocrit and SaO_2 are measured through a capillary blood sample and peripheral pulse oximeter, respectively. Organ mass is determined by segmenting a series of scout images. This leaves the key parameters of BFR and SvO_2, both of which can be noninvasively determined through quantitative MRI methods.

Measurements of Venous Oxygenation and Blood Flow Rate

MRI oximetry exploits the magnetic properties of deoxyhemoglobin to quantify SvO_2. Specifically, hemoglobin undergoes a conformational change upon deoxygenation, which, in turn, perturbs the local magnetic field around red blood cells. The chemical exchange and diffusion of nearby water molecules through the magnetic gradients thereby modulate the overall signal. This signal then serves as the basis for noninvasive measurements of SvO_2, i.e., the magnetic property of blood depends on its oxygenation level. In general, there are two classes of MRI-oximetric methods to quantify SvO_2: susceptometry and T_2-based.

Susceptometry

Susceptometry is a field-mapping technique that quantifies the magnetic susceptibility of venous blood water protons relative to the surrounding tissue. The tissue serves as a reference to compute SvO_2 because its magnetic property is indistinguishable from fully oxygenated arterial blood. "OxFlow" is an example of a susceptometric technique previously developed in the authors' laboratory that interleaves a RF-spoiled multi-echo gradient recalled echo sequence with a phase-contrast sequence to simultaneously measure intravascular magnetic susceptibility (and in turn SvO_2) and blood flow velocity [3]. Susceptometry is a calibration free method that requires surrounding reference tissue for phase-correction and is best suited when the vein is relatively straight and oriented in a direction close to the main magnetic field. When a subject is positioned supine or prone in the scanner bore, the renal vessels are oriented nearly perpendicular to the main magnetic field (exceeding 30°). Further, in the abdomen, reference tissue is often unavailable, and the accuracy of field maps suffers from the presence of several tissue interfaces with different susceptibilities. As a result, T_2-based oximetry is the preferred method to determine SvO_2 in the renal vein.

T_2-Based Oximetry

T_2-based oximetry determines the T_2 relaxation time or the decay constant of the transient MR signal of venous blood water protons. Thulborn et al. reported that the T_2 of water protons in blood depends on oxygen saturation. Wright et al. later demonstrated that in vivo quantification of oxygen saturation by measuring T_2 is feasible. In this method, the T_2 relaxation time is derived by fitting a mono-exponential decay to the venous blood signal intensities, followed by conversion to SvO_2 via a calibration model. Wright's group reported the oxygen saturation in major vessels, including the superior vena cava, aorta, and pulmonary trunk [4]. Another established T_2-based method, "T_2 Relaxation Under Spin Tagging" (TRUST), has quantified the SvO_2 in the superior sagittal sinus of the brain [5]. Targeting the kidney in a preliminary study, Daniel et al. have implemented TRUST in the

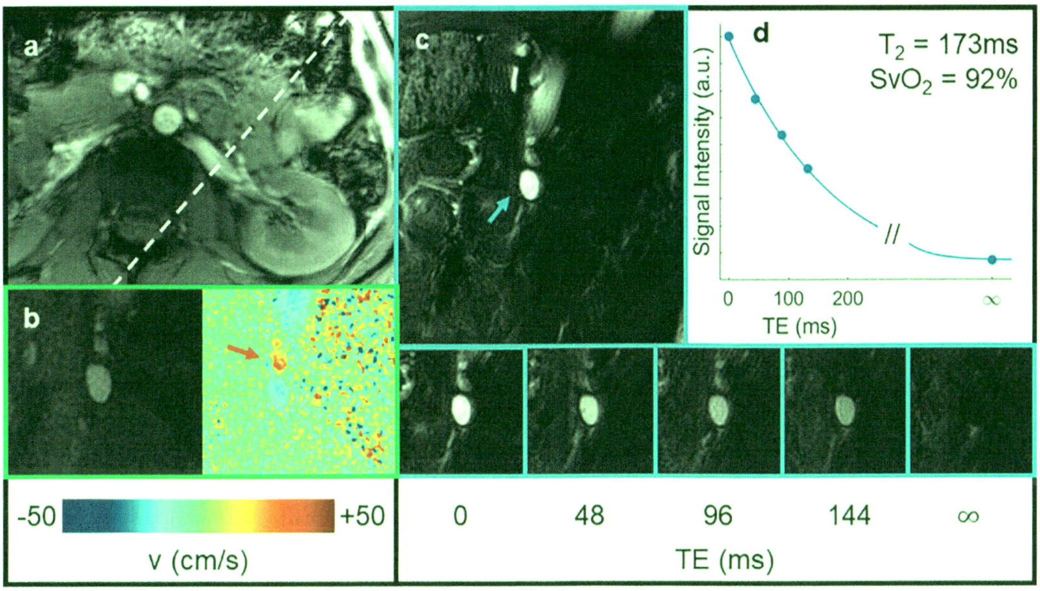

Fig. 30.1 (**a**) Axial image of the kidneys and renal vasculature. (**b**) Phase-contrast magnitude image and velocity map with renal artery in red arrow. (**c**) Background-suppressed magnitude balanced steady-state free precession image where left renal vein is marked in blue. The blue box shows the renal vein at increasing echo times (TEs). (**d**) T_2-decay curve, reporting T_2 and SvO_2

renal vein and reported an SvO_2 of 89 ± 2%. However, TRUST requires two scans, a control and label, to isolate intravascular signal. As a result, this approach is susceptible to motion artifacts, particularly when imaging the renal vessels. In addition, TRUST does not measure blood flow velocity, thereby necessitating a separate measurement for MRO_2 quantification.

To overcome these limitations, a new imaging pulse sequence named "Kidney Metabolism of Oxygen via T_2 and Interleaved Velocity Encoding" (K-MOTIVE) has recently been developed in the authors' laboratory and has been used to quantify whole-organ renal MRO_2 in humans [6, 7]. The K-MOTIVE pulse sequence interleaves a radial phase-contrast module before a background-suppressed T_2-prepared readout to simultaneously measure blood flow velocity and T_2. Background-suppression significantly attenuates the signal from static tissue to isolate intravascular blood. Importantly, background-suppression eliminates the need for two scans, making K-MOTIVE a more convenient approach than a method such as TRUST. Thus, the pulse sequence is more robust to motion and measures blood flow rate and SvO_2 from a single pass, enabling quantification of MRO_2. Another advantage of the K-MOTIVE sequence is that its duration is under 22 seconds, which permits a breath-held acquisition at the kidney.

Representative images from K-MOTIVE applied to the kidney in a healthy human subject are shown in Fig. 30.1. Quantitative parameters from our recent work [4] were found to be the following: average SvO_2 = 92 ± 6%, BFR = 400 ± 110 mL/min, and renal MRO_2 = 114 ± 117 (μmol O_2/min)/100 g. In comparison, De Keijzer et al. performed catheter-based measurements of SvO_2 in the renal vein in healthy subjects and reported values of 92–93% [8].

Conclusion

Noninvasive quantification of renal oxygen consumption by magnetic resonance imaging is feasible. The method may be clinically useful in monitoring or diagnosing early-stage kidney disease, such as during the pathogenesis of diabetes. The preliminary T_2-based results are plausible given that SvO_2 in the renal vein is known to be higher than in other organ systems. Of note is that the MRI-based oximetric methods discussed here exploit the endogenous magnetic contrast properties of deoxyhemoglobin. Accordingly, there is no need for exogenous agents, including gadolinium, whose use may be contraindicated in patients with kidney disease. Future directions include further technique development and quantification of renal metabolism in patients with diabetes.

Acknowledgments This work was supported by NIH grants T32EB020087, P41EB029460, UL1TR001878, and F30DK130510.

Reference

1. Hesp, et al. The role of renal hypoxia in the pathogenesis of diabetic kidney disease: a promising target for newer renoprotective agents including SGLT2 inhibitors? Kidney International. 2020;98(3):579–89. https://doi.org/10.1016/j.kint.2020.02.041.
2. Yablonskiy DA, Sukstanskii AL, He X. Blood oxygenation level-dependent (BOLD)-based techniques for the quantification of brain hemodynamic and metabolic properties—theoretical models and experimental approaches. NMR Biomed. 2013;26(8):963–86.
3. Jain V, Langham MC, Wehrli FW. MRI estimation of global brain oxygen consumption rate. J Cereb Blood Flow Metab. 2010;30(9):1598–607. https://doi.org/10.1038/jcbfm.2010.49.
4. Graham A, Wright Bob S, Hu Albert, Macovski (1991) Estimating oxygen saturation of blood in vivo with MR imaging at 1.5 T Journal of Magnetic Resonance Imaging 1(3) 275-283 https://doi.org/10.1002/(ISSN)1522-2586 10.1002/jmri.v1:3 https://doi.org/10.1002/jmri.1880010303
5. Hanzhang, Lu Yulin, Ge (2008) Quantitative evaluation of oxygenation in venous vessels using T2-Relaxation-Under-Spin-Tagging MRI Magnetic Resonance in Medicine 60(2) 357-363 https://doi.org/10.1002/mrm.v60:2 https://doi.org/10.1002/mrm.21627
6. Deshpande RS, Langham MC, Cheng C-C, Wehrli FW. Metabolism of oxygen via T_2 and interleaved velocity encoding: A rapid method to quantify whole-brain cerebral metabolic rate of oxygen. Magnetic Resonance in Medicine. 2022;88(3):1229–43. https://doi.org/10.1002/mrm.29299.
7. Deshpande RS. Langham MC. Wehrli FW. MRI-based Quantification of Whole-Organ Renal Metabolic Rate of Oxygen. NMR in Biomedicine: Susztak; 2023. (In Press).
8. Keijzer D, et al. Agreement of somatic and renal near-infrared spectroscopy with reference blood samples during a controlled hypoxia sequence: a healthy volunteer study Abstract. Journal of Clinical Monitoring and Computing. 2023;37(3):805–14. https://doi.org/10.1007/s10877-022-00944-9.

Index

S. D. Serai, K. Darge (eds.), *Advanced Clinical MRI of the Kidney*,
https://doi.org/10.1007/978-3-031-40169-5

C

D

E

GPSR Compliance

The European Union's (EU) General Product Safety Regulation (GPSR) is a set of rules that requires consumer products to be safe and our obligations to ensure this.

If you have any concerns about our products, you can contact us on ProductSafety@springernature.com

In case Publisher is established outside the EU, the EU authorized representative is:

Springer Nature Customer Service Center GmbH
Europaplatz 3
69115 Heidelberg, Germany

Batch number: 10732807

Printed by Printforce, the Netherlands